LAST MINUTE PREPARATION
SURGERY
KARNATAKA

SHASHANK BAID

AF810055

Peepee Publishers and Distributors Private Limited®

LMP Surgery Karnataka

Published by
Pawaninder P. Vij and Anupam Vij

Peepee Publishers and Distributors Private Limited
Head Office: 160, Shakti Vihar, Pitam Pura, Delhi-110 034 (India)

Correspondence Address:
7/31, First Floor, Ansari Road, Daryaganj
New Delhi-110 002 (India)
Ph: 41512412, 9811156083
e-mail: peepee160@yahoo.co.in
e-mail: peepee160@gmail.com
www.peepeepub.com
join us on facebook.com/pp.publishers

First Edition: 2025

ISBN: 978-81-9720-723-5

PREFACE

While preparing for my university exams as an MBBS student, I always felt the need for an exam-oriented book that would help cope with the stress experienced by students. This book strives to fill that void, providing just the right amount of material to help students excel. The content is neither too lengthy to reproduce during the exam nor too brief; it hits the sweet spot.

I have compiled 'Last Minute Preparation' using only the latest editions of standard surgical texts: Bailey and Love's Short Practice of Surgery (28th edition), Sabiston's Textbook of Surgery (21st edition), and Schwartz's Principles of Surgery (11th edition). For questions no longer covered in these editions, I referred to older editions of Bailey and Love, as well as Harrison's Principles of Internal Medicine (21st edition) and Essential Pediatrics by Ghai (10th edition) to supplement some answers.

Chapters are divided into topics for student convenience. I have used headings and sub-headings extensively to aid understanding, and important topics are highlighted in bold to emphasize key points. Efforts have been made to simplify complex topics thoroughly.

Most importantly, 'Last Minute Preparation' covers all topics from the past 12 years. Additionally, I have included "Other Important Topics" at the end of each chapter, discussing topics not yet asked but likely to be featured in future exams. A student who reads this book from cover to cover is virtually guaranteed to pass their exams with ease.

Shashank Baid

HOW TO USE THIS BOOK

In every chapter, questions have been divided according to topics in a sequence that would best help them understand the subject.

There are some questions where they ask you two topics at the same time. If a topic has been covered in an earlier question, it has not been discussed again, even if asked in a subsequent question.

For example, if indications of splenectomy have been asked in a question, it has been discussed. Now, if in a subsequent section, they have asked both indications and complications of splenectomy, I have discussed only the complications.

ACKNOWLEDGEMENTS

First and foremost, I would like to express my heartfelt gratitude to my family for their unwavering support and encouragement throughout this endeavor. I am also deeply grateful to my students, whose valuable inputs have not only helped me become a better teacher but have also significantly shaped the content of this book.

LIST OF ABBREVIATIONS

5D	–	5 % Dextrose
ABG	–	Arterial Blood Gases
ACTH	–	Adreno Cortico Trophic Hormone
AFP	–	Alpha Feto Protein
aka	–	Also Known As
AKI	–	Acute Kidney Injury
ARDS	–	Acute Respiratory Distress Syndrome
ARF	–	Acute Renal Failure
ATN	–	Acute Tubular Necrosis
β-hCG	–	Beta Human Chorionic Gonadotrophin
BCC	–	Basal Cell Carcinoma
b/l	–	Bilateral
BOO	–	Bladder Outflow Obstruction
BP	–	Blood Pressure
BPH	–	Benign Prostatic Hyperplasia
b/w	–	Between
Ca	–	Carcinoma
CBC	–	Complete Blood Count
CBD	–	Common Bile Duct
CD	–	Crohn's Disease
CECT	–	Contrast Enhanced Computed Tomography
chr	–	Chromosome
CKD	–	Chronic Kidney Disease
c/l	–	Contralateral
cm	–	Centimetre
c/o	–	Complains of
c/s	–	Culture and Sensitivity
CSF	–	Cerebrospinal Fluid
CT	–	Computed Tomography
CXR	–	Chest X-ray
CVP	–	Central Venous Pressure
DCR	–	Damage Control Resuscitation
DCS	–	Damage Control Surgery
DD	–	Differential Diagnosis
Defn	–	Definition
DIR	–	Deep Inguinal Ring
DRE	–	Digital Rectal Examination
DVT	–	Deep Vein Thrombosis
ECG	–	Electro Cardio Gram
EDH	–	Extra Dural Haematoma
e.g.	–	Example
FAST	–	Focussed Assessment with Sonography for Trauma
FFP	–	Fresh Frozen Plasma
FNAC	–	Fine Needle Aspiration Cytology
Fr	–	French
FTSG	–	Full Thickness Skin Graft
F/U	–	Follow up
G	–	Gauge
GA	–	General Anaesthesia
GCS	–	Glasgow Coma Score
GCT	–	Germ Cell Tumour
GEJ	–	Gastro Esophageal Junction
GIT	–	Gastro Intestinal Tract
GPE	–	General Physical Examination
GSV	–	Great Saphenous Vein
GUT	–	Genito Urinary Tract
Hb	–	Haemoglobin
HIV	–	Human Immunodeficiency Virus
h/o	–	History of
HPE	–	Histo Pathological Examination
hpf	–	High Power Field
HR	–	Heart Rate
IBD	–	Inflammatory Bowel Disease
IBS	–	Irritable Bowel Syndrome
ICD	–	Inter Costal Drain
ICP	–	Intra Cranial Pressure
ICU	–	Intensive Care Unit
i.e.	–	That is
IHC	–	Immunohistochemistry
i/l	–	Ipsilateral
IM	–	Intramuscular
I/O	–	Input/ output
IV	–	Intravenous

K – Potassium
KCl – Potassium Chloride
LA – Local Anaesthesia
LDH – Lactate Dehydrogenase
L/E – Local Examination
LFT – Liver Function Tests
LLQ – Left Lower Quadrant
LOC – Loss of Consciousness
LSV – Long Saphenous Vein
LUQ – Left Upper Quadrant
LUTS – Lower Urinary Tract Symptoms
mc – Most common
MEN – Multiple Endocrine Neoplasia
mets – Metastases
mm – Millimetre
MODS – Multiple Organ Dysfunction Syndrome
MRI – Magnetic Resonance Imaging
Na – Sodium
NaCl – Sodium Chloride
NACT – Neo Adjuvant Chemo Therapy
NGT – Naso Gastric Tube
NPM – Nil Per Mouth
NPO – Nil Per Oral
NS – Normal Saline
NSAID – Non Steroidal Anti Inflammatory Drug
o/e – On examination
OT – Operating Theatre
PDA – Patent Ductus Arteriosus
PFT – Pulmonary Function Tests
PPI – Proton Pump Inhibitor
PR – Per Rectal
PR – Pulse Rate
PRBC – Packed Red Blood Cells
PSA – Prostate Specific Antigen
pt – Patient
PTE – Pulmonary Thrombo Embolism
PTFE – Poly Tetra Fluoro Ethylene
PUJO – Pelvi-Ureteric Junction Obstruction
RAAS – Renin Angiotensin Aldosterone System
RBC – Red Blood Cells
RFA – Radio Frequency Ablation
RFT – Renal Function Tests
RIF – Right Iliac Fossa
RL – Ringer's Lactate
RLQ – Right Left Quadrant
RPLND – Retro Peritoneal Lymph Node Dissection
RR – Respiratory Rate
RT – Radiation Therapy
RUQ – Right Upper Quadrant
SA – Spinal Anaesthesia
SAB – Sub Arachnoid Block
SAH – Sub Arachnoid Haemorrhage
sc – Subcutaneous
SCC – Squamous Cell Carcinoma
SDH – Sub Dural Haemorrhage
SIR – Superficial Inguinal Ring
SIRS – Systemic Inflammatory Response Syndrome
SLN – Sentinel Lymph Node
SLNB – Sentinel Lymph Node Biopsy
SSG – Split Thickness Skin Graft
SSI – Surgical Site Infection
SSV – Short or Small Saphenous Vein
STSG – Split Thickness Skin Graft
TACO – Transfusion Associated Circulatory Overload
TBSA – Total Body Surface Area
TLC – Total Leukocyte Count
TRALI – Transfusion Related Acute Lung Injury
U – Units
UC – Ulcerative Colitis
u/l – Unilateral
USG – Ultra Sono Gram
UTI – Urinary Tract Infection
VAC – Vacuum Assisted Closure
VATS – Video Assisted Thoracoscopic Surgery
VIP – Vasoactive Intestinal Peptide
WBC – White Blood Cells
wks – Weeks
yrs – Years

CONTENTS

1.	Shock, Blood Transfusion and Fluids	1
2.	Wound Healing	16
3.	Infections and Infestations	23
4.	Diagnostic Imaging	38
5.	Endoscopy	41
6.	Minimal Access Surgery	44
7.	Tissue and Molecular Diagnosis	46
8.	Principles of Oncology	48
9.	Pediatric Surgery	51
10.	Day Care Surgery	55
11.	Anesthesia, Pain Relief and Perioperative Care	58
12.	Trauma	62
13.	Neurosurgery	76
14.	Lungs	81
15.	Cardiothoracic and Vascular Surgery (CTVS)	83
16.	Skin and Subcutaneous Tissue	85
17.	Common Cysts and Swellings	95
18.	Ulcers	100
19.	Burns	101
20.	Plastic Surgery	110
21.	Hand	113
22.	Cleft Lip and Palate	117
23.	Pharynx, Larynx and Neck	122
24.	Oral Cavity and Swellings of Jaw	128
25.	Salivary Glands	140
26.	Thyroid and Parathyroid Glands	147
27.	Adrenals	164
28.	Breast	169
29.	Arteries	183
30.	Veins	193
31.	Lymphatics	205
32.	Liver	212
33.	Gall Bladder and Biliary Tree	226
34.	Pancreas	237
35.	Spleen	251
36.	Abdominal Wall, Umbilicus and Hernia	257
37.	Peritoneum, Omentum and Mesentery	272
38.	Esophagus	278
39.	Stomach and Duodenum	289

40.	Bariatric Surgery	310
41.	Small Intestine	312
42.	Large Intestine and Rectum	315
43.	Inflammatory Bowel Disease	328
44.	Intestinal Obstruction	334
45.	Appendix	345
46.	Anus	353
47.	Urinary Symptoms and Investigations	361
48.	Kidney and Ureter	366
49.	Urinary Bladder	383
50.	Prostate	389
51.	Penis and Urethra	397
52.	Testes and Scrotum	406
53.	Transplantation	419
54.	Miscellaneous	423

1

Shock, Blood Transfusion and Fluids

SHOCK

[10] Define and classify shock. How will you manage a case of hypovolemic shock? ***Sep 21***

[10] Classify shock. Describe the pathophysiology, clinical features, assessment and management of hypovolemic shock. ***July 18***

[10] Define shock. Discuss the clinical features, presentations and management of various types of shock. ***June 16***

[10] Define shock. Describe pathophysiology and classification of shock. Discuss the management of hypovolemic shock. ***Dec 12***

[10] Define shock. Describe the pathophysiology, types and principles of management of shock. ***March 24***

[5] Enumerate types of shock and principles of resuscitation. ***CBME March 24***

- **Definition:** Shock is a **systemic state of low tissue perfusion** that is inadequate for normal cellular respiration.
- Shock is the **most common cause of death of surgical patients.** Death may occur rapidly because of a profound state of shock or may occur later because of the consequences of organ ischemia and reperfusion injury.

Pathophysiology

Insufficient delivery of oxygen and glucose

↓

Cells switch from aerobic to anaerobic metabolism

↓

Cell death

A. Cellular

- Due to anaerobic metabolism, **lactic acid** is produced, which **accumulates and produces systemic metabolic acidosis.**
- Failure of Na/K pumps.
- Cell lysis causes release of intracellular contents including potassium into bloodstream. This results in **hyperkalemia.**

B. Microvascular

- **Activation of immune and coagulation systems.**
- Oxygen free radicals and cytokines injure the capillary endothelial cells.
- Endothelial cells become leaky resulting in **tissue oedema.**

C. Cardiovascular System

- As preload and afterload decrease, there is a compensatory increase in sympathetic activity.
- This results in **tachycardia and systemic vasoconstriction.**

D. Respiratory System

- The metabolic acidosis and increased sympathetic response result in an increased respiratory rate and minute ventilation to increase the excretion of carbon dioxide.
- This produces a **compensatory respiratory alkalosis.**

E. Renal System

- Shock causes decreased urine output. RAAS is stimulated, resulting in further vasoconstriction and **increased sodium and water reabsorption by the kidney.**

F. Endocrine

- **Vasopressin (anti-diuretic hormone) is released** which results in vasoconstriction and resorption of water in the renal collecting system.
- **Cortisol is released from the adrenal cortex,** contributing to sodium and water resorption and sensitizing cells to catecholamines.

CLASSIFICATION OF SHOCK

Shock is classified **based on the initiating mechanism.** All states are characterized by systemic tissue hypo-perfusion and **different states may coexist within the same patient.**

- **Hemorrhagic and Hypovolemic shock.**
- **Cardiogenic shock.**
- **Obstructive shock.**
- **Distributive shock.**
- **Endocrine shock.**

Hemorrhagic and Hypovolemic Shock

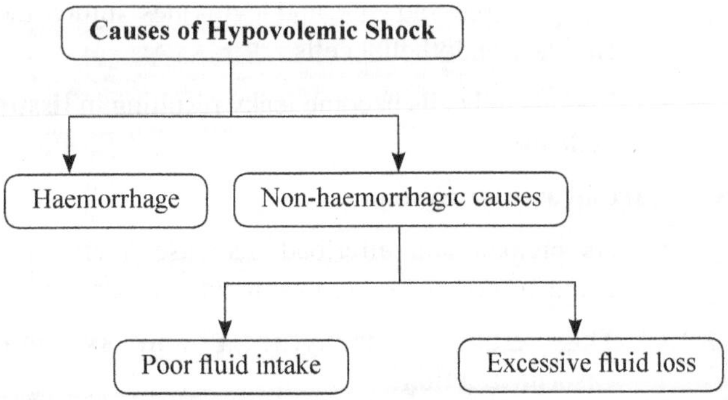

- Hypovolemic shock is the **most common form of shock** and is a component of all other forms of shock.
- Hypovolemic shock is **due to reduced circulating volume** and its causes are:
  - o **Hemorrhage.**
  - o **Non-hemorrhagic causes:**
    - ♦ **Poor fluid intake,** i.e., dehydration.
    - ♦ **Excessive fluid loss:** Vomiting, diarrhea, urinary loss (e.g., diabetes), evaporation, third spacing. Third spacing means loss of fluid into the GIT and interstitial spaces, e.g., bowel obstruction, pancreatitis.

Cardiogenic Shock

- It is due to **primary failure of the heart to pump blood** to the tissues.
- **Causes:**
  - o Myocardial infarction.
  - o Cardiac dysrhythmias.
  - o Valvular heart disease.
  - o Blunt myocardial injury.
  - o Cardiomyopathy.
  - o Myocardial depression. It is due to:
    - ♦ Endogenous factors – Bacterial and humoral agents released in sepsis.
    - ♦ Exogenous factors – Drugs.
- Along with the classical signs of shock, there is also evidence of venous hypertension with pulmonary or systemic oedema.

Obstructive Shock

- There is a **reduction in preload due to mechanical obstruction of cardiac filling.**
- The reduced filling of the left and/or right sides of the heart, leads to **low cardiac output.**
- **Causes:**
  - o Cardiac tamponade.
  - o Tension pneumothorax.
  - o Massive pulmonary or air embolism.

Distributive Shock

- **Features of distributive shock are as follows:**
  - o Inadequate organ perfusion.

- **Vascular dilatation.**
- **Hypotension.**
- Low systemic vascular resistance.
- Inadequate afterload.
- **Abnormally high cardiac output.**

- **Causes:**
  - **Anaphylaxis:** Vasodilation is due to histamine release.
  - **Spinal cord injury or neurogenic shock:** Vasodilation is due to failure of sympathetic outflow and inadequate vascular tone.
  - **Septic shock:** Vasodilation is related to the release of bacterial products (endotoxins) and the activation of cellular and humoral components of the immune system.

Endocrine Shock

- May present as a combination of hypovolemic, cardiogenic or distributive shock.
- **Causes:**
  - Hypothyroidism.
  - Thyrotoxicosis.
  - Adrenal insufficiency.

Characteristics of Shock

	Hypo-volemic	Cardio-genic	Obstruc-tive	Distribu-tive
Cardiac Output	Low	Low	Low	High
Systemic Vascular Resistance	High	High	High	Low
Venous Pressure	Low	High	High	Low
Mixed Venous Saturation	Low	Low	Low	High
Base Deficit	High	High	High	High

Stages of Shock

- Shock can clinically be divided into **2 stages:**
  - Compensated (mild).
  - Decompensated (moderate, severe).

Compensated Shock (Mild Shock)

- As shock progresses, the body's compensatory responses **reduce flow to non-essential organs (skin, muscle, GIT)** to preserve preload and **maintain flow to the essential organs (lungs, brain, kidneys).**
- The non-essential organs are under-perfused: their cells respire anaerobically and sustain ischemic damage.
- There is **systemic metabolic acidosis** and **activation of humoral and cellular inflammation.**
- Although **clinically occult,** this state will **lead to MODS and death if prolonged.**

Decompensated Shock (Moderate, Severe)

- Further loss of circulating volume **overloads the body's compensatory mechanisms** and there is progressive renal, respiratory and cardiovascular decompensation.

Clinical Features

A. Mild (Compensated) Shock

- **Tachycardia.**
- **Tachypnoea.**
- Mild reduction in urine output.
- Mild anxiety.
- **BP is maintained**, although there is a decrease in pulse pressure.
- **Peripheries are cool and sweaty** with prolonged capillary refill times (except in septic shock).

B. Moderate (Decompensated) Shock

- As shock progresses, the renal compensatory mechanisms fail, renal perfusion falls and **urine output decreases below 0.5 ml/kg/hour.**
- There is further tachycardia.
- **BP starts to fall.**
- Patient becomes **drowsy and mildly confused.**

C. Severe (Decompensated) Shock

- Profound tachycardia.
- Profound hypotension.
- **Urine output falls to zero.**
- Patients are **unconscious.**
- **Labored respiration.**

	Compensated	Decompensated	
	Mild	**Moderate**	**Severe**
Lactic Acidosis	+	++	+++
Urine Output	Normal	Reduced	Anuric
Conscious Level	Mild anxiety	Drowsy	Comatose
Respiratory Rate	Increased	Increased	Labored
Pulse Rate	Increased	Increased	Increased
Blood Pressure	Normal	Mild hypotension	Severe hypotension

Clinical Consequences/Complications of Shock

- Unresuscitatable shock.
- Ischemia reperfusion syndrome.
- Systemic Inflammatory Response Syndrome (SIRS).
- **Multiple Organ Dysfunction Syndrome (MODS):**
    - o ≥ 2 failed organ systems:
        - ♦ **Heart:** Cardiovascular failure.
        - ♦ **Lungs:** Acute respiratory distress syndrome.
        - ♦ **Kidney:** Acute renal insufficiency.
        - ♦ **Liver:** Liver failure and coagulopathy.
        - ♦ **Brain:** Cerebral swelling and dysfunction.

Investigations/Monitoring for Patients in Shock

A. Minimum

- ECG.
- Pulse oximetry.
- Blood pressure.
- Urine output.

B. Additional Modalities

- Central venous pressure.
- Invasive blood pressure.
- Cardiac output.
- Base deficit and serum lactate.

Treatment of Shock

- Once **airway and breathing are controlled,** attention is directed to cardiovascular resuscitation.
- The **treatment of shock is resuscitation** and consists of the following:
    - o Fluid therapy.
    - o Vasopressor and inotropic support.

A. Fluid Therapy

- Fluids should be given before other therapy such as inotropic or chronotropic agents are given.
- **1st line therapy is IV access and administration of IV fluids.**
- **Green IV** cannula (**18 G**) is the cannula of choice.
- The **ideal replacement fluid is one that approximates the fluid lost** by the underlying cause of shock.

  Therefore, if blood is being lost, the ideal replacement fluid is whole blood.
- However, due to obvious reasons, **blood** cannot always be used and **is transfused only when specifically indicated.**

Fluids used are:

- **Crystalloids**
    - o E.g., **normal saline, Hartmann's solution, Ringer's lactate.**
    - o Crystalloids are **routinely used for resuscitation along with appropriate electrolyte supplementation.**
    - o Cheaper and easily available.
- **Colloids**
    - o E.g., human **albumin**, other commercially available products.
    - o More expensive.
    - o Worse side effect profiles.
- **Hypotonic solutions**
    - o E.g., **dextrose.**
    - o Poor volume expanders.
    - o Used in the treatment of shock when the deficit is free water loss (e.g., diabetes insipidus) or when patients are sodium overloaded (e.g., cirrhosis).

B. Vasopressor and Inotropic Support

- **Phenylephrine, noradrenaline**
    - o They are vasopressors.

  - o Indicated in **distributive shock states,** e.g., sepsis, neurogenic shock.
- **Vasopressin**
  - o Used as an alternate vasopressor.
  - o Used **when vasodilatation is resistant to catecholamines**, e.g., absolute or relative steroid deficiency.
- **Dobutamine**
  - o It is an inotrope.
  - o Used in cardiogenic shock, or where myocardial depression has complicated a shock state, e.g., severe septic shock with low cardiac output.

Principles of Resuscitation

- Resuscitation is guided by measures of tissue perfusion.
- Resuscitation should not be delayed in order to definitively diagnose the source of the shocked state.
- Timing and nature of resuscitation will depend on the type of shock and also on the timing and severity of the insult.
- Rapid clinical examination will provide adequate clues to make an appropriate first determination, even if a source of bleeding or sepsis is not immediately identifiable.
- If there is initial doubt about the cause of shock, it is safer to assume the cause is hypovolemia and begin with fluid resuscitation and then assess the response.
- Correction of shock is important in the pre- and peri-operative period for all cases of urgent surgery, e.g. a patient with bowel obstruction and hypovolemic shock must be adequately resuscitated before undergoing surgery.
- In all cases of shock, regardless of classification, hypovolemia and inadequate preload must be addressed (i.e. fluids must be given) before other therapy is instituted.
- Administration of inotropic or chronotropic agents or vasopressors to an empty heart will rapidly and permanently deplete the myocardium of oxygen stores and dramatically reduce diastolic filling and thus the coronary perfusion.
- The ideal replacement fluid is one that approximates the fluid lost by the underlying cause of shock. Therefore, if blood is lost, the ideal replacement fluid is whole blood or its equivalent in components. However, crystalloids may be required while awaiting blood products.
- Resuscitation is very different if patients are actively bleeding or if they are not bleeding:
  a. In patients who are bleeding, the priority is to stop bleeding.
  b. In patients who are not bleeding, priority shifts to normalising end-organ perfusion, i.e. correcting the shock state.

End Points of Resuscitation

- The easiest and best parameter for monitoring resuscitation in shock is urine output.
- Resuscitation is continued till global perfusion end points are corrected, i.e., base deficit and lactate, mixed venous oxygen saturation.

[MCQ] Which solution is preferred in the initial management of hypovolemic shock? ***CBME June 24***

A. Normal Saline B. Ringer Lactate*

C. Albumin D. Blood

Ringer's Lactate is generally preferred for initial resuscitation in hypovolemic shock because it better mimics the body's plasma electrolyte composition and helps buffer acidosis.

HEMORRHAGIC SHOCK

[10] Define shock. Discuss the management of hemorrhagic shock. Discuss the role of blood products. ***August 22***

[3] Secondary Hemorrhage. ***March 22***

Types of Hemorrhage

Hemorrhage is of the following types:

A. Revealed and Concealed Hemorrhage

- **Revealed**
  - o Obvious external hemorrhage.
  - o E.g., exsanguination from an open arterial wound, massive hematemesis from a duodenal ulcer.
- **Concealed**
  - o Contained within the body cavity.

- o Must be suspected and actively investigated.
- o E.g., hemorrhage within a body cavity (pleura, peritoneum, pelvis), non-traumatic concealed hemorrhage (occult GI bleeding or ruptured aortic aneurysm).

B. Primary, Reactionary and Secondary Hemorrhage

- **Primary hemorrhage**
  - o Occurs immediately due to an injury or surgery.
- **Reactionary hemorrhage**
  - o Occurs within 24 hours of surgery.
  - o It is caused by:
    - ♦ Dislodgement of a clot by resuscitation.
    - ♦ Normalization of BP.
    - ♦ Vasodilation.
    - ♦ Technical failure, such as slippage of a ligature.
- **Secondary hemorrhage**
  - o Occurs after 1 week of surgery.
  - o It is due to sloughing of the wall of a vessel and is precipitated by factors such as infection, pressure necrosis (from a drain) or malignancy.

C. Surgical and Non-Surgical

- **Surgical hemorrhage**
  - o Due to a direct injury.
  - o It is amenable to surgical control or other techniques such as embolization.
- **Non-surgical hemorrhage**
  - o General bleeding from raw surfaces and mucous membranes due to coagulopathy.
  - o It cannot be stopped by surgical means (except packing).
  - o Treatment: Correction of coagulation abnormalities.

Grades or Classification of Hemorrhagic Shock

- Hemorrhage is classified into four grades on the basis of the percentage of total blood volume lost.

Class	Blood volume lost as percentage of total
1	< 15%
2	15 – 30%
3	30 – 40%
4	> 40%

Treatment of Hemorrhagic Shock

- The treatment of hemorrhagic shock **depends on whether the patient is actively bleeding or not.**
- If the patient is **actively bleeding**, treatment focuses on achieving rapid hemostasis and maintaining the ability of the blood to clot. This paradigm is called **damage control resuscitation.**
- If the patient is **not actively bleeding**, has stopped bleeding or the cause of the shock is not hemorrhage, then resuscitation is directed at **correcting the shock state and restoring perfusion** to end organs.
- It consists of:
  - A. Identify hemorrhage:
    - o Immediate resuscitative measures.
    - o Large bore I.V. access.
    - o Blood is drawn for cross matching.
    - o Emergency blood transfusion (O negative).
  - B. Damage Control Resuscitation:
    - o Rapid hemorrhage control.
    - o Permissive hypotension.
    - o Avoid dilutional coagulopathy.
    - o Treat existing coagulation deficits.
  - C. After hemorrhage control.

A. Identify Hemorrhage

- External hemorrhage may be obvious.
- The diagnosis of concealed hemorrhage may be more difficult.
- The aim of identifying the site of hemorrhage is not to identify the exact location definitively, but rather **to define the next step in hemorrhage control**, i.e., operation, angioembolization or endoscopic control.
- This is done with the help of the following:
  - o History

- ♦ Previous episodes, known aneurysm, NSAID use.
- o Examination
  - ♦ External signs of injury may suggest internal hemorrhage.
- o CXR, pelvis X-ray, USG, FAST scan.

B. Damage Control Resuscitation (DCR)

- Also known as hemostatic resuscitation.
- It is a paradigm that **prioritizes hemorrhage control** in patients who are still actively bleeding.
- **No aspect of the shock state** (end organ perfusion, blood pressure, temperature, lactic acidosis) **can be corrected while patients are still bleeding**.
- Repeated cycles of volume resuscitation will exacerbate coagulopathy, hypothermia and acidosis.
- DCR **reduces mortality**.
- DCR is based on 4 key principles:

1. **Rapid hemorrhage control**
   - o Direct pressure over the site of external hemorrhage.
2. Temporary bleeding control with tourniquets, balloon occlusion or other techniques.
3. Damage control surgery is done, where **surgical intervention is limited** to the minimum necessary **to stop bleeding** and control sepsis.
4. **Definitive repairs are delayed** until the patient is hemodynamically stable and physiologically capable of sustaining the procedure.
   - o **Permissive hypotension**
     - ♦ Allows the patient to set their own BP while bleeding and **avoids continued volume resuscitation** in the vain attempt to normalize perfusion while bleeding.
     - ♦ This **reduces blood loss from bleeding sites** and **reduces dilutional coagulopathy and hypothermia induced by fluids.**
   - o **Avoid dilutional coagulopathy**
     - ♦ This is done by **avoiding clear fluids (crystalloids or colloids) and by giving a transfusion that approximates whole blood**–usually administered as equal volumes of **PRBCs and plasma.**
   - o **Treat existing coagulation deficits**
     - ♦ This is done either empirically or by regular coagulation testing and acting on the results.
     - ♦ E.g., **tranexamic acid, cryoprecipitate, platelet transfusion.**

C. After Hemorrhage Control

- Patients should be **definitively resuscitated and warmed**.

SEPTIC SHOCK

[10] 60 year old diabetic male came with history of ulcer in left leg for 1 month, h/o fever, oliguria, drowsiness for 2 days. On examination, temp - 102 °F, PR - 110/min, BP - 70/40 mm Hg, RR - 25/min, sPO_2 - 85% at room air, left leg – 8 × 6 cm ulcer with copious purulent foul smelling discharge with pitting oedema in left lower limb.

(a) Classify various types of shock.

(b) Write in detail pathophysiology, clinical features and management of this patient. ***CBME June 24***

[10] Define shock. Enumerate classification of shock. Discuss clinical features and management of septic shock. ***Oct 20***

[5] Systemic Inflammatory Response Syndrome. ***July 23***

SEPTIC SHOCK OR ENDOTOXIC SHOCK

Cause

- Most frequently triggered by Gram-positive bacterial infections, followed by Gram-negative bacteria and fungi.

Pathophysiology

- It is due to a **dysregulated immune response.**
- Bacterial or fungal pathogens (i.e., source of infection).

↓

- **Immune system** and other cells (e.g., endothelial cells) **release inflammatory mediators**, which have the following effects:
  a. Enhanced macrophage and neutrophil killing effector mechanisms.
  b. Increased procoagulant and fibroblast activity to localize invaders.
  c. Increased microvascular blood flow to enhance delivery of the inflammatory mediators.

↓

When this **response is overly exuberant.**

OR

When this **response becomes systemic rather than localized.**

↓

Septic shock.

- There is **peripheral vasodilation seen in septic shock** as opposed to other types of shock (where peripheral vasoconstriction) is seen. This is **due to:**
  1. Maldistribution of blood flow at a microvascular level with arteriovenous shunting.
  2. Dysfunction of cellular utilization of oxygen.
  3. Upregulation of iNOS (inducible Nitric Oxide Synthase) in the vessel wall.

     This causes large quantities of **nitric oxide** to be produced which is a potent vasodilator and renders the vasculature resistant to the effects of vasoconstricting agents.
- Because of (1) and (2), there is **high mixed venous saturation (>70%).** Less oxygen is presented to the cells, and those cells cannot utilize what little oxygen is presented. Thus, venous blood has a higher oxygen concentration than normal.
- Leakage of fluid into the interstitial spaces occurs due to an **increase in vascular permeability.**
- In the later phases of septic shock, there is **hypovolemia** (due to fluid loss into interstitial spaces) and **myocardial depression.** Therefore, cardiac output which was initially high in septic shock becomes low in the later phases of septic shock.

Definitions and Clinical Features

- **Infection:** Identifiable source of microbial insult.
- **SIRS or Systemic Inflammatory Response Syndrome:** Shows ≥ 2 of the following:
  - o Temperature ≥ 38°C (100.4°F) or ≤ 36°C (96.8° F).
  - o Heart rate ≥ 90 beats per minute.
  - o Respiratory rate ≥ 20 cycles per minute or $PaCO_2$ ≥ 32 mm Hg or patient is on mechanical ventilation.
  - o WBCs ≥ 12,000/µl or ≤ 4,000/µl or ≥ 10% band forms.
- **Sepsis:** Identifiable source of infection + SIRS.
- **Severe sepsis:** Sepsis + organ dysfunction.
- **MODS or Multiple Organ Dysfunction Syndrome:** ≥ 2 organ systems are in dysfunction.
- **Septic shock:** Sepsis or cardiovascular collapse (requiring vasopressor support).

Scores Used to Diagnose Sepsis and Septic Shock

1. **SOFA, i.e., Sequential Organ Failure Assessment:**
   - **Sepsis:** Organ dysfunction as represented by an increase in **SOFA score of ≥ 2.**
   - **Septic shock:** Sepsis with hypotension despite fluid resuscitation.

     and/or

     Serum lactate >2 despite a lack of hypovolemia.
   - SOFA score is cumbersome to calculate and requires lab test results.
2. **q SOFA or quick SOFA score:**
   - It is simpler to calculate.
   - It consists of:
     a. Respiratory rate ≥ 22.
     b. Altered mental status.
     c. Systolic BP ≤ 100 mm Hg.

- If the patient meets any 2 of these criteria and they are at risk for sepsis; an aggressive search for infection, including a thorough physical examination, inspection of all wounds, evaluation of intravascular catheters or other foreign bodies, obtaining appropriate cultures and adjunctive imaging studies are needed.

Treatment

This consists of a 6-hour protocol of early goal-directed therapy.

A. Monitoring

- **Lactate** and other lab values which measure tissue hypoperfusion are **used as a guide to resuscitation.**
- **Central venous catheterization is done to monitor CVP and central venous oxygen saturation**. These guide the use of I.V. fluids, vasopressors, PRBC transfusions and dobutamine.
- **Swan Ganz catheter** can also be used to accurately measure hemodynamic variables.
- Dynamic parameters are also used in monitoring: passive leg raise, fluid challenges, pulse pressure variation in response to mechanical ventilation.
- The target mean arterial pressure is 65 mm Hg.

B. Treatment

- Severely obtunded patients and patients whose work of breathing is excessive, require **intubation and ventilation** to prevent respiratory collapse.
- Empirical **fluid bolus of crystalloids** is given (up to 2 liters). Incremental fluids are continued based on the end points of resuscitation, including clearance of lactate.
- Empirical antibiotics and early source control of infection are associated with positive outcomes.
  - o **Initially, broad spectrum antibiotics** are given.
  - o Later, **antibiotics are tailored as per c/s.**
  - o **Source control:** Percutaneous drainage of abscesses and other surgical methods to target a source of infection.
- If crystalloids are not effective at raising blood pressure, vasopressors are given. The **vasopressor of choice is noradrenaline.**
- If blood pressure still does not rise and the requirements of noradrenaline increase significantly (> 5 mcg/min), **low dose vasopressin** is added. High dose vasopressin is not recommended.
- If high dose noradrenaline + low dose vasopressin are not enough, **adrenaline** is added.
- If cardiac output is low, **dobutamine** may also be used to augment tissue perfusion.
- The use of corticosteroids is controversial:
  - o **Hydrocortisone is not recommended** as routine adjuvant therapy.
  - o **Low dose steroids can be given** in vasopressor dependent, volume-replete septic shock.
  - o If systolic blood pressure remains < 90 mm Hg despite appropriate fluids and vasopressor therapy, corticosteroids can be used.
- **Marik protocol – bundle of Vitamin C, thiamine and hydrocortisone.**
- **Intensive insulin treatment:**
  - o Hyperglycemia and insulin resistance are typical in critically ill and septic patients without underlying diabetes mellitus.
  - o Tight glucose management has a significantly positive impact on outcome, in critically ill patients.

BLOOD TRANSFUSION

[5] Blood transfusion, its indications and complications. *Sept 21*

[5] Complications of blood transfusion. *Oct 20, Dec 15, March 24, CBME March 24*

[3] Mention complications of blood transfusion. *June 17, Dec 13*

[3] Mention indications of blood transfusion. *Dec 14*

[5] Indications of blood transfusion and its complications. *July 23*

[MCQ] Complications of blood transfusion includes all except: *CBME March 24*

A. Febrile reaction B. Allergic reaction
C. AIDS D. Leukemia*

[5] Enumerate indications and complications of blood transfusion. *CBME June 24*

Indications of Blood Transfusion

- Blood transfusions should be avoided if possible, and many previous uses of blood and blood products are now no longer considered appropriate.

The indications for blood transfusion are as follows:

- **Acute blood loss:** To replace circulating volume and maintain oxygen delivery.
- **Perioperative anemia:** To ensure adequate oxygen delivery during the perioperative phase.
- **Symptomatic chronic anemia:** In this, blood transfusion is indicated even when there is no hemorrhage or impending surgery.

Perioperative RBC transfusion criteria are as follows:

- **Hb < 6g/dl:** Patient will benefit from transfusion.
- **Hb 6 - 8g/dl:** Transfusion unlikely to be of benefit in the absence of bleeding or impending surgery.
- **Hb > 8g/dl:** No indication for transfusion in the absence of other risk factors.
  - o A Hb level of 6g/dl is acceptable in patients who are not actively bleeding, those who are not about to undergo major surgery and those who are not symptomatic.

Complications of Blood Transfusion

These can be categorised as:

A. Complications from a Single Transfusion

a. Incompatibility hemolytic transfusion reactions:

- It happens when antibodies present in the recipient's serum are incompatible with the donor's cells.
- It usually takes the form of an acute hemolytic reaction.
- Severe immune related transfusion reactions due to ABO incompatibility result in potentially fatal complement mediated intravascular hemolysis and multiple organ failure. Transfusion reactions from other antigen systems are usually milder and self-limiting.

b. Febrile transfusion reactions:

- Non-hemolytic.
- Usually caused by a graft versus host response from leukocytes in transfused components.
- Associated with fever, chills or rigors.
- Transfusion should be stopped immediately.
- It is rare with leukodepleted blood.

c. Allergic reaction.

d. Infection:

- Bacterial (usually due to faulty storage).
- Hepatitis.
- HIV.
- Malaria.

e. Air embolism.

f. Thrombophlebitis.

g. Transfusion related acute lung injury (TRALI):

- Usually from FFP.

B. Complications from Massive Transfusions

- Coagulopathy.
- Hypocalcemia.
- Hypokalemia.
- Hyperkalemia.
- Hypothermia.
- Iron overload (seen in patients with thalassemia).

[MCQ] Which of the following is not a complication of massive transfusion? ***CBME June 24***

A. Hypercalcemia* B. Coagulopathy

C. Hypothermia D. Hyperkalemia

[3] Massive Blood Transfusion. ***June 14***

- **Definition:** Massive blood transfusion is defined as transfusion of 10 units of packed red blood cells (PRBCs) within a 24-hour period **OR** transfusion greater than or equal to the patient's own blood volume within a 24-hour period.

Indications

- The primary indication for massive transfusion is **any situation resulting in an acute blood loss and hemodynamic instability.**
- Indications include, but are not limited to:
  - o Bleeding due to trauma.
  - o Obstetrical catastrophes.
  - o Surgery.
  - o Gastrointestinal bleeding.

Complications

The complications of massive blood transfusion are as follows:

- Metabolic alkalosis.
- Hypocalcemia.
- Hypothermia.
- Hyperkalemia.
- TRALI or transfusion related acute lung injury.
- TACO or transfusion associated circulatory overload.

BLOOD PRODUCTS AND BLOOD SUBSTITUTES

[3] Fresh Frozen Plasma. ***July 23***

Blood Products

- Blood products are derivatives of whole blood.
- Blood is collected from donors who have been previously screened before donating, to exclude:
  - o Any donor whose blood may have the potential to harm the patient.
  - o To prevent possible harm that donating a unit of blood may have for the donor.
- The following are available:

A. Whole Blood

- It is now rarely available because it is seen as an inefficient use of a limited resource.
- Whole blood transfusion has significant advantages over packed cells as it is coagulation factor rich and if fresh, more metabolically active than fresh blood.

B. Packed Red Blood Cells (PRBC)

- These are spun down and concentrated packs of red blood cells.
- **Each unit is ~330 ml and has a hematocrit of 50-70%.**
- Stored in a SAG-M (Saline Adenine Glucose Mannitol) solution to increase shelf life to 5 weeks at 2-6°C.

C. Fresh Frozen Plasma (FFP)

- Rich in **coagulation factors**.
- **Used as first line therapy in the treatment of coagulopathic hemorrhage.**
- It is removed from fresh blood and stored at -40°C to -50°C with a 2-year shelf life.
- RhD positive FFP may be given to a RhD negative woman.
- However, Rhesus-D immunization should be considered when large volumes are being transfused.

D. Cryoprecipitate

- It is a supernatant precipitate of FFP and is rich in fibrinogen, factor VIII and factor XII.
- Stored at -30°C with a 2-year shelf life.
- **Given in low fibrinogen states or factor VIII deficiency.**

E. Prothrombin Complex Concentrates

- Highly purified concentrates which are prepared from pooled plasma.
- Contains factors II, IX and X.
  - o Factor VII may be included OR produced separately.
  - o **Indicated for the emergency reversal of anti-coagulant (Warfarin) therapy in uncontrolled hemorrhage.**

F. Platelets

- Platelets are supplied as a pooled platelet concentrate.
- Contain about 250 × 10^9 platelets per litre.
- Stored on a special agitator at 20-24°C and have a shelf life of only 5 days.
- **Platelet transfusions are given to patients with thrombocytopenia or with platelet dysfunction who are bleeding or undergoing surgery.**

G. Autologous Blood

- Patients undergoing elective surgery can pre-donate their own blood.

[5] Blood Substitutes. ***July 15***

Blood Substitutes

- In contrast to volume expanders, blood substitutes **refer to fluids that can carry oxygen.**
- Blood substitutes are an alternative to the costly process of donating, checking, storing and administering blood.
- The properties of an ideal blood substitute are:
  - o Delivers oxygen.
  - o Be compatible with all blood types.

- o Have few side effects.
- o Have prolonged storage capabilities.
- o Persist in the circulation (i.e., it should not get excreted).
- o Cost-effective.

- Blood and blood products can cause immunogenic and infectious complications. These are not seen with blood substitutes.

Types of Blood Substitutes

A. Biomimetic

- Hemoglobin based.
- Mimic the standard oxygen carrying capacity of blood.

B. Abiotic

- Perfluorocarbon based.
- Synthetic oxygen carriers.
- Hb is seen as the obvious candidate for developing an effective blood substitute.
- Various engineered molecules are under clinical trials; and are based on human, bovine or recombinant technologies.
- The Hb for blood substitutes comes from a variety of sources, such as outdated donated human blood, bovine or porcine blood and transgenic *Escherichia coli*.

ELECTROLYTES AND ACID-BASE IMBALANCE

[5] Hyperkalemia. ***July 18***

- **Definition:** Hyperkalemia is defined as a serum potassium concentration **higher than the normal range of 3.5 – 5.0 mEq/l.**

Causes

- The **most common cause of hyperkalemia is acute onset of renal dysfunction or failure.**
- **Cellular injury (seen in sepsis or ischemia-reperfusion):** This releases potassium from its intracellular source, which overwhelms the kidney's ability to excrete it.
- **Drugs:** Triamterene, spironolactone, beta blockers, cyclosporine, tacrolimus, succinylcholine.

Clinical Features

- Cardiac arrhythmia, which can be lethal.
- **Other CVS features:** Low heart rate with irregular beats, low blood pressure, poor peripheral circulation, cyanosed skin.
- **GI symptoms:**
  - o Nausea and vomiting.
  - o Intermittent intestinal colic.
  - o Diarrhea.
- Mental confusion.
- Apathy.
- Sensory disturbances.
- Weakness of limbs.

Investigations

- Serum potassium.
- ECG shows following changes:
  - o Tall T waves.
  - o Wide QRS complex.
  - o Increased PR interval.
  - o Depressed ST segment.

Treatment

- **Intravenous sodium bicarbonate:**
  - o It shifts the potassium intracellularly.
- Sodium bicarbonate is administered before reperfusion to prevent ischemia reperfusion injury.
- IV calcium chloride or calcium gluconate: used as a cardiac stabiliser.
- **Short acting insulin:** Drives the potassium into the cells.
- **Beta 2 agonists such as albuterol:** Drives the potassium into the cells.
- **Furosemide:** It is a loop diuretic which causes excretion of potassium.

[5] Hypokalemia. ***Dec 18***
[3] Hypokalemia. ***July 23, Aug 22, Dec 13***

- **Definition:** Hypokalemia is defined as a serum

potassium **concentration below the normal range of 3.5-5.0 mEq/l.**

- Hypokalemia is much more common than hyperkalemia in the surgical patient.

Aetiopathogenesis

Hypokalemia can be broadly divided into 2 types:

A. Sudden Hypokalemia

- Unlikely to be encountered in surgical practice.
- **Causes:**
  - o Diabetic coma treated by insulin.
  - o Prolonged infusion of saline solution.

B. Gradual Hypokalemia

- Commonly encountered in surgical practice.
- **Causes:**
  - o **Inadequate intake:**
    - ♦ Dietary.
    - ♦ Potassium free IV fluids.
    - ♦ Potassium deficient TPN.
  - o Excessive potassium excretion **(potassium lost in the urine):**
    - ♦ Hyperaldosteronism.
    - ♦ Drugs (e.g., diuretics, amphotericin, aminoglycosides, cisplatin, ifosfamide).
  - o **GI losses:**
    - ♦ Direct loss of potassium from GI fluids: E.g., **Diarrhea, ulcerative colitis, villous tumours of rectum, loss from external fistulae of GIT (duodenal fistula, ileostomy).**
    - ♦ Prolonged gastroduodenal aspiration with fluid replacement by IV isotonic saline solution.
    - ♦ Post-op period following extensive resections for carcinoma of the alimentary tract (because often the operation has to be undertaken after months of weight loss and potassium depletion).
    - ♦ Vomiting.

Clinical Features

- Patient lies listlessly in bed: **Weakness, fatigue.**
- **Speech is slurred and slow**, often the patient fails to complete a sentence.
- Intense **drowsiness**.
- **Muscular hypotonia** is the outstanding physical sign.
- Loss of deep tendon reflexes.
- Incontinence of urine.
- Abdominal distension due to **paralytic ileus.**
- **Weakness of respiratory muscles** results in rapid, shallow, gasping respirations. This can cause post-op pulmonary complications.
- Diastolic blood pressure is low.
- Bounding pulse.
- **ECG changes: Prolonged QT interval, depression of ST segment, lowering or inversion of T-wave.**
- In severe hypokalemia, cardiac arrest may happen.

Investigations

- Serum potassium levels.
- ECG.

Treatment

- **Oral potassium:**
  - o Potassium chloride tablets or syrup.
  - o Milk, meat extracts, fruit juices and honey.
- **Intravenous potassium:**
  - o If oral route is inadequate or contraindicated, IV route must be used.
  - o The dangers of giving potassium IV are:
    - ♦ Administration should be properly controlled and the level of potassium should be checked at least daily.
    - ♦ If too much potassium is given too quickly, especially when renal function is impaired, it may raise the serum concentration to dangerous levels and cause cardiac arrest.
    - ♦ **Urine output must be adequate:** 1000 ml/24 hours or 40 ml/hour.

[3] Metabolic Acidosis. *July 23*

- **Definition:** Metabolic acidosis is a clinical disturbance defined by **a pH < 7.35 and a serum bicarbonate < 24 mEq/l.**

Aetiology

This results from an **increased intake of acid, an increased generation of acids, or an increased loss of bicarbonate.**

A. Increased Anion Gap Metabolic Acidosis

- Exogenous acid ingestion:
  - o Ethylene glycol, salicylates, methanol.
- Endogenous acid production:
  - o Ketoacidosis, lactic acidosis, renal insufficiency.

B. Normal Anion Gap Metabolic Acidosis

- Acid administration.
- Loss of bicarbonate.
- GI losses (diarrhea, fistulas).
- Ureterosigmoidostomy.
- Renal tubular acidosis.
- **Carbonic anhydrase inhibitor**
- Anion Gap (AG) is an index of unmeasured anions:

  AG = (Na) – (Cl + HCO_3).
  - o The normal anion gap is < 12 mmol/l and is due primarily to the albumin effect, so that the estimated anion gap must be adjusted for albumin. Therefore, hypoalbuminemia reduces the anion gap.
  - o Corrected anion gap = actual AG – [2.5 (4.5 – albumin)].

Clinical Features

- **Kussmaul's respiration:**
  - o Rapid, dry, noisy respirations which are continuous, except when the patient unsuccessfully tries to moisten his dry lips with his parched tongue.
  - o Increased ventilation/hyperpnea is due to overstimulation of the respiratory centre by the reduction of pH of the blood, and the physiological purpose of overbreathing is to eliminate as much as possible of the acid substance (carbonic acid).
- **Pulse rate and blood pressure are raised:**
  - o Except in renal acidosis.
- **Urine is strongly acidic.**
- **Standard bicarbonate level is lowered and there is a base deficit:**
  - o Therefore, body responds by increasing renal reabsorption and generation of bicarbonate.
  - o Kidney increases the secretion of hydrogen and thus increases the urinary excretion of ammonium.
  - o The body produces buffers (extracellular bicarbonate and intracellular buffers from bone and muscle).

Treatment

- Normal anion gap metabolic acidosis is treated by the **administration of RL solution or slow infusion of dilute sodium bicarbonate solution.**
- If patient is dehydrated, rapid infusion of sufficient isotonic saline solution (0.9% NS) is given, to restore the extracellular fluid volume **before** treatment with sodium bicarbonate solution.
- In lactic acidosis due to circulatory shock, the treatment is **to restore volume resuscitation rather than to attempt to correct the abnormality with exogenous bicarbonate.**

MISCELLANEOUS

[5] Hematoma. *July 18*

- **Definition:** A hematoma is a collection of blood clot and blood at the surgical site. It includes not only the subcutaneous tissues but may also be found in a deeper tissue space where surgery was performed.

Causes

- Incomplete surgical hemostasis.
- **Medical conditions that impair clotting:**
  - o Coagulation disorders.
  - o Platelet disorders.
  - o Other conditions that impair hemostasis, e.g., uremia, cirrhosis or sepsis.
- **Drugs:**
  - o **Antiplatelet agents:** Aspirin, Clopidogrel, Ticagrelor, Abciximab, Rivaroxaban, Apixaban, Dabigatran.

Clinical Features

A hematoma can occur in various spaces and the clinical features vary depending on the space affected.

A. Superficial Hematoma

- Skin discolouration.
- Subcutaneous swelling.
- Pain at the affected area due to pressure.

B. Abdominal Cavity

- Abdominal compartment syndrome or ileus.

C. Forearm or Leg

- Compartment syndrome.

D Anterior Neck

- Airway compromise.
- When clotting disorders are present, the bleeding may persist and patients with large hematomas can present with anemia or hypovolemia.
- Infected hematomas may cause fever, leukocytosis, or sepsis.

Prevention

- Appropriate evaluation of bleeding disorders and anticoagulant drugs in the pre-op period.
- Attention to hemostasis during surgical procedures.

Treatment

- The treatment of choice is **evacuation of hematoma.**

[3] Venesection. *Dec 17*

- Also known as **phlebotomy.**
- It is a procedure in which blood is withdrawn from a patient's body for therapeutic purposes.

Indications

- Blood disorders such as:
  - o Hemochromatosis.
  - o Polycythemia vera.
  - o Porphyria.
- These conditions involve an excess of iron, RBCs or certain metabolic by-products in the blood respectively.
- By removing blood, venesection helps to reduce these elevated levels and manage the associated symptoms.

Veins Used

- The vessel most commonly punctured during venesection is the median cubital vein, which is located in the antecubital fossa of the arm.
- Other veins such as basilic vein and cephalic vein can also be used.

[3] Virchow's triad. *July 23*

- Virchow's triad describes the 3 primary abnormalities which lead to thrombus formation:
  1. Endothelial injury.
  2. Stasis or turbulent blood flow.
  3. Hypercoagulability of blood.
- Endothelial injury is the most important factor.
- Abnormal blood flow (stasis or turbulence) can lead to hypercoagulability directly and also indirectly through endothelial dysfunction.

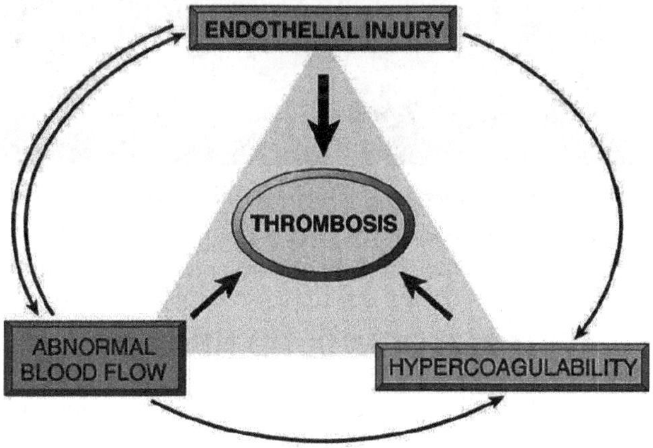

Figure: Mechanism of blood coagulation

2

Wound Healing

[10] What is wound? Describe the phases of wound healing and the factors affecting wound healing. *Feb 23*

[5] Factors which influence wound healing. *August 22, June 13, CBME March 24*

[3] Mention factors which influence wound healing. *Dec 12*

[3] Enumerate various factors affecting wound healing. *CBME June 24*

[MCQ] In remodelling phase of wound healing, it is characterized by maturation of collagen in which type III collagen is replaced by ? *CBME June 24*

A. Type I*	B. Type II
C. Fibroblasts	D. Type IV

- A wound refers to a physical injury or damage to the body's tissues, typically involving a break or disruption in the integrity of skin and/or other tissues.

PHASES OF WOUND HEALING

- Wound healing is described in **3** overlapping but distinct **stages**:
  1. Inflammation.
  2. Proliferation.
  3. Remodelling.
- An **additional stage, hemostasis**, is often described as the immediate stage occurring before inflammation.

Hemostasis

- Disruption of the vascular endothelium following injury causes **vasoconstriction** and **exposure of the subendothelial extracellular matrix.**
- This encourages platelets to adhere, activate and aggregate, resulting in a platelet plug, which also helps limit further blood loss.

Inflammation

A. Early Inflammatory Phase (Days 1-2)

- Platelet activation causes an **influx of inflammatory cells** led by polymorphonuclear leukocytes, **particularly neutrophils.**
- Neutrophils minimise bacterial contamination.
- Platelets and local injured tissue release **vasoactive amines** (histamine and serotonin) which **increase vascular permeability**, thereby helping the infiltration of inflammatory cells (diapedesis).

B. Late Inflammatory Phase (Days 2-3)

- **Monocytes** appear in the wound and **differentiate into macrophages.**
- Macrophages function as **phagocytic cells** and **release proteolytic enzymes** to help debride the wound.
- They also produce cytokines and growth factors which promote **fibroblast proliferation** and **angiogenesis.**

Proliferation

- Starts around day 3 and **lasts for 2-4 weeks.**

- Consists mainly of **fibroblast activity** with the production of **ground substance, collagen, angiogenesis and re-epithelialisation** of the wound.
- **Granulation tissue is formed** which has a pink and granular appearance.
- There is an **increase in the tensile strength** of the wound due to increased collagen synthesized by fibroblasts.
- Fibroblasts differentiate into **myofibroblasts** which **contract** to bring the edges of the wound together.

Remodelling

- Begins 2-3 weeks after injury and lasts for > 1 year.
- **Maturation of collagen** occurs.
- **Type III collagen is replaced by type I**, until the normal ratio of **4 : 1** is achieved.
- **Collagen** becomes more **cross-linked** and uniformly aligned.
- **Tensile strength increases** and is 80% of uninjured skin strength.

FACTORS WHICH INFLUENCE WOUND HEALING

Wound healing is influenced by local and systemic factors.

A. Local Factors

- The presence of these factors impair wound healing:
  - o Skin tension.
  - o Hypoxia and ischemia.
  - o Vascular insufficiency.
  - o Lymphedema.
  - o Contamination.
  - o Infection.
  - o Presence of foreign bodies.
  - o Radiotherapy.

B. Systemic Factors

- These factors impair wound healing:
  - o **Advancing age:** As age advances, protein turnover reduces, which impairs wound healing.
  - o Obesity.
  - o Malnutrition.
  - o Smoking.
  - o Diseases (e.g., diabetes mellitus, connective tissue diseases).
  - o Immunocompromised (e.g., AIDS).
  - o Drugs (e.g., steroids, immunosuppressants, chemotherapy).

[10] Classify wounds. Describe the principles of management of severely injured person. *Dec 19*

CLASSIFICATION OF WOUNDS

- Wounds are diverse and there is **no standard classification system** that incorporates all relevant aspects for different clinical contexts.
- A **wide variety of classifications** are used.

A. Based on Aetiology

- Clean or surgical.
- Shearing or degloving.
- Crush.
- Blast.
- Burn (Thermal, electrical, chemical, radiation, mechanical).
- Cold injury.
- Avulsion or traction.
- Low or high energy.
- Bite.

B. Based on Depth

- Epidermal.
- Dermal (Superficial or deep).
- Full thickness.

C. Based on Contamination

- Clean.
- Clean-contaminated.
- Contaminated.
- Dirty.
- Implant or non-implant.

D. Based on Complexity

1. Simple.
2. **Complex:**

- o Significant soft tissue loss.
- o Open fracture or joint involvement.
- o Visceral involvement.

3. **Complicated:**
   - o Infection.
   - o Necrosis.
   - o Hematoma.
   - o Gas gangrene.
   - o Compartment syndrome.

PRINCIPLES OF WOUND MANAGEMENT

- **Clinical judgement** is crucial in managing wounds.
- Some general principles of wound management are as follows:

A. **Preparation**

- **Antibiotic prophylaxis**
  - o Needed for clean-contaminated, contaminated and dirty wounds.
  - o May also be used in clean wounds when there is a high risk of infection or when the sequelae of infection are potentially disastrous.
- **Tetanus prophylaxis**
  - o Should be given based on the type of wound and immunization status.
- **Adequate analgesia/anesthesia**

B. **Wound Care**

- **Irrigation**
  - o All wounds should be irrigated **to reduce bacterial contamination** and **to wash away debris or dirt.**
  - o It also allows better visualization for **wound assessment.**
  - o **Warm NS** is typically used, although other irrigation fluids are available such as water and antiseptic solutions.
  - o Can also be performed with a **soft brush or sponge to clear particulate matter.**
- **Debridement**
  - o It is essential to **remove any devitalized tissue** and **foreign material** from the wound.
  - o Non-viable tissue must be excised **until healthy bleeding occurs at the wound edges.**
  - o Sometimes, **multiple sittings** are required before definitive repair and closure, e.g., blast injuries, necrotizing fasciitis.
  - o **Types of debridement:**
    - ♦ **Surgical:** Using surgical instruments such as a scalpel, curette or scissors.
    - ♦ **Mechanical:** Using irrigation, wet-to-dry dressings and hydrotherapy.
    - ♦ **Autolytic:** Using dressings such as hydrocolloids or transparent films to retain moisture and allow wound enzymes to selectively liquefy non-viable tissue.
    - ♦ **Enzymatic:** Chemically liquefy necrotic tissue with enzymes using topical agents such as collagenase or papain-urea.
    - ♦ **Biological:** Medical grade larvae of *Lucilia sericata* release proteolytic and antimicrobial substances to remove necrotic tissue. They also directly promote wound healing.
- **Exploration**
  - o Wounds should be explored **to determine the extent of injury**, including any damage to underlying neurovascular structures, tendons, joints and bones.
- **Repair structures**
  - o Repair of all damaged structures may be attempted once the wounds are clean.
  - o Repair of nerves and vessels should be performed under magnification using loupes or a microscope.
- **Hemostasis.**

C. **Closure**

- **Skin closure without tension**
  - o Skin closure should always be without tension.
  - o Direct closure is not always possible and other reconstruction methods should be considered.
- **Consider reconstruction options**
  - o Skin graft or flaps can be used.
- **Suture choice**
  - o Finer sutures are more cosmetic.

- **Consider drains**
  - o Prevents hematoma formation.
- **Optimal dressings**
  - o **Negative pressure wound therapy** (NPWT) or **vacuum assisted closure** (VAC) helps draw the wound edges together, removes exudate, reduces oedema, and promotes granulation tissue formation.

D. Follow-Up

- Removal of sutures.
- Sutures on the head and neck are removed earlier than sutures on other parts:
- Physiotherapy.
- Monitoring for complications.
- Scar management.
- Hypertrophic scar, keloid, contractures are all examples of abnormal wound healing and should be dealt with.

[5] Keloid. ***Sept 21, Dec 13***

[3] Keloid. ***June 19, Dec 14***

- **Definition:** A keloid scar is defined as **excessive scar tissue that extends beyond the boundaries** of the original incision or wound.
- Keloids are rare compared to hypertrophic scars.

Cause

- The exact cause is **unknown.**
- However, it is **associated with** the following:
  - o Increased growth factors.
  - o Deeply pigmented skin.
  - o Inherited tendency.
  - o Certain areas of the body are predisposed: **triangle formed by both tips of shoulders and xiphisternum.**

Clinical Features

- May be seen in the ear lobe following piercing.
- May appear years after injury.
- Does not regress.
- Complains of pain, itching, hyperesthesia.

HPE

- Excessive collagen with hypervascularity.
- Collagen fibers are in random orientation.

Treatment

- **Pressure:** Local moulds or elasticated garments.
- Silicone gels or sheets.
- Intralesional steroid injection (Triamcinolone).
- Excision + steroid injection.
- Excision + post-op radiation (External beam or brachytherapy).
- Intralesional excision.
- **Laser:** To reduce redness.
- Vitamin E.
- Palm oil massage.

[3] Hypertrophic Scar. ***July 15***

HYPERTROPHIC SCAR

- **Definition:** A hypertrophic scar is defined as excessive scar tissue that does not extend beyond the boundary of the original incision or wound.
- A hypertrophic scar is common.

Cause

- Prolonged inflammatory phase of wound healing.
- Unfavourable scar location, i.e., across the lines of skin tension.

Clinical Features

- Occurs anywhere in the body.
- Usually appears 4-6 weeks after injury.
- Frequently undergoes spontaneous regression.
- Patient may complain of itching.

HPE

- Excessive collagen with hypervascularity.
- Parallel orientation of collagen fibres.

Treatment

- **Pressure:** Local moulds or elasticated garments.
- Silicone gels or sheets.
- Intralesional injection of steroid (triamcinolone).
- Excision + steroid injection.
- Excision + post-op radiation (external beam or brachytherapy).
- **Laser:** To reduce redness.
- Vitamin E.
- Palm oil massage.

[5] Difference between hypertrophic scar and keloid. *March 24*

[3] Differentiate between hypertrophic scar and keloid. *CBME June 24*

	Hypertrophic Scar	**Keloid**
Incidence	Frequent	Rare
Ethnic groups	No predilection	African, American, Asian, Hispanic
Prior injury	Yes	Yes
Site predilection	Anywhere	Neck, chest, ear lobes, shoulders, upper back
Genetics	No	Autosomal dominant with incomplete penetration
Timing	4–6 weeks post injury	Symptom-free interval; may appear years after injury
Symptoms	Raised, some pruritus, respects wound confines	Pain, pruritus, hyperesthesia, growth beyond wound margins
Regression	Frequent, spontaneous	No
Contracture	Frequent	Rare
Histology	Parallel orientation of collagen fibres	Hypocellular, thick, wavy collagen fibres in random orientation

[5] Marjolin's Ulcer. ***Dec 17, June 14***

[3] Marjolin's Ulcer. ***July 15, July 23***

[MCQ] Malignancy arising from a chronic scar is called what? ***CBME June 24***

A. Meleney's ulcer B. Melanoma

C. Marjolin's ulcer * D. Rodent ulcer

- **Definition:** It is the name given to a **squamous cell carcinoma** or **basal cell carcinoma** which **arises in chronically inflamed wounds or scars.**

Causes

- It was originally described to occur in **chronic burn scars.**
- However, it can occur in **any chronically inflamed wound:**
  - o Long-standing venous ulcer.
  - o Chronic sinus tracts.
  - o Pre-existing scars.
  - o Chronic osteomyelitis.
  - o Vaccination points.
  - o Pressure sores.
  - o Hidradenitis suppurativa.

Pathogenesis

- Any wound that **does not heal for a prolonged period of time** is prone to malignant transformation.
- Such wounds may first exhibit **pseudoepitheliomatous hyperplasia which is a pre-malignant condition**, before transforming into SCC or BCC.
- **Other rare tumours are:** Sarcoma, neurotropic malignant melanoma, malignant fibrous histiocytoma.
- Typically **appear decades after the original injury.**
- However, burn scar carcinoma may be encountered within the first year.

Clinical Features

- Burn scar carcinomas **most commonly** occur in the **head and neck** region.
- **Slow growing malignant lesion**, probably due to less vascularity of the region.
- Edges may be raised and everted.
- Usually painless.
- It is less malignant than a typical SCC, but more malignant than SCC occurring in immunocompromised patients.
- **Lymphatic mets is less** because lymphatics are destroyed or occluded by the previous chronic lesions.

Investigations

- An **edge-wedge** or an **incisional biopsy** is used in diagnosing Marjolin's ulcer.
- **Indications:**
  - o A chronic ulcer which is unresponsive to dressings and simple treatments.
  - o Chronic wounds that appear atypical clinically.

Treatment

- **Wide local excision** of the lesion ± **reconstruction** of the defect with a split-thickness or full-thickness skin graft.
- Burn scar carcinoma in **head and neck** can be treated with **excision followed by radiotherapy.**

[3] Granuloma Pyogenicum. *August 22*

- **Definition:** Exuberant outburst of highly vascular granulation tissue at the site of previously trivial trauma.
- Also known as granuloma pyogenicum.

Pathology

- It is a **benign proliferation of capillary blood vessels** of the skin.
- Histologically **similar to hemangioma.**

Clinical Features

- Occur at the sites of **previously trivial trauma.**
- Common on **fingertips.**
- Small (0.5 - 1.5 cm).
- Raised or pedunculated.
- Soft.
- Painless.
- Red fleshy nodule.
- Grows rapidly over several weeks.
- Bleeds easily.
- Friable.

Treatment

- Topical silver nitrate or corticosteroids.
- **Surgical options:**
  - o Curettage.
  - o Simple excision with cauterization of base.
  - o Reconstruction of defect.

[5] Pressure Sore. *Dec 14*

- Also known as pressure ulcer, pressure injury, bed sores, decubitus ulcer.
- Pressure ulcers are ulcers which **occur over pressure points.**

Sites

- Pressure ulcers occur over a **bony prominence:**
  - o Ischium.
  - o Greater trochanter.
  - o Sacrum.
  - o Heel.
  - o Malleolus.
  - o Occiput.

Aetiopathogenesis

- An **increase in local tissue pressure above that of perfusion pressure produces ischemic necrosis.**
- Due to a result of **friction or persisting pressure** on soft tissues.
- **Risk factors** which predispose to pressure ulcers are:
  - o Severely ill patients.
  - o Impaired mobility.
  - o Prolonged immobility.
  - o Those with a significant loss of sensation.
  - o Elderly patients.
  - o Spinal injury patients.
  - o Malnutrition.
  - o Anemia.
  - o Injury.
  - o Moisture.

Clinical Features

- Occur over pressure points.
- Easy to prevent and difficult to treat.
- **On Examination:** Have a punched out edge.

Staging of Pressure Injuries

1. **Non blanchable erythema** of intact skin.
2. **Partial thickness skin loss with exposed dermis**, i.e., appear as a shallow open ulcer with a red-pink wound bed or an intact or ruptured serum filled blister.
3. **Full thickness skin loss**, i.e., subcutaneous fat is visible in the wound; but not bone, tendon or muscle.
4. **Full thickness skin and tissue loss**, i.e., exposed bone, tendon or muscle.

Risk Assessment Scales

- The following are used to assess the risk of development of bed sores:
  - o Braden scale.
  - o Waterlow score.
  - o Norton scale.

Prevention

- Avoidance of pressure over bony prominences.
- Regular turning/Repositioning of the patient.
- Use of pressure redistribution beds: Water bed, air bed.
- Regular inspection of pressure points.
- Optimise nutrition.
- Correction of anemia.
- Prevent infection.

Treatment

- Nutrition.
- Debridement.
- Regular dressing.
- Antibiotics are given if there are signs of infection.
- Surgery is considered only as a last option:
  - o Primary closure and skin grafting should be avoided as they are likely to fail.
  - o **Reconstruction options:** Fasciocutaneous or musculocutaneous flaps.

OTHER IMPORTANT TOPICS

Types of Wound Healing

A. Primary Healing or Healing by First Intention

- There is **direct approximation of wound edges** (suturing or stapling).
- Wound heals well.
- Minimal or best scar.

B. Secondary Healing or Healing by Secondary Intention

- Wounds are left open.
- Wound heals by granulation, contraction and re-epithelialisation.
- There is increased inflammation and proliferation.
- Poor scar.

C. Tertiary or Delayed Primary Healing

- It is indicated in contaminated or untidy wounds.
- Wound is **initially left open**, i.e., wound edges are not opposed.
- Non-viable tissue is debrided.
- When the wound becomes clean and the healing **conditions become favourable, the wound edges may be surgically approximated** (secondary suturing).
- Split-thickness skin grafting is also an example of tertiary healing.

3

Infections and Infestations

[10] Aetiopathogenesis, clinical features, diagnosis and management of tuberculous lymphadenitis. ***March 21***

[10] Discuss the clinical features, investigations and treatment of tuberculous cervical lymphadenopathy. ***Dec 15***

[5] TB lymphadenitis. ***March 24***

[3] Cold abscess. ***July 18, Dec 16***

[3] Mention the stages of tubercular lymphadenitis. ***Dec 14, June 13 (paper I and II)***

[3] Collar stud abscess. ***June 23***

- Common in the Indian subcontinent.
- Most common cause of cervical lymphadenopathy in the Indian subcontinent is tuberculosis.

Aetiopathogenesis

- **Causative organism:** *Mycobacterium tuberculosis.*
- **Source of infection:**
  - o Those in contact with **open human TB.**
  - o Those who drink **infected milk.**
- **Lymph nodes affected:**
  - o The **deep upper cervical nodes** are most commonly affected.
  - o But any of the cervical group of lymph nodes may be affected.
- **Route of entry:**
  - o Tubercle bacilli gain **entry through the i/l tonsil** of the corresponding side.

Stages of Tuberculous Lymphadenopathy

1. **Stage of lymphadenitis:**
   - o Tubercles form within the cortex of the lymph node.
2. **Stage of perilymphadenitis/matting:**
   - o As disease spreads, several lymph nodes become involved.
   - o Capsule of the lymph node is breached and neighbouring lymph nodes get matted.
3. **Stage of cold abscess:**
   - o Several **lymph nodes coalesce** and break down to form **caseous tuberculous pus.**
   - o The caseating material gradually **liquefies** and a cold abscess forms.
   - o A cold abscess is a **painless, fluctuant** mass which is not warm. It is **not associated with any signs of inflammation** and is therefore called a cold abscess.
   - o A cold abscess is a clinical manifestation of underlying caseation.
4. **Stage of collar stud abscess:**
   - o **Initially**, cold abscess remains **deep to deep cervical fascia**.
   - o In a few weeks time, the deep cervical **fascia becomes eroded at one point** and the **pus flows through the small opening into the superficial fascia**.

- o The pus deep to the deep cervical fascia becomes continuous with the pus in the superficial fascia through a small opening in the deep cervical fascia.
- o This is called a collar stud abscess.
- o It is a **cross fluctuant swelling** and is **bilocular**.

5. **Stage of chronic sinus/ulceration:**
   - o In untreated cases, the skin gradually becomes indurated, breaks down and forms a tuberculous sinus which **discharges pus** and, if ignored, the sinus remains unhealed for years.
   - o The lesion may **eventually ulcerate**. It gives a watery discharge. A tuberculous ulcer has **undermined edges** as the tubercle bacilli destroys the subcutaneous tissue faster than the skin and thrives in the relatively anoxic environment.

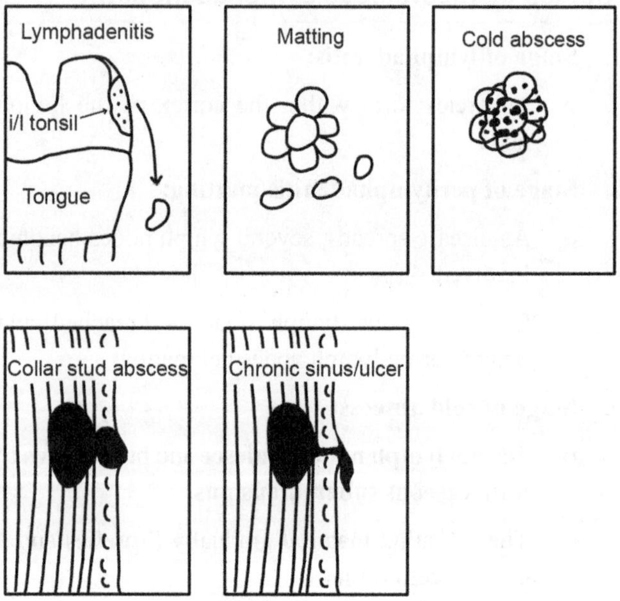

Figure: Stages of TB lymphadenitis

- o From each of these stages, **resolution may take place with:**
  - ♦ **Calcification:** If caseation has occurred.
  - ♦ **Scarring:** If sinuses have formed.
- o In 80% of the cases, the tuberculous process is limited to the clinically affected group of lymph nodes: but, a **primary focus in the lungs must always be ruled out.**

Clinical Features

- It can occur in any age group, but it is common in **children and young adults.**
- **General manifestations of tuberculosis:**
  - o Evening rise of temperature.
  - o Night sweats.
  - o Malaise.
  - o Cough (may be from pulmonary TB).
  - o Loss of weight.
  - o Failure to thrive in children.
- Swelling in the neck.
- Cold abscess.
- Collar stud abscess.
- Chronic tuberculous sinus.

Investigations

- **FNAC** can be done of the enlarged lymph node and it is tested for acid fast bacilli.
- If mass is still in early stages of adenitis, **excision biopsy** should be done. Part of the lymph node is then sent fresh and unfixed to the lab, which should process it immediately.
- **Mantoux test or Tuberculin skin test:**
  - o Now being superseded by **interferon-gamma (IFN-ϒ) release assay.**
  - o Mantoux is not useful in the following patient groups:
    - ♦ Patients from an endemic area.
    - ♦ Immunocompromised patients.
    - ♦ Patients with prior BCG vaccination.
- **Interferon gamma (IFN-ϒ) release assay:**
  - o Also called **quantiferon gold assay.**
  - o Gold standard test.
  - o It is a blood test which **measures the cellular immune response to antigens** derived from *Mycobacterium tuberculosis.*
- Sputum for:
  - o C/S (Results take several weeks).
  - o ZN staining.
- Aspiration of pus from a cold abscess for C/S.
- **Chest X-ray:** To look for pulmonary TB.
- **Blood tests:**
  - o Increased ESR.
  - o Increased CRP.
  - o Low Hb.

- Patients should also be **tested for HIV**, as the two often **coexist**.

Treatment

A. Anti Tubercular Therapy (ATT)

Type of TB case	Intensive phase	Continuous phase
New case	(2) HRZE	(4) HRE
Previously treated	(2) HRZES + (1) HRZE	(5) HRE

- The number in brackets indicates the number of months that it should be taken:

  H – Isoniazid.

  R – Rifampicin.

  Z – Pyrazinamide.

  E – Ethambutol.

  S – Streptomycin.

B. General Measures

- High protein diet.
- Vitamin supplements.

C. Surgery

- A small cold abscess resolves with general treatment and ATT, and no special treatment is required.
- **Aspiration of cold abscess**: The needle should be **inserted through healthy skin** from above (avoiding the dependent part) to prevent chances of sinus formation.
- Sometimes, **excision of the abscess and its surrounding fibrous capsule** is necessary, together with the relevant lymph nodes.
- Matted nodes are associated with significant fibrosis, which makes surgery difficult.

[5] Abdominal tuberculosis. ***August 22, March 21, Dec 18, Dec 17, Dec 15***

[5] Ileocecal tuberculosis. ***June 17***

Aetiology

- **Causative organism:** *Mycobacterium tuberculosis.*
- **Route of infection:**
  - o **Swallowing of infected sputum** in a patient with pulmonary TB.
  - o By **drinking infected unpasteurised milk.**
  - o **Hematogenous** spread.
- The increased prevalence of HIV infection has made TB more common.

Pathology

- There are 2 types:
  1. **Ulcerative** type.
  2. **Hyperplastic** type.
- In both types, there may be marked **mesenteric lymphadenopathy.**

Ulcerative	Hyperplastic
Denotes a severe form of the disease in which the **virulence of the organism overwhelms host resistance**	Occurs when **host resistance has the upper hand** over the virulence of the organism
The organism **colonises the lymphatics of the terminal ileum**, which results in: • **Transverse ulcers** with typical undermined edges • Serosa is usually studded with tubercles	There is marked inflammatory reaction causing **hyperplasia and thickening of the terminal ileum** because of its abundance of lymphoid follicles, which results in: • Narrowing of the lumen • Obstruction
HPE: Caseating granuloma with giant cells	
Terminal ileum is affected	Ileocecal area is affected
Sequelae: • Ulcers heal by **fibrosis** • Transverse ulcers lead to **multiple strictures**	**Sequelae:** • As a result of **fibrosis**, there is shortening of the bowel • **Cecum gets pulled up** into a subhepatic position • Resultant widening of ileocecal angle beyond 90°
Presents with: • Strictures • Intestinal obstruction	**Presents with:** • Right iliac fossa mass • Obstructive symptoms

Clinical Features

- Patient stays in an endemic area with a history of TB in the neighbourhood.
- **Constitutional symptoms of TB:**
  - o Weight loss.
  - o Chronic cough.
  - o Malaise.

- o Evening rise of temperature with sweating.
- Complains of vague abdominal pain.
- Distension.
- Alternating constipation and diarrhoea.
- Patients may present to the emergency with **distal small bowel obstruction.**
- Rarely, patients present with features of **peritonitis from perforation of a tuberculous ulcer** in the small bowel.
- Some patients may present with **fistula-in-ano** which is typically **multiple** with undermined edges and **watery discharge.**

On Examination

- Abdomen has a **doughy feel**, due to areas of localised ascites.
- In the hyperplastic type, a **mass** may be felt in the **right iliac fossa.**

Investigations

A. Contrast X-rays

- Barium meal, barium follow through.
- **Findings:**
  - o **Strictures** of the small bowel, particularly the ileum.
  - o Pulled up or high **subhepatic cecum.**
  - o The narrow **ileum enters the cecum** directly from below upwards **in a straight line** rather than at an angle.

B. Diagnostic Laparoscopy

- Tubercles on the bowel serosa.
- Multiple strictures.
- High cecum.
- Enlarged lymph nodes.
- Areas of caseation.
- Ascites.

C. CBNAAT

- Tissue or tubercle can be sent for CBNAAT, culture.

D. CXR

- If pulmonary TB is suspected.

Treatment

A. Anti-TB Drugs

- **New case:** 2 months of HRZE (intensive phase) + 4 months of HRE (continuous phase).
- **Previously treated:** 2 months of HRZES and 1 month of HRZE (intensive phase) + 5 months of HRE (continuous phase).

  H: Isoniazid.

  R: Rifampicin.

  Z: Pyrazinamide.

  E: Ethambutol.

  S: Streptomycin.

B. Surgery

- **Ileocolic resection** + anastomosis between terminal ileum and ascending colon.
  - o Done for ileocolic hyperplastic disease.
- **Strictureplasty:**
  - o For single ileal stricture.
- **Bowel resection:**
  - o For multiple closely-placed strictures.
- **Right hemicolectomy:**
  - o For extensive ileocolic disease.

C. Patient Presenting to Emergency

- Vigorous **resuscitation** should be done before the operation.
- At laparotomy, the **minimum life-saving procedure is carried out:**
  - o Resection of diseased segment with **proximal ileostomy** and distal ileal or colonic mucus fistula to avoid anastomosis.
  - o Perforation is treated by appropriate local resection and anastomosis or ileostomy.
- After emergency surgery, the patient is given anti-tubercular drugs.

[5] TB peritonitis. *Dec 14*

Aetiology

- **Causative organism:** *Mycobacterium tuberculosis, Mycobacterium avium intracellulare.*
- An increased prevalence of HIV infection has made TB more common.

- **Route of infection:**
  - o From ileocaecal TB via mesenteric lymph nodes.
  - o Hematogenous route from pulmonary TB.
  - o From Fallopian tubes.

Pathology

There are 2 types of TB peritonitis:

1. **Wet, ascitic type (90%):**
   - o Most common type.
   - o It is characterized by **generalized or loculated ascites.**
   - o Multiple **tubercle deposits** are present on both layers of the peritoneum (parietal and visceral).
2. **Dry, plastic type (10%):**
   - o Less common.
   - o Fibrotic fixed loops of **bowel and omentum** are **matted together.**
   - o Bowel may be encased in a fibrotic sac **(cocoon).**
   - o Ascites is not seen.

Clinical Features

- Presentation is often insidious.
- **Constitutional symptoms of TB:**
  - o Weight loss.
  - o Chronic cough.
  - o Malaise.
  - o Evening rise of temperature with sweating.
- The most common symptom is abdominal distension due to ascites.
- Poorly localized, vague abdominal pain.
- Patients may present with subacute intestinal obstruction.

Investigations

- **USG of abdomen.**
- **CT abdomen:**
  - o These detect ascites and lymphadenopathy with/without diffuse thickening of the peritoneum, mesentery and/or omentum.
- **Analysis of ascitic fluid:**
  - o Straw coloured.
  - o Exudates (protein > 25-30 g/l).
  - o WBCs > 500/ml.
  - o Lymphocytes > 40%.
  - o Adenose deaminase is present.
- **Diagnostic laparoscopy:**
  - o The parietal and visceral peritoneum is studded with tubercles.
  - o Peritoneal and/or omental biopsy can be taken.
- **Xpert MTB/RIF assay:**
  - o It rapidly and simultaneously detects *Mycobacterium tuberculosis* complex and resistance to rifampicin.

Treatment

A. **Supportive**
   - Nutrition.
   - Hydration.

B. **Medical**
   - Oral anti-TB therapy.

C. **Surgery**
   - May be required for specific complications such as intestinal obstruction.

[10] Describe the aetiopathogenesis, clinical features, prophylaxis and management of tetanus. ***June 23***

[10] Discuss the aetiology, clinical features and management of tetanus. ***July 15, June 14***

[10] Describe the aetiology, clinical features and treatment of tetanus. ***June 13***

[5] Tetanus. ***June 16***

[3] Risus sardonicus. ***Dec 13***

[5] Write in detail about types, clinical features and management of tetanus. ***CBME June 24***

- Also known as lockjaw.
- The range of injuries and accidents which may lead to tetanus, comprise a trivial pin prick, skin abrasion, puncture wounds, burns, human bites, animal bites, unsterile surgery, etc.

Aetiopathogenesis

- **Causative organism is *Clostridium tetani*:**
  - o It is a gram-positive spore-forming bacillus which **occurs naturally in the intestines of humans** and in the **soil.**
  - o **Incubation period:** 4-14 days.

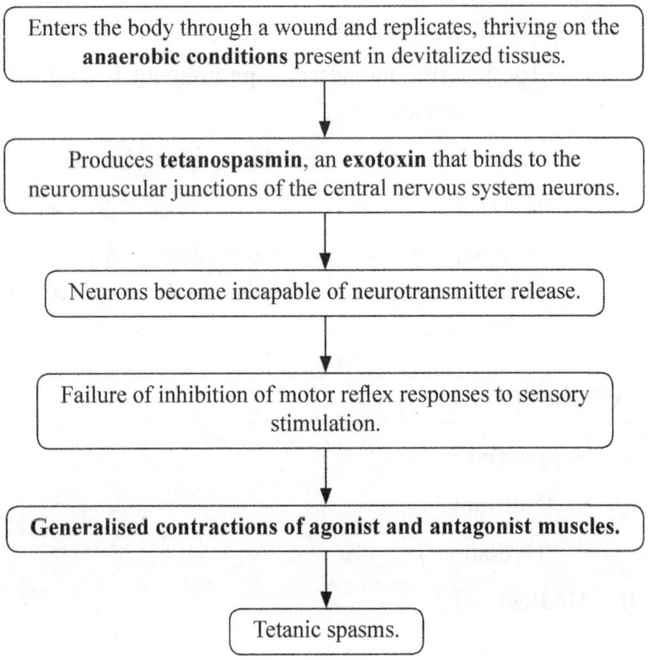

Clinical Features

- Entry wound may show a **localized** small area of **cellulitis.**
- Dysphagia, jaw stiffness and severe pains in the neck, back and abdomen precede the tonic muscle spasms.
- Early symptoms are **painful spasms of the facial muscles resulting in risus sardonicus**, i.e., sardonic smile.
- Spasms spread to involve the respiratory and laryngeal musculature.
- **Laryngeal muscle spasm** leads to apnoea and if prolonged; to asphyxia, cyanosis and respiratory arrest.
- Swallowing becomes progressively more difficult.
- Spasms of the paravertebral and extensor limb musculature produce **opisthotonus**, an arching of the whole body.
- Spasms can be **brought on by the slightest of sensory stimuli** such as noise or movement.
- Spasms can cause great **pain** and even **muscle rupture.**
- Between the reflex convulsions, the tonic muscular spasm remains, thus distinguishing tetanus from strychnine poisoning.
- Temperature is elevated.
- Pulse is rapid.
- If untreated, **respiratory failure and death** during a **cyanotic attack** result.

Tetanus Prone Wounds

- Puncture type injuries in a contaminated environment.
- Bites.
- Compound fractures.
- Wounds containing foreign bodies.
- Wounds or burns with systemic sepsis.

High Risk Tetanus Prone Wounds

- **Any tetanus prone wound with:**
  - o Heavy contamination, e.g., soil or manure.
  - o Wound requiring surgery with > 6 hours delay.
  - o Extensive devitalized tissue.

Investigations

- It is a clinical diagnosis.
- **Exudates** or aspirates from the wound may show **Gram-positive rods.**

Prognosis

- The shorter the interval between the first symptom and the first reflex spasm, the poorer is the prognosis. If the interval is < 48 hours death is likely.
- Once the exotoxin (tetanospasmin) is fixed in the nerve tissue, it can no longer be neutralized by antitoxin.

Treatment

- **There are 3 aspects of management:**
  - o Prevention.
  - o Local wound care.
  - o Supportive care for established disease.

Prevention

- Active immunization is given by administering **0.5 ml of tetanus toxoid (TT) intramuscularly.**
- Patients with **gross contamination** of cavitating wounds should also receive **250-500 U of human anti-tetanus globulin (ATG) IM** to provide passive immunization and to neutralise the circulating toxins.
- In full-blown clinical tetanus 3000-10,000 U of ATG should be administered.
- **Wound manipulation** should be **avoided** for 2-3 hours after ATG administration to minimize tetanospasmin release.
- General measures of **routine wound care**, such as **washing and debridement** prevent and reduce the incidence of tetanus.

Local Wound Care

- Thorough wound debridement to eliminate the anaerobic environment.
- Wounds should be closed using the delayed primary or secondary closure techniques.
- **IV penicillin G** 10-24 × 10^6 U per day for 10-14 days.
- **If** patient is **allergic** to penicillin, give **erythromycin.**

Supportive Care for Established Disease

- Shift patient to **ICU**, free from strong sensory stimuli.
- **IV diazepam** is given to prevent the onset of spasms.
- If spasms become sustained, the patient is paralyzed, intubated and placed on a ventilator.
- The patient is then gradually weaned off the ventilator under cover of anticonvulsants.
- In full-blown clinical tetanus 3000-10,000 U of ATG should be administered IM.

Tetanus Vaccination or Active Immunization

- Tetanus is **best prevented by active immunization** with TT or Tetanus Toxoid.
- It stimulates the production of the protective antitoxin.
- The aim should be to **vaccinate the entire community.**
- All persons should be immunized regardless of age.
- Individuals sustaining tetanus-prone wounds should be immunized if their vaccination status is incomplete or unknown or if their last booster was given > 10 years ago.
- Two preparations are available for active immunization:
  1. **Combined vaccine – DPT.**
  2. **Monovalent vaccines:**
     - Plain or fluid (formal) toxoid.
     - Tetanus vaccine, adsorbed (PTAP, APT).

Combined Vaccine

- According to the National Immunization Schedule, 3 doses of DPT are given, at intervals of 4-8 weeks, starting at 6 weeks of age.
- This is followed by a booster at 18 months of age and a second booster at 5-6 years of age and a third booster (only TT) after 10 years of age.
- At present, pentavalent vaccine is being given at 6th, 10th and 14th weeks of age instead of DPT vaccine. The DPT vaccine is used for booster dose.

Monovalent Vaccines

- Adsorbed tetanus toxoid has replaced plain toxoid because it stimulates a higher and longer lasting immunity response.
- But, plain toxoid is given for booster injection when rapid protection is indicated.
- **A primary course of immunization consists of 2 doses of adsorbed TT given at intervals of 1-2 months.**
- Each dose is 0.5 ml and is injected into the arm.
- The longer the interval between the 2 doses, the better is the immune response.
- The first booster dose (the third in order) should be given a year after the initial 2 doses.
- No more than one additional booster dose (a total of 4 doses altogether) given 5 years after the 3rd dose is required.
- Frequent boosters must be avoided.

[3] Intestinal amoebiasis. ***August 22***

- It is common in the Indian subcontinent.

Aetiology

- **Causative organism:** *Entamoeba histolytica.*
- **Mode of transmission: Faeco-oral route.**
- It occurs as a result of substandard hygiene and sanitation and **contaminated drinking water.**
- The majority of the patients remain **asymptomatic carriers.**

Pathology

- It causes **ulcers**, which are most commonly seen in **distal sigmoid colon and rectum.**
- Called **bottle-necked ulcers** or **flask-shaped ulcers**, as it has an undermined edge.
- Ulcers typically also have a **yellow necrotic floor**, from which blood and pus exude.

Clinical Features

- Bloody diarrhoea.
- Severe colonic complications can occur:
  - o Haemorrhage.
  - o Stricture formation.
  - o Perforation.
  - o A **pericolitis** may occur which results in **adhesions** that may cause **intestinal obstruction.**
  - o If perforation of the intestinal wall is followed by secondary infection, it can cause **paracolic abscess, ischiorectal abscess and fistula.**

Investigations

- **Fresh stool sample**
  - o Amoebae are seen.
- **Endoscopy**
  - o Typical flask-shaped ulcers are seen.
  - o Biopsy can be taken.
- **Serological tests**
  - o Indirect haemagglutination assay, antibody detection.

Treatment

- **Metronidazole** is given in the acute phase.
- **Diloxanide furoate** is effective against chronic infection associated with the passage of cysts in stools.

[3] Gas gangrene. ***Dec 18, Sept 21, March 24***

[5] Gas gangrene. ***June 17***

[MCQ] Gas gangrene, following is true except: ***CBME, March 24***

A. Caused by *clostridium tetani**

B. Occurs in immunocompromised patients

C. Antibiotic prophylaxis is necessary

D. Gas in soft tissue

- It is a **rapidly progressive, potentially fatal** condition characterised by **widespread necrosis of the muscles** and soft tissue destruction.

Causative Organisms

- *Clostridium perfringens* is the most common.
- **Others:** *Clostridium bifermentans, Clostridium septicum, Clostridium sporogenes.*

Aetiopathogenesis

- Wounds which **contain necrotic or foreign material**, resulting in anaerobic conditions are at highest risk, e.g., military wounds.
- **Alpha toxin (lecithinase)** is the most important toxin. It destroys RBCs, WBCs, platelets, fibroblasts and muscle cells.
- **Other toxins: Phi-toxin, Kappa toxin.**
- The toxins act locally as well as systemically.
- Causes **spreading necrosis of muscles** and **thrombosis of blood vessels.**
- The typical feature is the **production of gas that spreads along the muscle planes.**
- **Systemic effects of the toxins:**
  - o Severe hemolysis.
  - o Rapid progression of the disease.
  - o Hypotension.
  - o Shock.
  - o Acute Kidney Injury.
  - o Acute Respiratory Distress Syndrome.

Clinical Features

- Pain that rapidly increases in severity is the earliest symptom.
- The limb swells up, i.e., oedema.
- Wound exudes a serosanguinous discharge which has a sickly sweet odour.
- Skin is involved secondary to muscle necrosis, turning brown and progressing to a blue-black colour with hemorrhagic bullae.
- Soft tissue crepitus, i.e., gas in the tissues.
- Pyrexia.
- Tachycardia.
- Tachypnoea.
- Altered mental status.

Investigations

- It is a clinical diagnosis.
- Gram stain of the exudate reveals large Gram-positive bacilli without neutrophils.
- X-rays will show gas in the soft tissues.
- ABG will show metabolic acidosis.
- RFT will show renal failure.

Treatment

- Admit patient to **ICU.**
- **IV antibiotics:** High dose penicillin G and clindamycin, along with 3rd generation cephalosporins.
- Surgery is the treatment of choice:
  - o **Amputation** of the involved extremity is life saving and should not be delayed.
  - o Amputation stumps are left open.
- **Hyperbaric oxygen.**

[5] Pyogenic abscess. ***Dec 12***
[3] Hilton's method of drainage. ***Dec 17***

- **Definition:** An abscess is a collection of pus.

Source of Infection

- Bacteria which cause pus (pyogenic bacteria) reach the infected area by:
  - o Direct infection from outside, e.g., penetrating wounds.
  - o Local extension from some adjacent focus of infection.
  - o Lymphatics.
  - o Blood stream, i.e., hematogenous.

Pathogenesis

- Pus is a collection of polymorphonuclear leucocytes (neutrophils), bacteria, dead cells.
- Neutrophils secrete proteolytic enzymes which cause liquefaction of the tissues.
- Tension within an abscess rises as plasma exudes into it.
- Unless the abscess is surgically drained, pus will eventually discharge along the line of least resistance.
- The area immediately around the abscess which is infiltrated with leucocytes and bacteria is called the pyogenic membrane.

Clinical Features

- Symptoms depend upon the site, size and tension of the abscess and the virulence of the bacteria causing it.

A. Generalized Features

- Fever.
- Bacteremia with rigors may occur.

B. Local Features

- The five classical signs of local inflammation are due to hyperemia and inflammatory exudates:
  - o Calor or heat.
  - o Rubor or redness.
  - o Dolor or pain.
  - o Tumour or swelling.
  - o Functio laesa or loss of function.

Treatment

An abscess is always treated surgically, with the aim of draining the pus.

- **Incision and Drainage:**
  - o A cruciate incision is made on the most dependent part.

- **Hilton's Method:**
  - o Used in high risk anatomical areas, as in the neck or axilla.
  - o This consists of incising the skin and superficial fascia and opening the abscess by thrusting a pair of sinus forceps or a haemostat into the cavity.
  - o By separating the blades, a sufficiently large opening can be made to insert, if necessary, a finger in order to convert loculi into a single cavity and to insert a drainage tube.
  - o Pus should be sent for C/S and antibiotics given accordingly.

[3] Erysipelas. *Dec 17*

- **Definition:** Spreading inflammation of the skin and subcutaneous tissues due to an infection by *Streptococcus pyogenes*.

Causes/Predisposing Factors

- Poor hygienic living conditions.
- Recurrent upper respiratory tract infections.
- Debilitating illnesses.
- Extremes of life.
- Lesion develops around a scratch or abrasion which is the site of inoculation of the streptococcus.

Clinical Features

- Starts as a **rose pink rash** which extends to the adjacent skin:
  - o **Vesicles** appear over the rash and rupture.
  - o **Serous discharge** comes out from these vesicles.
  - o Rash has a very **clear edge**, which is **better felt than seen.**
  - o Once the rash fades, a **brown discolouration remains.**
- When it affects skin below which there is loose areolar tissue, e.g., orbit, scrotum; there is considerable edema. This resembles cellulitis.
- **Milian's ear sign:**
  - o Used to differentiate between erysipelas and cellulitis.
  - o In case of the face, erysipelas can spread into the pinna (being a cuticular infection), whereas cellulitis cannot spread to the pinna due to close adhesion of skin to the cartilage of the ear (i.e., there is no areolar tissue).

Treatment

- **Antibiotics:**
  - o IV penicillin, ceftriaxone, flucloxacillin.
- Local application of ice-bags.

[3] Necrotising fasciitis. *June 17, Dec 15*
[5] Necrotising fasciitis. *March 24*

- Also known as synergistic spreading gangrene, subdermal gangrene.
- Also named according to the area involved:
  - o **Abdominal wall:** Meleney's gangrene.
  - o **Scrotum:** Fournier's gangrene.
- **Definition:** It is a severe, rapidly progressive, bacterial infection of soft tissue and fascia (which produces necrosis of subcutaneous tissues and overlying skin) which is associated with significant morbidity and mortality.

Causative Organisms

- Synergistic polymicrobial bacterial infection:
  - o *Streptococcus pyogenes.*
  - o *Staphylococcus aureus.*
  - o *Escherichia coli.*
  - o *Pseudomonas.*
  - o *Clostridium.*
  - o *Bacteroides.*

Predisposing Conditions

- Diabetes mellitus.
- Smoking.
- Penetrating trauma.
- Immunosuppression.

Pathogenesis

- Wound initiating the infection may be minor, but severely contaminated wounds are more likely to be the cause.

- **Spreads via deep fascia**, therefore called fasciitis.
- Aerobic bacteria destroy the living tissue, allowing anaerobic bacteria to thrive.
- **Subdermal spread** of gangrene is always much more extensive than appears from initial examination.
- **Spreads contiguously**, but occasionally produces skip lesions that later coalesce.

HPE

- **Obliterative vasculitis** of subcutaneous vessels.
- Acute inflammatory infiltrate.
- Extensive tissue necrosis.

Clinical Features

- There is usually a history of trauma or surgery with wound contamination.
- Complains of severe pain which is disproportionate in relation to the affected area.
- **Systemic features:**
  - o Fever.
  - o Tachycardia.
  - o Tachypnoea.
- **Rapid progression to:**
  - o Septic shock.
  - o Coagulopathy.
  - o Multiple organ dysfunction syndrome (MODS).

On Examination

- Erythema of skin.
- Oedema which stretches beyond visible skin erythema.
- Localized raise of temperature.
- Crepitus.
- Blisters, bullae.
- Discharge of greyish material ('dishwater pus').
- Necrosis and gangrene.
- Subcutaneous tissues have a woody hard texture.
- Inability to distinguish fascial planes and muscle groups on palpation.

Treatment

- Admit patient and shift to **ICU.**
- **Fluid resuscitation with aggressive circulatory support.**
- **IV antibiotics:** High dose penicillin G + third generation cephalosporins + metronidazole.
- **Urgent radical surgical debridement:**
  - o It is the cornerstone of treatment.
  - o Wide excision of necrotic tissue, going beyond the area of induration.
  - o Affected areas are laid open.
- A **second look operation** is usually done in 24-48 hours depending on the clinical response.
- **Multiple debridements** may be required.
- **Vacuum assisted dressings.**
- Once the wound starts to heal, **reconstruction** is planned using skin grafts or flaps.
- Use of **Hyperbaric Oxygen (HBO)** reduces mortality.

[5] Carbuncle. ***June 16, Dec 14***

- **Definition:** It is an infective gangrene of the subcutaneous tissue due to *Staphylococcus aureus* infection.
- Gram-negative bacilli and *Streptococci* may be found coincidentally.

Pathology

- **Sites:** Occurs most commonly in the **nape of the neck**. The other sites are back and shoulders.
- The subcutaneous tissues become painful and indurated, and the overlying skin is red.
- After a few days, areas of softening appear, the skin gives way and there is discharge of thick pus and slough.
- Usually there is **one central large slough, surrounded by a 'rosette' of smaller areas of necrosis.**
- Infection may extend widely and fresh openings appear on the surface and coalesce with those previously formed.

Clinical Features

- M > F.
- Age > 40 years.
- More common in diabetics and immunosuppressed patients.

- Constitutional symptoms and toxemia vary according to the degree of the resistance of the individual and efficiency of treatment.

On Examination

- Starts as a **painful and stiff swelling** which spreads very rapidly with marked induration.
- Overlying **skin becomes red, dusky and edematous.**
- Central part softens and **multiple vesicles appear** on the skin.
- Vesicles transform into **pustules.**
- Pustules burst, allowing the **discharge** to come out through several openings in the skin.
- **Sieve-like or cribriform appearance** (pathognomonic of carbuncle).
- Openings enlarge and ultimately coalesce to produce an **ulcer.**
- There is **ash-grey slough** at the floor of the ulcer.
- Finally, the slough separates leaving an excavated granulation tissue, which heals by itself.

Investigations

- It is a clinical diagnosis.
- Pus or tissue is sent for C/S.

Treatment

- Treatment is mainly surgical:
  - o Incision and drainage.
  - o Excision of the carbuncle.
  - o Reconstruction using split skin graft, after granulation tissue appears.
- **I.V. antibiotics:** Penicillin, amoxicillin – clavulanic acid, cloxacillin.
- Glycemic control.

[3] Actinomycosis. *June 16*

[5] Madura foot. *June 13*

- Also known as Mycetoma, Madura mycosis.
- It is a chronic, specific, granulomatous, progressive, destructive inflammatory disease that involves the skin, subcutaneous tissues and deeper structures.

Aetiology

- When the causative organism is true fungi, it is called eumycetoma.
- When it is caused by bacteria, it is called actinomycetoma.
- Occurs in the 'Mycetoma belt'.
- **Route of infection:** The organism which is present in the soil enters through a traumatised area in the foot.
- Common in bare-footed people walking in a terrain full of thorns.

Pathology

- Granulomatous inflammation.
- Once the granuloma forms, it increases in size.
- The overlying skin becomes stretched, smooth, shiny and attached to the lesion.
- It invades deeper structures.
- Tendons and nerves are spared until later in the disease.

Clinical Features

- The most common site affected is the foot.
- The pathognomonic feature is the triad of:
  1. Painless subcutaneous mass/swelling.
  2. Multiple sinuses.
  3. Seropurulent discharge.
- It presents as a slowly progressive, painless, subcutaneous swelling commonly at the site of trauma.
- Multiple secondary nodules develop, which suppurate and drain through multiple sinus tracts.
- During the active phase of the disease, the sinuses discharge grains, the colour of which can be black, yellow, white or red depending upon the organism.
- Sinuses may coalesce and form abscesses.
- Lymphadenopathy is common, with lymph nodes being small and shotty.
- The condition remains localized.
- Constitutional symptoms are due to secondary bacterial infection.
- It causes tissue destruction, deformity and disability and even death in extreme cases.

Investigations

A. Plain X-ray

- Soft tissue shadows with calcification and obliteration of the fascial planes.
- Bone scalloping.
- Periosteal reaction causes sun ray appearance and Codman's triangle.
- Multiple punched-out cavities throughout the bone.

B. USG

- **Eumycetoma:** Grains produce numerous sharp bright hyperreflective echoes.
- **Actinomycetoma:** Grains are less distinct.

C. MRI

- Dot-in-circle sign.

D. CT

E. FNAC

F. Culture-Sensitivity

Treatment

Medical Management

A. Actinomycetoma

- **Treatment of choice:** Combined drug therapy with amikacin and cotrimoxazole in the form of cycles.
- **2nd line drugs:** Amoxicillin-clavulanic acid, rifampicin, sulphonamides, gentamicin and kanamycin.

B. Eumycetoma

- **Drugs of choice:** Ketoconazole, itraconazole, voriconazole.

Surgery

- **Indications:**
  - o Small, localised lesions.
  - o Resistance to medical treatment.
  - o For a better response after medical treatment in patients with massive disease.
- **Surgical options are:**
  - o **Wide local and debulking excisions.**
  - o **Amputations:**
    - ♦ Amputation is used as a life-saving procedure and is indicated in advanced mycetoma refractory to medical treatment with severe secondary bacterial infection.

[3] Mention universal precautions during surgery with HIV patients. ***Dec 14***

[3] An HIV positive patient is posted for hernia surgery. What are the universal precautions to be followed? ***CBME June 24***

- Universal precautions are taken by surgeons who are involved with HIV/AIDS or hepatitis patients.
- These patients may present to surgeons for operative treatment of a surgical disease, for biopsy or for vascular access.
- Particular care should be taken when there is a risk of splashing/aerosol formation, particularly with power tools.
- Centre for Disease Control, USA came up with universal precautions to protect surgeons from HIV/AIDS, hepatitis or at risk patients.
- These consist of the following:
  - o Use a full face mask ideally, or protective spectacles.
  - o Use of fully waterproof, disposable gowns and drapes, particularly during seroconversion.
  - o Wear boots to avoid injury from dropped sharps.
  - o Double gloving.
  - o Allow only essential personnel in theatre.
  - o Avoid unnecessary movement in theatre.
  - o Sharps should be respected and passed around in a kidney tray only.
  - o Operate slowly and meticulously with minimised bleeding.
- Needle stick injuries are most common on non-dominant index finger during operative surgery.
- Hollow needle injury carries the greatest risk of viral transmission.
- Injured part should be washed under running water.
- Incident should be reported.
- Post exposure anti-retroviral treatment depends on local policies.

- After high risk exposure, the surgeon is advised on the following:
  - o Occupational health advice.
  - o Need for HIV testing.
  - o Option for continuation in a non-operative specialty.

[MCQ] The following may be associated with HIV except: ***CBME March 24***

A. Pneumocystis carinii pneumonia
B. Kaposi's sarcoma
C. Drug treatment is most effective in late phase*
D. Drug treatment is most effective in early phase

Opportunistic Infections in HIV

- Bacterial infections, multiple or recurrent.
- Candidiasis of bronchi, trachea or lungs.
- Candidiasis of esophagus.
- Cervical cancer, invasive.
- Coccidioidomycosis, disseminated or extrapulmonary.
- Cryptococcosis, extrapulmonary.
- Cryptosporidiosis, chronic intestinal (>1 month duration).
- Cytomegalovirus disease (other than liver, spleen or nodes), onset at age >1 month.
- Cytomegalovirus retinitis (with loss of vision).
- Encephalopathy attributed to HIV.
- **Herpes simplex:** Chronic ulcers (>1 month duration) or bronchitis, pneumonitis, or esophagitis (onset at age >1 month).
- Histoplasmosis, disseminated or extrapulmonary.
- Isosporiasis, chronic intestinal (>1 month duration).
- Kaposi's sarcoma.
- Lymphoma, Burkitt's (or equivalent term).
- Lymphoma, immunoblastic (or equivalent term).
- Lymphoma, primary, of brain.
- *Mycobacterium avium* complex or *Mycobacterium kansasii*, disseminated or extrapulmonary.
- *Mycobacterium tuberculosis* of any site, pulmonary, disseminated, or extrapulmonary.
- *Mycobacterium*, other species or unidentified species, disseminated or extrapulmonary.
- *Pneumocystis jirovecii* (previously known as *Pneumocystis carinii*) pneumonia.
- Pneumonia, recurrent.
- Progressive multifocal leukoencephalopathy.
- *Salmonella* septicemia, recurrent.
- Toxoplasmosis of brain, onset at age >1 month.
- Wasting syndrome attributed to HIV.

[5] Sterilisation methods. ***July 18***
[3] Gas sterilisation. ***June 14***
[3] Disinfectant. ***March 24***

- Sterilisation is the process of completely destroying all microorganisms including bacteria, viruses, fungi and spores from surfaces, equipment or substances.
- Disinfection is the process of eliminating or reducing microorganisms such as bacteria, viruses, fungi and protozoa from surfaces, water or air.

Classification of Sterilisation/ Disinfection Methods

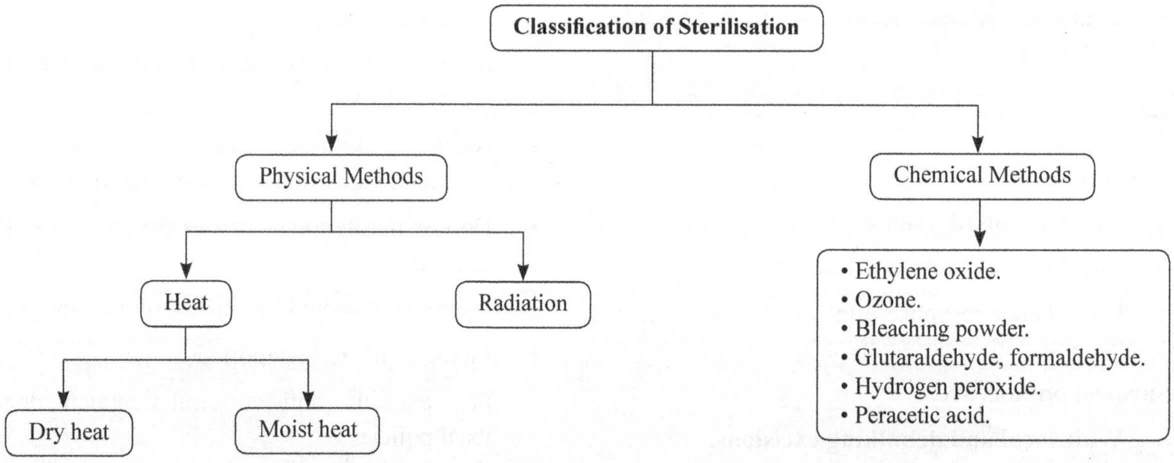

A. Physical Methods

- **Heat:**
  - o Dry heat:
    - ♦ Coagulates proteins in any organism and causes oxidative free radical damage and dying of cells.
    - ♦ E.g., hot air oven, radiation, microwave.
  - o Moist heat, i.e., steam under pressure:
    - ♦ Destroys microorganisms by the irreversible denaturation of enzymes and structural proteins.
    - ♦ Water vapour has high penetrating property and also causes damage through the formation of oxidative free radicals.
    - ♦ E.g., autoclaving, boiling, steam sterilisation.
- **Radiation:**
  - o E.g., electron beams, X-rays, gamma rays.

B. Chemical Methods

- Ethylene oxide.
- Ozone.
- Bleaching powder.
- Glutaraldehyde, formaldehyde.
- Hydrogen peroxide.
- Peracetic acid.

[3] Sterilisation methods for surgical instruments. *Dec 13*

- No matter which sterilisation process is deemed most appropriate, thorough cleaning is essential; otherwise dirt or biological matter may shield microorganisms.
- Physical scrubbing with detergent and water is recommended.
- Cool water is needed to clean organic matter from instruments, as warm or hot water may cause coagulation of organic debris.
- Alternative cleaning methods include ultrasound or pulsed air.
- The sterilisation methods for surgical instruments are as follows:
  - o **Steam under pressure using autoclaves**
    - ♦ It is the most commonly used method for sterilisation of instruments.
  - o **Ethylene oxide**
    - ♦ Used to sterilise heat and moisture sensitive materials, including electrical equipment.
    - ♦ E.g., laparoscopic instruments, heart-lung machine, suture materials, respirators.
  - o **Hot air ovens**
    - ♦ Ophthalmic instruments.
  - o **Glutaraldehyde**
    - ♦ Endoscopes, cystoscopes, bronchoscopes, laparoscopic instruments.
  - o **Peracetic acid**
    - ♦ Flexible endoscopes.
  - o **Beta propiolactone, formaldehyde gas**
    - ♦ Used in the fumigation of labs, wards, operation theatres.

[MCQ] Which virus is associated with nasopharyngeal carcinoma? ***CBME June 24***

A. Epstein Barr virus* B. Varicella Zoster

C. HPV 6 and 11 D. Rhinovirus

Virus	Associated Cancers
Human Papillomavirus (HPV)	Cervical cancer, anal cancer, some oropharyngeal cancers
Hepatitis B Virus (HBV) and Hepatitis C Virus (HCV)	Hepatocellular carcinoma
Epstein-Barr Virus (EBV)	Burkitt lymphoma, Hodgkin lymphoma, nasopharyngeal carcinoma
Human T-cell Lymphotropic Virus type 1 (HTLV-1)	Adult T-cell leukemia/ lymphoma (ATLL)
Kaposi's Sarcoma-associated Herpesvirus (KSHV), also known as Human Herpesvirus 8 (HHV-8)	Kaposi's sarcoma, primary effusion lymphoma and multicentric Castleman disease

4

Diagnostic Imaging

[3] PET Scan. *July 18*

- Positron Emission Tomography.
- It is an extension of nuclear medicine.

Principle

- A radioactive element or radionuclide is administered to the patient as part of a **radiopharmaceutical agent**, and a detector such as a **gamma camera** is then **used to record and localize the emission from the patient**, thus forming the image.
- The radionuclide is chosen and coupled with other compounds such that it is **distributed and taken up in the tissues of interest.**
- A positron-emitting substance such as F18 is tagged.
- **Most commonly used radiolabelled tracer is ^{18}F-2-fluoro-2-deoxy-D-glucose (FDG).**
- Tracers are **used to assess metabolic functions such as oxygen and glucose consumption, blood flow.**
- Radioisotope decay causes the emission of a positron, which subsequently, within a few mm, collides with and annihilates an electron to produce a pair of annihilation photons.

Disadvantages

- High cost.
- Very limited availability.
- Relatively **low special resolution**; this has been **improved by combining simultaneous PET imaging and CT.**

Uses

- PET-CT can accurately stage cancer for a range of malignancies.
- Inflammatory conditions.
- Pyrexia of unknown origin.

[3] Double Contrast Study. *July 18*

- Also known as double contrast examination or double contrast radiography.

Method

- **It involves administration of a contrast medium and air:**
  - o 1st contrast – barium.
  - o 2nd contrast – gas/air.
- **Upper GI:**
  - o **Barium is ingested, after which the patient may be given effervescent crystals or a solution to drink. This produces gas bubbles within the GI tract, which helps to distend the organs and improve the visibility of the inner lining.**
- **Lower GI:**
  - o Barium enema is given, after which air is injected.
- After contrast administration, a series of X-ray images are taken at different angles while the patient changes position, allowing for a comprehensive evaluation of the GIT.

Advantages

- The combination of the contrast medium and gas helps to create a **double contrast effect**. The barium coats the inner lining of the GIT, while the gas bubbles provide contrast by separating the folds and highlighting any abnormalities.

Uses

- It **visualizes the inner lining of the GIT**. This highlights any abnormalities such as ulcers, tumors, polyps or inflammation.

[3] MRI Scan. *Dec 13*

- Magnetic Resonance Imaging.

Principle

- Nuclei containing an odd number of protons have a characteristic motion in a magnetic field (called **precession**).
- A **magnetic moment** is produced as a result of this motion.
- In a strong uniform magnetic field such as an MRI scanner, these nuclei align themselves with the main magnetic field and result in a net magnetic moment.
- A brief **radiofrequency pulse** is then applied to alter the motion of the nuclei.
- Once the radiofrequency pulse is removed, the nuclei realign themselves with the main magnetic field (called **relaxation**).
- In this process, they emit a radiofrequency signal then can be recorded, spatially encoded and used to construct a **grey-scale image.**
- The **specific tissue characteristics define the manner and rate at which the nuclei relax.**
- **This relaxation is measured in two ways:** T1 and T2 relaxation times.

Images

- **T1** weighted images give details about **anatomy.**
- **T2** weighted images give details about **pathology.**
- IV gadolinium may be given for tissue contrast.

Advantages

- No ionizing radiation.
- Excellent soft tissue contrast.
- **Multiplanar Imaging:** Images can be acquired in any plane prescribed.

Disadvantages

- **Absolute contraindications:**
  - o Ocular metallic foreign bodies.
  - o Cochlear implants.
  - o Cranial aneurysm clips.
- **Relative contraindications:**
  - o Pacemakers.
  - o First trimester of pregnancy.
- **Claustrophobia:**
  - o Long scan times, so patients may not be able to keep still, especially if in pain.
- **Limited availability.**
- **Expensive.**

Uses

- **It is the best imaging technique for:**
  - o Intracranial lesions.
  - o Spine.
  - o Bone marrow and joint lesions.
- **Oncological imaging:**
  - o Staging of rectal carcinoma.
  - o Staging of gynecological malignancies.
  - o Identification and characterization of hepatic masses.
  - o Breast malignancy.
- Assessment of the biliary tree by MRCP (Magnetic Resonance Cholangiopancreatography).
- Imaging of small bowel, e.g., Crohn's disease, where repeated imaging with ionizing radiation can incur a significant radiation dose over time (MR enterography).
- **MR Angiography:** Cranial and peripheral circulation.
- **Cardiac imaging.**
- **Diffusion Weighted Imaging:** Used to distinguish benign and malignant or inflammatory lesions in a variety of organs.

[5] MRCP. *March 24*

- Magnetic resonance cholangiopancreatography (MRCP) is a non-invasive modality that provides excellent images of the gallbladder, biliary system and pancreas.

Method

- Magnetic resonance imaging (MRI) **uses the water in bile to delineate the biliary tree** and thus provides superior anatomic definition of the intrahepatic and extrahepatic biliary tree, and the pancreas.
- By use of the water content of bile, a **cholangiopancreatogram** can be created, which makes it an excellent modality for cross-sectional imaging of the biliary tree.
- Using the technique in conjunction with **IV secretin, emptying of the pancreatic duct** can be demonstrated to show the absence or presence of obstruction.

Uses

- They can demonstrate **ductal abnormalities** (pancreatic and bile duct), including obstruction/stricture, stones and tumours.
- It is the **gold standard for complete morphological evaluation of the biliary tree** as it offers detailed information about the integrity of the biliary tract. It is helpful in determining the level and degree of injury.
- Extremely useful in **planning resection of biliary or pancreatic neoplasms** or management of complex biliary disease.

Advantages

- Non-invasive.
- Less expensive compared to ERCP.
- No radiation exposure.

Disadvantages

- Not available easily.
- Expensive.

5

Endoscopy

[5]	Gastroscopy. ***Dec. 14***
[3]	Mention indications for gastroscopy. ***Dec. 13***
[3]	Endoscopy. ***June 14***

- **Definition:** Endoscopy is a procedure in which an instrument (endoscope) is introduced into the body to give a view of its internal parts.

Types

A. Upper Gastrointestinal Endoscopy or Esophago-gastroduodenoscopy

- It is the most commonly performed endoscopic procedure.
- Excellent visualization of the **esophagus, gastro-esophageal junction, stomach, duodenal bulb (first part) and second part of the duodenum** can be obtained.
- **Retroversion** of the gastroscope in the stomach is essential to obtain complete **views of the gastric cardia and fundus.**
- A **side-viewing scope** is used to visualize the **ampulla of Vater.**
- A **longer enteroscope** is required to view **beyond the ligament of Treitz**.
- Diagnostic + Therapeutic.

B. Capsule Endoscopy

- Used for assessment of **small bowel.**
- A **capsule** is ingested, which **contains a camera** that **transmits images to a recorder** unit worn outside the body.
- **Captures images from the mouth to the colon** as it passes the entire length of the GIT via peristalsis and is ultimately excreted in the stools.
- Useful in the localization of **occult GI bleeding** and the diagnosis of **small bowel Crohn's.**
- **Only diagnostic**.

C. Single/Double Balloon Enteroscopy

- Allows the direct visualization of and therapeutic intervention for the **small bowel.**
- May be attempted via either the **oral or rectal route.**

D. Endoscopic Retrograde Cholangiopancreatography (ERCP)

- **Diagnostic ERCP is obsolete** and has been **replaced by MRCP.**
- ERCP is currently performed for **therapeutic purposes only.**
- However, there is still a **role for accessing cytology/biopsy specimens.**
- Involves the use of a side-viewing duodenoscope to visualize the ampulla of Vater.
- By altering the angle of approach, **one can selectively cannulate the pancreatic duct or biliary tree.**

E. Colonoscopy

- Visualizes the **entire colon and the terminal ileum.**
- Diagnostic + Therapeutic.

Indications for Oesophagogastro-duodenoscopy

- Patient's **symptoms are persistent** despite appropriate empirical therapy.
- Symptoms are **associated with warning signs** such as intractable vomiting, anemia, weight loss, dysphagia or bleeding.
- Part of the **diagnostic work up** for patients with anemia, symptoms of malabsorption and chronic diarrhea.
- **Surveillance of neoplasia development** in high-risk patient groups, such as those with **genetic conditions** like familial adenomatous polyposis.
- **Surveillance of neoplasia development in pre-malignant conditions** such as Barrett's esophagus.

Indications of Colonoscopy

- **Per rectal bleeding** unexplained after proctoscopy/ sigmoidoscopy.
- **Abdominal pain related to bowel actions.**
- **Iron deficiency anemia.**
- **Right iliac fossa mass**, if imaging suggests it is of **colonic origin.**
- Unexplained **alteration in bowel habit.**
- **Chronic diarrhea (> 6 weeks)** after sigmoidoscopy/ rectal biopsy and negative celiac serology.
- **Follow-up of colorectal cancer and polyps.**
- **Screening** of patients with a **family history** of colorectal cancer.
- **Assessment/removal of a lesion** seen on radiological examination.
- **Assessment of ulcerative colitis/Crohn's extent and activity.**
- Surveillance of inflammatory bowel disease.
- Surveillance in patients with acromegaly or following ureterosigmoidostomy.

Uses of Upper GI Endoscopy

- Gives clear mucosal views which allows a **diagnosis** to be made.
- **Mucosal biopsies** can be taken, which may:
  - o Undergo processing for **HPE** (e.g., Barrett's esophagus).
  - o Be used for near-patient detection of *Helicobacter pylori* infection using a commercial **urease-based kit.**
- **Brushings** may be taken for **cytology.**
- **Aspirates** may be taken for microbiological **C/S.**
- The **most common therapeutic endoscopic procedure performed as an emergency is the control of upper GI hemorrhage of any etiology, e.g., band ligation of varices.**
- **Dilation** of benign esophageal and pyloric **strictures.**
- **POEM** or per oral endoscopic myotomy in the treatment of **achalasia cardia.**
- **BOTOX injection** in the treatment of **achalasia cardia.**
- **Endoscopic techniques to reduce gastroesophageal reflux by plication, radiofrequency ablation or mucosal resection.**
- Endoscopic mucosal resection **(EMR)** and endoscopic submucosal dissection **(ESD)** in the treatment of **early Ca esophagus and gastric cancer.**
- **Endoscopic bariatric therapy**, e.g., intragastric balloons, sleeve gastroplasty and duodenal resurfacing.
- Percutaneous Endoscopic Gastrostomy **(PEG)** tube enhances nutritional and functional outcome in patients unable to maintain oral nutritional intake.
- Self-expanding metallic stents **(SEMS)** is used in malignant esophageal and gastric outlet obstruction.
- Endoscopic treatment of Barrett's high grade dysplasia, e.g., **radiofrequency ablation.**

Uses of ERCP

- The **most common indication for therapeutic ERCP is relief of biliary obstruction due to gallstone disease or benign or malignant biliary strictures.**
- **Biliary sphincterotomy allows clearance of CBD stones < 1 cm in diameter.**
- **Dilation** of benign biliary **strictures** using balloon catheters; a temporary plastic stent is used to maintain drainage.
- **Self-expanding metal stents** are most commonly used for the **palliation of malignant biliary obstruction.**
- **Pancreatic duct stone extraction.**
- Dilatation of pancreatic duct strictures.
- **Transgastric drainage of pancreatic pseudocysts.**

- **Pancreatic sphincterotomy** is most safely performed after the placement of a temporary pancreatic stent to prevent stasis within the pancreatic duct.
- **Assessment of biliary dysmotility** (Sphincter of Oddi dysfunction) **using manometry**.
- Visualization and sampling of biliary lesions is becoming easier and more effective due to the development of newer scopes that allow direct visualization and instrumentation of the biliary and pancreatic ducts.

Uses of Colonoscopy

- Gives clear mucosal views which allows a diagnosis to be made.
- Mucosal biopsies can be taken, which is sent for HPE.
- Screening of colorectal cancer in high risk groups.
- Resection of colonic polyps.
- EMR and ESD of non-pedunculated polyps.
- Argon Plasma Coagulation and other thermal therapies are used in the treatment of symptomatic angioectasias of the colon.
- Laser photocoagulation may be used to debulk colonic tumors not suitable for resection.
- Balloon dilation of short colonic strictures.
- Placement of self-expanding metal stents provide excellent palliation of inoperable malignant strictures and is also used in decompressing an obstructed colon to allow planned, as opposed to emergency surgery.

Complications of Upper GI Endoscopy

- **Perforation** can occur at any point in the upper GIT, including the oropharynx and is more common with therapeutic procedures than diagnostic procedures.
- **Hemorrhage**.
- Appropriate patient selection and safe sedation practices reduce complications.
- Particular caution showed be exercised in patients with recent unstable cardiac ischemia and respiratory compromise.

Complications of ERCP

- Duodenal perforation.
- Hemorrhage after sphincterotomy.
- Pancreatitis.
- Sepsis.

Complications of Colonoscopy

- Perforation risk is higher with therapeutic procedures than diagnostic procedures.
- Hemorrhage.

[MCQ] Standard upper GI endoscopy includes examination of all except: ***CBME June 24***

A. Pharynx*　　B. Esophagus

C. Duodenum　　D. Jejunum

6

Minimal Access Surgery

[5] Principles of laparoscopy. *Dec 13, July 15, June 17, July 23, CBME March 24*

- The core principles of minimal access surgery (independent of procedure or device) can be summarised by the acronym **I-VITROS**.

  I for **Insufflate:** Create space, to allow surgery to take place in the minimal access setting.

  V for **Visualise:** The tissues, anatomical landmarks and the environment for the surgery to take place.

  I for **Identify:** The specific structures for surgery.

  T for **Triangulate:** Surgical tools (such as port placement) to optimise the efficiency of their action, and ergonomics by minimizing overlap and clashing of the instruments.

  R for **Retract:** And manipulate local tissues to improve access and gain entry into the correct tissue planes.

  O for **Operate:** Incise, suture, anastomose, fuse.

  S for **Seal:** Haemostasis.

[5] Advantages and disadvantages of minimally invasive surgery. *CBME March 24*

[5] Advantages and limitations of Minimal Access Surgery. *Dec 16*

Advantages of Minimal Access Surgery

- Smaller incisions with less post-op pain and disability.
- Improved cosmesis.
- Decreased wound related pathology, such as wound infection, hernia and nerve entrapment.
- Decreased tissue trauma.
- Decreased physiological insult.
- Earlier return to full activity.
- Significantly reduced hospital stay, improving cost effectiveness.
- Improved visualization of the operative field for the whole surgical team including trainees and students.
- Decreased contact with pathogens such as HIV for the surgical team.
- Decreased heat loss during the procedure.
- Use of video records aids communication with patients and their families.

Disadvantages/Limitations of Minimal Access Surgery

- Loss of tactile feedback from tissues and instruments.
- Potential difficulty in controlling major bleeding which may be associated with a rapidly deteriorating visual field.
- Longer procedure times, especially initially during the learning curve.
- Requirement for specialist instrumentation and an appropriate surgical skill set, increases the cost.
- Greater potential for iatrogenic damage either through surgical disorientation (e.g., common bile duct injury) or unrecognized visceral injury (e.g., missed bowel perforation).
- Lack of three dimensional vision.
- Tissue extraction, especially of large specimens such as lung or colon may be difficult.

[3] Mention the complications of laparoscopy. ***Dec 18, Dec 14, June 13***

- Vascular/Visceral injury.
- **Respiratory complications:**
  - o Subcutaneous emphysema.
  - o Pneumothorax.
  - o Pneumomediastinum.
  - o Pneumopericardium.
- Gas embolism.
- **Cardiovascular complications:**
  - o Arrhythmias.
  - o Bradycardia/Tachycardia.
  - o Hypotension/Hypertension.
  - o Circulatory collapse.
- Aspiration of gastric contents.
- Nerve injury due to patient positioning.
- Hypothermia.

OTHER IMPORTANT TOPICS

Pneumoperitoneum in Laparoscopy

- There are 2 fundamental ways to access the abdomen laparoscopically:
  1. Open technique (Hasson's or modified Hasson's).
  2. Closed technique (Veress needle and/or visual entry trocar).

Open Hasson's Technique

- Umbilicus is the preferred site for a 10-12 mm initial port placement.
- Umbilical cicatrix is everted with an Allis or Littlewood's forceps, revealing the stalk of the umbilicus.
- A curved subumbilical incision is made.
- The skin is retracted to reveal the junction of the stalk and the linea alba.
- A small vertical incision is made in the junction using an 11 bladed scalpel.
- A blunt, long haemostat is used to enter the peritoneum and enlarge the incision in the umbilical stalk.
- A blunt primary trocar and cannula are inserted and their position is confirmed with camera.

Closed Technique

- Veress needle can be inserted in the umbilical region or in other regions of the abdomen, such as Palmer's point.
- A 10 mm incision is made in the umbilical region or Palmer's point.
- The needle is advanced until it reaches the muscle.
- The abdominal wall is then lifted and the needle advanced through the oblique muscles.
- A 'pop' is heard and a 'give' is felt on successful insertion into the peritoneal cavity.
- Intraperitoneal placement is confirmed using a combination of following techniques:
  - o Hanging drop method.
  - o Free flow of saline into the peritoneal cavity.
  - o Abdominal pressure reading of < 10 mm Hg.
- Once the position is confirmed, CO_2 insufflation is started at a slow pace until the target pressure is reached.
- Veress needle is now removed.
- Primary port is placed after Veress needle insufflation (optical port may be used for this purpose).
- Remaining ports are inserted under vision.

Triangles in Laparoscopy

Azimuth Angle

- The azimuth angle refers to the angle between the working axis of the laparoscopic instrument and the viewing axis of the laparoscope.

Manipulation Angle

- It refers to the angle at which the surgeon manipulates or manoeuvres surgical instruments.
- It should ideally be 45° to 60° for best ergonomics.

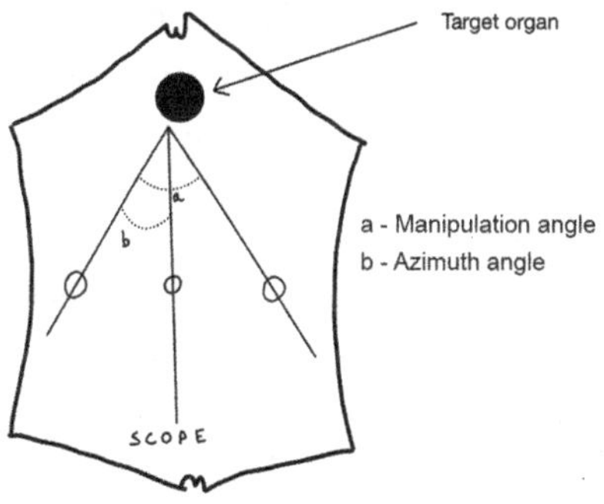

Figure: Angles in laparoscopy

7

Tissue and Molecular Diagnosis

- No questions have been asked from this chapter since Dec 12 session.
- However, I am including some important topics from this chapter, which can probably be asked in the future.

CORE NEEDLE BIOPSY

- It is a technique where a thin, hollow needle is used to extract a small, cylindrical core of **tissue** from a suspicious area.

Method

- Performed with trigger devices requiring multiple entries (e.g., gun) or with vacuum-assisted devices that require only a single insertion.
- The size ranges from 8-14 G.
- Can be performed directly or under guidance (mammographic or stereotactic, ultrasound, CT or MRI).
- Image-guided localization is required if the lesion cannot be adequately sampled by core needle biopsy or if there is discordance between the imaging abnormality and pathologic findings.
- Under LA, a small skin incision is made, and a core biopsy needle is inserted into the lesion to obtain the tissue sample.
- The number of samples obtained depends on the tumour, e.g., in Ca breast, 6 samples are taken.

Uses

- It is the method of choice to sample breast tumours, soft tissue tumours.

Advantages

- If a malignancy is detected, histologic subtype, grade and receptor status can be determined.
- Immunohistochemistry can be determined.
- It is a minimally invasive procedure.
- Can be performed under LA.

Disadvantages

- It is expensive.
- Requires a trained pathologist to interpret the results.
- There may be seeding of malignant cells along the track of the core needle biopsy.

FNAC

- A cytological preparation consists of a sample of cells only. Assessment relies on the characteristics of the individual cells and assessment of architecture is not usually possible because intact tissue is absent or sparse.

Method

- The procedure involves aspirating cells and attendant fluid with a small-bore needle (usually 21-23 G).
- The needle is repeatedly inserted into the mass while constant negative pressure is applied to the syringe.
- Samples for cytology can be smeared immediately onto glass slides, fixed (usually in alcohol) or air dried and stained immediately or later.

- The process usually produces several slides, some of which are stained with a Papanicolaou (Pap) stain and some with another method such as May–Grünwald–Giemsa (MGG), H&E or Romanowsky.

Uses

- FNAC takes a sample from accessible sites such as the breast, thyroid and superficial lymph nodes.
- Ultrasound or CT guidance is used to assist FNAC from deeper and less accessible structures, e.g., liver, pancreas, kidney and lung.
- Ultrasound-guided transbronchial FNAC may allow sampling of mediastinal masses.
- Transmucosal FNA may be appropriate for submucosal gastrointestinal lesions or perivisceral lesions (taken via endoscopy).

Advantages

- Obtaining a specimen may be easier, less traumatic and less invasive compared to a biopsy.
- The area of sampling may be wider.
- It is faster as processing times are usually shorter.
- Non-medical staff can report some cases.
- Cheap.

Disadvantages

- FNAC assesses individual cells and not tissue architecture. Accordingly, diagnosis of malignancy is often difficult because the pathologist cannot assess certain features that support a diagnosis of malignancy such as invasiveness.
- Less amenable to further tissue studies.

FROZEN SECTION SPECIMEN

- A frozen section means that a fresh tissue sample (i.e., without the usual formation or any other fixative) which is taken and supplied to the lab for assessment.

Method

- Surgeons are the main users.
- It is done intraoperatively.
- The surgeon takes a small representative fresh tissue sample of the area of interest and sends it to the lab.
- A biomedical scientist freezes the tissue quickly in the pathology laboratory and can produce sections for microscopic examination within several minutes.
- The report facilitates intra-op decision making of the surgeon.

Advantages

- Quick diagnosis.

Disadvantages

- **Poorer quality sections** results in a potential **reduction in accuracy** and precision of histological diagnosis.
- Labour intensive.
- Process is time-consuming and disruptive.
- Risk of infection.
- Small but representative sample required.
- Some tissue types are difficult to process (e.g., fat).

Uses

- It facilitates intra-op decision making. E.g.,:
    - o Whether tissue sent is malignant or not, this helps decide the limit of resection.
    - o During parathyroidectomy, it confirms whether the tissue excised is indeed the parathyroid gland.

8

Principles of Oncology

[3] Tumour markers in surgery. *Dec 16, June 14*
[5] Tumour markers in surgery. *Dec 14, Dec 13*

- Tumour markers are indicators of cellular, biochemical, molecular or genetic alterations by which neoplasia can be recognized.

Uses

- They are surrogate measures of the biology of the cancer and thus provide an insight into the **clinical behaviour of the tumour**.
- It is particularly **useful when the cancer is not clinically detectable.**
- It helps to **distinguish benign from malignant** disease.
- It may **correlate** with the amount of tumour present (**tumour burden**).
- It may **allow subtype classification to more accurately stage the patient.**
- It may be **prognostic** – either by the presence or absence of the marker or by its concentration.
- It may **guide choice of therapy.**
- It may **predict response to therapy.**

Properties of An Ideal Tumour Marker

- It should be **expressed exclusively** by the particular tumour.
- **Collection** of the **specimen** for the tumour marker assay **should be easy**.
- The assay itself should be **reproducible, rapid and inexpensive.**

Currently, there is no one marker that fulfils all these criteria for any cancer, nor is there any specific cancer for which there are biomarkers that completely describe its behaviour.

Examples

- **Carcinoembryonic Antigen (CEA):** Colorectal cancers.
- **Alpha-fetoprotein (AFP):** Hepatocellular carcinoma.
- **Carbohydrate antigen 19-9 (CA 19-9):** Pancreatic ductal adenocarcinoma, biliary tree cancers.
- **Prostate Specific Antigen (PSA):** Carcinoma of the prostate.
- **Carbohydrate Antigen 125 (CA-125) or MUC 16:** Ovarian cancer.
- **Human Chorionic Gonadotropin (HCG):** Chorio-carcinomas.

[3] Brachytherapy. *March 24*

RADIOTHERAPY

Mechanism of Action

- Ionising radiation **causes** single- and double-stranded **DNA breaks.**
- Cells most sensitive to radiotherapy are in mitosis or late G2 in the cell cycle.

- Damage may be caused by the **direct effect of the ionising radiation** on the DNA.
- However, the **predominant therapeutic effect** is **indirect**, and is achieved by ionising radiation causing the creation of **oxygen free radicals**, which then damage the DNA.
- **Hypoxic cells** are relatively **resistant** to radiotherapy.
- Cancer types differ greatly in their sensitivity to radiotherapy.

Five 'R's of Radiotherapy

1. **Repair**
   - If given sufficient time between fractional doses of radiation, cells will repair the radiation-induced damage.
2. **Reoxygenation**
   - Hypoxic cells are, compared with well-oxygenated cells, relatively radioresistant.
   - Normal tissues are well oxygenated, tumours are often hypoxic.
   - This is an obvious therapeutic disadvantage.
   - The problem may be mitigated if a sequence of daily treatments is used.
3. **Repopulation**
   - As radiotherapy kills cancer cells within a tumour it may provide a stimulus for proliferation of tumour cells.
   - Thus, during protracted treatment, production of cells by the tumour may equal, or even exceed, radiation induced cell loss.
   - Overall treatment time should therefore be as short as possible.
4. **Redistribution**
   - Fractions of radiotherapy should be timed to coincide with vulnerable phases of the cell cycle (late G2 and M).
5. **Radiosensitivity**

Types of Radiotherapy

- Aim is to provide a **uniform therapeutic radiation dose** to the target area, while sparing adjacent structures from significant damage.
- The **target area is defined** by anatomical imaging, such as **CT and MRI**, to identify the tumour mass, neighbouring structures and landmarks for radiotherapy planning.
- Sometimes functional imaging, such as **PET**, is used to further define structures that should be included in the radiation field such as lymph nodes containing small volumes of tumour, whose metabolic signature is detected by PET.
- The planning and technical setup of radiotherapy is a highly specialised subject.
- Therapeutic radiation is delivered in three ways:
  1. **Teletherapy or External Beam Radiotherapy (EBRT):**
     - o Focused beams of radiation are **generated at a distance and aimed at the tumour** within the patient.
     - o This is the **most common form of treatment**.
     - o Where necessary, modern radiotherapy can employ sophisticated computer programs and algorithms to sculpt the shape of the treatment volume.
     - o It is **now possible to irradiate irregularly shaped target volumes using techniques such as intensity-modulated radiation therapy (IMRT) and image-guided radiation therapy (IGRT)**.
     - o The ability to give high fractional doses in this way has led to the development of **stereotactic ablative radiotherapy (SAbR)**, in which a small number of fractions can be used to treat primary tumours, or isolated metastases, to curative dose levels.
  2. **Brachytherapy:**
     - o Encapsulated sources of radiation are implanted directly into or adjacent to tumour tissues, e.g., radioactive seeds.
     - o Used in prostate cancer, cervical cancer.
  3. **Systemic therapy:**
     - o Radionuclides are administered, for example, intravenously but perhaps targeted by some means to a tumour site.

Complications of Radiotherapy

A. **Systemic Effects**
   - Systemic effects may develop that are related to:
     - o The volume of tissue irradiated.
     - o Dose fractionation.

- o Radiation fields.
- o Individual susceptibility.

- Injured tissues release cytokines that act systemically to produce:
  - o Fatigue.
  - o Anorexia.
  - o Nausea and vomiting.

B. Local Effects

- Bone is among the most radioresistant organs, with radiation effects being manifested mainly in children through premature fusion of the epiphyseal growth plate.
- By contrast, the male testis, female ovary, and bone marrow are the most radiosensitive organs. Any bone marrow in a radiation field will be eradicated by therapeutic irradiation.
- Organs with less need for cell renewal, such as heart, skeletal muscle, and nerves, are more resistant to immediate radiation effects.
- In radioresistant organs, the vascular endothelium is the most sensitive component.

C. Acute Toxicities

- These include:
  - o Mucositis.
  - o Skin erythema (ulceration in severe cases).
  - o Bone marrow toxicity.
- These can be alleviated by periodic interruption of treatment.

D. Chronic Toxicities

- Chronic toxicities are more serious.
- Radiation of the head and neck region produces:
  - o Thyroid failure.
  - o Cataracts.
  - o Retinal damage can lead to blindness.
  - o Salivary glands stop making saliva, which leads to dental caries and poor dentition.
- Mediastinal irradiation increases myocardial vascular disease.
- Other late vascular effects include:
  - o Chronic constrictive pericarditis.
  - o Lung fibrosis.
  - o Viscus stricture.
  - o Spinal cord transection.
  - o Radiation cystitis.
  - o Radiation enteritis.
- Development of second solid tumours in or adjacent to the radiation fields. Such tumours can develop in any organ or tissue in the second decade after treatment.

9

Pediatric Surgery

[5] Imperforate anus. ***July 23, March 24***

[3] Imperforate anus. ***Oct 20, July 18***

- Also known as anal agenesis or anal atresia.
- It is an anorectal malformation.
- The spectrum of anorectal malformations ranges from simple anal stenosis to the persistence of a cloaca.
- Imperforate anus is the most common anorectal malformation.

Aetiology/Embryogenesis

- Failure of the urorectal septum to form results in a fistula.
- Complete or partial failure of the anal membrane to resorb results in an anal membrane or stenosis.
- Breakdown of the cloacal membrane anywhere along its course results in the external anal opening being anterior to the external sphincter (i.e., anteriorly displaced anus).

Clinical Features

- M > F.
- There is **no anal opening.**
- In boys, the rectum ends either blindly or with a fistula to the bulbar urethra, prostate or bladder neck.
- In girls, there is a fistula between the distal colon and vestibule of the vagina.
- Occasionally, in both boys and girls, a **rectoperineal fistula** may be present.
- May be associated with **VACTERL** anomalies:
  - o V: Vertebral defects.
  - o A: Anal atresia.
  - o C: Cardiac defects.
  - o TE: Tracheo-esophageal fistula.
  - o R: Renal anomalies.
  - o L: Limb abnormalities.
- **Vesicoureteral reflux and hydronephrosis** are the most common renal anomalies.
- In girls, a single orifice called cloaca may be present in the perineum. It is a defect in which the rectum, vagina and urethra all fuse to form a single common channel.

Classification

- An anatomic classification of anorectal anomalies is based on the level at which the rectal pouch ends, in relationship to the levator ani musculature:
  - o Low.
  - o Intermediate.
  - o High.

Investigations

- **Invertogram:**
  - o It is a lateral pelvic X-ray taken after the infant is held upside down for several minutes.
  - o It helps determine the **most distal point of the rectal pouch** by looking at the **rectal gas shadow.**
- **ECHO** is done to look for cardiac anomalies.

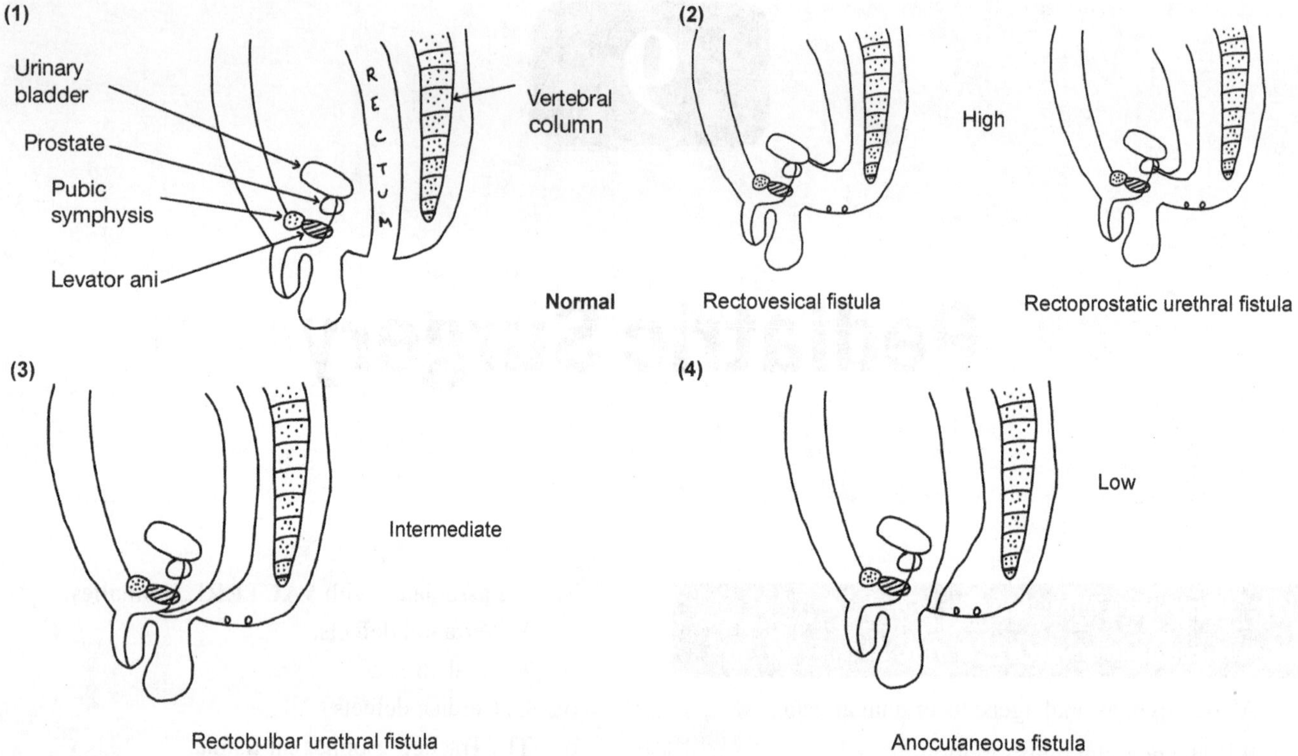

Figure 1-4: Anorectal malformations in males

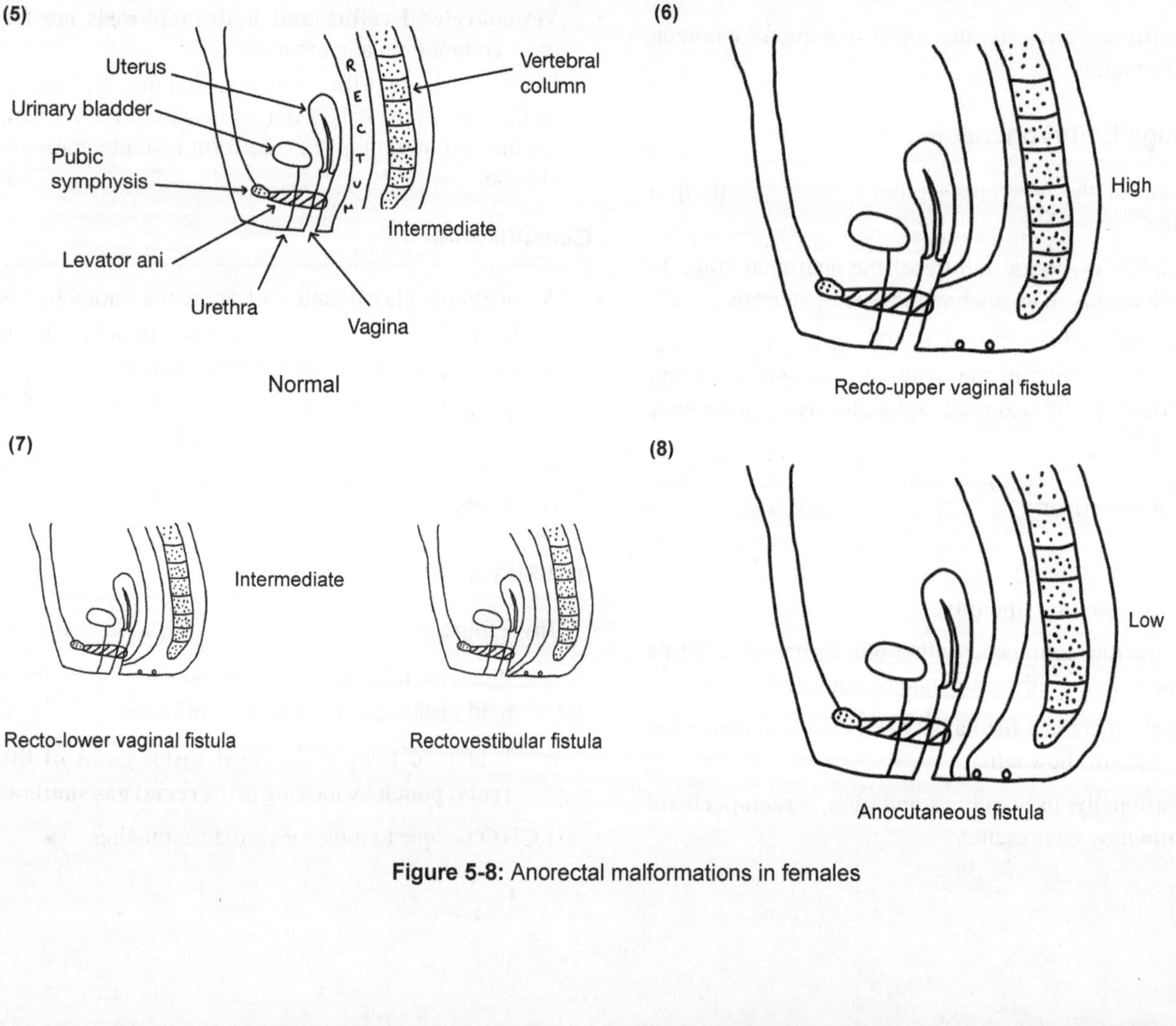

Figure 5-8: Anorectal malformations in females

- **Renal USG and micturating cystourethrography.**

Treatment

- The treatment is different for boys and girls.
- It depends on the position of the rectal gas and whether any fistula is present.

A. Boys

1. Perineal fistula
    - Anoplasty.
2. Rectal gas below coccyx
    - Posterior Sagittal Ano Recto Plasty (PSARP) ± colostomy.
3. Rectal gas above coccyx
    - Colostomy.

B. Girls

1. Single perineal orifice (cloaca)
    - Colostomy.
    - Drain hydrocolpos.
    - Urinary diversion (if necessary)
2. Perineal fistula
    - Anoplasty.
3. Vestibular fistula
    - Colostomy.
- The fistula may need to be repaired with a combined abdominal and perineal approach.

[5] Meconium ileus. *June 19*

- It is a cause of intestinal obstruction **seen in neonates due to the inspissation of meconium** in the distal ileum.

Aetiopathogenesis

- **Cystic fibrosis** is almost always the underlying cause of this condition.
- Since cystic fibrosis is inherited in an autosomal recessive manner, a **family history** may be present.
- Meconium is normally kept fluid by the action of pancreatic enzymes.
- In meconium ileus, the **meconium inspissates and the terminal ileum becomes filled with thick viscid meconium, resulting in progressive intestinal obstruction.**
- A sterile meconium peritonitis may occur in utero.

Clinical Features

- Visibly dilated loops of bowel are often palpable.
- Child does not pass stools after birth and may vomit.
- **Complications**
    - o Intestinal perforation.
    - o Segmental ileal volvulus.
    - o Ileal atresia.
- If the ileum perforates, it may seal and cause a large meconium pseudocyst.

Investigations

A. Abdominal X-ray

- Dilated small intestine with mottling.
- Ground glass appearance.
- Fluid levels are generally not seen.
- Peritoneal calcification indicates an antenatal perforation.
- Unlike ileal atresia there is no abrupt termination of the gas filled intestine.

B. Contrast Enema

- An unused microcolon is seen.

C. Gene Mutation Analysis

D. Sweat Test

- Used to diagnose cystic fibrosis.
- Shows elevated sodium and chloride levels.

Treatment

A. Hyperosmolar Gastrograffin Enema

- Used to treat uncomplicated meconium ileus.
- It draws fluid into the gut lumen and also has detergent properties, which help to liquefy the meconium.
- Infants treated in this way need extra IV fluids to compensate for fluid shifts.
- Diatrizoate which is a water-soluble hyperosmolar contrast enema can also be used.
- Fluoroscopy may be used concomitantly.

B. Surgery

- Indicated in complicated cases.
- **Options are:**
  - o Enterotomy and irrigation of the bowel.
  - o Intestinal resection and temporary stoma formation.
  - o Resection and primary anastomosis.
  - o Bishop Koop operation.
- **Bishop Koop operation:**
  - o The grossly distended ileum is resected.
  - o The distal end is brought out as an irrigating stoma.
  - o The proximal end is anastomosed to the distal loop as an end-to-side ileoileostomy.
  - o Intestinal continuity is maintained.

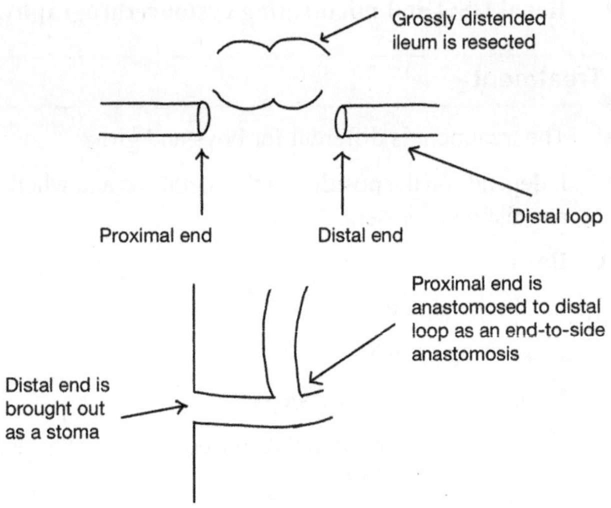

Figure 9: Bishop Koop operation

- Post-operatively, N-acetyl cysteine can be given by nasogastric tube and as enemas to loosen residual meconium.

10

Day Care Surgery

[5]	Day care surgery. *March 24*
[3]	Indications for day care surgery. *CBME March 24*

- **Definition:** The admission of selected patients to hospital for a planned surgical procedure, **returning home on the same day.**
- Surgery that requires a **23-hour stay, including an overnight stay, is *not* classed as day surgery.**

Selection Criteria

A. Surgical Criteria

- Traditionally, day surgery was limited to cases that lasted < 1 hour, but surgical **procedures lasting 3–4 hours are now being routinely performed** as successful day cases.
- Day surgery surgical criteria include the following:
  - o Low risk of significant immediate post-op complications, e.g., catastrophic bleeding or airway compromise.
  - o Patient should be able to eat and drink or take oral nutrition post-op.
  - o Post-op pain needs to be managed by oral painkillers, which may be in conjunction with local anaesthetic infiltration or peripheral nerve block.
  - o Patient should be able to mobilise post-op with or without aid.

B. Medical Criteria

- **Medical exclusions to day surgery:**
  - o Unstable ASA 3.
  - o ASA 4 or 5.
  - o Any poorly controlled abnormality/comorbidity.
- A patient's suitability for day surgery should be judged on their comorbidities and functional status.
- Patients with well-controlled diabetes (HbA1c < 6.9) can be safely managed as a day case.
- Patients with well-controlled epilepsy can be taken for day care surgery.
- Even morbidly obese patients can be safely managed in expert hands, with appropriate resources.
- Risk factors that may make day surgery unsuitable in obese patients are:
  - o Poor functional capacity.
  - o Oxygen saturation < 94% on air.
  - o STOP-BANG ≥ 5.

C. Social Criteria

- Adequate housing conditions, an inside toilet and access to a phone.
- Patient should live within a 1-hour drive of a hospital.

- A responsible adult should be able to stay with the patient for 24 hours after a regional anaesthetic/general anaesthetic.

Delivery of Day Care Surgery

Facilities

- Should be performed in a **dedicated unit** with its own admission area, operating theatres and discharge ward.
- A dedicated **day surgery ward** is required.
- Appropriate equipment, drugs and expertise are essential.

Pre-op Assessment

- Should follow the same principles as for any other patient.
- Should be nurse-led.
- Pre-anaesthetic check.

Admission and List Planning

- Day care surgery patients should follow the **same starvation guidance** as any other elective patient.
- Patients should be encouraged to **walk to the theatre.**
- Put operations with longer recovery times or patients who take longer to recover early on the lists.
- This needs to be balanced with patients who would benefit from being first on the list, such as patients with insulin-dependent diabetes.

Anesthesia and Surgery

- Surgical technique should be the same as non-day care surgeries.
- Any specific post-op care or discharge information should be documented in the theatre itself to avoid delay in discharge.
- **Appropriate day surgery anaesthesia requires:**
  - o Ensuring good pain relief.
  - o Avoidance of post-op nausea and vomiting.
  - o Should include premedication and a multimodal approach.
  - o Short-acting GA agents, day care spinals or regional anaesthesia should be used to enable rapid recovery.
  - o Use of long-acting opioids is discouraged because they can delay recovery owing to increased sleepiness or nausea.

Discharge

- Patient is discharged on the same day.
- There should be no time restriction except for certain procedures, e.g., patients should remain in hospital until 6 hours after tonsillectomy.
- Patient should receive written and verbal post-op instructions.
- SOS phone number to contact in case of emergency.
- All patients should be telephoned the day after surgery to check that they have no problems.
- **Discharge criteria:**
  - o Vital signs stable for at least 1 hour.
  - o Correct orientation as to time, place and person if appropriate.
  - o Adequate pain control with supply of oral analgesia.
  - o Understands how to use oral analgesia supplied.
  - o Ability to dress and walk where appropriate.
  - o Minimal nausea, vomiting or dizziness.
  - o Has taken oral fluids.
  - o Minimal bleeding or wound drainage.
  - o Has passed urine (if appropriate).
  - o Has a responsible adult to take them home.
  - o Written and verbal instructions given about postoperative care.
  - o Knows when to come back for follow-up (if appropriate).
  - o Emergency contact number supplied.

Advantages

- Patients often prefer to recover in the comfort of their own home.
- Causes less disruption to their domestic situation.
- Reduces risk of hospital-acquired infection.
- For the hospital, it increases the number of available inpatient beds. Therefore, activity can continue even during a time of pressure on inpatient beds.

- **All members of the team are focused on day surgery:**
  - o Nurses with expertise in day surgery.
  - o Nurses not distracted by inpatients.
- Fewer cancellations.
- Can be made a COVID secure area – protected from COVID-positive areas of hospital.
- Higher patient satisfaction.
- Higher quality outcomes.

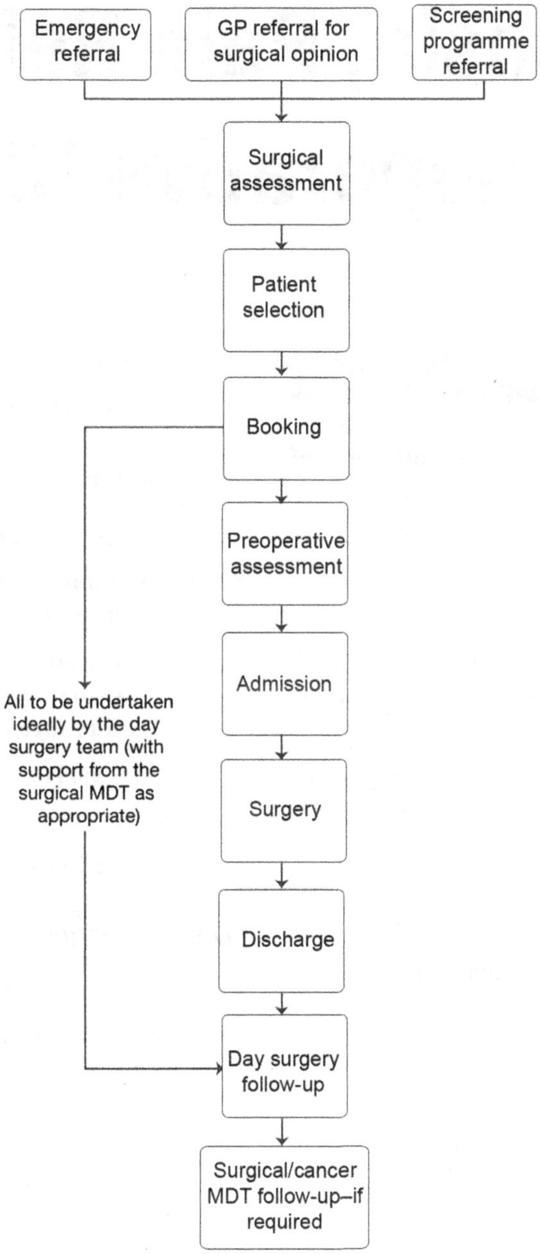

Day surgery pathway. GP, general practitioner; MDT, multidisciplinary team

Figure: Day surgery pathway

11

Anesthesia, Pain Relief and Perioperative Care

[5] Epidural anesthesia. ***March 21, Dec 12***

- Epidural anesthesia is induced by the **injection of local anaesthetics into the epidural space**.

Method

- **25 G or 27 G** needle is used.
- Epidural anesthesia is administered in the epidural space at **lumbar or thoracic level**, depending on the surgery.
- A catheter is threaded over the needle, which can be used for repeated dosing as well as for post-op analgesia.

Drugs

- Local anesthetics – Lidocaine, bupivacaine.
- Opioids – Fentanyl, morphine.

Uses

- Placement of an epidural catheter in the high thoracic region provides excellent analgesia for a wide variety of **upper abdominal and thoracic surgeries**.
- **Post-op analgesia.**
- The remaining uses are same as for spinal anesthesia:
  - **Lower limb surgeries.**
  - **Lower abdominal surgeries.**
  - **Perineal surgeries.**
  - **Pelvic surgeries.**
  - **Urologic surgeries.**
  - **Obstetric surgeries.**

Advantages

- **Prolonged analgesia by multiple dosing.**
- **Continuous infusion** through a catheter placed in the epidural space.
- Since it is slower in onset, the **resulting hypotension from sympathetic blockade can be better controlled and can reduce blood loss.**
- Enables **early mobilization.**
- **Reduces respiratory complications.**
- **Decreased post-op ileus** after abdominal surgeries.

Disadvantages

- **Slower in onset than spinal** anesthesia.
- **Technically more difficult** than spinal anesthesia.
- **Higher failure rate.**

Side Effects

- Nerve damage.
- Spinal injuries.
- Accidental spinal injection of a large volume of local anesthesia.
- Infection at site of injection.
- Epidural hematoma.
- Epidural abscess.

Contraindications

- Sepsis.
- Bacteremia.
- Infection at site of injection.
- Severe hypovolemia.
- Coagulopathy.
- Therapeutic anticoagulation.
- Increased intracranial pressure.
- Patient refusal.

[3] Spinal anesthesia. *Dec 17*

[3] Mention complications of spinal anesthesia. *Dec 13*

- Also known as subarachnoid block.
- Spinal anesthesia is induced by the **injection of local anaesthetic, with or without opiates, into the subarachnoid space.**

Method

- **25 G or 27 G** needle is used.
- Administered in the **subarachnoid space.**
- **L3 - L4 or L4 - L5 interspace.**
- Provides excellent **sensory and motor blockade below the level of block.**
- Generally has a relatively **rapid and predictable onset.**

Drugs Given

- **Local Anaesthetics:**
  - o Lidocaine, bupivacaine, tetracaine.
  - o Injection of a single shot LA agent produces intense and rapid block for surgery.
- **Opioids:**
  - o Fentanyl, morphine.
  - o Prolongs the duration of analgesia.
- **Vasoconstrictors:**
  - o Epinephrine, phenylephrine.
  - o Increases the duration of action.

Uses

- Spinal anesthesia can be **used alone or in combination** with general anesthesia or sedation.
- **Lower limb surgeries.**
- **Lower abdominal surgeries.**
- **Perineal surgeries.**
- **Pelvic surgeries.**
- **Urologic surgeries.**
- **Obstetric surgeries.**

Advantages

- Avoids manipulation of airway.
- Avoids potential complications of tracheal intubation.
- Avoids side effects of general anaesthetics.
- Intrathecal opiate administration can provide high quality post-op analgesia.
- Patient is awake, which can be of value for intra-op assessment and monitoring.
- Less/no post-op confusion and delirium.

Complications

- Hypotension (sometimes refractory).
- Bradycardia.
- Post-dural puncture headache.
- Transient radicular neuropathy.
- Backache.
- Urinary retention.
- Infection.
- Epidural hematoma.
- Excessive cephalad spread, resulting in cardio-respiratory compromise.

Contraindications

- Sepsis.
- Bacteremia.
- Infection at site of injection.
- Severe hypovolemia.
- Coagulopathy.
- Therapeutic anticoagulation.
- Increased intracranial pressure.

[3] Propofol. *March 24*

- For most adult patients and many older children, IV induction is preferable to inhalational induction; as it is rapid and pleasant.
- Propofol is the **most widely used agent for IV induction of anesthesia.**
- **Other agents:** Sodium thiopental, ketamine, methohexital, etomidate and midazolam.
- Propofol is a **short-acting induction agent.**
- Associated with smooth, nausea-free emergence.

Mechanism of Action

- It is a short-acting induction agent.
- **Enhances the activity of the inhibitory neurotransmitter GABA** in the brain, leading to sedation and anesthesia.
- **Binds to GABA-A receptors, facilitating the opening of chloride channels**, which hyperpolarises neurons, resulting in inhibition of neuronal activity.

Uses

- Used for IV induction of anesthesia.
- Small doses are also useful for short-term sedation during brief procedures such as retrobulbar or peribulbar eye blocks.
- Continuous infusion during total IV anesthesia.
- For sedation during less invasive procedures such as gastrointestinal endoscopy.

Advantages

- Associated with low incidence of post-op nausea and vomiting.
- Produces excellent bronchodilatation, therefore it is useful in asthmatics and smokers.

Side Effects/Limitations

- Pain on injection.
- Blood pressure reduction.
- Should be used with caution in patients who may be hypovolemic or who may tolerate hypotension poorly, such as those with severe coronary artery disease.

[MCQ] Pain caused by irritation of nerves: ***CBME March 24***

A. Psychogenic pain

B. Nociceptive pain

C. Neuropathic pain*

D. Inflammatory pain

Types of Pain	
Allodynia	**Pain due to a stimulus that does not normally provoke pain.** Allodynia involves a change in the quality of a sensation, whether tactile, thermal or of any other sort.
Hyperalgesia	**Abnormally heightened sensitivity to pain.** For pain evoked by stimuli that usually are not painful, the term allodynia is preferred, while hyperalgesia is more appropriately used for cases with an increased response at a normal threshold or at an increased threshold.
Hypoalgesia	**Decreased sensitivity to painful stimuli.** Hypoalgesia can be caused by exogenous chemicals such as opioids, as well as by chemicals produced by the body in phenomena such as fear- and exercise-induced hypoalgesia.
Neuropathic pain	Neuropathic pain is defined as pain caused by a lesion or disease of the somatosensory nervous system. **Due to irritation of nerve endings.**
Nociceptive pain	Pain that **arises from actual or threatened damage to non-neural tissue and that is due to the activation of nociceptors.**
Paraesthesia	**Abnormal cutaneous sensations such as tingling, tickling, pricking or burning with no apparent physical cause.** Often described as 'pins and needles' or of a limb 'falling asleep'.

[MCQ] Which of the following is not part of the anaesthetic triad used during surgery? ***CBME June 24***

A. Unconsciousness B. Pain relief

C. Amnesia D. Muscle relaxation*

TRIAD OF ANESTHESIA

- The "triad of anesthesia" refers to a set of three overlapping effects that general anaesthetic agents produce on the body:

1. Hypnosis.
2. Amnesia.
3. Analgesia.

Hypnosis

- Hypnosis refers to the induction of a reversible state of unconsciousness.
- It is the primary effect sought during surgical procedures to ensure that the patient is unaware and unresponsive to surgical stimuli and does not experience pain or discomfort.
- Anaesthetic agents act on the brain to suppress consciousness. This involves decreasing the activity of excitatory neurotransmitters and neural pathways that regulate wakefulness and arousal.

Amnesia

- Amnesia refers to the inability to recall events that occurred during the surgical procedure.
- Ensuring that patients do not remember the details of their surgical experience helps reduce psychological trauma and anxiety associated with medical procedures.
- Anaesthetic agents interfere with memory formation by affecting regions of the brain involved in encoding and storing memories.
- This effect is particularly important because patients might still respond physiologically to surgical stimuli even if they do not consciously perceive or remember them.

Analgesia

- Analgesia refers to the absence of pain sensation or the reduction of sensitivity to painful stimuli.
- It ensures that patients do not experience pain during surgical procedures, enhancing patient comfort and allowing surgeons to perform interventions without causing distress.
- Anaesthetic agents act on the peripheral and central nervous systems to inhibit the transmission of pain signals and alter pain perception.
- Involves blocking nociceptive pathways and modulating neurotransmitter activity involved in pain sensation.

12

Trauma

[3] Enumerate components of triage. ***CBME June 24***

- The word triage means 'to sort'.
- It is the cornerstone of the management of mass casualties.

Aims

- To identify those patients who will benefit the most by being treated the earliest.
- To ensure 'the greatest good for the greatest number'.
- By sorting out the minor injuries, triage lessens the immediate burden on medical facilities. This is because numerous studies show that only 10-15% of disaster casualties are serious enough to require hospitalization.

Who Does it?

- Triage should be undertaken by someone senior, who has the experience and authority to make these critical decisions.

How Many Times is it Done?

- Triage is done twice.
- 1st : In the field, before evacuation.
- 2nd : At the hospital.

Categories

- All methods of triage use simple criteria based on vital signs.
- A rapid clinical assessment is made taking into account:
    - o The patient's ability to walk.
    - o Mental status.
    - o Presence or absence of ventilation or capillary perfusion.
- There are 4 categories:
    1. Red – Immediate
    2. Yellow – Urgent
    3. Green – Non-urgent
    4. Black – Unsalvageable

Priority	Colour	Medical Need	Clinical Status	Examples
First (I)	Red	Immediate	Critical, but likely to survive if treatment given early	Severe facial trauma, tension pneumothorax, hemothorax, flail chest, profuse external bleeding, major intra-abdominal bleed, EDH

Contd.

Second (II)	Yellow	Urgent	Critical, likely to survive if treatment given within hours	Compound fracture, degloving injuries, ruptured abdominal viscus, pelvic fracture, spinal injuries
Third (III)	Green	Non-urgent	Stable, likely to survive even if treatment is delayed for hours to days	Simple fracture, sprains, minor lacerations
Last (0)	Black	Unsal-vageable	Not breathing, pulseless. Medical care is unlikely to help	Severe brain damage, extensive burns

CHEST TRAUMA

[5] Flail chest. *March 22, June 13*

- **Definition: ≥ 3 ribs fractured in two or more places.**

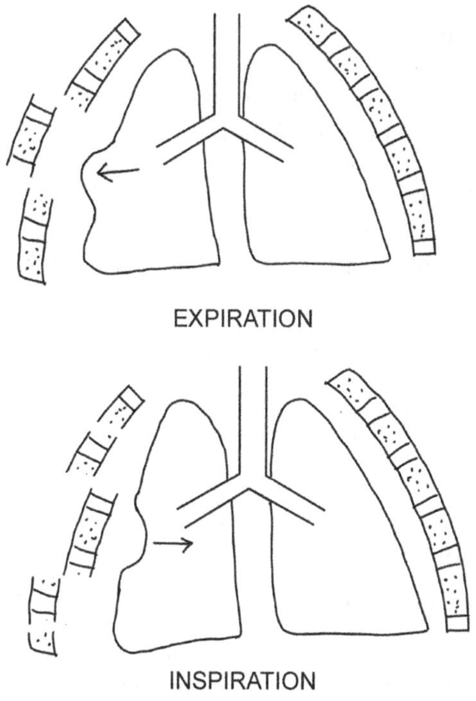

Figure 1: Paradoxical movements in flail chest

Mechanism

- Usually results from **blunt trauma.**
- Blunt force typically also produces an **underlying pulmonary contusion.**

Clinical Features

- Chest wall is observed for **paradoxical motion** of a chest wall segment:
  - o **On inspiration,** the **loose segment of the chest wall is displaced inwards** and therefore less air moves into the lungs.
  - o **On expiration, segment moves outwards** (paradoxical respiration).
- **Voluntary splinting of the chest wall** occurs as a result of pain.
- **Hypoxia** (because of mechanically impaired chest wall movement and associated lung contusion).
- Pneumothorax.
- Haemothorax.

Investigations

- CT scan is the gold standard.
- In patients who are intubated, diagnosis is made clinically and not radiologically.

Treatment

- **Oxygen** administration.
- Adequate **analgesia** (including opiates).
- Physiotherapy.
- If a chest tube is in place, **topical intrapleural local analgesia introduced via the tube** can also be used.
- **Ventilation** is reserved for patients developing respiratory failure despite adequate analgesia and oxygen.
- **Internal fixation of ribs** may be useful in patients with isolated or severe chest injury and pulmonary contusion.

[3] Stove-in chest. *March 22*

- A stove-in chest develops from the **extensive localized crushing force, which produces multiple rib fractures.**
- This results in **depression of the chest wall** in that region.
- Relative immobility leads to **accumulation of bronchopulmonary secretions.**
- If associated with depressed fracture of clavicle, it becomes a serious condition.
- It has a **high mortality** at the scene of the trauma itself, and therefore it is rarely seen in the hospital.

[5] Enumerate clinical features and write a note on management of tension pneumothorax. *CBME March 24*

[3] Tension pneumothorax. *March 22, Sept 21, March 24*

- It is an **immediate life-threatening chest injury.**

Causes

- **Penetrating chest trauma.**
- **Blunt chest trauma** with a parenchymal lung injury and **air leak that did not spontaneously close.**
- **Iatrogenic lung injury** (e.g., due to central venepuncture).
- **Mechanical positive pressure ventilation.**

Pathogenesis

- A tension pneumothorax develops when a **one-way valve air leak** occurs either from the lung or through the chest wall.
- Air is sucked into the thoracic cavity without any means of escape, completely collapsing and then compressing the affected lung.
- The **mediastinum is displaced** to the opposite side, decreasing venous return and compressing the opposite lung.

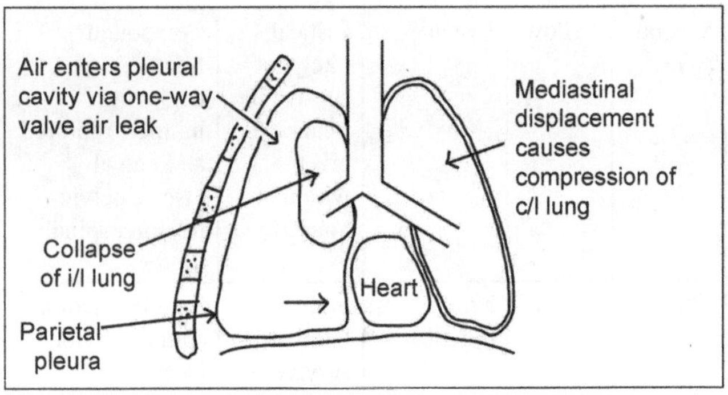

Figure 2: Pathogenesis of tension pneumothorax

Clinical Features

- The clinical **presentation is dramatic.**
- Patient is increasingly **restless** with:
  - o Tachypnea.
  - o Dyspnea.
  - o Distended neck veins.
- **Hyperresonance** over the affected hemithorax.
- **Decreased or absent breath sounds** over the affected hemithorax.
- **Tracheal deviation** is a late finding and is not necessary to clinically confirm the diagnosis.

Investigations

- It is a **clinical diagnosis** and treatment should never be delayed by waiting for radiological confirmation.

Treatment

The treatment consists of **immediate decompression.**

A. Conventional Teaching

- Rapid insertion of a **large bore cannula** into the **2nd intercostal space in the mid-clavicular line** of the affected side.
- This is followed by **insertion of a chest tube** through the **5th intercostal space in the anterior axillary line.**

B. Current Teaching

- Decompression by insertion of ICD in the **triangle of safety** (defined posteriorly by latissimus dorsi, anteriorly by the lateral border of pectoralis major and inferiorly by a line perpendicular to the nipple going to the back, just anterior to the mid-axillary line).

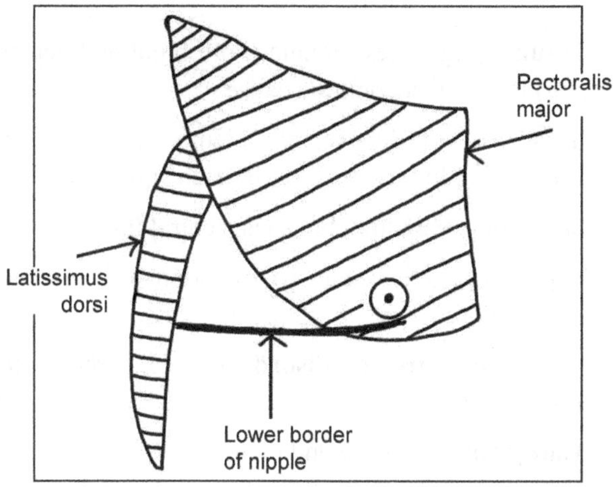

Figure 3: Triangle of safety

- **In extremis:** A finger thoracostomy at the **same location.**

[10] Discuss causes and pathophysiology of flail chest. How do you manage a case of hemothorax? ***July 18***

[5] Hemothorax. ***Dec 13***

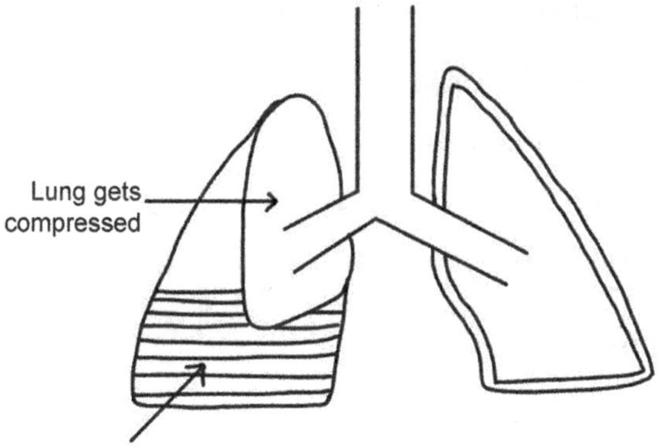

Figure 4: CXR findings in hemothorax

- **Collection of blood in the pleural cavity** is called hemothorax.
- It is often **associated with air, called hemo-pneumothorax.**

Causes

- **Trauma:**
  - o Chest wall, lung, heart and great vessels may be the source of the bleeding.
  - o The **most common cause of massive hemothorax in blunt trauma is continuing bleeding from torn intercostal vessels or occasionally from the internal mammary artery secondary to rib fracture.**
- **Postoperatively:**
  - o Following pulmonary, cardiac or esophageal surgeries.
  - o After central line insertion.
- **Malignancy:**
  - o Both primary (lung, mediastinum or pleura) and metastatic.
- **Leaking aneurysms.**
- **Spontaneous.**

Pathogenesis

- Respiratory and cardiac **movements defibrinate the blood** as it reaches the pleural cavity, so the **collection remains fluid.**
- Massive **clotting occurs only occasionally.**
- **Blood is a pleural irritant** and its presence produces:
  - o **Early stages – pain and shock.**
  - o **Later stages** – excites the formation of a considerable **effusion.**
- Blood is an excellent culture medium and **infection** is relatively common.
- It can **compromise respiratory efforts**, compressing the lung and preventing adequate ventilation.

Clinical Features

- Complains of pain.
- Difficulty in breathing.
- Drop in saturation (sPO_2).

On Examination

- Dull note on percussion.
- Weak breath sounds on auscultation.
- Cyanosis.

Investigations

- **Chest X-ray:**
  - o It is **confirmatory.**
  - o **Obliteration of costophrenic angle.**
  - o **About 400-500 ml of blood needs to be collected for detection on X-ray.**
- **eFAST scan:**
  - o Can be done in the emergency itself,
- **CT scan:**
  - o Other diseases/pathology can also be seen.
  - o **Done in** trauma cases only if patient is **hemodynamically stable.**

Treatment

- **Correcting** the hypovolemic **shock.**
- **Small** hemothorax requires **simple aspiration.**
- **Insertion of an intercostal drain** in the triangle of safety.
- **Intubation** may be necessary **in massive hemothorax.**
- **Urgent thoracotomy** is indicated in:
  - o Initial drainage of > 1500 ml blood.
  - o Ongoing hemorrhage of > 200 ml/hr over 3-4 hours.
- **Physiotherapy** and **active mobilization** should begin as soon as possible.

[5] Hydropneumothorax. *June 19*

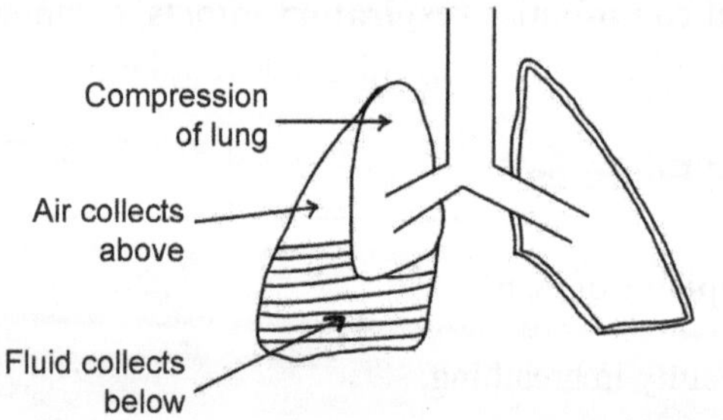

Figure 5: CXR findings in hydropneumothorax

- **Definition:** Hydropneumothorax is the **presence of air along with serous fluid** in the pleural cavity.

Causes

- **Trauma**, e.g., chest trauma (both blunt and penetrating) is the most common cause.
- **Infections** of lungs and pleura, e.g., bacterial pneumonia, lung abscess, empyema, TB.
- **Iatrogenic**, e.g., lung biopsies, central line.
- Ruptured lung bullae in combination with infection, malignancy.
- **Connective tissue disorders**, e.g., rheumatoid arthritis, SLE.
- **Malignancies** of lung and pleura.

Clinical Features

- Dyspnea or shortness of breath.
- Chest pain.
- Cough.
- Fever and signs of infection.
- Chest wall mass or swelling.

On Examination

- Decreased breath sounds.
- Diminished chest wall movement.
- Tachypnea.
- Cyanosis.

Investigations

- Chest X-ray.
- CT scan.
- Pleural fluid analysis.

Treatment

- To **treat** the **underlying cause.**
- **ICD** insertion and drainage in the triangle of safety.
- **Simple aspiration** of the fluid.
- Thoracoscopy or thoracotomy.
- **Chest physiotherapy** and **early ambulation.**

[3] Surgical emphysema – Its Causes. *June 13*

- Also known as subcutaneous emphysema.
- **Definition:** It is the **presence of air in the subcutaneous tissues.**

Causes

- **Blunt chest trauma**.
- In case of **extraperitoneal injuries of the ascending or descending colon or rectum, there may be surgical emphysema in the loin.**
- **Ruptured oesophagous or bronchus** causes mediastinal emphysema, which causes surgical emphysema in the neck.
- **Fractures of paranasal sinuses** causes surgical emphysema in the face.

Mechanism

- **Fractured ends of ribs are forced in** due to the injuring force and **injure the underlying lung.**
- This **causes air to come out** into the muscles and subcutaneous tissue of chest wall.

Clinical Features

- Complains of pain in chest.

On Examination

- Bruised skin.
- Affected area around fractured ribs may be seen slightly swollen with air.
- Such swelling may extend into the neck or to the upper limb of corresponding side.
- Crepitus.
- Decreased/absent breath sounds due to associated pneumothorax.

Investigations

- Chest X-ray.
- CT scan.

Treatment

- Surgical emphysema itself **does not require any treatment as air is usually absorbed from the subcutaneous tissue.**
- The **underlying** fractured ribs and pneumothorax need to be treated.

[3] Cardiac tamponade. *June 19*

- It is an **immediate life threatening chest injury.**
- Accumulation of **blood in the pericardial cavity** is called tamponade.

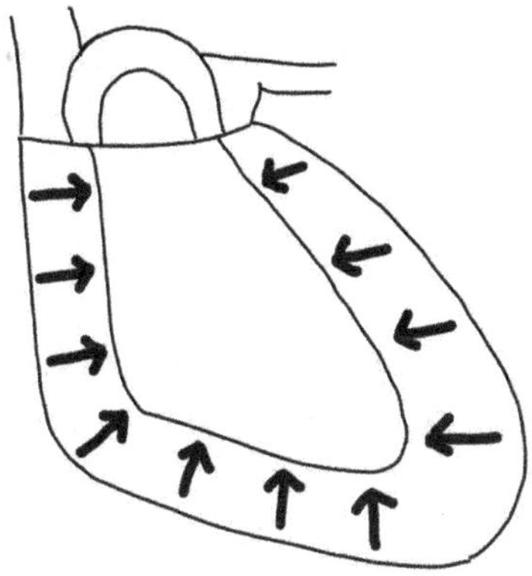

Blood collects in the non-distensible pericardial sac, causing compression of the heart

Figure 6: Pathogenesis of cardiac tamponade

Causes

- Penetrating trauma (most common cause).

Pathogenesis

Accumulation of even a relatively small amount of blood (50 ml) into the non-distensible pericardial sac

↓

Compression of the heart

↓

Obstruction of the venous return

↓

Decreased filling of the cardiac chambers during diastole

↓

Cardiac output decreases

↓

Cardiogenic shock

Clinical Features

- All patients with penetrating injury anywhere near the heart + shock must be considered to have a cardiac injury until proven otherwise.
- Classically, the presentation consists of **Beck's triad:**
  1. **Central venous pressure elevation** (causing jugular venous distension).
  2. **Hypotension** (with tachycardia).
  3. **Muffled heart sounds.**
- In cases in which major bleeding from other sites has taken place, the neck veins may be flat.

Investigations

- **eFAST scan:**
  - o Shows fluid in the pericardial sac.
  - o It is the fastest and most reliable diagnostic tool.
- **Chest X-ray:**
  - o An enlarged heart shadow is seen.

Treatment

- **Pericardiocentesis has no role** in the management of cardiac tamponade secondary to penetrating myocardial injury.
- The **correct immediate treatment of tamponade is operative, with repair of the heart in the operating theatre if time allows or otherwise in the emergency department.**
- **Approach to the heart:**
  - o Subxiphoid window.
  - o Open surgery (sternotomy or left anterolateral thoracotomy).
- In penetrating injury to the heart, there is usually a substantial clot in the pericardium, which may prevent aspiration.

HEAD TRAUMA

[5] Extradural hematoma. ***June 14, Dec 13***

[3] Lucid interval. ***June 13***

- It is a **neurosurgical emergency** due to the accumulation of blood in the extradural space.
- It **results from rupture of an artery, vein or venous sinus, in association with a skull fracture.**

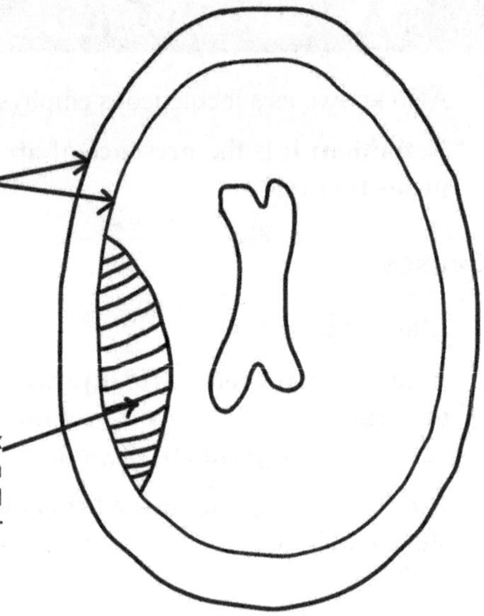

Figure 7: CT findings in EDH

Aetiopathogenesis

- The classical injury is a **fracture of the thin squamous temporal bone**, with associated damage to the **middle meningeal artery (most common).**
- **Mechanism of Injury:**
  - o Road traffic accident.
  - o Sometimes, the injuring force, which comes from a lateral direction, is often relatively trivial, such as a blow from a golf or a cricket ball.
- Although it is most common due to injury to an artery, it **can also occur from injury to a vein or a venous sinus**, e.g., fractures which injure the major sinuses or by tearing of a meningeal vein.
- **Monro Kellie doctrine** states that the cranium is a rigid box containing a nearly incompressible brain. Any expansion in the contents, especially hematoma and brain swelling, may be initially accommodated by exclusion of fluid components, venous blood and CSF. Further expansion is associated with an exponential **rise in intracranial pressure.**
- Uncontrolled increases in ICP result in **cerebral herniation.**
- Typically, herniation of the **uncus of the temporal lobe over the tentorium** results in **pupil abnormalities**, usually **occurring first on the side of any expanding hematoma.**
- Cerebellar tonsillar herniation through the foramen magnum compresses medullary vasomotor and

respiratory centres, classically producing **Cushing's triad: hypertension + bradycardia + irregular respiration.**

- The patient is then said to be **'coning'** and **brainstem death will result** without immediate intervention.

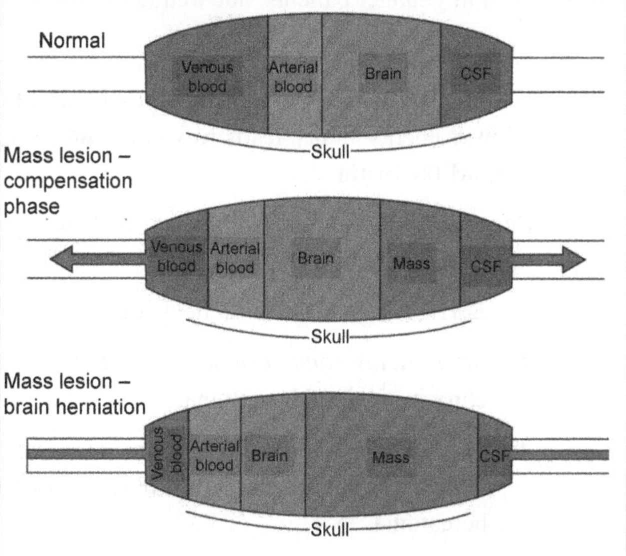

Figure 8: Monro-Kellie doctrine

Clinical Features

- History of trauma to the head with swelling under the temporal muscle.
- Transient loss of consciousness.
- Headache.
- **Lucid Interval:**
  - o After a short period of loss of consciousness, the patient recovers completely and continues to do what they were doing prior to the injury.
  - o This period of normalcy is known as the lucid interval.
  - o It is the **time taken by the hemorrhage to become big enough to cause cerebral compression**.
  - o E.g., an unconscious footballer who was carried off the field but later recovered sufficiently to finish the match; headache and drowsiness supervened so that he retired to bed early and was later found dead.
  - o There is **no neurological deficit** during the lucid interval.
  - o GCS is 15/15.
- In certain cases, the lucid interval may not be seen and the patient remains unconscious throughout.
- As the hematoma expands, compensation is exhausted with rapid deterioration.
- Level of consciousness reduces.
- The pupillary changes are referred to as **Hutchinson's pupil** and consists of the following:

a. **Ipsilateral Pupil**

- When the medial part of the temporal lobe herniates through the tentorial hiatus, it first stretches the oculomotor nerve and then paralyses it.
- **Initially:** The pupil will be constricted due to irritation of oculomotor nerve.
- **Later:** The pupil becomes dilated due to paralysis of the oculomotor nerve.

b. **Contralateral Pupil**

- When the uncus has been sufficiently herniated to cause the midbrain to be pushed to the opposite side and to be pressed against the tentorial edge, the opposite oculomotor nerve gets compressed.
- The same sequence of changes is then seen in the contralateral pupil.

Finally, the pupils of both sides become dilated, fixed and not reacting to light. This characteristic pupillary change is known as Hutchinson's pupil.

- **Contralateral hemiparesis:**
  - o It occurs due to pressure on the ipsilateral motor cortex.
  - o **Paralysis occurs in descending order:** First the face, then the upper limbs and lastly, the lower limbs.
- **Ipsilateral hemiparesis:**
  - o Seen after contralateral hemiparesis.
  - o Due to pressure on contralateral motor cortex.
- Paralysis is preceded by a short phase of twitching.
- Decerebrate rigidity.
- **Cushing's sign:**
  - o Pulse rate decreases and blood pressure increases.
  - o This is an attempt to maintain cerebral circulation against cerebral compression.
- **Cheyne Stokes** respiration.
- Temperature is slightly higher on the paralyzed side (**Victor Horsley's sign**).

Investigations

- **Non Contrast CT of Brain:**
  - o EDH appears as a **lentiform (lens-shaped or biconvex) hyperdense lesion** between the skull and the dura mater.
  - o A mass effect may be seen, with **compression of the surrounding brain and midline shift**.
  - o Areas of **mixed density suggests active bleeding.**
  - o **Skull fracture** will usually be evident.
- **ICP Monitoring:**
  - o In patients with abnormal findings on CT scan and GCS scores of ≤ 8, ICP should be monitored using:
    - ♦ Fiber-optic intraparenchymal devices.
    - ♦ Intraventricular catheters.

Treatment

- **Burr hole:**
  - o Decompresses the extradural hematoma as a life saving measure.
  - o **Made on the side of the dilated pupil** to decompress the intracranial space.
  - o **After stabilization**, patient is transferred to a facility with neurosurgery for **formal craniotomy**.
- **Open craniotomy:**
  - o For evacuation of congealed clot and hemostasis.

[5] Subdural hemorrhage. ***Feb 23, Oct 20***

ACUTE SUBDURAL HEMATOMA

- It is more common than extradural hematoma.
- It is the collection of blood between the dura and arachnoid mater.
- It is a neurosurgical emergency.

Aetiopathogenesis

- Acute SDH is **usually due to venous bleeding**.
- Most SDH occurs over the cerebral hemispheres.
- **High Energy Injury:**
  - o Results in the **rupture of cortical surface vessels with significant associated primary brain injury**.
  - o Results in an **expanding hematoma** with rapid deterioration and development of signs of raised ICP.
  - o Resembles EDH, without the lucid interval.
  - o Seen in younger patients, due to trauma.
- **Lower Energy Injury:**
  - o In **older patients who are on anticoagulants**, a lower energy injury leads to **venous bleeding around the brain.**
  - o Depending on the total volume of bleeding, the resulting hematoma may present:
    - ♦ *Early:* As acute subdural hematoma.
    - ♦ *After delay and osmotic expansion:* As chronic subdural hematoma.
    - ♦ *May remain silent:* May present much later with a further 'acute on chronic' subdural hematoma.

Clinical Features

- As subdural hematoma is often **accompanied with severe primary brain damage** (e.g., laceration), there is **initial as well as persisting loss of consciousness.**
- A truly lucid interval is unusual.
- Headache.
- Deterioration tends to occur sooner than in EDH.
  - o Acute SDH may be:
    - ♦ **Coup**: Craniocerebral damage occurs on the side of the blow to the head.
    - ♦ **Contre-coup**: Opposite (and often diagonally opposite) to the position of the blow.
  - o Hematoma is often extensive and may cover an entire hemisphere.
  - o Signs and symptoms of cerebral compression.

Investigations

- **Non Contrast CT Scan:**
  - o Seen as a **crescent shaped (lunate) opacity.**
  - o Clot is bright (indicating fresh blood) or mixed density (hypodense material represents old blood and higher density indicates more recent bleeding).

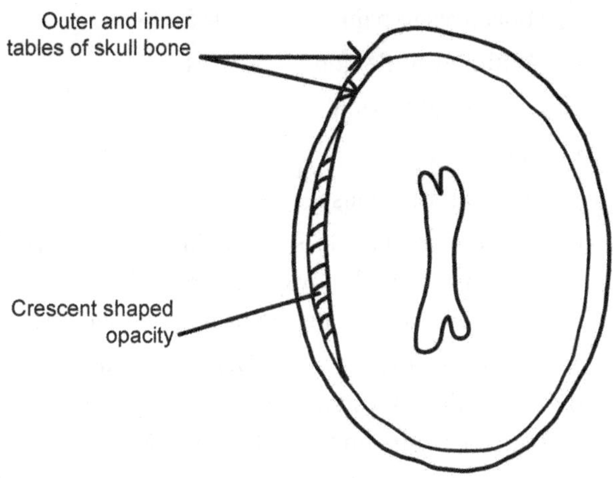

Figure 9: CT findings in acute SDH

- Clot may have a less distinct border.
- Does not cross the midline due to the presence of the falx.
- Since the dura is not as adherent to the brain as it is to the skull, subdural blood is free to expand across the brain surface, giving a diffuse concave appearance.
- Also visualizes the associated brain injury.

- **PT-INR:**
  - Should always be checked as acute SDH is associated with anticoagulants.

Treatment

- **Clotting function should be corrected** wherever possible.
- **Urgent evacuation via craniotomy**, is indicated in the following:
  - Bleeds of significant size, with significant associated midline shift.
  - Deteriorating neurology.
- **Conservative management ± Burr hole:**
  - Smaller bleeds in neurologically stable patients may be managed conservatively, at least initially.
  - Liquefaction of the clot over 7-10 days after the bleed may allow for a much less invasive evacuation through burr holes.

CHRONIC SUBDURAL HEMATOMA

- Chronic SDH is a **collection of blood breakdown products that is at least 2-3 weeks old.**
- It is a common cause of acute neurological deterioration in the elderly.

Aetiopathogenesis

- In the elderly, **cerebral atrophy** results in stretching of the cortical-dural **bridging veins**, which are then **vulnerable to rupture.**
- The resulting **hematoma can expand** over days or weeks by **osmosis**, ultimately producing symptoms of raised intracranial pressure or focal deficits.
- There is usually a **history of recent injury**.
- In patients who are on anticoagulants, even apparently trivial impacts may be responsible.

Clinical Features

- Often occurs in patients without a clear history of head trauma as they may arise from minor head injury.
- Patients may be alcoholics, elderly or on antiplatelets/anticoagulants.
- Patients may present with the following:
  - Headache.
  - Seizure.
  - Confusion.
  - Contralateral hemiparesis.
  - Coma.
  - Focal deficits.
- On presentation, it is important to exclude coexisting electrolyte disturbances and infections, which may contribute to clinical impairment.

Investigations

- **Non-Contrast CT Scan:**
  - Acute hematomas are bright white (hyperdense) for 3 days, after which they fade to isodensity with the brain, and then to hypodensity after 2-3 weeks.
  - A true chronic SDH will be nearly as dark as CSF on CT.
  - Traces of white are often seen due to small, recurrent hemorrhages into the collection (acute on chronic SDH).

- These small bleeds may expand the collection enough to make it symptomatic.
- Mass effect may be seen.

- **PT-INR.**

Treatment

- **Reverse the anticoagulation:**
  - Vitamin K.
  - Transfusion of recombinant clotting factors.
- **Conservative management:**
  - Can be considered **for small bleeds** without symptoms or with headache alone.
  - **Corticosteroids** are given.
- **Drainage via burr holes:**
  - Done for the majority of the patients.
  - Urgency is dictated by the clinical condition of the patient and imaging evidence of mass effect.
  - If clinically stable, a delay of 7-10 days to allow platelet function to normalize, after withdrawal of aspirin/clopidogrel may be considered.
- **Open Craniotomy:**
  - Done if the collection of blood cannot be drained via a Burr hole.

[5] GCS. ***July 15, March 24***

[3] GCS. ***August 22, CBME March 24***

GCS score is the sum of scores of 3 components:

A. Eyes open (E)

- Spontaneously – 4
- To verbal command – 3
- To painful stimulus – 2
- Do not open – 1

B. Verbal (V)

- Normal – 5
- Confused – 4
- Inappropriate/words only – 3
- Sounds only – 2
- No sounds – 1
- Intubated patient – NT (Non Testable)

C. Motor (M)

- Obeys commands – 6
- Localizes to pain – 5
- Withdrawal/flexion – 4
- Abnormal flexion – 3
- Extension – 2
- No motor response – 1

- Breakdown of the GCS score in to E, V and M components should always be recorded and used when communicating the status to other doctors.
- It **represents the best performance elicited**, so a patient flexing in response to a painful stimulus on the left and localizing on the right scores M5.
- **Severity of head injury** is classified according to the **post resuscitation GCS score.**
- GCS score, and in particular the motor score, is the **best predictor of neurological outcome.**
- Alcohol and drug effects often complicate the classification.

Head Injury Severity

- Minor head injury – GCS 15 with no LOC.
- Mild head injury – GCS 14 or 15 with LOC.
- Moderate head injury – GCS 9-13.
- Severe head injury – GCS 3-8.

[MCQ] A patient who was admitted after a road traffic accident is put on mechanical ventilation. He opens his eyes on verbal command and moves all four limbs spontaneously. Calculate his GCS. ***CBME June 24***

A. Eyes - 2, Verbal - 1, Motor - 5

B. Eyes - 2, Verbal - NT, Motor - 5

C. Eyes - 3, Verbal - 1, Motor - 6

D. Eyes - 3, Verbal - NT, Motor - 6*

[5] Diffuse axonal injury. ***Dec 17***

- It is a form of **primary brain injury** seen in high energy accidents.
- It usually renders the patient comatose.
- Associated with **poor outcomes.**

Causes

- **Damage to axons** throughout the brain, due to **rotational acceleration and then deceleration.**

Pathology

- Axons may be completely disrupted and then retract, forming **axon balls.**
- Hemorrhagic foci in the corpus callosum and dorsolateral rostral brainstem.

Clinical Features

- Patient is comatose/impaired arousal.
- It is considered to be a severe form of a concussion, often with irreversible consequences.

Differential Diagnosis

- Basilar thrombus.

Investigations

- **It is strictly a pathological diagnosis made at post-mortem.**
- **CT scan:**
    - o **Hemorrhagic foci in the corpus callosum and dorsolateral rostral brainstem is suggestive of diffuse axonal injury.**
    - o **Loss of gray and white matter differentiation.**
- MRI.

Treatment

- **Goals of treatment are:**
    - o To stabilize the patient.
    - o To prevent further brain damage.
    - o To manage secondary complications that may arise.
- **Intubation and ventilation** are required for airway control.
- **Intracranial pressure management:**
    - o Elevate head end of the bed.
    - o Mannitol, hypertonic saline, diuretics, sedatives, analgesics, muscle relaxants.
    - o External ventricular drain inserted into lateral ventricle.
- **Drugs:**
    - o **Antiepileptics:** Phenytoin.
    - o **Routine use of corticosteroids** is associated with increased mortality and **is no longer recommended.**
- **Nutrition:**
    - o Enteral nutrition > TPN.
    - o Prokinetics (e.g., metoclopramide, erythromycin) promote absorption.

LIMB TRAUMA

[3] Compartment syndrome. ***June 16***

[MCQ] Fasciotomy is indicated in compartment syndrome, if compartment syndrome is higher than how many mm of Hg? ***CBME June 24***

A. 20 B. 22

C. 25 D. 30*

- **Definition:** Compartment syndrome is raised interstitial pressure in a closed osteofascial compartment to a level that compromises tissue perfusion.
- It is a **surgical emergency** as delayed treatment may lead to **irreversible muscle ischemia and significant long-term morbidity.**

Causes

- The **most common cause is fractures**, most common in lower limb.
- Soft tissue contusion.
- Bleeding disorders, including anti-coagulation drugs.
- Arterial injuries.
- **Burns:** Particularly **circumferential third degree burns.**
- **Post ischemic swelling:** Reperfusion injury.
- Tight casts/dressing.
- Extravasation of IV infusions (contrast under pressure).
- **Acute post-op compartment syndrome:** Due to under perfusion during prolonged surgery, often with elevation of leg.

Pathophysiology

- Compartment syndrome **occurs in muscles enclosed in a fascia, such as calf and forearm muscles and intrinsic muscles of hand and foot.**

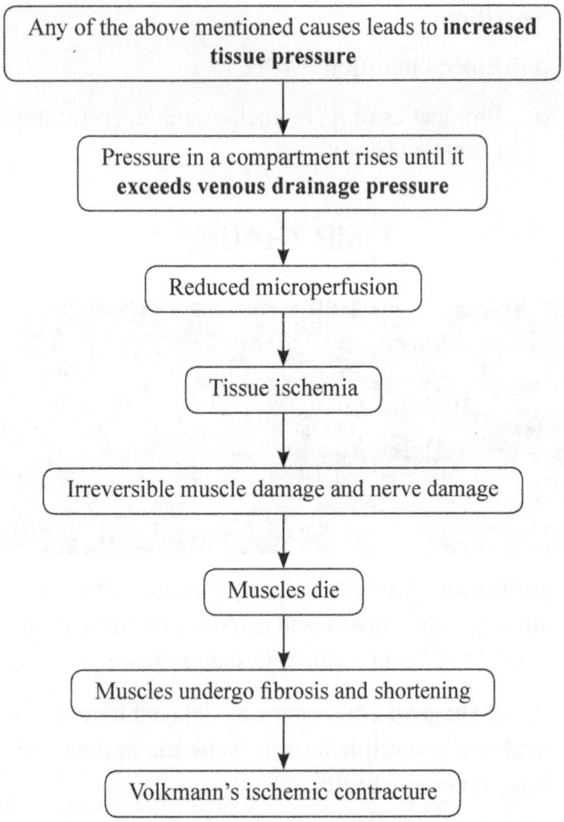

Clinical Features

- Severe pain/pain that is out of proportion to expected pain.
- Pain on passive movement of affected compartment muscles.
- Swelling of the affected limb.
- **Pressure on nerves:** Numbness, tingling, paralysis, paresthesia.
- **Pressure on blood vessels:** Pallor and pulselessness.
- The **absence of distal pulses is an extremely late sign**.

Investigations

- It is a **clinical diagnosis.**
- Compartment pressures can be measured using a **pressure monitor with a catheter placed in the muscle compartment.**
- Pressure studies are not reliable.
- Pressures indicative of compartment syndrome:
  - o Absolute pressure ≥ 30 mm Hg.
  - o Pressure difference (diastolic pressure – compartment pressure) ≤ 30 mm Hg.

Treatment

A. Conservative Measures

- Circumferential casts can be split.
- Dressings are cut down to the skin.
- Elevate the limb.

B. Fasciotomy

- This is the **treatment of choice** and should be done whenever in doubt.
- It means making a **surgical opening in the fascia which encloses the affected compartment.**
- Done via longitudinal incisions of skin, fat and fascia.
- Healthy muscle is seen bulging out through the fasciotomy opening.
- In **crush injuries** which present several days later, late fasciotomy can be dangerous because of the risk of crush syndrome. In these cases, it may be **safer to amputate the limb.**

[MCQ] Metabolic response to trauma includes all except: *CBME March 24*

A. Increased energy requirement
B. Decreased energy requirement*
C. Increased nitrogen (protein) requirement
D. Increased gluconeogenesis

Metabolic Changes After Surgery and Trauma

- The reason for metabolic changes is to:
  - o Provide essential substrates for survival from tissue breakdown.
  - o Postpone anabolism.
  - o Optimise host defence.
- These changes may be helpful in the short-term, but may be harmful in the long-term, especially to the severely injured or critically ill patient.
- Broadly, the following changes in body metabolism occur:
  - o Adipocyte lipolysis increases.
  - o Hepatic gluconeogenesis increases.
  - o Skeletal muscle protein degradation increases.
  - o Increased synthesis of hepatic acute phase proteins.

- o Pyrexia.
- o Hypermetabolism.

A. Catabolic Phase

- Catabolic phase begins at the time of injury and lasts for approximately 24–48 hours.
- Is characterised by:
    - o Hypovolemia.
    - o Decreased basal metabolic rate.
    - o Reduced cardiac output.
    - o Hypothermia.
    - o Lactic acidosis.
- The main physiological role of the catabolic phase is to conserve both circulating volume and energy stores for later recovery and repair.

B. Hypermetabolic Flow Phase

- Following resuscitation, the catabolic phase evolves into a hypermetabolic flow phase, which corresponds to SIRS.
- Involves the mobilisation of body energy stores for recovery and repair.
- Is characterised by:
    - o Tissue oedema (from vasodilatation and increased capillary leakage).
    - o Increased basal metabolic rate (hypermetabolism).
    - o Increased cardiac output.
    - o Raised body temperature.
    - o Leukocytosis.
    - o Increased oxygen consumption.
    - o Increased gluconeogenesis.
    - o Fat and protein mobilisation, leading to significant weight loss and increased urinary nitrogen excretion.

13

Neurosurgery

[MCQ] Obstructive hydrocephalus is caused by: *CBME June 24*

A. Post-hemorrhagic state

B. CSF infection

C. Choroid plexus carcinoma

D. Lesion in the ventricle*

HYDROCEPHALUS

- **Definition:** Hydrocephalus refers to an increase in CSF volume with ventricular enlargement, often presenting with symptoms of raised ICP.

Physiology of Cerebrospinal Fluid Flow

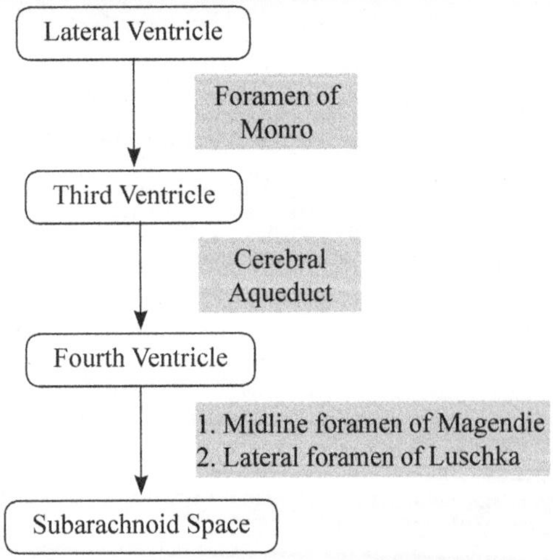

- CSF flows from the lateral ventricles through the foramen of Monro to the third ventricle, then down the cerebral aqueduct to the fourth ventricle, where it exits to the subarachnoid space via the midline foramen of Magendie and the lateral foramina of Luschka.
- CSF is reabsorbed into the arachnoid villi along the superior sagittal sinus.
- The total volume of CSF is normally about 150 mL.
- Production from the walls of the ventricles and the choroid plexus is about 20 mL/h.

Aetiology

A. Obstructive Hydrocephalus

- Lesions within the ventricle.
- Lesions in the ventricular wall.
- Lesions distant from the ventricle but with a mass effect.

B. Communicating Hydrocephalus

- Post hemorrhagic.
- CSF infection.
- Raised CSF protein.

C. Excessive CSF Production (Rare)

- Choroid plexus papilloma/carcinoma.

Pathophysiology

- Hydrocephalus almost always reflects obstruction to circulation (an obstructive hydrocephalus) or failure of reabsorption (a communicating hydrocephalus).

- The distinction is important since obstructive hydrocephalus especially can cause very sudden deterioration with coma and death.
- Lumbar puncture in obstructive hydrocephalus carries a risk of herniation of the brainstem and cerebellar tonsils owing to the resulting differential pressure changes (sometimes termed 'coning').
- On the other hand, lumbar puncture is of diagnostic value in communicating hydrocephalus, deriving an opening pressure and assessment of the CSF contents.
- It is also therapeutic: drainage of typically between 10 and 30 mL of CSF can relieve hydrocephalus temporarily.

Clinical Features

- Acutely raised ICP is a neurosurgical emergency.
- A high pressure headache that is worse on coughing or bending forward.
- Nausea and vomiting.
- Diplopia.
- Blurred vision.
- Cranial nerve compression can result in eye movement and pupil abnormalities.
- Drowsiness then coma.
- Before closure of the skull sutures in infancy, raised ICP presents differently with an increase in head circumference, prominent scalp veins and a tense bulging fontanelle.
- In infants and older children, raised CSF pressure results in dorsal midbrain compression with a loss of upgaze known as sunsetting, a feature of **Parinaud's syndrome**.

Investigations

- Fundoscopy can detect papilloedema, but this takes time to develop so may be absent in the acute phase.
- CT is a first-line investigation to identify causes of raised ICP, including mass lesions, bleeds, cerebral oedema and hydrocephalus and to guide treatment.
- Outside the emergency setting many pathologies, as well as the anatomy relating to potential treatments such as third ventriculostomy, may be better visualised on MRI.
- The gold standard for quantifying ICP and monitoring in real time is by transducing CSF pressure through an external ventricular drain or insertion of a pressure monitor into the brain substance.

Treatment

- The aim is to delay progression to cerebral herniation which can result in death.
- Raise the head end of the bed.
- Administer hypertonic saline or mannitol.
- Treatment of hydrocephalus in the emergency setting usually involves CSF diversion, for example using an external ventricular drain.

ACUTE OBSTRUCTIVE HYDROCEPHALUS

- Acute obstructive hydrocephalus is an emergency because of the risk of rapid progression to coma and death.
- It may be relieved by addressing the underlying pathology, e.g., by excision of a tumour responsible for an obstructive hydrocephalus.
- Most often, however, temporary ventricular drainage is required as a precaution in the preoperative and perioperative period or as an emergency in an obtunded or deteriorating patient.

A. External Ventricular Drain

- Is an effective temporary measure to relieve hydrocephalus.
- Most commonly inserted through a burr hole at Kocher's point (right of midline, anterior to the coronal suture), perpendicular to the brain surface, so that the catheter tip rests adjacent to the foramen of Monro in the lateral ventricle.
- Intrathecal antibiotics may also be given through it.
- Lumbar drains are an alternative means of temporary CSF diversion.

B. Ventriculoperitoneal Shunts

- Comprises the insertion of a proximal or ventricular catheter into the lateral ventricle, while a distal catheter is tunnelled subcutaneously to the abdomen.

- A shunt valve inserted between the proximal and distal catheters regulates flow through the system by opening at a predetermined pressure.

C. Endoscopic Third Ventriculostomy

- Especially useful in obstructive hydrocephalus due to aqueduct stenosis.

[3] Surgical anatomy of Circle of Willis. ***CBME June 24***

- The Circle of Willis is a critical anatomical structure located at the base of the brain, specifically at the junction between the anterior and posterior circulations.
- It forms a circular arterial network that provides redundancy and collateral circulation to the brain, ensuring continuous blood flow even if one of the arteries becomes blocked or compromised.

Components

A. Anterior Circulation Contributions

Anterior Cerebral Arteries (ACA):

- These arise from the internal carotid arteries and travel along the midline of the brain, supplying blood to the frontal lobes and medial aspects of the parietal lobes.

Anterior Communicating Artery (ACoA):

- This small artery connects the left and right ACAs.
- It serves as a crucial link in the circle, allowing blood to flow from one ACA to the other.

B. Posterior Circulation Contributions

Posterior Cerebral Arteries (PCA):

- These branches arise from the basilar artery, which is formed by the fusion of the two vertebral arteries.
- PCAs supply blood to the occipital lobes and the inferior aspect of the temporal lobes.

Posterior Communicating Arteries (PCoA):

- These arteries connect the posterior cerebral arteries to the internal carotid arteries, contributing to the posterior part of the circle.

Anatomy and Structure

Basilar Artery:

- Formed by the fusion of the vertebral arteries, it ascends along the brainstem and bifurcates into the posterior cerebral arteries.

Internal Carotid Arteries:

- Each ICA bifurcates into the middle cerebral artery (MCA) and anterior cerebral artery (ACA), contributing to the anterior part of the circle.

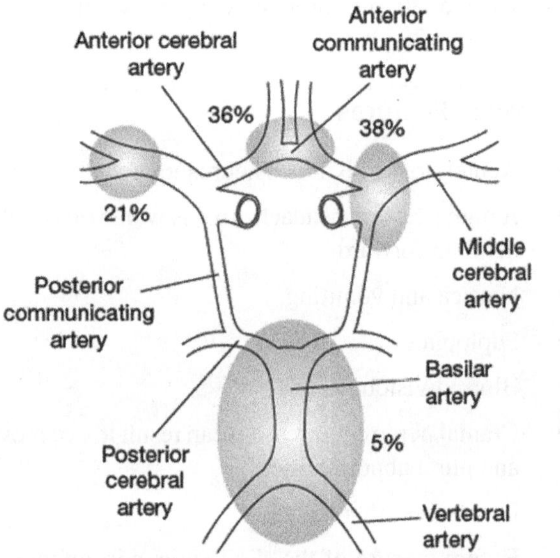

Figure 1: Common sites of aneurysm in the Circle of Willis

[3] Berry aneurysm. ***Sept 21***

- Also known as cerebral or intracranial aneurysm.
- It is a saccular aneurysm.

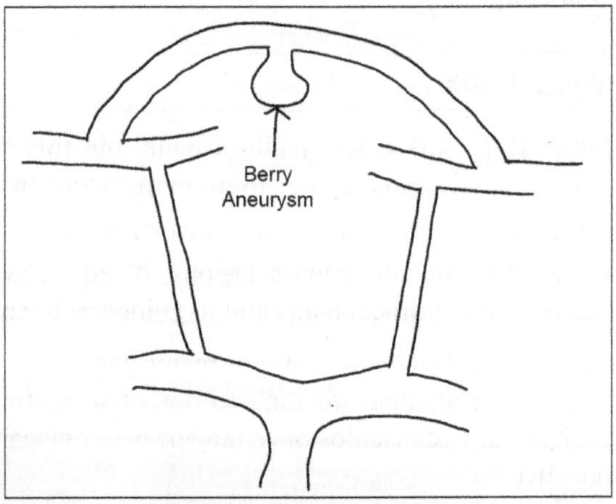

Figure 2: Berry aneurysm

Site/Location

- The **most common location is the circle of Willis** at the base of the brain.
- Commonly occurs at **arterial bifurcations** or branch points.

Causes

- F > M.
- Elderly.
- Family history.
- Hypertension.
- Smoking.
- Connective tissue disorders.

Clinical Features

- Found **incidentally** on neuroimaging.
- May present with **subarachnoid hemorrhage.**
  - o Sudden onset of headache described as the **'worst headache of my life', called thunderclap headache.**
  - o High fatality rate.
  - o Survivors have varying degrees of neurological disability.

Investigations

- NCCT scan of brain.
- CT angiography of brain.

Complications

- Rebleeding.
- Hydrocephalus.
- Seizures.
- Hyponatremia.
- Vasospasm of cerebral arteries.

Predictors of Outcome

- Hunt and Hess clinical grading scale.
- World Federation of Neurological Surgeons clinical grading scale.
- Fisher's grading for appearance of subarachnoid hemorrhage on CT scan.

Treatment

Treatment of Berry Aneurysm

Endovascular Techniques
- Coiling.
- Coiling through a stent.
- Flow diversion stent.
- Surgical clipping.

Open Surgery
- Open craniotomy and clipping

A. Endovascular Techniques

- Coiling.
- Coiling through a stent.
- Flow diversion stent.
- Surgical clipping.

B. Open Surgery

- Open craniotomy and clipping is indicated when endovascular techniques is not feasible or if it fails.

[MCQ] A 65-year-old patient presented in the casualty with two hours history of sudden onset of severe headache associated with nausea and vomiting. On clinical examination, the patient had neck stiffness and right-sided ptosis. The rest of the neurological examination was normal. What is the clinical diagnosis? ***CBME June 24***

A. Hypertensive brain hemorrhage

B. Migraine

C. Aneurysmal subarachnoid hemorrhage*

D. Arteriovenous malformation

[3] Horner's Syndrome. ***Dec 18, July 15***

- Also known as oculosympathetic palsy.

Cause

- **Injury to cervical sympathetic nerve:**
  - o Trauma.
  - o Tumours.
  - o Infections.

Components

- There can be easily remembered by the mnemonic PAMELA.

  P - Ptosis.

  A - Anhidrosis, i.e., decreased sweating on the affected side of the face.

  M - Miosis.

  E - Enophthalmos.

  L - Loss of ciliospinal reflex on affected side.

  A - Anisocoria.

[3] Hypothalamopituitary axis. *June 14*

- The hypothalamus is closely linked with the pituitary gland, both anatomically and functionally.
- The connection between hypothalamus and pituitary is called hypothalamopituitary axis.
- Hypothalamus is connected separately and differently with anterior and posterior pituitaries.
  - o **The connection with anterior pituitary is by means of blood vessels:** Portal-hypophyseal vessels.
  - o **The connection with posterior pituitary is through the neurons:** Hypothalamo-hypophyseal tract.

Importance

- It plays a crucial role in maintaining homeostasis and regulating various physiological processes in the body:
  - o Growth and development (via growth hormone).
  - o Thyroid gland (via TSH).
  - o Cortisol secretion (via ACTH).
  - o Lactogenesis (via prolactin).
  - o Reproduction (via FSH and LH).

14

Lungs

[3] Empyema necessitans. *Dec 19*

- Also known as empyema necessitatis.
- It is a **rare and serious complication** of empyema, which is a condition characterized by the collection of pus in the pleural cavity. **When an empyema perforates the chest walls, it is called empyema necessitans.**

Aetiopathogenesis

- It is caused by an empyema perforating the chest wall.
- It presents with a **subcutaneous collection of pus communicating**, often by a tortuous channel, **with the main pleural collection.**
- The site of the subcutaneous abscess does not always correspond to the site of pleural perforation, as the abscess may track along the intercostal spaces before becoming superficial.

Cause

- Neglected or undiagnosed empyema.
- Following aspiration of thin, highly infective pus from an empyema.

Clinical Features

- Diffuse, fluctuant, tender swelling or an open wound on the chest wall.
- Impulse on cough may be present.
- Associated with the clinical and radiological signs of an underlying empyema.
- Draining pus may have a foul odour.
- Skin around the area may be red, swollen and inflamed.

Investigations

- Chest X-ray.
- CT scan.
- USG guided aspiration/drainage.
- Pleural fluid analysis.
- CBNAAT, Gene Xpert (to rule out tuberculosis).

Treatment

- Treatment is primarily aimed at the empyema, which should be **aspirated and drained.**
- The superficial abscess may disappear as a result of aspirating the empyema, or may itself require separate aspirations or drainage.
- IV antibiotics as per C/S.

[3] Differential Diagnosis for Mediastinal Tumours. *CBME March 24*

A. Anterior Mediastinum

- Thymoma.
- Lymphoma.
- Germ cell tumour.

B. Middle Mediastinum

- Cystic lesions.

- Lymphoma.
- Mesenchymal tumours.

C. Superior Mediastinum

- Lymphoma.
- Thyroid tumours.
- Parathyroid tumours.

D. Posterior Mediastinum

- Neurogenic tumours.
- Cystic lesions.
- Mesenchymal tumours.

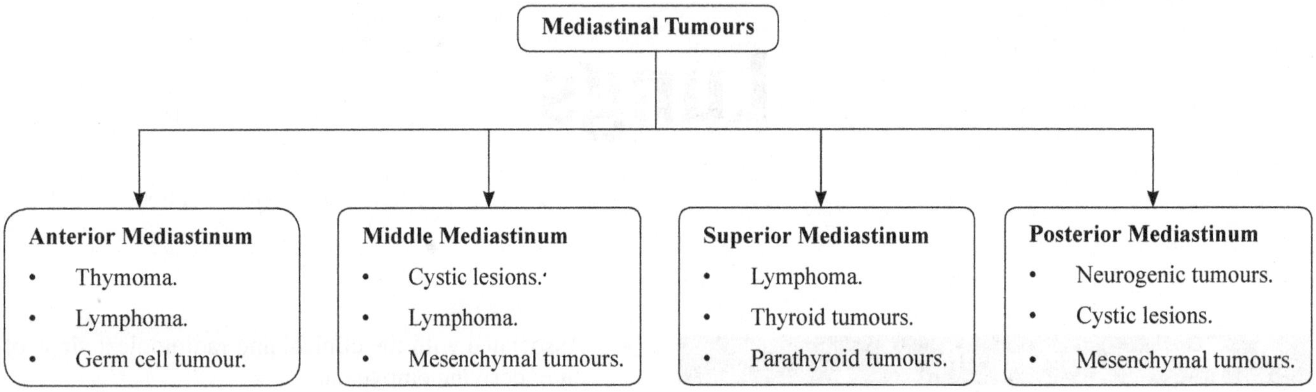

15

Cardiothoracic and Vascular Surgery (CTVS)

[3] Patent Ductus Arteriosus. *Sept 21*

- It is a congenital heart defect where the **ductus arteriosus**, a blood vessel that allows blood to bypass the lungs in a developing foetus, **fails to close after birth.**
- It is a **left to right shunt.**

Pathophysiology

- The ductus arteriosus is a normal fetal communication, which facilitates the shunting of oxygenated blood from the pulmonary artery to the aorta, away from the lungs.
- Normally, **functional closure begins within minutes to hours after birth**, and the **anatomical closure is typically completed within the first few days to weeks of life.**

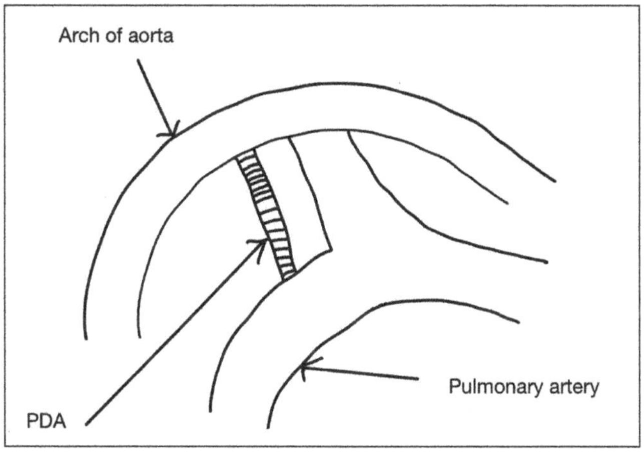

Figure: Patent ductus arteriosus

- It involves a combination of functional constriction and eventual anatomical sealing of the ductus.
- The ductus **closes in response to an increase in peripheral oxygen saturation and a drop in the resistance of the pulmonary circulation as the lungs expand**; this causes the ductal tissue to contract through a prostaglandin inhibition mechanism.
- **In premature babies**, the ductus is more likely to **remain patent** for a longer duration or even permanently.
- It is a left to right shunt.
- It results in **high pulmonary blood flow.**

Clinical Features

- The severity of the symptoms depends on the size of the ductus and the age of the individual.
- **Respiratory Symptoms:**
  - o In newborns and young infants, respiratory distress may be evident.
  - o They might have tachypnoea, shortness of breath and difficulty in feeding.
- Recurrent respiratory infections.
- Failure to thrive.
- Fatigue and weakness.
- Palpitations.
- **Eisenmenger syndrome** occurs in severe cases.

On Examination

- **Continuous machinery murmur** in left second intercostal space.
- Bounding pulse.
- Larger ducts can sometimes lead to shunt reversal with cyanosis and clubbing.

Complications

- Heart failure (left ventricular failure).
- Infective endocarditis.
- Pulmonary hypertension.
- Eisenmenger syndrome.

Investigations

- The diagnosis is confirmed by **echocardiography** with colour flow doppler imaging.

Treatment

A. Medical Treatment

- A **COX inhibitor (e.g., indomethacin)** may be used therapeutically to close the ductus in the first few weeks of life.

B. Surgical Treatment

- **Timing of Repair:**
  - o After 6 months of age, spontaneous PDA closure is rare.
  - o Most **should be closed by preschool age**, regardless of symptoms.
- **Indications of Surgery:**
  - o Most should be closed by pre-school age, regardless of symptoms.
  - o In the adult, surgical treatment is indicated if there is a persistent left-to-right shunt even in the presence of reversible pulmonary hypertension.
- **Methods of Surgical Closure:**
  - o **Percutaneous** interventional cardiology **techniques using an umbrella or coil duct occlusion device.**
  - o **If the PDA is very large: Surgical closure via a left thoracotomy** is preferred. This can be accomplished by either ligation or division of the PDA.

16

Skin and Subcutaneous Tissue

BASAL CELL CARCINOMA

[10] Discuss aetiology, pathology, clinical features and management of Basal Cell Carcinoma. ***Dec 12***

[5] Basal Cell Carcinoma. ***March 22, March 21, Oct 20, Dec 16, July 15***

[5] Rodent ulcer. ***June 19***

[3] Rodent ulcer. ***July 18***

[3] Basal Cell Carcinoma. ***June 16***

- Also known as **rodent ulcer.**
- It is usually a **slow growing, locally invasive, malignant tumor of pluripotent epithelial cells arising from basal epidermis and hair follicles.**
- It affects the pilosebaceous skin.
- It is the **most common non melanoma** skin cancer.

Causes/Risk Factors

- **Ultraviolet radiation**, i.e., excessive sun exposure:
  - o **Strongest predisposing factor**.
  - o Incidence of BCC rises with proximity to the equator.
  - o **1/3rd arise in parts of the body not usually exposed to the sun**.
- Occurs almost exclusively in **white skinned people**.
- M > F.
- **Exposure to chemicals:**
  - o Arsenical compounds.
  - o Coal tar.
  - o Aromatic hydrocarbons.
- Exposure to **ionizing radiation.**
- **Genetic skin cancer syndromes.**

Pathogenesis

- Have **no apparent precursor lesions.**
- **Development is proportional to the initial dose of the carcinogen, but not duration of exposure.**
- Most likely model of pathogenesis involves **mesodermal factors as intrinsic promoters** coupled with an initiation step.
- Local infiltration is common.
- **Metastasizes extremely rarely:**
  - o Mets are associated with advanced age and large, neglected lesions.

Types

A. Localised

- Nodular.
- Nodulocystic.
- Cystic.
- Pigmented.

- Naevoid
  - o Nodular and nodulocystic are most common (90% of BCCs).

B. Generalized

- Superficial
  - o Multifocal.
  - o Superficial spreading.
- Infiltrative
  - o Morphoeic.
  - o Ice pick.
  - o Cicatrizing.

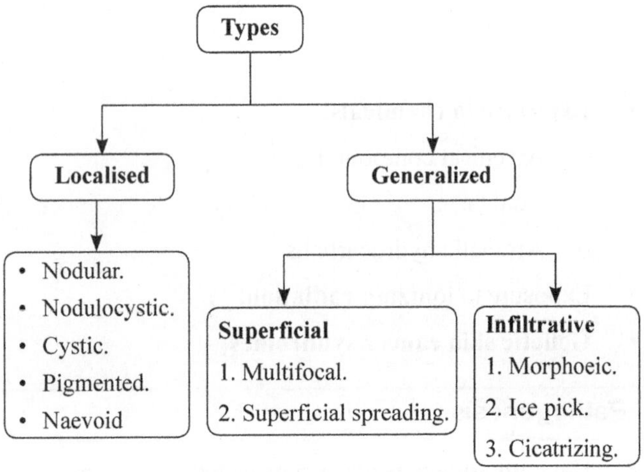

HPE

- **26 histologic subtypes** have been described.
- Characteristic finding is of **ovoid cells in nests with a single palisading layer**.
- **Only the outer layer of cells activity divide:**
  - o This is why tumor growth rates are slower than their cell cycle speed would suggest and why incompletely excised lesions are more aggressive.
- **Morphoeic BCCs** synthesize Type 4 collagenase and so **spread rapidly**.

Clinical Features

- There are **no precursor skin lesions** (unlike SCC and actinic keratoses).
- **Appearance varies:**
  - o Nodules in the skin.
  - o Large non-healing sore with discharge and crusting.
- **Slow growth rate:** Some tumors grow at so slow a rate that they are, for all practical purposes, benign.
- **Nodular growth pattern (classical BCC):**
  - o **Well defined, elevated lesion with a waxy appearance.**
  - o As the lesion grows, **pearly opalescent nodules** develop along the margins.
  - o A **central depression with umbilication or ulceration and raised edges** is a classic sign.
  - o **Distinct blood vessels (telangiectasia)** may be seen across the surface or along the edges of the lesion.

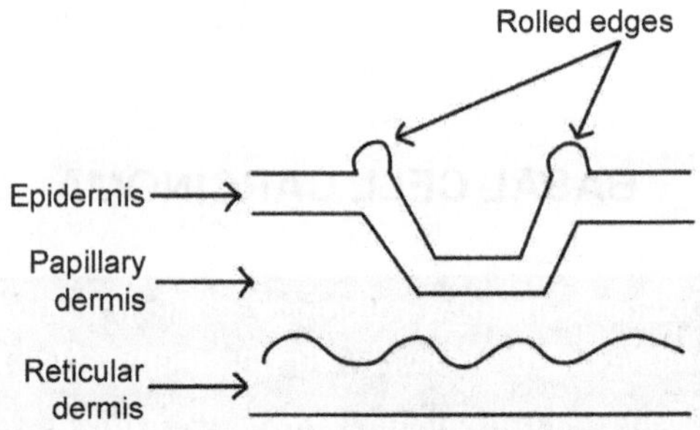

Figure 1: Rolled edges of Basal Cell Carcinoma

  - o **Most are pink or skin-coloured,** but may also have shades of brown or black.
- **Cystic type** is less common but has a distinctive **translucent appearance.**
- **Superficial type:**
  - o Has a more **macular** growth pattern.
  - o May extend over the surface of the skin in a **multicentric** pattern.
  - o **Centre can ulcerate.**
  - o **Margins** are often **irregular** and ill-defined.
- **Morpheaform/morphoeic type (cicatricial BCC):**
  - o White **scarring** growth pattern.
  - o These lesions are among the **most locally invasive** subtypes and can penetrate deep into the underlying dermis.
- **Rodent ulcer:**
  - o Also known as Jacobi ulcer.
  - o Neglected BCC that has formed an ulceration.
  - o Pearly border of the lesion may not be recognized.
  - o Indurated edge.

- o Advanced lesion.
- 80% of all BCC occur on the head and neck.
- **Ohngren's line:**
  - o Connects the medial canthus of the eye to the angle of the mandible.
  - o Tumors below it have a better prognosis than those above the line.

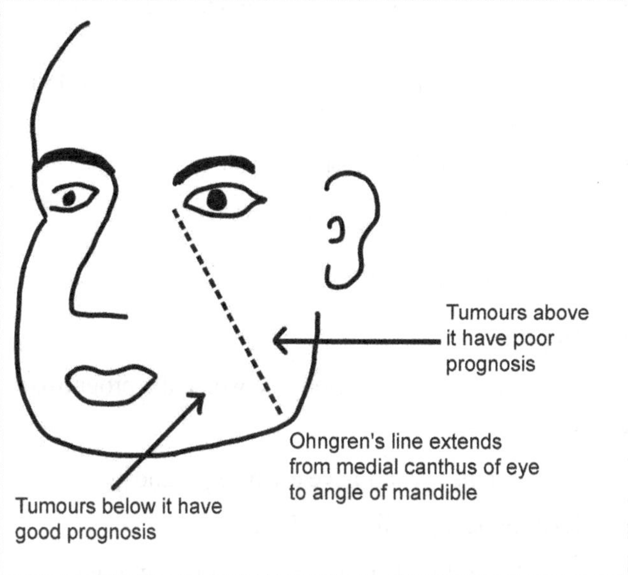

Figure 2: Ohngren's line

Prognosis

- **High risk tumours are:**
  - o Large (> 2 cm).
  - o Located at sites where direct invasion gives access to the cranium (near the eye, nose and ear).
  - o Recurrent tumors.
  - o Tumors forming in the presence of immunosuppression.
  - o Micronodular or infiltrating histologic subtypes.

Investigations

- Edge wedge biopsy.
- Excision biopsy.

Treatment

A. Surgical

- **Excision** of the tumor/lesion is the treatment of choice:
  - o **Loupe magnification** is used.
  - o **Margins: 2 mm to 15 mm** (depending on macroscopic variant).
  - o If margins are ill-defined or tissue is at a premium (nose, eyes):
    - ♦ **Two-staged surgical approach with subsequent reconstruction** after confirmation of clear margins.
    - ♦ **Moh's micrographic surgery**, i.e., excision under microscopic control.

B. Non-Surgical

- **Indications:** Elderly, infirm.
- **Options are:**
  - o Radiotherapy.
  - o **Topical treatment:** 5-fluorouracil, imiquimod.

SQUAMOUS CELL CARCINOMA

[10] Discuss aetiology, pathology, clinical features and management of SCC skin. ***June 17***

[3] How do you arrive at a diagnosis of SCC of skin? ***CBME March 24***

- It is a malignant tumour of keratinizing cells of the epidermis or its appendages.
- Arises from the **stratum basalis** of the epidermis.
- Expresses **cytokeratins 1 and 10.**

Cause/Risk Factors

- **Cumulative sun exposure and damage (UV radiation):**
  - o Especially in **white-skinned** individuals living nearer the equator.
- M > F.
- Middle aged to elderly.
- **Chronic inflammation** (chronic sinus tracts, pre-existing scars, osteomyelitis, burns, vaccination points).
- **Immunosuppression**, particularly with the suppression of cell mediated immunity **after solid organ transplantation.**
- Ionising radiation.
- **Chemical carcinogens:**
  - o Arsenicals, tar.

- **Human Papilloma Virus:**
  - o Subtypes 5 and 16.
- Tobacco.
- **Actinic Keratoses:**
  - o When an actinic keratosis has a keratinous surface with a height greater than its base diameter, it is termed as keratin horn. 10% of these will have an underlying SCC.
- **Keratoacanthomas:**
  - o They are currently considered to be self-healing SCCs.
- **Bowen's Disease and Erythroplasia of Queyrat:**
  - o It is SCC in situ.

HPE

- Characteristic **irregular masses of squamous epithelium which proliferate and invade the dermis** from the basal layer.
- Tumour stains **positive for cytokeratins 1 and 10.**
- Can be graded histologically according to **Broders grading**, which describes the proportion of dedifferentiated cells in the tumour.

Staging

- TNM staging.

Clinical Features

- SCC frequently **begins at the site of actinic keratoses** on sun exposed areas (face, back of hand).
- Appearance varies from **smooth nodular, verrucous, papillomatous to ulcerating** lesions.
- All lesions **eventually ulcerate** as they grow:
  - o Ulcers have a characteristic **everted or rolled out edge.**
  - o Ulcers are **surrounded by inflamed, indurated skin.**
  - o Ulcer is at first superficial and **hidden by a crust**.
  - o When the crust is removed, a **well-defined papillary base** is seen, and on palpation, a discrete hard disk is felt.

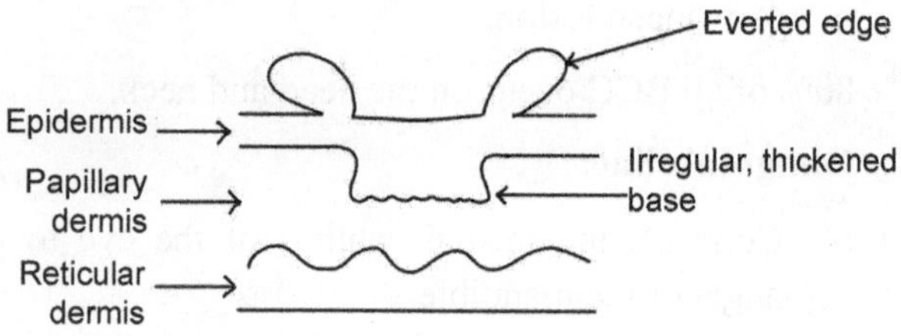

Figure 3: Everted edges of Squamous Cell Carcinoma

- In advanced lesions, the **surface is usually cauliflower like.**
- Local symptoms may wax and wane for a period of many months.
- It metastasizes to regional lymph nodes.
- Malignant potential varies between subtypes.

Prognostic Factors

- **Depth:**
  - o The deeper the lesion, the worse the prognosis.
- **Surface size:**
  - o Lesions > 2 cm have a worse prognosis.
- **Histological grade:**
  - o Higher the Broders grade, worse the prognosis.
- **Lymphovascular or perineural invasion:**
  - o Carries a high risk of mets.
- **Site:**
  - o Tumour on lips and ears have higher local recurrence rates.
  - o Tumours at the extremities have worse prognosis than those on the trunk.
- **Aetiology:**
  - o SCCs that arise in burn scars, osteomyelitis, skin sinuses, chronic ulcers, irradiated skin have higher metastatic potential.
- **Immunosuppression:**
  - o SCCs invade further in those with impaired immune response.

Investigations

- Edge wedge biopsy.
- Excision biopsy.

Treatment

- **Treatment must address the following:**
  - o Lesion.
  - o Tumour's tendency for lymphatic mets.
  - o Possibility of *in-transit* mets.
- **Surgical excision is the treatment of choice:**
  - o It is the only means of providing accurate information on histology and clearance.
- **Margins:**
  - o Assessed using Loupe magnification.
  - o Margins for primary excision should be tailored to surface size in the first instance.
  - o **< 2 cm:** 4 mm clearance margin.
  - o **> 2 cm:** 1 cm clearance margin.
- **Field therapies:**
  - o Treats a generalized area but does not define the status of the margin.
  - o E.g., radiation therapy, cryosurgery, photodynamic therapy, electrodesiccation and curettage, topical agents like imiquimod.
- **Sentinel lymph node biopsy:**
  - o Done in high risk lesions because of the presence of clinically occult lymph node mets.
  - o Subsequent nodal management strategy is: Completion lymphadenectomy ± radiation.
- Adjuvant radiation to the primary tumour is recommended for any SCC with extensive perineural or large nerve involvement.
- **Locally advanced or metastatic SCC:**
  - o Rare.
  - o Difficult to treat.
  - o Systemic cytotoxic chemotherapy: Cisplatin, carboplatin.
  - o Targeted therapy with epidermal growth factor receptor antagonists.
- **New drug:** Cemiplimab.

MALIGNANT MELANOMA

[10] Discuss the types, clinical features and management of Malignant Melanoma. ***June 19***

[10] Discuss aetiology, pathology, clinical features, and management of Malignant Melanoma. ***Dec 14***

[5] Malignant Melanoma. ***June 16***

[5] Enumerate clinical features and management of Malignant Melanoma. ***CBME June 24***

- Melanoma is a **cancer of melanocytes** and can therefore arise in skin, mucosa, retina and the leptomeninges.
- It is the **most common cancer in young adults** (20-39 years) and is the most likely cause of skin cancer-related death.

Cause/Risk Factors

- Exposure to **ultraviolet radiation**, i.e., sun exposure:
  - o Recreational activity in the sun.
  - o Emigration among white skinned people not suited to sun exposure.
- Common in **white skinned** people with **light** (blonde or red) **hair and light coloured eyes** (blue eyes).
- People who **sunburn easily.**
- People with tendency to develop **freckles.**
- **Inability to tan.**
- Predominantly seen in middle-age adults, although it occurs across all ages.
- **Genetic risk factors:**
  - o High risk skin types (**Fitzpatrick skin types 1 and 2**).
  - o **Family history** of melanoma.
  - o **Xeroderma pigmentosum.**
- **Pre-existing naevi:**
  - o Only 10-20% of MM form in pre-existing naevi, with the reminder arising de novo in previously normally pigmented skin.

- Most likely naevi to form malignant melanoma are: **Atypical naevi, atypical junctional lentiginous naevi (usually facial) and giant pigmented congenital naevi.**
- Patients who have **> 30 sun acquired naevi.**

- **Immunosuppression.**

Types

- **There are 4 main types:**
  1. Superficial spreading melanoma.
  2. Nodular melanoma.
  3. Lentigo maligna melanoma.
  4. Acral lentiginous melanoma.
- **Miscellaneous types:**
  - Amelanotic melanoma.
  - Desmoplastic melanoma.

HPE

- Malignant change occurs in the melanocytes in the basal epidermis.
- In situ atypical melanocytes are limited to the dermo-epidermal junction and show no evidence of dermal involvement.
- During the horizontal growth phase, cells spread along the dermoepidermal junction and their migration is predominantly radial.
- During the vertical growth phase, the dermis may be invaded.
- The greater the depth of invasion, the greater the metastatic potential of the tumour.

Clinical Features

- Commonly presents as an **irregular pigmented skin lesion** that has grown or changed over time.
- **ABCDE criteria** are used to guide diagnosis in suspicious skin lesions.

  A – Asymmetry.

  B – Irregular borders.

  C – Colour variegation.

  D – Diameter > 6 mm.

  E – Evolution or changes over time.
- Other features in naevi which are suggestive of malignant melanoma are:
  - **Thickness** (elevation/nodularity or ulceration).
  - **Satellite lesions** (pigment spreading into surrounding areas).
  - **Late signs – Tingling, itching, serosanguinous discharge.**

Superficial Spreading Melanoma

- Most common presentation.
- Usually **arises in pre-existing naevus.**
- **Nodularity** within this type **heralds** the onset of the **vertical growth** phase.

Nodular Melanoma

- More **aggressive** than superficial spreading type, with a shorter clinical onset.
- Often **arises de novo** in skin.
- M > F.
- Middle age.
- **Sites:** Trunk, head or neck.
- Typically appear as blue/black papules which are 1-2 cm in diameter.
- Because they lack the horizontal growth phase, they tend to be **sharply demarcated.**

Lentigo Maligna Melanoma

- Previously known as **Hutchinson's melanotic freckle.**
- Presents as a **slow growing, variegated, brown macule** on the face, neck or hands of the elderly.
- Have **lesser metastatic potential** than other variants as they take longer to enter a vertical growth phase.
- However, once they enter the vertical growth phase, their metastatic potential is the same as any other melanoma.

Acral Lentiginous Melanoma

- Affects the **soles and palms.**
- Presents as a **flat, irregular macule.**
- May mimic a fungal infection or pyogenic granuloma.
- History and clinical examination should be directed

at discovering the primary lesion and identification of local, regional or distant spread.

- It metastasizes through lymphatics.
- **Distant mets:** Liver > lung.

Staging

- **Breslow Thickness:**
  - o It is **measured to the nearest 0.1 mm from the granular layer to the base of the tumour.**
  - o It is the **most important prognostic indicator** in the absence of lymph node mets.
  - o The likelihood of metastatic spread to regional lymph nodes is proportional to the Breslow thickness.
- **AJCC Staging:**
  - o It takes into account the following factors:
    - ♦ Primary tumour.
    - ♦ Lymph node involvement.
    - ♦ Distant mets.
    - ♦ Other evidence based prognostic factors.

Prognostic Factors

- Breslow thickness.
- **Mitotic index:** Higher the mitotic index, poorer the prognosis.
- **Lymph node mets:**
  - o The presence of lymph node mets is the single most important prognostic factor.
  - o Once regional lymph nodes are involved, there is a higher chance of occult distant mets.

Investigations

- **Excision biopsy:**
  - o With a 2-3 mm margin of skin and a cuff of subdermal fat.
- **Incision biopsy:**
  - o Occasionally indicated, e.g., in large lesions on the face where an excision biopsy of the whole lesion would be disfiguring.
- **Serial clinical and dermoscopic photography** every 2 months may avoid biopsies in equivocal cases.
- **Sentinel node biopsy:**
  - o Offered to patients with ≥ T2a.
  - o Based on the fact that lymphatic mets proceed in an orderly fashion and can be predicted by mapping the lymphatic drainage from a primary tumour to the first (or sentinel node) in the regional lymphatic basin.

Treatment

- **Surgical excision of the primary tumour:**
  - o Excision with a margin of normal tissue is the only cure for malignant melanoma.
  - o **Margins:**
    - ♦ Melanoma in situ: 5 mm margin.
    - ♦ Melanoma < 1 mm deep: 1 cm margin.
    - ♦ Melanoma > 1 mm deep: 2 cm margin.
- **Regional lymph nodes:**
  - o Management of regional lymph nodes is controversial.
  - o Some surgeons advocate simultaneous lymph node clearance at the time of wide local excision of the primary melanoma.
  - o Other surgeons favour a therapeutic lymphadenectomy only if regional lymph nodes become clinically evident.
  - o Sentinel node biopsy can be done:
    - ♦ Completion lymphadenectomy after positive sentinel node biopsy is the best method for regional control.
- **Drugs:**
  - o **Targeted therapy:** Dabrafenib, vemurafenib, trametinib, ipilimumab, nivolumab.

PRE-MALIGNANT CONDITIONS OF SKIN

[3] Mention pre-malignant conditions of skin. *Dec 14*

[10] List the pre-malignant lesions of skin. Discuss the clinical features and management of malignant melanoma. *Dec 13*

The pre-malignant conditions of the skin are as follows:

1. Extra mammary Paget's disease or intraepidermal adenocarcinoma.
2. Giant congenital pigmented naevus or giant hairy naevus.
3. Atypical or dysplastic naevus.
4. Actinic or solar keratosis.
5. Cutaneous horn.
6. Bowen's disease (squamous cell carcinoma in situ).

HAEMANGIOMA

[3] Haemangioma. *Dec 16*

[5] Haemangioma. *June 14*

[3] Types of haemangioma and their differences. *Dec 12*

- **Definition:** Benign vascular tumours that arise from the **proliferation of endothelial cells that surround blood filled cavities**.
- Many of these lesions are considered to be **vascular malformations.**
- It can occur in any tissue of the body, but is **most common in the skin and subcutaneous tissues.**

Clinical Features

- F : M = 3:1.
- 30% have a **herald patch at birth**, which then **grows rapidly in the first year of life and slowly involutes over several years**, with 70% having resolved by 7 years of age.
- Occasionally, **during the rapid growth phase**, the lesions **can obstruct** the airway, GI tract, vision and musculoskeletal function. In these cases, surgical resection is indicated prior to the involution phase.
- Hemangiomas can sometimes consume a large percentage of cardiac output, resulting in **high output heart failure.**
- Large hemangiomata can trap platelets, leading to thrombocytopenia (**consumptive coagulopathy**). This is called **Kasabach-Merritt Syndrome**.
- Lesions which cause high output heart failure or consumptive coagulopathy, characteristically express the GLUT-1 glucose transporter protein, which is absent in cells of the normal cutaneous vasculature.

Treatment

- **Indications of Resection:**
  - o Lesions which cause obstructive symptoms during the rapid growth phase.
  - o Lesions which cause high output heart failure.
  - o Lesions which cause consumptive coagulopathy.
  - o Tumours which persist into adolescence, leaving a cosmetically undesirable defect.
- When surgical resection or debulking is considered, **upfront selective embolization** can help with planned resection.
- **First-line therapy for infantile hemangiomas is propranolol.** This causes cessation of growth, and in most cases, actual regression of the lesions.
- Drugs which slow down tumour progression:
  - o Systemic corticosteroids.
  - o Interferon alpha.
- Laser Therapy.

Types of Hemangioma

A. Capillary Hemangioma:

1. Salmon patch.
2. Port-wine stain.
3. Strawberry angioma or strawberry naevus.

B. Venous Hemangioma or Cavernous Hemangioma.

C. Arterial Hemangioma or Plexiform Hemangioma.

Salmon Patch

- Pinkish macule.
- Usually found at the nape of the neck.
- Caused by an area of persistent fetal dermal circulation.
- Usually disappears at 1 year of age.

Strawberry Naevus

- Most common birthmark.
- Occurs most frequently on the head and neck.
- Usually resolves by early childhood.

Port-wine Stain

- **Cause: Defective maturation of the cutaneous sympathetic innervation during embryogenesis,** leading to localized intradermal capillary vasodilatation.
- Appears at birth as flat, smooth, intensely purple-stained areas.
- Situated **most frequently on the head and neck**, often within the maxillary and mandibular dermatomes of the trigeminal nerve.
- May be associated with various syndromes.
- **Treatment: Intense pulsed light and pulsed-dye laser**.

Venous or Cavernous Hemangioma

- Present at birth.
- Consists of a multiplicity of venous channels of varying caliber.
- Shows **no tendency to involution.**
- May become larger or more troublesome later on in life.
- Sometimes, the whole of one limb and the adjacent part of the trunk is affected.
- Arteriovenous communications may sometimes be present.
- Skin overlying the hemangioma may be atrophic, which puts it in danger of severe hemorrhage from trauma.

OTHERS

[3] Café au lait macules. *June 17*

- Also known as café au lait spots.

Description

- Café au lait describes the colour of the spots, which **resembles the colour of coffee when mixed with milk.**
- Light brown to dark brown in colour.
- They are **macules**, i.e., flat.
- Typically oval or round in shape and have a **well-defined border.**
- **Painless** and do not cause any physical discomfort.
- Can vary in size and number, and their appearance can change over time, especially in childhood and adolescence when new spots may develop.

Aetiology

- Caused by an **excess of melanin** in the affected areas.
- Sporadic.
- As part of certain genetic conditions, such as **neurofibromatosis type I**.

Clinical Significance

- As a **marker of neurofibromatosis:**
  - o > 5 CALM can be a skin manifestation of neurofibromatosis.

[5] Cylindroma. *June 13*

- Also known as **turban tumour.**
- It is a variant of **eccrine spiradenoma.**
- Can occur as part of an inherited syndrome called **Brooke-Spiegler syndrome.**

HPE

- There are **cylindrical masses of epithelial cells** which are surrounded and segmented by thick bands of a hyaline material. This is why it is called a cylindroma.

Clinical Features

- Cutaneous cylindroma occurs predominantly on the **scalp and face** as a solitary lesion.
- When **multiple cylindromas** are present on the scalp, it **coalesces and the tumor gradually forms an extensive, turban like swelling** extending over the scalp.
- It is firm but **rubber like** in consistency.
- Ranges in size from a few mm to several cm.
- May be mistaken for pilar cyst, but the distinctive appearance and consistency make diagnosis easy, especially in the multiple type.
- Ulceration is uncommon.

Treatment

- Surgical excision.
- Laser ablation.

[5] Xeroderma Pigmentosum. *Dec 12*

- It is a **disorder of photosensitivity**, caused by **mutations in genes involved in nucleotide excision repair**.

Cause

- Abnormality on the **patched gene of chromosome 9q**, resulting in **aberrant nucleotide repair** during cellular DNA maintenance.
- **Autosomal recessive.**

Clinical Features

- Patients have a **> 2000 fold increase in skin cancer risk.**
- Patients are **intolerant of UV radiation** which leads to premature skin ageing:
  - o Sun sensitivity.
  - o Freckling.
  - o Lentigines.
  - o Skin cancers often appear < 10 years of age.
  - o Most of the skin tumours occur on the head and neck in sun exposed areas.
- **Increase in internal cancers,** i.e., non-skin cancers.
- Most affected individuals die in early adulthood from metastatic disease.
- **Ocular abnormalities:**
  - o Photophobia.
  - o Ectropion.
  - o Corneal opacity.
  - o Blepharospasm.
  - o Neoplasms.
- Progressive neurologic degeneration.
- Loss of high-frequency hearing.

Treatment

- The main intervention that is vital is extremely diligent **photoprotection.**
- Vitamin D.
- Nicotinamide.
- Zinc supplementation.
- Retinoids can prevent the appearance of new cancers.
- Individual tumours may be excised or destroyed with cryotherapy.
- **Topical creams:** Imiquimod, 5-Fluorouracil.

17

Common Cysts and Swellings

[3] Classification of cysts. *July 18*

- Two types of classifications are in use:

Based on the Cyst Wall

A. True Cysts

- Lined by epithelium or endothelium.
- If infected, it may be lined by granulation tissue, e.g., sebaceous cyst.

B. False Cysts or Pseudocysts

- These are not lined by epithelium.

1. Exudation cyst:

- Develop from exudation of fluid and are limited to anatomical spaces, e.g., pseudopancreatic cyst, vaginal hydrocele.

2. Degeneration cyst:

- Develop as degeneration in the centre of a malignant tumour due to hemorrhage or ischemic necrosis or colliquative necrosis, e.g., apoplectic cyst.

Based on Whether it is Congenital or Acquired

A. Congenital Cysts

a. Sequestration cyst:

- Develops at the line of closure of embryonic clefts due to burial of dermal cells in the fusion line, e.g., angular dermoid, branchial cysts.

Based on Whether it is Congenital or Acquired

- **Congenital**
  - a. Sequestration cyst
  - b. Tubulo-embryonic or Tubulo-dermoid cyst
  - c. Cysts of embryonic remnants
- **Acquired**
  - a. Retention cysts
  - b. Distension cyst
  - c. Exudation cyst
  - d. Degeneration cyst
  - e. Cystic tumours
  - f. Implantation dermoid
  - g. Traumatic cyst
  - h. Parasitic cyst

b. Tubulo-embryonic or Tubulo-dermoid cyst:

- Develop in the tract of an ectodermal tube, e.g., thyroglossal cyst, post anal dermoid, ependymal cyst in the brain.

c. Cysts of embryonic remnants:

- Develop from embryonic tubules or ducts which normally disappear, e.g., cysts of urachus and vitellointestinal duct.

B. Acquired Cysts

a. Retention cysts:

- Develops due to retention of secretion of a gland due to obstruction of its duct, e.g., sebaceous cysts, cysts of the breast.

b. Distension cyst:

- Develops from distension of normal acini or follicles of a gland, e.g., thyroid cyst, ovarian cyst.
- Develops due to distension of lymph sacs or lymphatics, e.g., lymphatic cyst, cystic hygroma.

c. Exudation cyst:

- Develops due to exudation of fluid into an anatomical space already lined by epithelium, e.g., vaginal hydrocele.

d. Degeneration cyst:

- Develops as degeneration in the center of a malignant tumour due to hemorrhage or ischemic necrosis or colliquative necrosis, e.g., apoplectic cyst.

e. Cystic tumours:

- E.g., dermoid cyst of ovary.

f. Implantation dermoid:

- Develop when squamous epithelium of the skin is driven in by a penetrating wound, e.g., seen in finger, hand.

g. Traumatic cyst:

- Sometimes, hematoma within the muscles, fascia or subcutaneous tissue may resolve into a cyst.

h. Parasitic cyst:

- E.g., hydatid cyst.

[5] Sebaceous cyst. ***August 22***
[3] Sebaceous cyst. ***Oct 20, Dec 19, July 18***
[5] Epidermal cyst. ***June 17***
[3] Epidermoid cyst. ***Dec 14***

- Sebaceous cyst is also known as epidermal cyst, epidermoid cyst.
- **Definition:** It is a cyst containing keratin and its breakdown products, surrounded by a squamous epithelial wall.

Pathology

- The duct of the sebaceous gland mainly opens into the hair follicle and rarely may open directly on to the skin.
- If the duct or mouth of the sebaceous gland becomes blocked, the gland becomes distended with its own secretions and forms a sebaceous cyst.
- It is therefore a **retention cyst**.
- Situated in the dermis, it raises the epidermis to produce a dome shaped protuberance.
- It is tethered to the epidermis at a **black spot** which is a keratin filled **punctum** and indicates the blocked opening of the duct.

Clinical Features

- It is very **common**, affecting young and old but it is rare in childhood.
- **Common sites:** Face, neck, **scalp**, shoulders, chest, **scrotum**. These are the parts where there are plenty of sebaceous glands.
- Lesions may be solitary but are commonly multiple, e.g., scrotum.

On Examination

- Spherical in shape.
- Fixed to the skin, but mobile over the deeper structures.
- Smooth surface which may contain a blackish spot or punctum.
- Cystic consistency.
- Due to presence of sebum, there may be indentation due to pressure with a finger-tip.
- Usually not tender.
- If tender, it means that the cyst is infected.

Complications

- **Infection:**
  - o Cyst becomes enlarged and painful.
  - o Overlying skin is red.
  - o Contents of an infected cyst become semi-liquid/purulent and usually very foetid.
  - o Recurrent attacks cause the cyst wall to become adherent to surrounding subcutaneous tissue and consequently more difficult to remove.
- **Ulceration:**
  - o An infected cyst may discharge its contents.
  - o If an ulcerated surface remains, it can resemble an epithelioma which is called Cock's peculiar tumour.

- **Sebaceous horn:**
  - o Contents of a cyst sometimes escape slowly from the duct orifice and dry in successive layers on the skin, forming a sebaceous horn.
- **Calcification:**
  - o It is a rare complication.
  - o Seen in sebaceous cyst of the scrotum.
- **Malignancy:**
  - o Very rarely, a long standing sebaceous cyst may turn malignant.

Treatment

- **Surgical excision:**
  - o The cyst is excised in toto.
  - o Unless the wall is completely removed, recurrence is probable.
  - o Incomplete removal is common if attempted in the presence of recent infection.
- **Incision and drainage:**
  - o Done in the case of infected cysts.

[3] Dermoid cyst. *March 22, July 15*

- Dermoid is a loose term given to cysts lined by squamous epithelium occurring in various parts of the body.
- It lies deep to the skin and is lined by skin.
- Contains pultaceous or toothpaste like material which contains desquamated epithelial cells.

Types

A. Teratomatous Dermoid

B. Sequestration Dermoid

C. Implantation Dermoid

D. Tubulo Dermoid

A. Teratomatous Dermoid

- Develops from totipotent cells with ectodermal predominance.
- Contains bone, cartilage, tooth, hair and cheesy materials.
- Found in ovary, testis, retroperitoneum, superior mediastinum and presacral area.
- Can change into malignancy.

B. Sequestration Dermoid

- It is a congenital dermoid.
- Formed by the inclusion of **epithelial 'nests'** beneath the surface at places where lines of developing skin meet and join, i.e., **along the lines of fusion** of the two embryonic segments.
- **Common sites:**
  - o Midline of body, e.g., neck, root of nose.
  - o External angular, i.e., just above the outer canthus of the eye at the line of fusion of the frontonasal and maxillary processes.
  - o Post-auricular, i.e., at the site of fusion of mesodermal hillocks.
- Cyst may be noticed at birth, but is usually seen few years later (the time taken to form the cyst).
- Slowly growing, painless swelling.
- Cosmetic disfigurement.
- Very rarely gets infected.
- **On Examination**
  - o Smooth surface.
  - o Soft in consistency.
  - o Skin is pinchable over the swelling.
  - o There may be **bony indentation when the bone lies exactly deep to the cyst**. This can be palpated by moving the base of the cyst with a finger.
  - o When lying above cranial bones, such cysts may have intracranial connections.
- **Investigations**
  - o **X-ray/CT scan:** May show a depression in the bone underlying the cyst. A gap may be present when there is an intracranial extension or a fibrous band may pass through this bony gap and connect the cyst with the underlying dura mater.
- **Treatment**
  - o **Complete excision** under GA, as the cyst has to be dissected from the sensitive pericranium and there may also be intracranial extension.
  - o **Osteoplastic flap** is required for reconstruction after excision of intracranial part.

C. Implantation Dermoid

- Acquired dermoid.
- Arises from puncture wounds (needle prick, thorn prick) when epithelial cells are indriven and thus implanted beneath the surface of the skin.
- **Common sites:** Palms, soles, fingers.
- Tense cyst with a previous history of a punctured wound.
- Firm to hard in consistency.
- **Treatment:** Excision.

D. Tubulodermoid

- Develops from an unobliterated portion of a congenital ectodermal duct or tube.
- Cyst is formed by accumulation of secretions of the lining ectodermal cells of the unobliterated portion of an embryonic duct.
- E.g., thyroglossal cyst, post-anal dermoid, ependymal cyst in the brain.

[3] Mention transilluminant swellings in the body. ***July 18, Dec 17, June 17, Dec 16, Dec 14, Dec 13***

- Also known as translucent swellings.
- This means that the **swelling can transmit light through it**. For this it must contain clear fluid.

Method

- To carry out this test, darkness is essential.
- This can be achieved by a roll of paper, which is held on one side of the swelling, while a torch light is held on the other side of the swelling.
- The torch light should not be kept on the surface of the swelling, but on one side of the swelling, while the roll of paper should be kept on the other side, so that the whole swelling intervenes between the light and the roll of paper.
- If the torch light is seen from the other side, i.e., from the roll of paper, it means that the swelling is transilluminant.
- For a swelling to be transilluminant, it must contain clear fluid; and, the wall of the swelling should allow the transmission of light.

Examples

1. Vaginal hydrocele.
2. Encysted hydrocele of the cord.
3. A cyst of the canal of Nuck.
4. Cystic hygroma.
5. Spinal meningocele.
6. Ranula.
7. Epididymal cyst.
8. Spermatocele.
9. Cyst of an appendix of the testis.

[3] Baker's cyst. ***June 14***

- **Definition:** A Baker's cyst is simply a herniation of the synovial cavity of the knee, with the formation of a fluid filled sac extending backwards and downwards.

Pathophysiology

- It is not a primary condition but is **always secondary to a disorder of the knee with persistent synovial effusion**, such as rheumatoid arthritis or osteoarthritis.

Clinical Features

- Occurs around joints, **most commonly** in the **knee.**
- **Soft cystic bulge** near the midline behind the knee or in the upper calf.
- In long-standing cases, the hernial sac is much elongated, and may extend a considerable distance down the calf.
- Occasionally, this may rupture and the resultant pain and local, tenderness **may be mistaken for a deep vein thrombosis.**
- The underlying abnormality of the knee, with synovial effusion, will usually be obvious.

Investigations

- USG or MRI establishes the nature and extent of the lesion.

Treatment

- In most cases, treatment should be **directed towards the underlying condition of the knee** rather than to the cyst itself.
- If the cyst is extensive, it is sometimes advisable to excise it.

[5] Pott's puffy tumour. *Dec 13*

- Pott's puffy tumour is a **rare but serious complication of frontal sinusitis**.

Pathophysiology

- The **infection spreads from the frontal sinuses** to the surrounding bone and soft tissues.
- This may result in **osteomyelitis of the frontal bone**.
- This can lead to the formation of a **subperiosteal abscess**, which is a collection of pus between the bone and the periosteum.

Causative Organism

- **Most commonly:** *Staphylococcus aureus*.
- **Others:** Streptococcus species, anaerobes.

Clinical Features

- Swollen and tender forehead.
- Headache.
- Fever.
- Sometimes, there is a visible swelling or mass on the forehead (**scalp edema**).

Complications

- Infection can spread to the brain:
  - o Meningitis.
  - o Brain abscess.
- If it spreads to the eye or optic nerve, it can cause vision problems.
- Sepsis.

Investigations

- CT scan.
- MRI.
- Pus for C/S.

Treatment

- **IV antibiotics:** Ceftriaxone, clindamycin.
- Surgical drainage of abscess.

18

Ulcers

[3] Classification of ulcers. *August 22*

1. Vascular (venous, arterial, mixed).
2. Trauma (bites, self-inflicted, burns).
3. Infection (bacterial, fungal, mycobacterial, syphilis).
4. Metabolic disorders (diabetes mellitus, gout, calciphylaxis).
5. Autoimmune disorders (vasculitis, systemic sclerosis, rheumatoid arthritis).
6. Neoplastic (squamous cell carcinoma, basal cell carcinoma).

19

Burns

[10] Classify thermal burns. Management of thermal burns. *Dec 18*

Classification of Burns According to Causative Agent

A. Thermal Burns

- **Flame.**
- **Contact burns:**
  - o E.g., fall against a radiator and an inability to extract oneself.
- **Scald.**
- **Acute cold injuries:**
  - o Industrial accidents.
  - o Frostbite.
- **Ionizing radiation injury:**
  - o Localized.
  - o Whole body.

B. Electrical Burns

- **Low tension injuries.**
- **High tension injuries.**

C. Chemical Burns

- Acid.
- Alkali.

Classification of Burns According to Depth

A. Superficial Partial-Thickness Burns

- **Epidermis + papillary dermis is destroyed.**
- Underlying dermis is pink and moist and will exudate fluid for ≤ 36 hours post burn injury.
- **Clinical Features:**
  - o **Blistering** and/or loss of the epidermis.
  - o **Capillary return is clearly visible** when blanched.
  - o Little or **no fixed capillary staining.**
  - o Pin-prick sensation is normal.
  - o **Heals without residual scarring** in 2 weeks.
- **Treatment:** Supportive.

B. Deep Partial-Thickness Burn

- **Epidermis + papillary dermis + deeper parts of reticular dermis.**
- Exposed dermis is not as moist as that in a superficial burn.
- **Clinical Features:**
  - o **Abundant fixed capillary staining**, especially if examined after 48 hours.
  - o Colour **does not blanch** with pressure.
  - o **Sensation is reduced** and the patient is unable to distinguish sharp from blunt pressure when examined with a needle.
  - o Takes ≥ 3 weeks to heal without surgery and usually leads to **hypertrophic scarring.**

C. Full Thickness Burns

- **Whole of dermis** is destroyed.
- **Clinical Features:**

- o Hard, leathery feel.
- o Appearance can vary from similar to the patient's normal skin to charred black, depending upon the intensity of the heat.
- o **No capillary return.**
- o **Thrombosed vessels** can be seen under the skin.
- o **Completely anesthetic** – a needle can be stuck deep into the dermis without any pain or bleeding.

Figure 1 (See below)

Concept of Two Burn Depths

- In treatment terms, there are two burn depths:

Group A

- Superficial burns which **heal spontaneously and quickly (within 14 days)** with optimal support and good wound management
- Heal with an **excellent functional and cosmetic result.**

Group B

- Burns are **sufficiently deep** and **undergo prolonged healing by secondary intention**.
- Takes **weeks or months** to heal.
- Involves the degradation and separation of the eschar (burned tissue), the formation of granulation tissue and the process of wound contraction.
- Course of healing by secondary intention must be aborted and replaced as closely as possible by a process of primary intention healing with direct closure, skin graft and skin substitutes.

[10] Discuss in detail the clinical features and management of burns. ***Dec 15***
[5] Fluid replacement in burns. ***July 23***
[3] Fluid replacement in burns. ***Dec 16***
[3] Parkland formula for burns. ***CBME March 24***

- **Definition:** A burn may be defined as dissolution in tissue continuity consequent to thermal damage.

Mechanism of Burns

- **Children:** Scalds caused by accidents with kettles, pans, hot drinks and bath water.
- **Adolescents:** Experiments with matches and flammable liquids.
- **Adults:** Flame burns.
- Scald burns and contact burns become more common with age.
- Electrical and chemical injuries occur in adults and are frequently associated with occupation.

Pathophysiology

- Burns cause a multisystem injury.
- Most common organ affected is the skin.

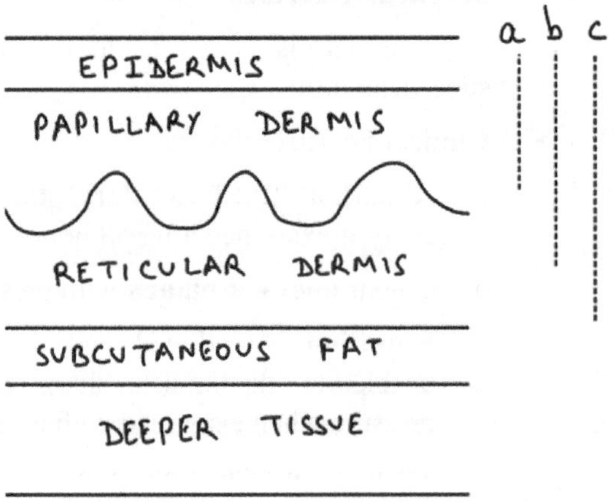

a - superficial partial thickness burn : epidermis + papillary dermis

b - deep partial thickness burn : epidermis + papillary dermis + deeper parts of reticular dermis

c - full thickness burn : whole of dermis

Figure 1: Depth of burns

A. Injury to Airway and Lungs

- Inhalation injury of hot, smoke-filled air has **3 components**, each of which can present alone or in any combination:
  1. Upper airway injury.
  2. Lower airway injury (true smoke inhalation).
  3. Metabolic poisoning.
- **Warning signs of burns to the respiratory system:**
  - o Burns around the face and neck.
  - o Blistering inside the mouth.
  - o History of being trapped in an enclosed space.
  - o Change of voice/hoarseness.
  - o Stridor.
  - o Singeing of facial and nasal hair.
- **Inhaled hot gases** cause **supraglottic airway burns and laryngeal edema.**
- **Inhaled steam** causes **subglottic burns and loss of respiratory epithelium.**
- **Inhaled smoke particles** cause **chemical pneumonitis and respiratory failure.**

B. Metabolic Poisoining

- **Carbon monoxide:**
  - o It is the most common immediate cause of death from fire.
  - o Produced by incomplete combustion of carbonaceous materials.
  - o CO + Hb ---> carboxy-hemoglobin (CO.Hb).
  - o Carboxyhemoglobin has the following effects:
    - ♦ Impairs O_2 delivery at tissue level.
    - ♦ Disrupts aerobic metabolism.
    - ♦ Decreases the capacity for cellular respiration.
  - o **Treatment:** High flow, high concentration oxygen.
- **Cyanide:**
  - o Produced by burning of nitrogen containing polymers.
  - o Inhibits electron transport chain and cellular respiration.

C. Mechanical Block on Rib Movement

- **Burns which extend across the chest** can physically stop rib expansion and compromise respiratory function, because:
  - o Full-thickness burned skin loses its elasticity and becomes stiff and leathery.
  - o Subcutaneous edema.

D. Circulatory Changes

Burns produce an inflammatory reaction.

↓

Vascular permeability increases→water, solutes and proteins move from intra to extravascular space.

- Volume of fluid lost is directly proportional to the area of the burn.
- **>15% burns:** Loss of fluid produces shock which requires resuscitation.

E. Immune System and Infection

- **Cell-mediated immunity decreases**, making the patient susceptible to bacterial and fungal infections.
- **Source of infection:** Burn wound, lungs (if injured), central lines, tracheostomies, urinary catheter.

F. Intestine

Inflammatory stimulus and shock.

↓

Microvascular damage.

↓

Ischemia of gut mucosa.

↓

Reduced gut motility.
1. Absorption of food decreases.
2. Translocation of gut bacteria increases.

- Gut mucosal swelling + gastric stasis + peritoneal edema causes abdominal compartment syndrome.
- This splints the diaphragm and increases the airway pressures needed for respiration.

G. Peripheral Circulation

- **Circumferential full-thickness burn** to a limb acts as a **tourniquet** which can cause **limb-threatening ischemia.**

Treatment

- Treatment of burns has the following components:
  1. **Fluid resuscitation.**
  2. **Treating the burn wound.**
  3. **Surgical treatment:**
     - o Escharotomy.
     - o Burn excision surgery/debridement:
       - ♦ Early excision.
       - ♦ Staged full thickness excision.
  4. **Additional aspects:**
     - o Analgesia.
     - o Energy balance and nutrition.
     - o Monitoring and control of infection.
     - o Nursing care.
     - o Physiotherapy and occupational therapy.
     - o Psychological care.
     - o Delayed reconstruction and scar management.

FLUID RESUSCITATION

- This **begins from the time of burn injury** and any delay in commencement must be caught up.
- **Indications of IV fluid resuscitation:**
  - o 15% TBSA in adults.
  - o 10% TBSA in children.

    (TBSA = Total Body Surface Area)
- **Extremes of age:**
  - o Children – Additional maintenance fluid is required.
  - o Elderly – Judicious monitoring is necessary because of concurrent comorbidities and the inherent physiology of ageing.
- Oral resuscitation is with **additional salt solutions** (e.g., dioralyte). This is required as **hyponatremia and water intoxication can be fatal**.
- **Fluid loss is maximum in the first 8 hours and slows by 24-36 hours,** by which stage normal fluid replacement is required.
- There are **3 main types of fluid** used in resuscitation:
  1. Crystalloids (most common).
  2. Colloids.
  3. Hypertonic saline.

A. Crystalloids

- Most commonly used crystalloid is **Hartmann's solution or Ringer's Lactate.**
- **Advantages:**
  - o Most closely replicates the osmolality of plasma.
  - o Cheaper than colloids.
  - o Can maintain intravascular volume.
- Administered by **modified Parkland formula**:

% burns of TBSA × weight in kgs × 4=volume in ml.

  - o This calculated volume is given over 24 hours. The first half is given in 8 hours and the second half over 16 hours.
- **In children, maintenance fluid** must also be given (over 24 hours). DNS is given as follows:
  - o 100 ml/kg for the 1st 10 kgs.
  - o 50 ml/kg for the next 10 kgs.
  - o 20 ml/kg for each kg over 20 kg body weight.

B. Colloids

- Most commonly used colloid is **human albumin** solution.
- Should be preferably **administered after the first 12 hours post-burns,** as the massive shift in fluids drives proteins out of the cells.
- Most common colloid based formula is the **Muir and Barclay formula,** which estimates the amount of fluid that needs to be infused during the first 36 hours post burn.
- The basic formula is:

% burns of TBSA × weight in kgs × 0.5 = one portion.

- **6 portions are given in total over 36 hours:**
  - o Give 1 portion every 4 hourly for 12 hours (3 portions in total).
  - o Then 1 portion every 6 hourly for 12 hours (2 portions in total).
  - o Then 1 portion over 12 hours (1 portion in total).
- **Disadvantages:**
  - o Albumin is expensive.
  - o Excessive use of albumin causes additional pressure on the renal system.

C. Hypertonic Saline

- Used in some centres.
- **Mechanism:** Produces hyperosmolality and hypernatremia which results in a reduction in the shift of intracellular water to the extracellular space.
- **Advantages:**
  - o Less tissue edema.
  - o Decreases in escharotomies and intubations.
- **Drawbacks:**
  - o Prolonged hypernatremia.

Monitoring of Resuscitation

- The key to monitoring of fluid resuscitation is urine output.
- Urine output should be between 0.5 and 1.0 ml/kg body weight/hour.
- If the urine output is > 2 ml/kg body weight/hour, fluid infusion should be decreased.
- If the urine output drops and the patient shows signs of hypoperfusion (tachycardia, cool peripheries and a high lactate or metabolic acidosis), then a bolus of 10 ml/kg body weight should be given.

TREATMENT OF THE BURN WOUND

A. Group A Burns – Superficial Dermal Partial Thickness Burns

- **There are 2 key concepts:**
  1. Prevent any factor that may result in the burn 'changing group,' predominantly infection, i.e., to prevent the borderline mid-dermal burns from progressing to deep dermal.
  2. Control pain, particularly during dressing changes and therapy.
- Clean the wound under GA.
- **Dressing options:**
  - o Silver sulphadiazine cream dressing.
  - o Permeable wound dressing (e.g., Mefix or Fixomull).
  - o Vaseline impregnated gauze (with or without an antiseptic such as chlorhexidine).
  - o Fenestrated silicone sheet (e.g., Mepitel).
  - o Acticoat dressings with silver nanocrystals provide antibacterial cover.
  - o Interactive dressings such as hydrocolloids and biological dressings.
- An ideal dressing should be easy to apply, non-painful, pain reducing, simple to manage and locally available.
- The simplest method of treating a superficial burn wound is by exposure, but this is usually only suitable for small burns on the face as this method is painful and requires an intensive amount of nursing support.

B. Group B Burns – Full Thickness and Deep Dermal Burns

- Management of burn wound remains the same, irrespective of the size of the injury.
- Burn needs to be cleaned and the size and depth need to be assessed.
- Escharotomy may be required.
- All but the very smallest of full-thickness burns are likely to involve excision.

SURGICAL TREATMENT

A. Escharotomy

- **Indications:**
  - o Circumferential full thickness burns to the limbs and torso.
- These burns have a tourniquet like effect which compromise respiration (torso) and peripheral circulation (limbs).
- Tourniquet effect of this injury is treated by incising the whole length of full thickness burns:
  - o **Chest:** Two longitudinal and two horizontal incisions are made which bring about an immediate improvement of respiration and, if intubated, the ventilation pressures.
  - o **Limbs:** Performed in the mid-axial line, avoiding major nerves.

B. Burn Excision Surgery/Debridement

- All burns except the smallest full-thickness burns need surgery.
- All burnt tissue needs to be excised.
- Surgeon needs to prepare for significant blood loss.

- Tumescence fluid and topical adrenaline reduces bleeding.
- Burn excision surgery can be done in 2 different ways:
  1. Early excision.
  2. Staged full-thickness excision.

EARLY EXCISION	STAGED FULL-THICKNESS EXCISION
Excision is done: On arrival at burns unit or as soon as logistically possible.	Serial debridement of the burn over several operating sessions in the first week of the burn.
Advantages: • To exploit the window before the overwhelming systemic response to the burn sets in. 3 windows are considered: Anesthetic, hemodynamic and bacterial window. • Excising a full thickness burn early, prior to the anesthetic and hemodynamic window results in less blood loss. • Removing the eschar results in less edema and lower fluid requirements. • Excising a full-thickness burn (which is essentially necrotic material), reduces bacterial load, thereby reducing risk of infection.	**Advantages:** • Shorter operating times. • Decreased requirement for blood transfusion.
Drawbacks: • It is dependent on the appropriate staff, resources, equipment and time which are not always available.	**Drawbacks:** • Relies on managing the remaining burn eschar until excision to prevent bacterial colonization and to prepare for surgery. This is achieved by using silver based dressing/creams containing anti-bacterial properties including against *Pseudomonas aeruginosa* and MRSA.

- The various dressings and creams used in staged full-thickness excision are:
  - o **Silver sulphadiazine cream 1%:**
    - ♦ Gives broad spectrum prophylaxis.
  - o **Mafenide acetate cream:**
    - ♦ Painful to apply.
    - ♦ Associated with metabolic acidosis.
  - o **Silver sulphadiazine and cerium nitrate:**
    - ♦ Induces a sterile eschar.
    - ♦ Boosts cell-mediated immunity.
  - o **Acticoat:**
    - ♦ Nanocrystalline silver barrier.
    - ♦ Broad spectrum action.
- The keystone of burns surgery is control, regardless of whether early or staged excision is the plan.
- Full-thickness burns require full-thickness excision of skin.
- In certain circumstances, we can excise down till the fascia, but, in most cases burn excision is done upto viable fat.
- Deep dermal burns need tangential shaving.
- Wherever possible, a split skin graft or a dermal substitute should be applied immediately.
- Graft application results in primary intention healing.
- Post-op management of these patients requires careful evaluation of fluid balance and levels of hemoglobin.
- Outer dressings will require attention and regular changing because of expected fluid leaks.
- Physiotherapy and splints maintain the range of movement and reduces chances of joint contracture.

Use of Skin Grafts and Skin Substitutes

- A number of methods are utilized to facilitate wound coverage by grafting:
  - o Serial episodes of grafting surgery.
  - o **Harvesting very thin autografts:**
    - ♦ Allows more rapid re-epithelialisation of donor sites.
    - ♦ Facilitates earlier re-harvest.
    - ♦ Allows a greater number of harvests from the same donor site.
  - o Widely meshing the grafts.
  - o **Meek wall technique:**
    - ♦ Minimizes graft wastage as even small pieces of graft can be meshed in this way.
  - o Cadaver skin.
  - o Dermal matrix strategy.

Additional Aspects

A. Analgesia

- **Acute:**
  - o **Small burns,** especially superficial burns: Simple oral analgesia, paracetamol, NSAIDs, topical cooling.
  - o **Large burns:** IV opiates.
  - o IM administration should be avoided as uptake is variable.
- **Subacute:**
  - o In patients with large burns, continuous analgesia is required, beginning with infusions and continuing with oral tablets.
  - o Powerful, short-acting analgesia should be administered before dressing changes.
  - o Dressing changes may be done under GA, midazolam, ketamine, morphine, nitrous oxide.

B. Energy Balance and Nutrition

- Children with > 10% and adults with > 15% burns have an increased nutritional requirement.
- Patients with > 20% burns require nasogastric or nasojejunal tube feeding which should start within 6 hours of injury to reduce gut mucosal damage.
- Burn injuries are catabolic in the acute episode. Therefore, excess energy requirements must be provided for and the nutritional balance monitored by measuring weight and nitrogen balance.

C. Monitoring and Control of Infection

- Burn patients are immunosuppressed.
- Infection can occur via the burn wound.
- There is compromised local defences in the lungs and gut owing to edema.
- Monitoring lines and catheters are portals of infection.
- **Infection control is achieved by:**
  - o Handwashing.
  - o Preventing cross contamination between patients.
  - o C/S from the wound, catheter tips and sputum.
  - o Empirical broad spectrum antibiotics or as guided by C/S.

D. Good Nursing Care.

E. Physiotherapy and Occupational Therapy.

F. Psychological Care.

G. Delayed Reconstruction and Scar Management.

[5] 30-year-old female suffered 60% burns due to gas cylinder explosion. Write about fluid and wound management of this patient. ***CBME June 24***

- An average healthy adult (both male and female) is considered to weigh 70 kg.
- Fluids are administered by **modified Parkland formula:**

% burns of TBSA × weight in kgs × 4 = volume in ml.

- 60% × 70 kg × 4 = 16,800 ml.
- This calculated volume is given over 24 hours.
- The first half, i.e., 8400 ml is given over 8 hours and the second half, i.e., 8400 ml over 16 hours.

[3] Rule of nine. ***Sept 21, June 19, Dec 12***

[5] Rule of nine. ***June 17***

ASSESSMENT OF SIZE OF BURN WOUND

A. Wallace rule of nines

- Each body area has a percentage depending on its size:
  - o Each upper limb – 9%.
  - o Each lower limb – 18%.
  - o Head and neck – 9%.
  - o Posterior torso and buttocks – 18%.
  - o Anterior torso – 18%
    (Chest and abdomen are 9% each).
  - o Genitalia – 1%.
- **Advantages:** It is quick and reliable.
- **Drawbacks:**
  - o It overestimates burn size.
  - o In the obese patient, the proportion of surface area of the arms and head decreases as the surface area of the torso and legs increase.
  - o Not suitable for children < 10 years.

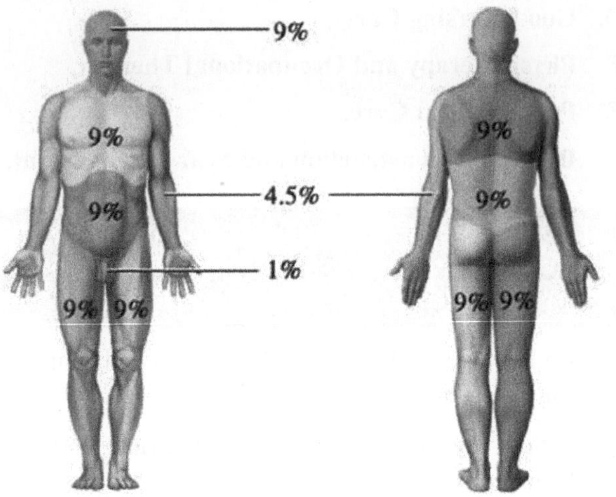

Figure 2: Rule of nines

B. Patient's Hand

- Distal wrist crease to fingertips of an adult patient's hand is approximately 1% of total body surface area (TBSA).
- Useful for small burns up to 10% TBSA.

C. Lund and Browder Chart

- Useful in larger burns.
- Compared to Wallace rule of nines, it further subdivides body areas and allows for differentiation of burn depth by shading.
- Can be completed at multiple points during a burn admission to document changes in burn size/ depth.

[3] Acid burns. ***July 15***

CHEMICAL INJURIES

Cause

- There are over 70,000 different chemicals in regular use within industry. Occasionally, these cause burns.
- Acid burns and alkali burns are more common.
- Burns affecting the fingers and caused by dilute acids are relatively common.

Pathogenesis

- There are 2 aspects to a chemical injury:
  1. Physical destruction of the skin (corrosion).
  2. Poisoning caused by systemic absorption.
- Acids cause coagulative necrosis.
- Alkalis cause liquefactive necrosis.
- Alkalis are more destructive and are especially dangerous if they have come into contact with the eyes.
- Acids chelate calcium and magnesium in tissues.

Management

- **Initial management:**
  - Ascertain whether the agent that caused burns is in a solid powder state or liquid state.
  - To assess the possibility of systemic damage, including threat to life.
- **If you are sure it is a solid powder:**
  - Remove with forceps.
  - Water irrigation should not be used as this will result in further reaction.
  - E.g., phosphorus (present in military devices), sodium (responsible for lab explosions).
- If agent is unknown, give copious lavage. After that, identify the chemical and its concentration.
- **Treatment of dilute acid burns (e.g., hydrofluoric acid):**
  - Apply calcium gluconate gel topically.
  - Severe burns or burns to large areas of hand: Bier's blocks containing calcium gluconate 10% gel.
- If concentration of acid is > 50%, it is an indication for acute early excision. This is because hypocalcemia can cause subsequent arrhythmias.
- SSG of acid burns should be done at a delayed stage.

[3] Electrical burns. ***July 23***

- These are divided into low and high voltage injuries, the threshold being 1000 V.

A. Low Voltage Injuries (< 1000 V)

- Caused by domestic appliances.
- It is not enough to cause significant damage to subcutaneous tissues.
- Contact point (fingers) suffers small deep burns.
- Underlying tendon and nerve damage is seen.
- There is a tetany within the muscles.

- The main danger is from the current interfering with the pacemaker activity of the heart, which can cause cardiac arrest.
- No significant underlying myocardial damage.
- Resuscitation, if successful, should be lasting.

B. High Voltage Injuries (> 1000 V)

- Can be caused by 3 sources of damage: The flash, the flame and the current itself:
  1. As current travels through the air, the air is heated and expands in an explosive manner, which can propel the victim. This is called the flash. It is the contact of superheated air with the skin for a short duration.
  2. The flash can ignite the patient's clothes and so cause a normal flame burn.
  3. **The current:**
     - o Not only are the entry and exit points damaged, but the subcutaneous tissue in between these points is also damaged.
     - o Muscle damage can cause the rapid onset of compartment syndrome, with myoglobinuria and subsequent renal dysfunction.
     - o Severe acidosis is common.
     - o Risk of myocardial damage as a result of direct muscle damage, rather than by interference with cardiac pacing. This gives rise to significant ECG changes, with raised cardiac enzymes. If there is significant damage, there is rapid onset of heart failure.

Treatment

- Maintain a high urine output of up to 2 ml/kg body weight/hour.
- IV fluids.
- IV bicarbonate.
- Fasciotomy.
- Amputation is done if limb injury is severe.

20

Plastic Surgery

[5]	Skin grafts. ***March 24***
[3]	Types of skin graft and its indications. ***June 17***

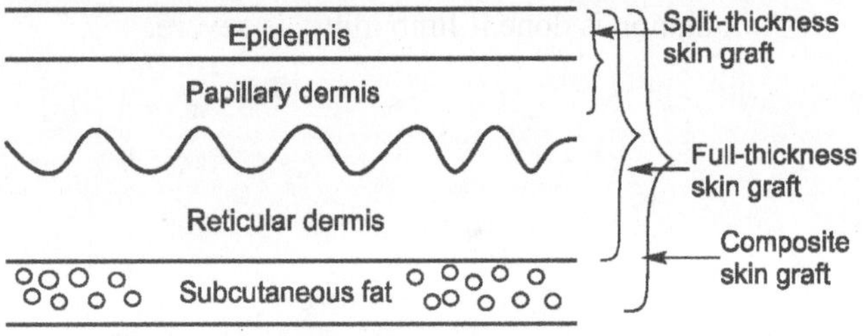

Figure: Types of graft

- Grafts are tissues that are **transferred without their blood supply** and therefore need to be revascularized through the recipient bed.
- Depending on the depth at which they are taken, skin grafts are of the following types:
  1. **Split thickness skin grafts:**
     - o Also known as Thiersch grafts.
     - o Consist of the **epidermis and a variable amount of dermis.**
     - o It is relatively simple to harvest.
     - o **Donor area usually heals by secondary intention within 2 weeks.**
  2. **Full Thickness Skin Grafts:**
     - o Also known as Wolfe graft.
     - o Consist of **epidermis and the entire thickness of dermis.**
     - o As they include the entire thickness of the dermis, they retain their elasticity and are **less prone to secondary scar contracture.**
     - o The **donor site needs to be closed by primary suturing**, which limits the size of the graft.
  3. **Composite Skin Grafts:**
     - o Combination of **skin and another tissue type**, such as fat or cartilage.
     - o **Examples:**
       - ♦ A skin/cartilage graft from the helical root of the ear to reconstruct the ala of the nose following skin cancer excision.
       - ♦ A hair-bearing composite scalp graft can be used to reconstruct an eyebrow.

[3]	Split Skin Grafting. ***Oct 20, July 23***
[3]	Thiersch Graft. ***Dec 19***

- Also known as Thiersch's grafts.
- It is an example of **delayed primary or tertiary** wound healing.
- **Definition:** A split thickness skin graft **consists of epidermis and a variable amount of dermis, that is transferred without its blood supply.**

Principle

- A split skin graft works on the principle that **skin is the best dressing.**
- Therefore, when conditions are favourable, an SSG is done to cover the recipient site.

- This ensures **quicker healing, is less morbid and is less tedious.**

Method of Harvesting SSG

- They are harvested using:
  1. Dermatome.
  2. Graft knife (Humby's knife).
- This gives it a consistent depth.
- Grafted skin can then be meshed or fenestrated to expand and cover a wider surface area.
- Graft is typically sutured, glued or stapled to the recipient site.
- Donor area usually heals by secondary intention within 2 weeks by means of simple dressing.

Anatomy of SSG

- SSG are harvested by taking all of the epidermis together with some dermis, leaving the remaining dermis behind to heal the donor site.
- The thicker the dermis that is taken:
  - o The more durable will be the graft once healed.
  - o The more difficult will be donor site healing.
- SSG inevitably contracts.

Nutrition of a SSG

- **For the 1st 48 hours:**
  - o Imbibition of plasma from the wound bed.
- **After 48 hours:**
  - o **Inosculation**, i.e., fine anastomotic connections between the blood vessels of graft and recipient bed.
- **Capillary in-growth** then completes the healing process with fibroblast maturation.

Donor Site

- Most commonly used donor site is thigh.
- The buttock is preferred in children and cosmetically sensitive individuals.
- For larger grafts, almost **any flat surface can be harvested**, including the scalp (if shaved).

Recipient Site

- Should contain clean and healthy granulation tissue.

Uses/Indications

- To **achieve wound closure in situations where the skin defects are too large** for primary closure and healing by secondary intention may be inappropriate or lead to an unreasonable delay in complete healing.
- To **reconstruct sizeable defects** such as those following a significant burn injury.
- To cover all sizes of wound.
- To provide valuable **temporary wound closure** before better cosmetic secondary correction after rehabilitation.

Contraindications

- It is contraindicated to use an SSG to cover **exposed tendons, cartilage or cortical bone.**
- Presence of **Group A beta hemolytic streptococci** in the recipient bed is a contraindication as it can destroy the SSG completely.
- SSG should not be placed where shearing forces act (e.g., **across a joint**). This is because shear forces disrupt the graft from the wound bed and can result in graft failure.
- Presence of pus, exudate, hematoma or residual dead tissue beneath the skin graft result in its failure.

OTHER IMPORTANT TOPICS

FULL THICKNESS SKIN GRAFTS

- Also known as Wolfe graft.
- **Definition:** A full thickness skin graft consists of **epidermis and the entire dermis**.

Advantages

- As it includes the entire thickness of the dermis, they **retain their elasticity.**
- It is **less prone to secondary contracture.**
- Older people can sustain larger harvests because of skin laxity.

Disadvantages

- The area harvested is limited as the **donor site needs to be closed primarily.**

Donor Sites

- A full thickness skin graft is usually harvested from sites which have adequate skin laxity as it enables easy direct closure of donor site:
  - o Supraclavicular skin.
  - o Groin crease.
  - o Posterior auricular region.

Uses

- A full thickness skin graft is **used for smaller areas of skin replacement** where good elastic skin that will not contract is required:
  - o **Syndactyly release** in the hand.
  - o **Reconstruction of facial defects** following skin cancer excision.
  - o **Contracture release** following burns.

COMPOSITE SKIN GRAFTS

- **Definition:** Composite skin grafts are a **combination of skin and another tissue type**, such as fat or cartilage.

Indications/Uses

- To harvest a skin/cartilage graft from the helical root of the ear to **reconstruct the ala of the nose** following skin cancer excision.
- A hair-bearing composite scalp graft can be used to **reconstruct an eyebrow.**

21

Hand

[5] Principles of treatment of hand infection. *July 18*

- The five principles in the treatment of infections of the hand can be summarized as follows:

1. **Provision of rest and elevation of the limb**
   - **Metacarpophalangeal joints are flexed to nearly 90°** and the interphalangeal joints are in a few degrees of flexion with the **wrist slightly dorsiflexed** and the thumb abducted.
   - This position can be maintained by a padded, **moulded plaster slab.**
   - In addition, the **forearm is supported in a sling** as high as possible towards the opposite shoulder in order to lessen oedema.
   - For in patients, **hand should be suspended from a drip stand** to provide full elevation.
2. **Early recognition of the presence of pus and its accurate localization**
   - This will follow if the swollen **hand is rested in elevation** and antibiotics are administered.
   - If given early, the **antibiotics** may cause complete resolution.
3. **Evacuation of pus and, in the case of fascial spaces, debridement of the walls of the abscess cavity**
   - Once the hand has changed from a 'whale flipper' to a more normal appearance, careful examination will indicate the site(s) for **exploration and evacuation of pus.**
4. **Antibiotic therapy**
   - Antibiotics will produce a response only if **given within 24-48 hours** of the onset of an infection.
   - Give high dose **intravenous** antibiotics.
   - After this time, because of the closed spaces and compartments in the hand, early and rapid sealing off of the infection takes place, which reduces the effectiveness of antibiotic action.
5. **Adequate after treatment**
   - Once the infection has settled and is quiescent, **active mobilization** of the stiff fingers and wrist must be started and actively pursued in order **to regain optimum function.**

[3] Pulp space infection. *June 13*

[3] Felon. *Dec 13, June 13*

- Also known as **terminal pulp space infection, whitlow.**
- Pulp space infection is the **2nd most common infection of the hand (after paronychia).**
- **Definition:** A felon is a **subcutaneous abscess of the fingertip** (terminal pulp space).

Aetiopathogenesis

- It is **most commonly caused by penetrating trauma** (e.g., a prick).
- **Staphylococcus aureus** is the most common pathogen.

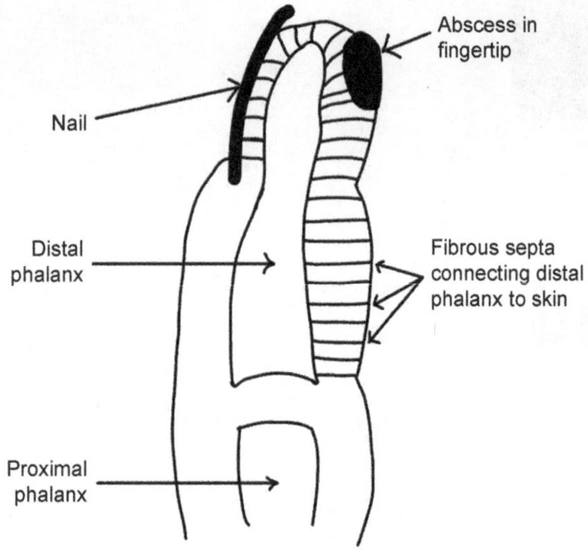

Figure 1: Felon aetiopathogenesis

- The fingertip contains multiple fibrous septa which connect the distal phalanx to the skin.
- These septa are poorly compliant, and presence of an abscess will increase pressure and may lead to tissue death.
- The **index finger and thumb** are most commonly affected.

Clinical Features

- **Dull pain**, which is worse when the hand is dependent, and **swelling** are the first symptoms.
- Severe **nocturnal exacerbations** of throbbing pain, which interfere with sleep.
- Light pressure over the affected pulp increases the pain.
- Regional **lymph nodes are enlarged** and tender.
- If the pulp is indurated and has lost its normal resilience, **pus** is present.
- Untreated, the abscess tends to point towards the centre of the pulp beneath a patch of devitalized skin.
- A **collar stud abscess** then occurs; if still untreated, the abscess bursts.
- Neglected cases suffer serious **loss of pulp tissue** leading to a markedly **scarred fingertip.**

Treatment

- **Oral antibiotics** (amoxicillin-clavulanic acid) may resolve the infection, if diagnosed very early.
- **Incision and drainage** is indicated when fluctuance is identified.
  - o Longitudinal incision over the point of maximal fluctuance.
  - o Transverse and lateral incisions should be avoided.
  - o Incision should never extend across the distal phalangeal joint crease.
  - o Deep incision should not be performed as this may cause seeding of bacteria into the flexor tendon sheath.

[3] Paronychia. ***Dec 19***

[3] Discuss clinical features and management of acute paronychia. ***CBME June 24***

- It is the **most common infection of the hand.**

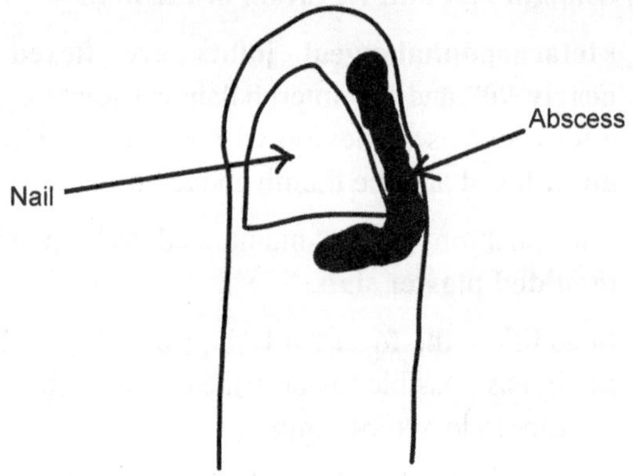

Figure 2: Acute paronychia

Causes

- **Hangnail** (a piece of torn skin at the root of a fingernail).
- **Careless nail paring.**
- **Unsterile manicure instrument.**

Pathogenesis

- Infection is **subcuticular and under the eponychium.**
- Suppuration usually follows.

- Pus is **confined** by the adherence of the eponychium to the base of the nail.
- Pus tends to **track around the cutaneous margin** and also, **under the nail.**

Clinical Features

- Diagnosis is obvious on inspection.
- **Redness and swelling** of the nail fold.
- Excruciatingly **painful.**
- Pus can sometimes be seen beneath the nail.

Treatment

- **Antibiotics** given early may resolve the infection (amoxicillin-clavulanic acid).
- If **pus** has formed, it **must be let out:**
  - o Only the **eponychium is stripped gently** and completely **away from the base of the nail.**
  - o All pus is wiped away.
  - o **Loose cuticle is cut** away.
  - o If there is any pus pocket under the corner of the nail fold, a **wedge of overlying skin is removed** to ensure healing from the bottom.
  - o The **loose and ragged eponychium is then excised.**
- When pus has extended beneath the nail, the undermined portion must be excised.
- **Floating nail is dead nail, all unattached nail must be excised.**

[3] Ganglion. *June 19, Dec 13, March 24*

- Also known as Ganglion Cysts.

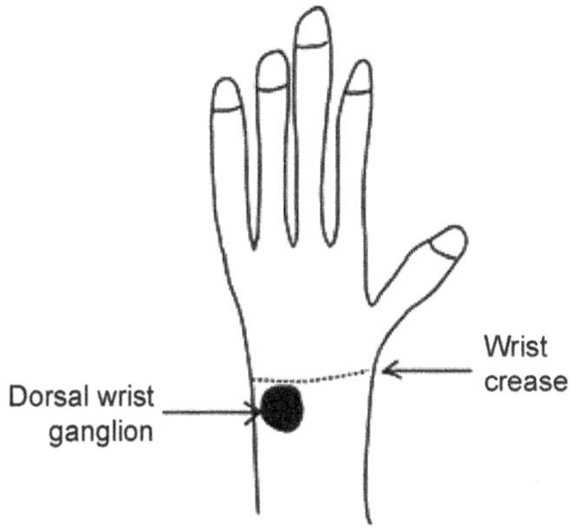

Figure 3: Ganglion

- **Definition:** It is a **localized, tense cystic swelling in connection with the joint capsule or tendon sheath.**

Aetiopathogenesis

- It is formed by an **outpouching of the synovial membrane from a joint or tendon sheath.**
- **Contains thick, jelly-like, mucinous material** similar in composition to synovial fluid.
- Occurs **most commonly on the dorsal aspect of the wrist**, arising in the region of the scapholunate ligament.
- **2nd most common site:** Volar wrist, arising from one of the scaphoid articulations.
- **Other sites:** Flexor tendon sheath, dorsum of distal interphalangeal joint.

Clinical Features

- Most common in women in the third decade of life.
- A **painless lump** is the most common presentation.
- Dorsal wrist ganglion **can sometimes be painful** as a result of pressure on the posterior interosseous nerve at that location.

Investigations

- MRI.

Treatment

- Ganglions are innocuous and can often be **left alone.**
- Treatment may be required for **cosmetic purposes** or to relieve **pressure effects** on adjacent structures.
- The following methods:
  1. A strike on the ganglion will cause rupture of the cyst with apparent relief/cure (historically done with Bible).
  2. **Aspiration** of the cyst and **injection of sclerosant** (3% sodium morrhuate or 5% phenol in almond oil).
  3. **Aspiration** of the cyst and **injection of hydrocortisone.**
  4. Surgical **excision** of ganglion.

[3] Compound palmar ganglion. *August 22*

- **Definition: Chronic inflammation sometimes distends the common sheath of the flexor tendons**

in front of the wrist both above and below the flexor retinaculum. This is known as compound ganglion.

Pathology

- **Common Causes:**
  1. Tuberculosis.
  2. Rheumatoid arthritis.
- **Ulnar bursa** which covers the flexor tendons of the fingers are usually affected.
- It is so named, because **there are 2 swellings: One above the flexor retinaculum and the other below it, almost in the hollow of the palm.**
- **Synovial membrane** is involved which **becomes thick and villous.**
- Amount of fluid is increased and it may contain fibrin particles in the shape of **melon seeds.**
- Lining membrane contains granulation tissue.
- Tendons eventually become frayed and may rupture.

Clinical Features

- Almost all patients are <40 years of age.
- Usually painless.
- There may be **paresthesia due to median nerve compression.**
- Swelling is shaped like an **hour-glass.**
- **Cross fluctuation test is positive.**
- There may be **wasting of muscles** of hand and fingers.
- **Cold abscess** may occasionally result.

Treatment

A. If the condition is tuberculous

- Anti-tubercular treatment is started.
- **Splinting** of the wrist.
- **Aspiration** of ganglion contents **and installation of streptomycin.**
- If there is no improvement, the entire flexor sheath is dissected out with excision of all the diseased synovial membrane.

B. If the condition is rheumatoid disease

- Complete excision of the affected synovial sheath and ulnar bursa keeping the flexor tendons intact.

22

Cleft Lip and Palate

[5] Cleft lip. *Dec 15, July 23*

- **Cleft lip and/or palate is the most common congenital abnormality affecting the orofacial region.**
- These conditions most commonly occur as isolated deformities but can also be **associated with other medical conditions, e.g., congenital heart disease.**

Incidence

- Cleft lip + palate > isolated cleft palate > isolated cleft lip.

Aetiology

- **Family history** in which a first degree relative is affected.
- **Genetic mutations.**
- Over **150 named syndromes** are associated: Stickler, DiGeorge, Down, Apert and Treacher Collins.
- **Environmental factors:**
  - o **Maternal epilepsy** and associated medications.
  - o **Drugs:** Steroids, diazepam, sodium valproate, phenytoin.
- **Pierre Robin sequence.**
- Most cases occur without a clear family history or known risk factors.

Embryology and Pathogenesis

- Clefts **occur at the points of fusion of facial processes.**
- **Normal anatomical structures are displaced and disrupted.**
- **Abnormal muscle insertion** results in aesthetic and functional sequelae.
- The **nasolabial, bilabial and labiomental muscle chains are disrupted.**

Clinical Features

A. Unilateral Cleft Lip

- The **muscle rings are disrupted** on one side, resulting in an **asymmetric upper lip and/or nose.**
- It **involves the external nasal cartilages, nasal septum and anterior maxilla (premaxilla).** This in turn influences the mucocutaneous tissues:
  - o Displacement of nasal skin onto the lip.
  - o Retraction of labial skin.
  - o Changes to the vermilion and lip mucosa.

B. Bilateral Cleft Lip

- The **disruption is greater, but often symmetrical.**
- Muscular continuity is disrupted bilaterally.
  - o **Flaring of the nose** (caused by a lack of nasolabial muscle continuity).

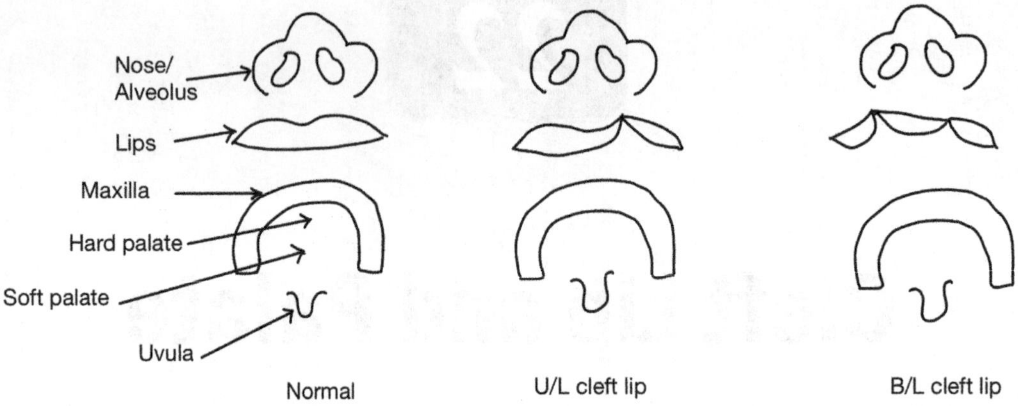

Figure 1: Unilateral and bilateral cleft lip

  - o A **protrusive premaxilla.**
  - o An area of skin in front of the premaxilla devoid of muscle, known as the **prolabium.**
- Defective dentition.

C. Airway

- Major **respiratory obstruction** is uncommon and occurs exclusively **in babies with Pierre Robbin sequence.**
- **Hypoxic episodes** during sleeping and feeding can be life threatening.
- **Intermittent airway obstruction** is more frequent.

Investigations

- An **antenatal diagnosis** of cleft lip (unilateral or bilateral) is possible by maternal **USG after 18 weeks of gestation.**

Treatment

A. Primary Management

a. Antenatal Diagnosis.

b. Feeding:

- Some mothers are successful in breastfeeding, particularly when the cleft is incomplete and confined to the lip.
- Good feeding patterns can be established with:
  - o Soft bottles (e.g., Mead Johnson).
  - o Modified teats (orthodontic, Nuyk).
  - o Enlarging the hole in the teat.
- Babies are provided with an active plate that aims not only to improve feeding but also to reduce the width of the cleft and improve the shape of the nose prior to surgery, called **nasoalveolar moulding (NAM).**

c. Airway:

- Intermittent airway obstruction is managed by **nursing the baby prone.**
- More severe and persistent airway compromise can be managed by **'retained nasopharyngeal intubation'** to maintain the airway.
  - o Surgical adhesion of tongue to lower lip (**labioglossopexy**) in the first few days after birth is an alternative, but is less commonly performed.
  - o Early mandibular surgery – **distraction osteogenesis**, is indicated in some cases and avoids the need for a tracheostomy.

B. Surgery

- **Principles of Cleft Surgery:**
  - o To **facilitate normal development** and well-being.

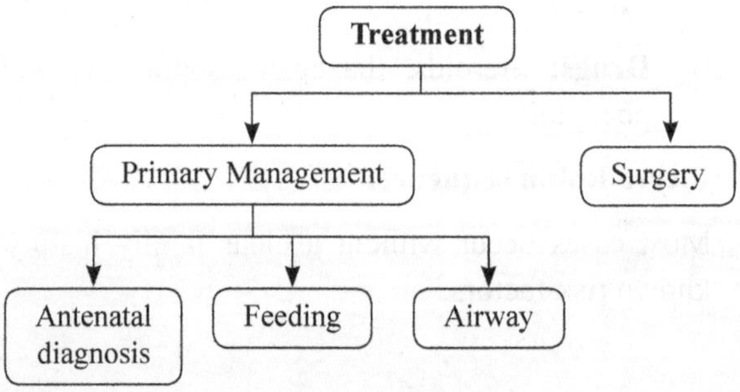

- o **Muscular reconstruction** of the lip, nose, face and soft palate to produce normal anatomy.
- o Normal or near-normal anatomy promotes normal function, thereby encouraging normal growth and development.

- **Timing of repair: between 3 and 6 months of age.**
- There are many techniques for repair of a cleft lip, but most are a variation of the **rotation-advancement repair, e.g., Millard's technique, Mirault-Blair operation.**
- **Muscle repair is more important than the skin incision.**
- **Millard's Technique:**
  - o Downward rotation of the medial portion of the lip and advancement of the lateral portion into the defect created by the rotation.
  - o The repair is based on the principle that existing elements need to be returned to their normal position to restore the normal anatomy while remaining cognizant of future growth and the effects of surgery on growth.
- **Secondary/Revision Surgery:**
  - o These procedures are undertaken **to improve aesthetics and/or function.**
  - o They may be considered as procedures that were unplanned at the time of primary surgery.
  - o Indications for revisional surgery to a previously repaired cleft lip are dependent on the site and severity of the residual deformity, e.g., misaligned vermilion, lip asymmetry.

[3] Types of cleft lip and timing of repair. ***Dec 12***

- A **minimum of three operations, and usually four,** will be required to correct the deformity.
- These are performed at specific times corresponding to the developmental stage of the patient.
- Commonly, the sequence is as follows:
  a. **Cleft lip repair at 3-6 months.**
  b. **Cleft palate repair < 1 year (or before speech development).**
  c. **Alveolar bone graft when permanent dentition begins and after orthodontic preparation.**
- Future surgeries are reserved for the end of skeletal maturity and include:
  a. Possible septorhinoplasty in the late teenage years.
  b. Possible lip revisions.
  c. Possible nose revisions.
  d. Le Fort 1 maxillary advancement.
  e. Secondary procedures for speech improvement.

[MCQ] Cleft palate occurs due to: ***CBME March 24***
A. Abnormal development of median nasal process
B. Abnormal development of maxillary process
C. Failure of fusion of palatine shelves*
D. Failure of fusion of nasal bones

- Cleft lip and/or palate is the most common congenital abnormality affecting the orofacial region.
- These conditions **most commonly occur as isolated deformities** but can also be **associated with other medical conditions**, e.g., congenital heart disease.

Incidence

- Cleft lip + palate > isolated cleft palate > isolated cleft lip.

Aetiology

- **Family history** in which a first degree relative is affected.
- Genetic mutations.
- **Over 150 named syndromes** are associated: Stickler, DiGeorge, Down, Apert and Treacher Collins.
- **Environmental factors:**
  - o **Maternal epilepsy and associated medications.**
  - o **Drugs**: Steroids, diazepam, sodium valproate, phenytoin.
- **Pierre Robin sequence**
- Most cases occur without a clear family history or known risk factors.

Embryology and Pathogenesis

- Clefts **occur at the points of fusion** of facial processes.
- Normal anatomical structures are **displaced and disrupted.**

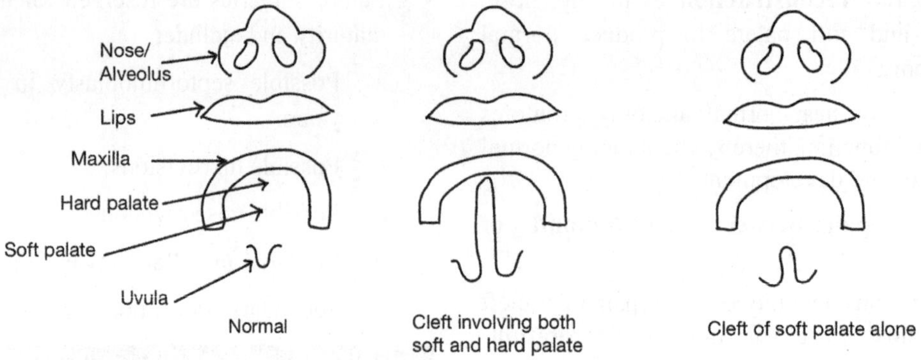

Figure 2: Embryology of cleft palate

- **Failure of fusion or descent of the two palatine shelves,** results in a cleft affecting any part of the palate.
- This failure may be confined to the **soft palate alone or involve both hard and soft palate.**
- **Complete Palate:**
  - o When the **nasal septum and vomer are completely separated from the palatine processes,** the cleft palate is termed complete.
  - o There is a **gap between the two halves of the palate** in its entire length.
  - o The **nose and mouth** become **interconnected.**
- **Incomplete Palate:**
  - o When the **cleft of the hard palate remains attached to the nasal septum and vomer,** the cleft is termed incomplete.
  - o The **two halves** of the palate **fuse** together in an **anterior to posterior direction,** such that the last parts to fuse are the two halves of the uvula.
  - o The anterior part of the palate is always normally formed.
  - o Incomplete fusion may be: bifid uvula, whole length of soft palate, whole length of soft palate + posterior part of hard palate.

Clinical Features

- Isolated cleft palate is more common in **females.**
- **Difficulties in suckling,** as the negative pressure which is required for suckling cannot be produced.
- **Difficulties in eating,** due to regurgitation of food into the nose.
- **Inability to pronounce** the palatal consonants (B, D, K, P, T).
- There is **nasal intonation** because air comes out through the nose while talking.
- Acute or chronic **otitis media** may develop, leading to difficulty in hearing.
- **Dental problems** due to irregular development of the alveolus.
- All the **incisors are badly displaced** in bilateral cleft palate.
- Relative **mandibular prognathism** may also result.
- Repeated **respiratory tract infections.**
- Chances of **aspiration bronchopneumonia.**

Investigations

- Isolated cleft palate cannot be diagnosed antenatally using routine scanning techniques.
- Doppler studies may help in diagnosing isolated cleft palate.

Treatment

A. Feeding

- Babies born with a cleft palate will feed well and thrive, provided that they receive the appropriate CNS input.
- **Expressed breast milk is best** and a range of modified bottles and teats are available.
- **Soft bottles** allow the parents to do much of the work of milk delivery for the child by synchronising their 'squeeze' to the baby's 'suck'.
- Babies are provided with an **active plate** that aims not only to **improve feeding** but also to reduce the width of the cleft and improve the shape of the nose prior to surgery, called **nasoalveolar moulding (NAM).**

B. Surgery

- **Principles of cleft surgery:**
  - o To facilitate normal development and well-being.
  - o Muscular reconstruction of the lip, nose, face and soft palate to produce normal anatomy.
  - o Normal or near-normal anatomy promotes normal function, thereby encouraging normal growth and development.
- **Timing of repair:**
  - o Varies across the world.
  - o The principle applied is that of closure during the early stages of speech development.
  - o Cleft lip/nose and anterior palate repair is performed between 3 and 6 months of age.
  - o Definitive cleft palate repair is carried out between 6 and 12 months.
- The most common surgical approach in cleft palate repair is the **intravelar veloplasty (IVVP),** in which incisions along the cleft edge provide access to the soft palate muscle. The **levator muscles are dissected free and sutured together in the midline to recreate a muscular sling**.
- **Other procedures:**
  - o Wardill's four flap operation.
  - o Langenbeck's operation.

23

Pharynx, Larynx and Neck

[3] Sternomastoid tumour. *March 21*

- Also known as congenital torticollis, fibromatosis coli.
- It is not a true congenital abnormality.

Aetiopathogenesis

- It is **due to infarction of central portion of one sternomastoid muscle** at the time of birth.
- The infarcted **muscle is gradually replaced by fibrous tissue which contracts.**
- As it does so, the **neck is turned** so that the face is directed away from the side of the lesion.

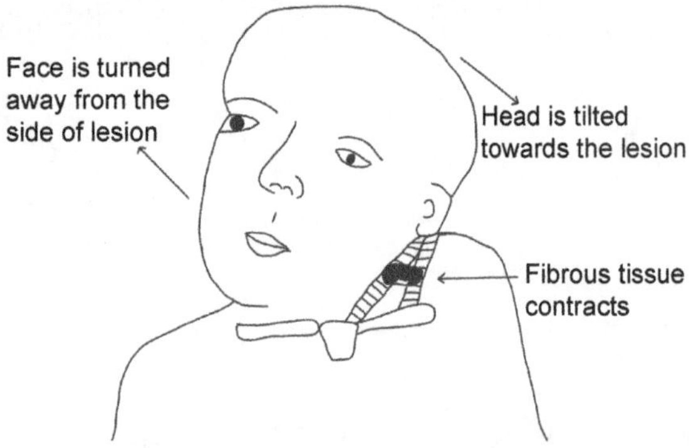

Figure 1: Sternomastoid tumour

Clinical Features

- A **lateral neck mass** may be palpated in the affected muscle.
- There is **rotation of the head towards the opposite side** of the mass.

Investigations

- The mass may be diagnosed by **USG**.

HPE

- Deposition of collagen and fibroblasts around atrophied muscle cells.

Treatment

- Physical therapy based on **passive stretching of the affected muscle** is usually all that is required.
- Rarely, **surgical transection** of the sternocleidomastoid may be indicated.

[5] Branchial cyst. *June 19*

[MCQ] Branchial cyst, following is true: *CBME March 24*

A. Sequestration dermoid
B. Presents at upper end of neck*
C. Seen at lower end of neck
D. Develops from 3rd branchial cleft

- During development, four branchial clefts are seen on either side of the neck. The first cleft persists as the external auditory meatus. The 2nd, 3rd and 4th clefts normally disappear. **Sometimes, the whole, or a portion, of one of the clefts that normally disappear may persist.**

Aetiopathogenesis

- A branchial cyst develops from the **vestigial remnants of the 2nd branchial cleft.**

- **Lined by squamous epithelium.**
- Contains **thick, turbid fluid**. Sometimes, it can also contain clear fluid.

Clinical Features

- **Age:** Early or middle adulthood.
- Usually present in the **upper neck.**
- Found at the **junction of upper 1/3rd and middle 1/3rd of the sternocleidomastoid muscle** at its anterior border.

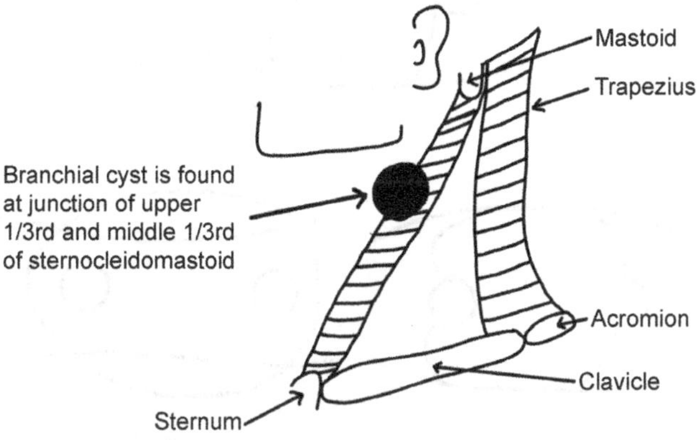

Figure 2: Branchial cyst

- It is a **fluctuant swelling.**
- If it **contains clear fluid**, it may transilluminate.
- It is often soft in its early stages so that it may be difficult to palpate.
- If the cyst becomes **infected**, it becomes **erythematous and tender**.

Investigations

- USG.
- FNAC.

Treatment

- The treatment of choice is complete **excision**, which is best undertaken when the lesion is quiescent.
- Care should be taken not to damage any nerves during excision.

[5] Branchial fistula. *Dec 12*

- A branchial fistula represents a **persistent 2nd branchial cleft.**

Aetiology

- During embryologic development, the **2nd branchial cleft** normally disappears.
- When it **persists**, it forms a branchial fistula.
- May also be **secondary to an incision in an infected branchial cyst.**

Clinical Features

- The **external orifice** is nearly always situated in the **lower 1/3rd of the neck near the anterior border of the sternocleidomastoid** muscle.
- The **internal orifice** is located on the **anterior aspect of the posterior faucial pillars** just behind the tonsils.
- History of small amount of **recurrent mucopurulent discharge** onto the neck.
- May be unilateral or bilateral.

Pathology

- The tract is **lined by ciliated columnar epithelium** until it is destroyed by recurrent attacks of inflammation.
- The track is **clothed with muscle.**

Treatment

- When causing troublesome symptoms, e.g., by a discharge of mucus, branchial fistulas should be **excised.**

[5] Carotid body tumour. *Dec 18, Feb 23*

- It is a rare tumour.
- It is a **paraganglioma.**
- Also known as **chemodectoma** or **potato tumour.**

Aetiology

- It has a **higher incidence in areas where people live at high altitudes because of chronic hypoxia leading to carotid body hyperplasia.**
- Familial cases are caused by **mutations in the genes for succinate dehydrogenate (SDH) enzyme.**
- **Associated with pheochromocytomas** in familial cases.

Pathology

- Tumours **arise from the chemoreceptor cells on the medial side of the carotid bulb** and, at this point, the tumour is adherent to the carotid wall.
- Usually **benign.**
- Only a small number of cases have produced proven metastases.

Sites

- Carotid body.
- Aortopulmonary bodies.
- Glomus jugulare.
- Tympanic bodies.

Clinical Features

- Usually **unilateral** and seen in **middle life.**
- There is often a long history of a slowly enlarging, **painless lump** at the carotid bifurcation.
- 1/3rd of patients present with a **pharyngeal mass that pushes the tonsil medially** and anteriorly.

On Examination

- Firm.
- Rubbery.
- Pulsatile.
- Mobile from side to side but not up and down.
- Can sometimes be **emptied by firm pressure**, after which it slowly **refills in a pulsatile manner.**
- A bruit may also be present.

Investigations

1. **Carotid angiogram:**
   - Carotid bifurcation is splayed.
   - A blush outlines the tumour vessels.
2. **MRI:**
   - Provides excellent detail.
   - Since it is of vascular origin, **FNAC and biopsy are contraindicated.**

Classification

- The **Shamblin classification** is used to determine the surgical resectability of these tumours:
  - o **Type I:** Tumours are localised and involve < 180° of carotid vessels.
  - o **Type II:** Tumours surround the vessel by > 180°.
  - o **Type III:** Tumours completely encase the vessels.

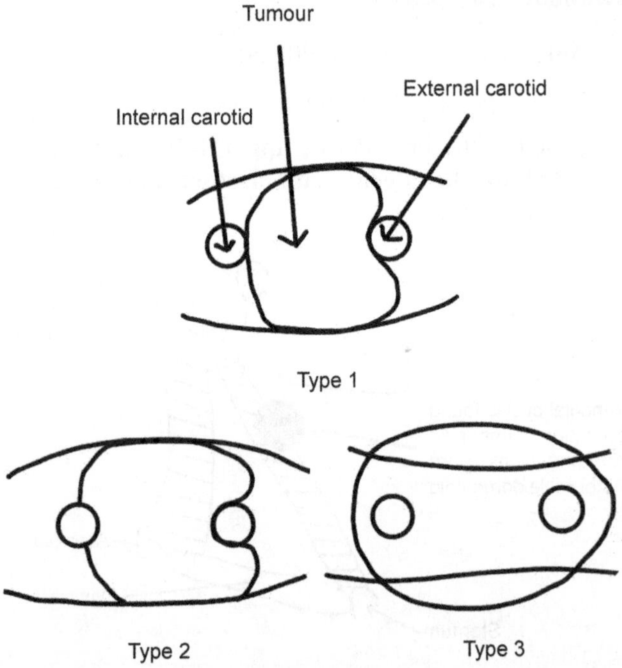

Figure 3: Shamblin classification of carotid body tumour

Treatment

- The treatment of choice of these tumours is **surgical resection.**
- Because these tumours rarely metastasize and their overall rate of growth is slow, the need for surgical removal must be carefully considered as complications of surgery are potentially serious.
- **Type III tumours are the most challenging to resect** with higher complications and a possible need for vessel reconstruction.
- Surgery is best avoided in elderly patients.
- In some cases it may be possible to dissect the tumour away from the carotid bifurcation.
- Resection will be necessary when the tumour is large. This is combined with **reconstruction with a vein autograft** (to restore arterial continuity).

[3] Mention complications of tracheostomy. *Dec 12*

- A tracheostomy is a procedure which relieves airway obstruction or protects the airway by fashioning a

direct entrance into the trachea through the skin of the neck.

Indications

a. **Acute upper airway obstruction:**
   - Inhaled foreign body.
   - A large pharyngolaryngeal tumour.
   - Acute pharyngolaryngeal infections in children.

b. **Potential upper airway obstruction:**
   - After or prior to major surgery involving the oral cavity, pharynx, larynx or neck.

c. **Protection of the lower airway:**
   - Protection against aspiration of saliva in unconscious patients as a consequence of head injuries, maxillofacial injuries comas, bulbar poliomyelitis or tetanus.

d. **Patients requiring prolonged artificial respiration:** Best performed within 10 days of ventilation.

Types

1. **Emergency tracheostomy:**
   - If a skilled anesthetist is unavailable, local anesthesia is employed, but in desperate cases when the patient is unconscious none is required.
   - Difficult to perform in small children and thick-necked adults as the landmarks are difficult to palpate.
   - The focus is on **establishing access to the airway as fast as possible.**
   - Heavy bleeding may be present (especially if the neck is congested as a result of the patients efforts to breathe around an acute upper airway obstruction).
   - **Hemostasis is secured only after an airway has been established.**
   - Any form of available tube should be inserted into the trachea as soon as possible. With the emergency under control, the **tracheostomy should be refashioned as soon as possible**.
   - Made via a **midline vertical skin incision.**

2. **Elective tracheostomy:**
   - The advantages of an elective surgical procedure are that there is **complete airway control at all times, unhurried dissection and careful placement of an appropriate tube.**
   - Done under GA, after endotracheal intubation.
   - A transverse skin incision is made.
   - The tracheostomy is made at the level of the 2nd to 4th tracheal ring.
   - A **Bjork flap** may be used in adults: It has the advantage of **allowing reintroduction of a displaced tube** with the minimum of difficulty.

3. **Percutaneous tracheostomy:**
   - It is an alternative to open tracheostomy.
   - It is **commonly performed in the critical care setting in an intubated patient**.
   - A **22G needle** is inserted between the 2nd and 3rd tracheal rings.
   - The **tracheostomy tube is introduced with the help of guidewire and dilator**.
   - It is rarely performed in children.

Tracheostomy Tubes

- Most modern tracheostomy tubes are made of plastic.
- They consist of an introducer, low pressure cuff and inner cannula.
- A **cuffed tube** is used initially. This **protects the airway from secretions or bleeding**. It is changed after 3-4 days to a non-cuffed tube.
- A **removable inner tube**, which is easily cleaned, should always be used to **prevent lumen occlusion by thickened, dried secretions** from the trachea.

Advantages

- Tracheostomy bypasses the upper airway and has the following advantages:
  1. The anatomical dead space is reduced by 50%.
  2. The work of breathing is reduced.
  3. Alveolar ventilation is increased.
  4. Level of sedation needed for patient comfort is decreased.
  5. Unlike endotracheal intubation the patient may be able to talk and eat with a tube in place.

Disadvantages

1. Loss of heat and moisture exchange in the upper respiratory tract.

2. Desiccation of tracheal epithelium, loss of ciliated cells and metaplasia.
3. The presence of a foreign body in the trachea stimulates production of mucus; where no cilia are present, the mucociliary stream is therefore impeded.
4. The increased mucus is more viscid and thick crusts may form and bock the tube.
5. Although many patients with a tracheostomy can feed satisfactorily there is some **splinting of the larynx which may prevent normal swallowing and lead to aspiration**, this aspiration may be silent.

Complications

a. **Intra-op complications:**
   - Hemorrhage.
   - Injury to carotid artery, recurrent laryngeal nerve and esophagous.
   - Damage to trachea.

b. **Early post-op complications:**
   - Apnea caused by a fall in the PCO_2.
   - Hemorrhage.
   - Subcutaneous emphysema, pneumomediastinum and pneumothorax.
   - Accidental extubation, anterior displacement of the tube, obstruction of the tube lumen and tip occlusion against the tracheal wall.
   - Infection.
   - Swallowing dysfunction.

c. **Late post-op complications:**
   - Difficult decannulation.
   - Tracheocutaneous fistula.
   - Tracheoesophageal fistula.
   - Tracheoinnominate artery fistula with severe hemorrhage.
   - Tracheal stenosis.

[3] Ludwig's angina. *Dec 19*

- **Definition:** It is a clinical entity characterized by a **brawny swelling of the submandibular region** combined with inflammatory edema of the mouth, with accompanying putrid halitosis.

Aetiology

- Often caused by a virulent **streptococcal infection associated with anaerobic organisms.**
- An **underlying oral cavity ulcer** may be present.

Pathogenesis

- Infection tracks deep to the mylohyoid muscle, causing edema and inflammation.
- **Tongue is displaced upwards and backwards**, giving rise to dysphagia and painful obstruction of the airway.
- Unless treated, **cellulitis may extend beneath the deep fascial layers of the neck to involve the larynx,** causing glottic edema and further airway compromise.

Clinical Features

- Brawny swelling of submandibular region.
- Inflammatory edema of the mouth.
- Putrid halitosis.
- Displacement of tongue results in dysphagia and painful obstruction of the airway.
- Glottic edema results in airway compromise.

Treatment

a. **Broad spectrum IV antibiotics with anaerobic cover:**
   - Penicillin, clindamycin, cephalosporins.

b. **Surgical drainage:**
   - Indicated if swelling does not subside with antibiotics or if pus is evident.
   - A curved submental incision may be used to drain both submandibular triangles.

[MCQ] Structure NOT preserved in modified radical neck dissection is: ***CBME June 24***

A. Spinal accessory nerve
B. Submandibular nerve*
C. Sternocleidomastoid muscle
D. Internal jugular vein

NECK DISSECTION

Radical Neck Dissection (RND)

- Sacrifice of the sternocleidomastoid, internal jugular vein and accessory nerve (CN XI).
- Removal of all lymphatic levels (levels I–V).

Modified Radical Neck Dissection (MRND)

- Any modification of the RND that preserves at least one of the non-lymphatic structures (i.e., CN XI, SCM, IJV) is defined as a MRND.

Selective Neck Dissection (SND)

- A neck dissection that preserves lymphatic compartments normally removed as part of a classic RND is called SND.
- The sternocleidomastoid, internal jugular vein and accessory nerve (CN XI) are preserved.
- E.g.:
  - Supra Omohyoid Neck Dissection (levels I–III).
  - Lateral Neck Dissection (levels II–IV).
  - Posterolateral Neck Dissection (levels II–V).

24

Oral Cavity and Swellings of Jaw

[3] Differential diagnosis of tongue ulcer. *June 13*

- The various types of tongue ulcers are as follows:

A. Aphthous or Dyspeptic Ulcer

- Small ulcer which is surrounded by a hyperemic zone.
- Painful.
- Seen in early adult life.
- F > M.

B. Dental or Traumatic Ulcer

- Caused by mechanical irritation either by a jagged tooth or dentures.
- Usually occur at periphery of tongue.
- Surrounded by a zone of erythema and induration.
- Painful.

C. Syphilitic Ulcer

- Snail-track ulcer.
- Seen in 2nd stage of syphilis.
- Syphilitic ulcers are rare in the tongue, but gumma and chronic superficial glossitis are more common.

D. Tuberculous Ulcers

- Shallow, often multiple with undermined edges.
- Usually seen at margins or tip.
- When seen in the anterior 2/3rd of tongue, it becomes very painful.
- Usually associated with TB of lungs and cervical lymphadenopathy.

E. Post-Pertussis Ulcer

- Occurs only in children with whooping cough.
- Usually seen at upper part of frenulum linguae.

F. Chronic Non-Specific Ulcer

- Usually occurs in the anterior 2/3rd of tongue.
- Idiopathic.
- Moderately indurated.
- Not very painful.

G. Carcinomatous Ulcer

- Malignant ulcers.

H. Herpetic Ulcer

- Common in children and young adults.
- Occurs due to herpetic affection of lingual nerve.
- Multiple superficial ulcers which are extremely painful.

I. Smokers Ulcer

- Occurs due to smoking.
- Superficial, multiple ulcers with hyperemia.

J. Ulcers Due to Glossitis

[3] Tongue tie. *Oct 20*

- Also known as ankyloglossia.

Pathophysiology

- The **lingual frenulum is short**, often **thicker** than normal and it is **fibrous.**
- It holds the tip of the tongue close to the edges of the lower central incisors, **preventing the tongue from protruding outside.**

Clinical Features

- Inability to protrude the tongue outside the oral cavity.
- Attempts to raise or protrude the tongue, causes:
  - o Eversion of lateral margin.
  - o Heaping up of mid-portion of dorsum.
- Most commonly, the deformity does not cause any problems and **remains asymptomatic.**
- **In newborns:**
  - o It is never responsible for any difficulty with suckling.
  - o May result in lisping in infancy.
- Difficulty in cleaning the backs of the lower front teeth.

Treatment

- Surgical division.

[3] Cancrum oris. *March 21*

- Also known as noma, gangrenous stomatitis.
- It is a **severe** and **rapidly progressive infectious disease** that primarily affects the soft tissues of the face, especially the lips, cheeks and jaw.

Aetiopathogenesis

- It occurs as a **complication of measles and other childhood illnesses like leukemia.**
- **Malnutrition** is a predisposing cause.
- Presence of erupted teeth appears necessary for the onset.
- Ulceration **starts on the gingivae** and spreads over and into the bone of the jaw.
- From the gum it **spreads onto the inside of the cheek** and then **through to the skin surface**, producing a large area of full thickness time loss.

Clinical Features

- Lesion begins as an area of **edema and induration** on the lip.
- It becomes ischemic and necrotic.
- The area of necrosis spreads steadily and large areas of lips, cheeks and jaws may be destroyed.
- Extremely **painful** condition.
- High fever.
- Patient is very ill and anorexic.
- Healing takes place with gross scarring which may prevent proper movement of the jaw.

Treatment

- **Antibiotics:** IV penicillin, metronidazole.
- High protein diet.
- Vitamin supplementation.
- Simultaneous treatment of underlying disease.
- Excision of scarred tissue with skin grafting is required if scarring is causing problems.

[3] Premalignant conditions of oral cancer. *Dec 15*

- Oral pre-malignant lesions are **mucosal abnormalities from which oral cancer can arise.**
- These are more accurately described as **potentially malignant** lesions.
- These are as follows:
  1. Leukoplakia.
  2. Erythroplakia.
  3. Erythroleukoplakia.
  4. Proliferative verrucous leukoplakia.
  5. Oral submucous fibrosis.
  6. Oral lichen planus.
  7. Lupus erythematosus.
  8. **Inherited conditions:**
     - o Epidermolysis bullosa.
     - o Dyskeratosis congenita.
  9. **Chronic infections:**
     - o Chronic hyperplastic candidiasis.
     - o Syphilitic glossitis.

Malignant Transformation

- The reported rates of malignant transformation vary widely between studies and countries.
- The following lesions carry the **highest risk for malignant transformation**:
  1. Erythroleukoplakia.
  2. Proliferative verrucous leukoplakia.
  3. Dyskeratosis congenita.
- The **following factors are associated with increased risk**:
  a. F > M.
  b. Size > 200 mm².
  c. Non-homogenous lesions.
  d. Smoker.
  e. Presence of multiple lesions.
  f. Location (e.g., lateral border of tongue/floor of mouth).

Investigations

- **Biopsy** gives the following information:
  - o Accurate pathological diagnosis.
  - o Degree of dysplasia (mild, moderate, severe).
  - o Presence of malignancy in a lesion.

Treatment

- The management is challenging because of an inconsistency with nomenclature and also because the natural history of these lesions remains unclear.
- Treatment is **surgical excision.**
- But, surgical excision does not completely remove the risk of transformation and surveillance is therefore necessary.

[3] Leukoplakia. *March 22, Oct 20*

- **Definition:** Leukoplakia is a clinical term used to describe any **white patch or plaque that cannot be rubbed off or characterized clinically or pathologically as another disease.**
- It is a **pre-malignant lesion** of the oral cavity.

Pathology

Gross

- It **varies** from a small, well-circumscribed, homogenous white plaque to an extensive lesion involving large surface areas of the oral mucosa.
- It may be **smooth or wrinkled or fissured.**
- It varies in white colouration, depending on the thickness of the lesion.

HPE

- Leucoplakia is a purely descriptive term and has **no histological correlation.**

Risk of Malignancy

- Malignant transformation in oral leukoplakia varies from 0.13 to 34%.
- **Erythroleucoplakia and proliferative verrucous leukoplakia have the highest risk for malignant transformation.**

Investigations

- **Biopsy** is done to rule out carcinoma.

Treatment

- There are various options:
  1. Surgical excision.
  2. Laser therapy.
  3. Cryotherapy.
  4. Photodynamic therapy.
- Monitoring of the lesion is essential.

[3] Speckled leukoplakia. *March 21*

- Also known as erythroleukoplakia.
- It is essentially a **combination of both leucoplakia and erythroplakia.**
- Some consider it to be a variation of leucoplakia arising on an erythematous base.
- It is a **premalignant lesion** of the oral cavity and carries the **greatest risk for malignant change.**
- A **biopsy** is taken to make an accurate diagnosis.
- The treatment is **excision.**

[10] Discuss aetiology, pathology, clinical features and management of carcinoma of buccal mucosa. *Dec 12*

- Oral cancer is one of the **most common cancers in India.**

Risk Factors

- Chewing tobacco/smoking.
- Alcohol.
- Betel quid (areca nut, catechu and slaked lime wrapped in a piper betel leaf).
- Gutka.
- Human Papilloma Virus.
- Previous exposure to radiation.
- Chronic infection.
- Immunosuppression.
- **Hereditary conditions:**
  - o Fanconi anemia.
  - o Li Fraumeni syndrome.
- **Potentially malignant/premalignant lesions:**
  - o Erythroleukoplakia.
  - o Proliferative verrucous leukoplakia.
  - o Dyskeratosis congenita.

Pathology

- The **vast majority** of oral cavity cancers **are squamous cell carcinomas (>95%).**
- In contrast to Western populations, **cancers of the buccogingival/ retromolar area are the most common sites.**
- **Alterations in p53 and CDKN2A are the two most frequent genomic mutations** noted in cancers of oral cavity.
- **Tumour grade (differentiation):**
  - o **G1** – Well differentiated.
  - o **G2** – Moderately differentiated.
  - o **G3** – Poorly differentiated.
  - o **Grade** is **based on how similar the tumour tissue appears relative to the normal tissue** from which it originated.
  - o Well differentiated tumours are less aggressive.
  - o Poorly differentiated tumours infiltrate and metastasize more readily and therefore carry a worse prognosis.
- Pattern of **invasion** is of **two types: Cohesive and non-cohesive.**
- **Metastases:** Most mets occur in **levels I and II** of the neck. Distant mets are rare.

Staging

- TNM staging is used.

Tx - Primary tumour cannot be assessed.

Tis - Carcinoma in situ.

T1 - Tumour size $\leq$ 2 cm.
Depth of invasion $\leq$ 5 mm.

T2 - Tumour $\leq$ 2 cm and DoI of 6 - 10 mm.

or

Tumour 2 - 4 cm and DoI of $\leq$ 10 mm.

T3 - Tumour > 4 cm (irrespective of DoI).

or

DoI > 10 mm (irrespective of tumour size).

T4 - Moderately advanced or very advanced local disease.

Nx - Regional lymph nodes cannot be assessed.

N0 - No regional lymph node mets.

N1 - Single i/l lymph node $\leq$ 3 cm and extra nodal extension negative.

N2 -

2a: Single i/l lymph node $\leq$ 3 cm and ENE positive.

or

Single i/l lymph node 3 - 6 cm and ENE negative.

2b: Multiple i/l lymph nodes, all < 6 cm and ENE negative.

2c: Bilateral or c/l lymph nodes, all < 6 cm and ENE negative.

N3 -

3a: Single i/l lymph node > 6 cm and ENE negative.

3b: Single i/l lymph node > 3 cm and ENE positive.

or

Multiple i/l, c/l or b/l lymph nodes with any lymph node being ENE positive.

M0- No distant metastases.

M1- Distant metastases present.

Clinical Features

- Incidence of oral cancer **increases with age**, mean age at presentation being 62 years.
- Strong correlation between **lower socio-economic status** and disease incidence.
- There is a **wide clinical presentation** of oral cavity cancers, which range from small areas of erythro/leukoplakia to larger erosive and cavitated lesions that invade surrounding tissues.
- Reduced tongue movement.
- Sensory nerve deficit.
- Trismus.
- Chronic otalgia.
- Dysphagia.

On Examination

- Non-healing ulcer (> 2 weeks) or ulceroproliferative growth.
- Persistent neck mass/lymphadenopathy.
- Lesion, pigmentation which progressively increases in size.
- Lesion with associated induration.
- Persistent, red or white lesion.
- Non-resolving 'inflammatory' lesion.
- Unexplained tooth mobility.

Investigations

A. Biopsy

a. Primary tumour:

- Histopathological diagnosis via a formal biopsy is the gold standard prior to further investigation and treatment.
- **Incisional biopsy** is preferred.
- A narrow deep biopsy is taken.

b. Neck lump:

- **FNAC** is the first line investigation.

B. Imaging

- **Aims of imaging are as follows:**
  1. **Outline the anatomical extent** of the primary tumour (T stage), **as well as the 'resectability'** of the tumour based on its relationship to vital structures.
  2. Detection of **locoregional mets.**
  3. Detection of **metastatic disease** precluding cure.
  4. Detection of **synchronous primary tumours** of the lung and upper aerodigestive tract.
  5. Monitoring of **disease response** following non-surgical treatment and for detection of disease recurrence.
- **CT and/or MRI are the gold standard** imaging modalities to stage a tumour of the oral cavity.
- **X-ray** is used mainly for evaluation of dentition.
- **USG** is used to **guide FNAC** sampling of suspicious **lymph nodes**.
- **PET-CT** is not a first line imaging investigation and its use is restricted to detection of distant mets or synchronous tumours.

C. Sentinel Lymph Node Biopsy

- Used for investigation and staging of early oral cancers that have no clinical or radiographic evidence for cervical mets.
- A positive SLNB necessitates subsequent management of the neck (typically with completion neck dissection).

Treatment

- **Surgery, with adjuvant radiotherapy (or chemoradiotherapy)** if indicated, remains the mainstay for management of oral cavity cancer.
- Nowadays, there is greater emphasis on **function sparing techniques** and a move away from more radical procedures.
- **Reconstruction** of post ablative defects is done.

A. Tumour Resection

- The gold standard treatment for oral cavity cancers is **resection with a 1 cm clinical margin circumferentially** (if vital structures permit such a resection).

a. Access procedure:

- o This is the procedure that is done to access the tumour.
- o While most tumours can be removed via a transoral approach, some cannot be resected safety without an access procedure.
- o The most commonly used access procedures are:

1. **Lip-split mandibulotomy.**
2. **Mandibular lingual release.**
3. **Visor flap.**
4. **Weber-Fergusson approach.**

b. **Tumour resection:**

- o The gold standard in oral cavity cancers is resection with a 1 cm clinical margin circumferentially (if vital structures permit such a resection).
  1. **Mandibular resection**
     - ♦ If there is evidence of infiltrative bone invasion, the following are done:
       - □ **Segmental resection** of mandible.
       - □ **Rim resection or 'marginal mandibulectomy'.**

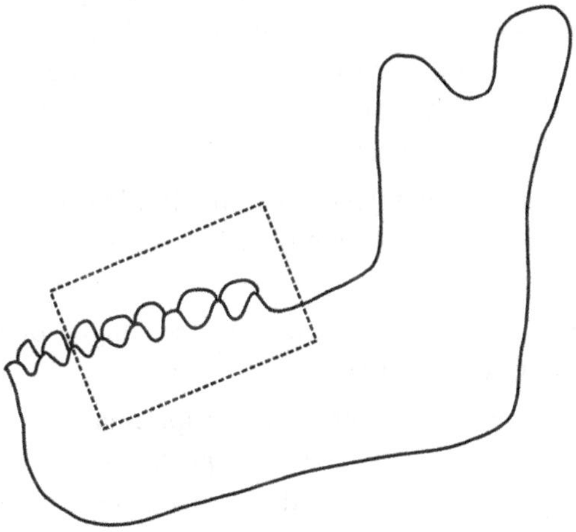

Figure 1: Rim resection or Marginal mandibulectomy

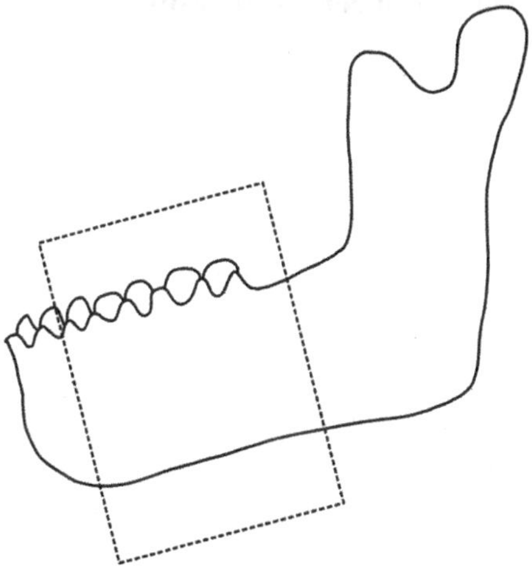

Figure 2: Segmental mandibulectomy

  2. **Maxillary resection**
     - ♦ Small tumours of the maxillary alveolus can be managed by transoral partial maxillectomy.
     - ♦ More extensive tumours involving the floor of maxillary sinus require wider access by a Weber Fergusson incision.
     - ♦ Tumours extending into the orbit require simultaneous orbital exenteration or a combined neurosurgical resection.

B. **Management of Neck**

1. **Therapeutic neck dissection**
   - Done in patients with clinical and/or radiographic evidence of cervical mets.
   - Involved lymph nodes are resected.
2. **Elective neck dissection**
   - Done in patients in whom there is no clinical or radiographic evidence for cervical mets.
   - A selective neck dissection involving levels I-III of the neck is done.

C. **Reconstruction**

- Post surgery defects are reconstructed with an aim to replace resected tissue with similar tissue.
- The reconstruction ladder is a useful algorithm that is commonly used:
  1. Healing by secondary intention.
  2. Primary closure.
  3. Skin grafting.
  4. Local flaps.
  5. Regional flaps.
  6. Microvascular free tissue transfer.
- Examples of flaps used are:
  - o Facial artery myomucosal flaps.
  - o Radial forearm flee flap.
  - o Anterolateral thigh flap.
  - o Pectoralis major myocutaneous flap.
- The fibula is the most commonly used bone-containing flap (composite flap).

D. Adjuvant Chemoradiotherapy

- It is given based on pathological features of the tumour.
- Cisplatin based chemotherapy.
- External beam radiotherapy.

[10] Describe the aetiology, pathogenesis, clinical features and management of carcinoma tongue. *Feb 23*

- Oral cavity cancers are very common in India.

Risk Factors

- Tobacco/smoking.
- Alcohol.
- Betel quid.
- Gutka.
- Human Papilloma Virus.
- Previous exposure to radiation.
- Chronic infection.
- Immunosuppression.
- **Hereditary conditions:**
  - o Fanconi anemia.
  - o Li Fraumeni syndrome.
- **Potentially malignant/pre-malignant lesions:**
  - o Erythroleukoplakia.
  - o Proliferative verrucous leukoplakia.
  - o Dyskeratosis congenita.

Pathology

- Most common cancer of tongue is **Squamous Cell Carcinoma.**
- Alterations in **p53 and CDKN2A** are the two most frequent mutations.
- **Tumour grade (differentiation):**

  G_1 : Well differentiated.

  G_2 : Moderately differentiated.

  G_3 : Severely differentiated.
- Well differentiated tumours are less aggressive.
- Poorly differentiated tumours infiltrate and metastasise more readily and therefore carry a worse prognosis.
- Most **mets** occur in **levels I and II** of the neck.
- Distant mets are rare.
- Occurs mostly on the **anterior 2/3rd of the tongue at or near the edges.**

Clinical Features

- M > F.
- Incidence increases with age, most cases are in patients > 50 years.
- **Most common complaint is a painless lump or an ulcer on the surface of the tongue.**
- Excessive salivation.
- In later stages, the saliva becomes blood stained.
- **Foetor oris** or foul smelling breath.
- **Ankyloglossia** or immobility of the tongue occurs due to extensive carcinomatous infiltration of the lingual musculature. It becomes even worse when the floor of the mouth is involved and ultimately this causes difficulty in speech.
- It is always painless to begin with, but in late stages the patient may complain of pain due to nerve involvement.
- **Pain** may be experienced in the tongue or may be **referred to the ear.**
- **Hoarseness of voice and dysphagia** may be seen when the growth is in the **posterior 1/3rd** of the tongue and has involved pharynx and larynx.
- Enlarged lymph nodes in the neck.
- Growth may be **ulceroproliferative** or warty.

Investigations

A. Biopsy

a. Primary tumour:

- Edge/wedge biopsy or incisional biopsy.
- It is the gold standard.

b. Neck swelling (lymph nodes):

- FNAC.

B. Imaging

- CT and/or MRI are the gold standard.
- USG is used to guide FNAC sampling of suspicious lymph nodes.

- PET-CT is used to detect distant mets or synchronous tumours.

Treatment

A. Excision of Primary Tumour

- The treatment of choice of the primary tumour is **surgical excision with a margin of 5 mm.**
- If the tumour is **restricted to one side**, a **partial or hemiglossectomy** is done.
- If the tumour **encroaches upon the floor of the mouth or mandible**, that needs to be **excised.**
- For tumours which **cross the midline**, **subtotal or total glossectomy** is done.

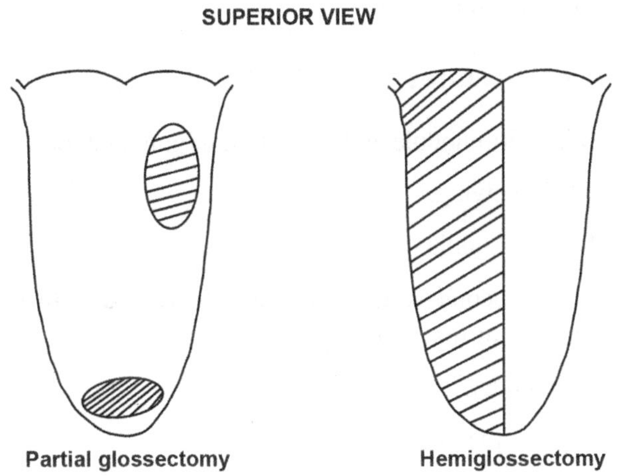

Figure 3: Partial glossectomy and hemiglossectomy

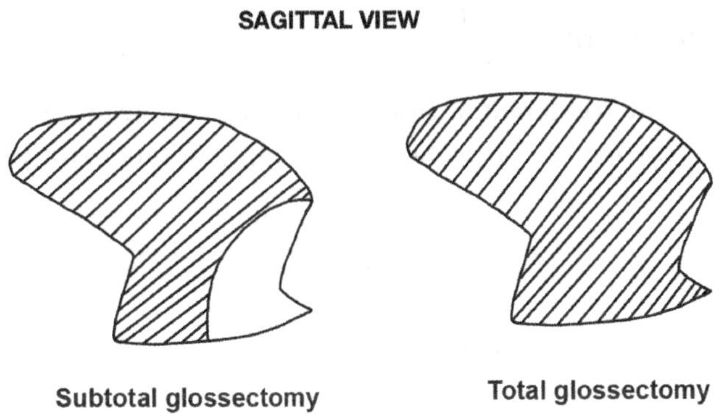

Figure 4: Subtotal and total glossectomy

B. Access

- There are various techniques of accessing the tumour:
  1. **Trans-oral:** For small to moderate sized anterior tumours.
  2. **Lip-split technique and paramedian or median mandibulotomy.**
  3. **Visor incision.**

C. Reconstruction

- The more **anterior** the **defect** in the oral cavity, the greater the **impact on speech.**
- The more **posterior** the **defect**, the more the impact on **swallowing.**
- Small defects of the lateral tongue can be managed by primary closure or be allowed to heal by secondary intention with little or no functional impairment.
- Larger defects require formal reconstruction:
  - o Radial forearm flap.
  - o ALT or anterolateral thigh flap.
  - o Rectus abdominis free flap.

D. Neck Dissection

- **Therapeutic neck dissection:**
  - o Indicated when there is evidence of cervical mets.
  - o Involved lymph nodes are resected.
- **Selective neck dissection:**
  - o Of levels I, II and III.
  - o May be done prophylactically, depending upon radiological or clinical findings.

[5] Ameloblastoma. *July 23*

- Also known as adamantinoma, Eve's disease.
- It is a rare tumour of the jaw.
- It is a **true neoplasm of the odontogenic epithelium.**

Pathology

- It **arises from ameloblasts**, i.e., enamel-forming cells.
- Pathologically, it **looks and behaves like a basal cell carcinoma.**
- It can also occur at other sites apart from the jaw:
  - o Stalk of pituitary gland.

- o Tibia.

- It is a **locally invasive tumour** and is not known for distant spread.
- It does not metastasize to lymph nodes.

Clinical Features

- Starts in early adult life.
- M > F.
- Usually found in the molar area of the mandible.
- Slow growing tumour.
- Painless.
- Causes expansion mostly of the outer table, so the swelling is more evident from outside than from inside the mouth.
- Cystic degeneration leads to areas of softening and egg-shell crackling on palpation.
- Not associated with any carious or missing tooth.

Investigations

- **X-ray:** Honeycomb appearance.
- CT scan.

Treatment

A. Small Tumour
- The treatment of choice is **resection of the tumour along with a margin of healthy bone.**
- The mandibular defect is filled with a **bone graft.**

B. Large Tumour
- A **hemi-mandibulectomy** may be necessary.
- The mandibular defect is substituted by a prosthesis and may be filled with a bone graft.

[3] Epulis. *June 13*

- **Definition:** Epulis is a swelling situated **on the gum.**
- It **arises from the alveolar margin** of the jaw. It can originate from the bone, the periosteum or the mucous membrane.

Types

1. Fibrous epulis.
2. Granulomatous or false epulis or pregnancy epulis.
3. Myeloid or giant cell epulis.
4. Carcinomatous epulis.

- The most common variety is the fibrous epulis.

FIBROUS EPULIS

- It is the most common type of epulis.

Aetiopathogenesis

- Arises from the periosteum at the **neck of an incisor or premolar tooth.**
- It is a **localized inflammatory hyperplasia** of the gum.
- Arises in response to **local irritation** from the sharp margin of a carious cavity.
- As it grows, it **separates the teeth and ultimately loosens them.**

Clinical Features

- It is a firm nodule at the junction of gum and tooth.
- Slow growing.
- Usually small.
- Some become larger and **may ulcerate due to the trauma of mastication.**
- Non tender.
- Adjacent teeth may become loose.
- Draining **lymph nodes are not enlarged.**
- May undergo malignant change.

Treatment

- **The treatment of choice is excision: Adjacent tooth (or teeth) + resection of a wedge of bone with its root** must be performed.

GRANULOMATOUS EPULIS

- Also known as **false epulis or pregnancy epulis or pyogenic granuloma.**
- It is a **mass of granulation tissue around a carious tooth or at the site of irritation by a denture.**
- A similar condition may be found temporarily during pregnancy called gingivitis gravidarum. It tends to regress after child birth.

Clinical Features

- **Bright red** swelling.
- Highly vascular and therefore it **easily bleeds on touch.**
- Often **associated with a carious tooth**, so it is found in those who don't maintain oral hygiene.
- **Halitosis.**
- Ill-fitting denture may cause such swelling.
- **Draining lymph nodes may be enlarged** and tender.

Treatment

- **Extraction of carious tooth** associated with the swelling.
- Ill-fitting dentures should be replaced.
- Maintain **oral hygiene.**
- Mass of **granulation tissue can be cauterised.**

OTHER IMPORTANT TOPICS

DENTAL CYST

- Also known as radicular cyst, periodontal cyst.
- This is the **most common of all the odontomes.**
- It is associated with **chronically infected pulpless tooth.**

Pathogenesis

- The **continued irritation of infection appears to stimulate the remaining nests of cells (epithelial debris) to proliferate.**
- The centre of the mass becomes necrosed, then liquefied and finally converted into a cyst.

Pathology

- Dental cyst is **lined by squamous epithelium.**

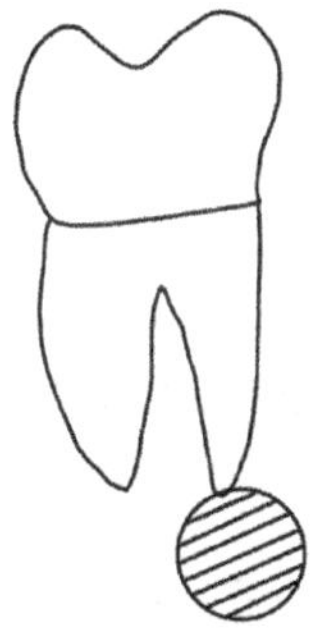

Figure 5: Dental cyst

- Contents may be fluid or semisolid containing cellular debris, cholesterol crystals and foreign body giant cells.
- The fluid is sterile unless secondary infection occurs.

Clinical Features

- Can appear at any age, but commonly seen in and around middle age.
- More common in the upper jaw.
- It is **always associated with a tooth that has normally erupted but has become chronically infected or carious.**
- Usually painless.
- Becomes painful when infected.
- When the bone is thinned out, there may be 'egg shell crackling'.
- If the bone is completely destroyed, fluctuation may be present.

Investigations

1. **X-ray:**
   - A circular radiolucent area is seen in relation to the root of the affected tooth.
   - Margin of the cyst is sclerosed.
2. **CT scan.**
3. **MRI.**

Treatment

- Maintain oral hygiene.
- Affected carious tooth should be removed.
- Deroofing of the cyst followed by curettage of cyst wall. The soft tissue is pushed in. The cyst is obliterated and the wound sutured.

DENTIGEROUS CYST

- Also known as follicular odontome or follicular cyst.

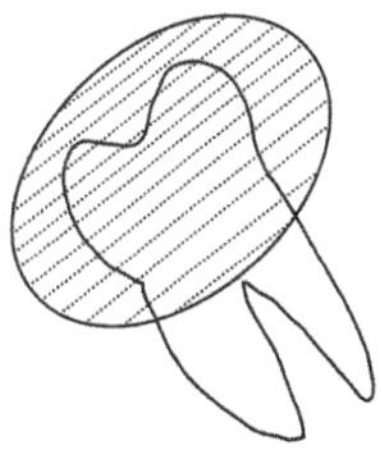

Figure 6: Dentigerous cyst

- This cyst is **usually associated with non-erupted permanent tooth.**
- It consists of a **cyst containing a tooth**, most commonly an **upper or a lower third molar tooth lying obliquely in the cyst with viscid fluid.**

Pathology

- The follicle consists of an **inner lining of squamous epithelium and an outer connective tissue** covering.
- Content is similar to that of the dental cyst, i.e., fluid or semi-solid content with cholesterol crystals and giant cells.
- Cyst continues to grow and **may attain a very large size.**
- May get infected.
- Within the cyst, the **tooth lies either free in the cavity obliquely or embedded in the wall of the follicle.**

Clinical Features

- **Age:** 20-30 years.
- **Most common sites: Mandibular 3rd molar, maxillary 3rd molar and mandibular 2nd premolar.**
- Cyst grows larger and expands the outer table of the jaw causing egg shell crackling.
- It is a painless swelling unless infected.
- Lower jaw is more often affected.
- Counting of teeth may help, as the non-erupted tooth causing dentigerous cyst will be missing.

Investigations

1. **X-ray:**
   - Appears as a well-defined radiolucency around the crown of the unerupted tooth.
   - Larger cysts are rarely multilocular.
   - Ridges of bone on the side walls cause pseudo-trabecular or soap-bubble appearance.
2. **CT scan.**
3. **MRI.**

Treatment

- **Total excision** of cyst wall is the treatment of choice.
- If the cyst is big and total excision is not possible, **marsupialisation** is done.

ORAL SUBMUCOUS FIBROSIS

- It is a **chronic insidious process** characterized by **juxta-epithelial deposition of fibrous tissue in the oral cavity and pharynx.**
- It is a **premalignant condition** and malignant transformation may be seen.

Aetiology

- Poor socioeconomic status.
- Tobacco chewing.
- Areca nut chewing.
- Alcohol.
- Deficiency of vitamin A, zinc and antioxidants.
- Immune mediated.

Pathogenesis

- It is considered a **cell-mediated immune reaction to arecoline in areca nuts.**
- It may also reflect a **localized collagen disorder or an autoimmune process in the oral cavity.**
- **Cytokines act on mesenchymal cells to produce fibrosis.**
- There is **upregulation of synthesis of collagen** and **downregulation of collagenase production** which further promotes **fibrosis.**

Clinical Features

- Mostly affects age group of 20–40 years.
- **Intolerance to chillies and spicy food.**
- Soreness of mouth with **constant burning sensation,** which worsens during meals.
- **Repeated vesicular eruption** on the palate and pillars.
- **Trismus**, i.e., difficulty to open the mouth fully.
- Trismus is progressive, so much so that patient may not be able to put his finger in the mouth or brush his teeth.
- **Difficulty to protrude the tongue.**
- Oral hygiene is affected badly and teeth become carious.
- There may be associated leukoplakia and squamous cell carcinoma.

On Examination

- In the initial stages, there is patchy redness of mucous membrane with formation of vesicles which rupture to form superficial ulcers.
- In later stages, when fibrosis develops in the submucosal layers, there is blanching of mucosa with loss of suppleness.
- Fibrotic bands can be seen and felt.

Treatment

Medical

- **Topical injection of steroids** into the affected area.
- It may be combined with **hyalase.**
- **Avoid irritant factors**, e.g., areca nuts, tobacco.
- **Treat existent anaemia or vitamin deficiencies.**
- **Encourage jaw opening exercises.**

Surgical

- It is **indicated in advanced cases to relieve trismus**
- **Various surgical techniques used are:**
  - o Simple release of fibrosis and skin grafting.
  - o Bilateral tongue flaps.
  - o Nasolabial flaps.
  - o Island palatal mucoperiosteal flap.
  - o Bilateral radial forearm free flap.
  - o Surgical excision and buccal fat pad graft.
  - o Superficial temporal fascia flap and split-skin graft.
  - o Coronoidectomy and temporal muscle myotomy.

25

Salivary Glands

[3] Classification of salivary gland tumours. *Dec 15*

WHO CLASSIFICATION OF SALIVARY GLAND NEOPLASMS

A. Malignant Epithelial Tumours

- Mucoepidermoid carcinoma.
- Acinic cell carcinoma.
- Adenoid cystic carcinoma.
- Polymorphous low-grade adenocarcinoma.
- Epithelial-myoepithelial carcinoma.

B. Benign Epithelial Tumours

- Pleomorphic adenoma.
- Warthin's tumour.
- Myoepithelioma.
- Basal cell adenoma.
- Ductal papillomas.
- Cystadenoma.

C. Soft Tissue Tumours

- Hemangioma.

D. Hematolymphoid Tumours

- Hodgkin's lymphoma.
- Diffuse large B-cell lymphoma.

E. Secondaries.

CLASSIFICATION OF SALIVARY GLAND TUMOURS

Based on Histological Grades

A. High Grade

- High grade mucoepidermoid carcinoma.
- Salivary duct carcinoma.
- Adenoid cystic carcinoma.
- Carcinoma ex pleomorphic adenoma.
- Squamous cell carcinoma.
- Anaplastic or undifferentiated carcinoma.
- Malignant mixed carcinoma.

B. Low to Intermediate Grades

- Low grade mucoepidermoid carcinoma.
- Acinic cell carcinoma.
- Polymorphous low-grade adenocarcinoma.
- Epithelial-myoepithelial carcinoma.

PAROTID GLAND

[10] Classify salivary gland tumours. Write about clinical features and management of mixed parotid tumour. *Dec 16*

[5] Mixed parotid tumour. *Sept 21*

[3] Pleomorphic adenoma. *Oct 20*

[5] Pleomorphic adenoma of parotid gland. *July 15*

[10] Classify parotid tumours. Discuss the clinical features and management of mixed parotid tumour. *July 15*

[10] Classify salivary tumours. Describe the etiology, pathogenesis, clinical features and management of pleomorphic adenoma. *July 23*

[10] Describe pathology, clinical features, investigations and treatment of pleomorphic adenoma. *March 24*

[5] Clinical features and management of pleomorphic adenoma. *CBME March 24*

- It is the **most common benign salivary gland tumour**.
- It is called **mixed tumour** as there is cartilage beside epithelial cells.

Site

- **Most commonly seen in parotid gland** (80%). Also seen in submandibular gland and hard palate.
- In the parotid gland, most tumours arise in the **superficial lobe in the tail of the gland.**

Aetiology

- **Radiation** exposure.
- **Viral infections.**
- Environmental and industrial exposure to **carcinogens**, e.g., rubber manufacturing, nickel compounds, hair dyes.

Clinical Features

- 20 to 60 years (average age is 45 years).
- F > M.
- **Painless** swelling.

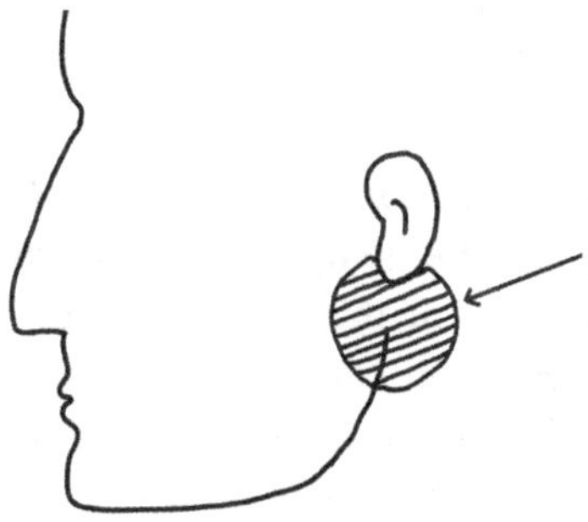

Figure 1: Pleomorphic adenoma

- **Location of swelling:**
  - o Superficial lobe tumours – below the ear, in front of the ear or in the upper aspect of the neck.
  - o Accessory lobe tumours – within the cheek.
  - o Deep lobe tumours – parapharyngeal mass, may present as a paratonsillar bulge.
- **Well defined, solitary, mobile mass.**
- **Slow growing** tumours with gradual progression over many years.
- Can reach enormous size.
- **Deep lobe parotid tumours may present with symptoms of difficulty in swallowing and snoring.**
- Can occasionally present as metachronous and synchronous tumours.
- If left untreated, ≤ 5% may become **malignant: called carcinoma ex pleomorphic adenoma** or malignant mixed tumours.

Symptoms of Malignant Transformation

- Sudden increase in size.
- Facial nerve palsy.

On Examination

- Parotid tumours may **obliterate the normal hollow just below the lobule of the ear.**
- **Surface** is usually **smooth** but can also be bosselated.
- Variable consistency.
- Bimanual examination is necessary to palpate the deep lobe.
- If tumour arises from the deep lobe, it **pushes the tonsils and the pillar of the fauces towards the midline.**

HPE

Gross Appearance:

- **Well circumscribed**, nodular, firm, mass which sometimes shows cartilaginous areas.
- **Marked morphological diversity with glandular areas, myxomatous areas and solid areas.**
- **Capsule is usually present** around the tumour but may be focally thin or absent in larger tumours.

Microscopic Appearance:

- It has **mixed epithelial, myoepithelial and stromal components.**
- They are called mixed tumours because of the **morphological and microscopic diversity.**

IHC

- Luminal cells – CK7.
- Myoepithelial cells – p63, S-100, SOX-10, SMA.

Investigations

1. **High frequency USG:**
    - It is an ideal tool for **examining the superficial lobe** of the parotid.
    - **Not useful if it involves deep lobe and when there is suspected involvement of skull base.**
    - Can also be used **to guide FNAC and core biopsies.**
    - Pleomorphic adenomas appear as **well defined and homogenous** lesions on USG. They are hypoechoic lesions with some calcifications.
2. **CT/MRI:**
    - Best tools for almost complete imaging of salivary glands as even the **deep lobe can be visualized.**
    - CT **can differentiate neoplasms from inflammatory conditions.**
    - **MRI**, especially, diffusion weighted MRI (DW-MRI) and Gadolinium enhanced dynamic MRI, can **differentiate between benign and malignant** lesions.
3. **FNAC:**
    - Often done under USG guidance.
    - Can differentiate between inflammatory, benign and malignant lesions.
    - **Milan system** is an effective tool to assess the adequacy of the cytopathology specimen and quantify the risk of malignancy.
4. **Core needle biopsy:**
    - It is a more invasive procedure than FNAC and is reserved as a supplement to FNAC for problem solving.

Treatment

- Because of the risk of malignant transformation, **surgical excision** is always advised.
- The choice of surgery depends on the following factors:
    - o Relation to the facial nerve plane (called Patey's faciovenous plane).
    - o Location of the tumour (superficial or deep lobe of the parotid).

The types of surgery done, are as follows:

A. Traditional Methods

1. **Superficial parotidectomy:**
    - Means removal of all the parotid gland superficial to the facial nerve.
2. **Partial superficial parotidectomy:**
    - Can be done in relatively small tumours.
    - The tumour is removed with a cuff of clinically normal parenchyma without removal of the entire superficial portion of the gland.
    - Cuff is removed all around the tumour, except where the tumour abuts the facial nerve.

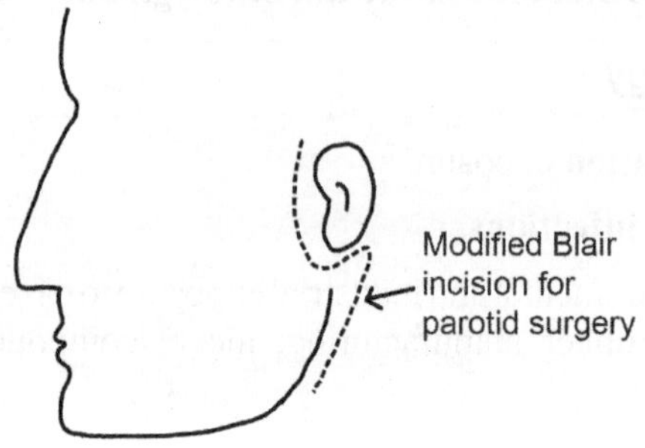

Figure 2: Modified Blair incision for parotid surgery

3. **Total conservative parotidectomy:**
    - Facial nerve is preserved.
    - Indicated in tumours where both lobes are involved, with the tumour straddling the superficial and deep lobes across the Patey's plane.
    - **Superficial lobe is removed + deep lobe is dissected off the temporal veins and terminal branches of the external carotid artery.** This results in complete removal of the suprafacial and subfacial parotid gland with preservation of the facial nerve.

4. **Radical parotidectomy:**
   - Facial nerve is sacrificed.
   - The facial nerve is excised en bloc with the tumour.
   - **Structures removed:** All parotid gland tissue + elective division of the involved facial nerve branches + structures involved (most commonly the masseter muscle).

B. Newer Methods

- Today, with a focus towards reducing morbidity and preserving gland function, variations of parotidectomy have evolved in the management of benign tumours of the parotid gland.

1. **Extra Capsular Dissection (ECD):**
   - In contrast to traditional methods which are basically dissection of the facial nerve, ECD focuses on the tumour itself as the principal procedure and not on facial nerve dissection.
   - **Since it does not require formal facial nerve dissection, it is a less invasive technique with reduced morbidity.**
   - This is a technically demanding procedure which requires the tumour to be mobile and large enough to allow digital manipulation.
2. **Adequate parotidectomy:**
   - Involves **removal of the tumour with a cuff of normal tissue in the tail of parotid lesions, preserving function.**
   - It may not be possible to excise the tumour with a cuff of normal tissue in all the cases, especially when the lump is abutting the facial nerve.
3. **Deep lobe parotidectomy:**
   - Deep lobe parotid tumours can be removed, preserving the entire superficial parotid gland, which is functional as well as cosmetic.

Enucleation

- May result in capsular breach and tumour spillage, increasing the possibility of local recurrence and should therefore be avoided.

[5] Warthin's tumour. *Dec 12*

- Also known as **adenolymphoma, papillary cystadenoma lymphomatosum.**
- It is the **second most common benign tumour of salivary glands.**
- It is **composed of oncocytic epithelial cells lining ductal, papillary and cystic spaces in a reactive lymphoid tissue.**

Cause

- Cigarette smoking.
- Radiation exposure.

Site

- Almost **exclusively seen in the parotid gland,** especially in the inferior pole, i.e., **tail of parotid gland.**
- Is also rarely seen in the **periparotid nodes.**
- Can occur **synchronously** or **metachronously** in the same or bilateral glands.
- May also occur **concurrently with other salivary gland neoplasms** such as pleomorphic adenoma and salivary duct carcinoma.

HPE

- Tumours have papillary and cystic structures lined by **bilayered oncocytic epithelial cells, in a lymphoid stroma with germinal centres.**
- Epithelium may show **metaplastic changes,** including squamous, sebaceous, ciliated and mucous cells.

Clinical Features

- Age > 60 years.
- M > F.
- Present as **painless, slow growing** swellings.
- The abundant **lymphoid tissue** in these tumours is **susceptible to acute inflammation.** Such inflammation may be preceded by an upper respiratory tract infection. This may lead to **marked swelling, tenderness and even ulceration** of the tumour.

On Examination

- **Multilobulated or multifocal** tumours on palpation.
- Is **soft or fluctuant in consistency,** but can also be firm depending on the extent of previous inflammation.

Investigations

- High frequency USG.
- CT/MRI.
- FNAC.
- Core needle biopsy.

Treatment

- **Simple excision** via **partial superficial parotidectomy.**
- **In elderly males with significant medical comorbidities, observation alone** is reasonable management. This is because malignant transformation is extremely rare.

[3] Mention complications of parotid gland surgery. *Dec 12*

[3] Complications of superficial parotidectomy. *CBME June 24*

1. **Hematoma formation:**
   - Uncommon.
   - Usually preventable with appropriate intra-operative hemostasis.
   - Small hematomas usually resolve without intervention.
   - Large hematoma suggests a possible bleeding diathesis that requires appropriate management and evacuation of the hematoma.
2. **Infection:**
   - Rare, because parotidectomy is a clean operation.
   - Post-op management of drains following aseptic precautions and their timely removal decreases the risk of infection.
3. **Deformity:**
   - Unsightly scar and retromandibular hollowing.
   - Hollowing of retromandibular area can be reduced with autologous fat grafts, which can be placed at the time of primary surgery.
4. **Temporary facial nerve weakness:**
   - Commonly seen in the lower branches, especially the marginal mandibular nerve.
   - Most patients tend to recover over time.
   - When the zygomaticotemporal division is affected, eye care is essential to protect the cornea.
5. **Transection of the facial nerve and permanent facial nerve weakness.**
6. **Sialocele:**
   - Cyst like structure that contains saliva.
   - Preventable by under-running the capsule, where possible, to avoid exposure of the main acinar ductal system.
   - **Treatment:**
     - o Anticholinergics to reduce salivary secretion.
     - o Aspiration.
     - o Pressure dressings.
     - o Long-standing salivary fistulae may require low dose radiation.
7. **Facial numbness.**
8. **Permanent numbness of the ear lobe associated with great auricular nerve transection.**
9. **Frey's syndrome.**

FREY'S SYNDROME

- Also known as gustatory sweating.

Aetiopathogenesis

- It is an inevitable consequence of parotidectomy, unless preventive measures are taken.
- It results from **damage to the autonomic innervation of the salivary gland with inappropriate regeneration of postganglionic parasympathetic nerve fibers of the auriculotemporal nerve.**
- This results in **cross innervation of the dermal sweat glands (of the overlying skin).**
- Even though it occurs in most patients, it is often not significant and patients rarely mention it, unless it is excessive.

Clinical Features

- **Sweating and flushing in the pre auricular region during meals.**
- Whenever there is parasympathetic stimulation of salivation by the smell or taste of food, there is sweating and flushing.

Investigations

- **Minor's starch iodine test:**
  - o Identifies the region affected.
  - o Iodine is painted in the preauricular region, dried and covered with starch.
  - o Salivary stimulation causes **sweating, which turns the starch blue**.

Prevention

1. By raising a **thick flap with all subcutaneous fat** over the parotid.
2. By **interposition of tissue** such as a sternocleidomastoid muscle flap, temporalis fascia flap, allodermal tissue or autologous fat between the skin and the surgical bed.
3. **Insertion of artificial membranes** between the skin and the surgical bed.
4. Incidence can be **reduced by extra capsular dissection** and careful closure of the superficial musculoaponeurotic system.

Treatment

- **Mild cases:**
  - o Anti-perspirants (usually containing aluminum chlorohydrate).
- **Severe cases:**
  - o Tympanic neurectomy.
  - o BOTOX injection at the site of perspiration.

[3] Ranula. ***Oct 20, Dec 17, March 24***
[5] Define ranula. What are the clinical features? How do you treat the same? ***CBME June 24***

- Ranula is an **extravasation cyst** arising from a damaged **sublingual salivary gland**.
- It is called ranula because it **resembles the belly of a frog** (*Tigris rana*).

Aetiology

1. Rupture of the main duct of sublingual gland.
2. Rupture of obstructed acini of sublingual gland.

Pathology

- It is **not a true cyst**.
- Wall is composed of a delicate capsule of fibrous tissue and is lined by a layer of macrophages.
- Contains clear ropy fluid or jelly like fluid which resembles thick sticky saliva.

Clinical Features

- Characteristic **bluish swelling** in the anterior floor of the mouth.
- May complain of **difficulty in speech and mastication** (depending on the size).
- Usually painless, unless infected.

On Examination

- Brilliantly transilluminant.
- Fluctuation test is positive.
- Overlying mucous membrane can be moved over the swelling.
- Cyst itself can be moved over the underlying structures, but such mobility is restricted due to lack of surrounding space.

Investigations

- MRI helps to corroborate the clinical diagnosis.
- Aspiration yields the thick sticky saliva that distinguishes it from a lymphangioma.

Treatment

- **Excision** of the sublingual gland as this gland has multiple ducts and ranula can recur if the gland is left behind.
- Local **injection of OK-432** produces inflammation and fibrosis.
- Local injection of **BOTOX.**
- Incision, drainage and **marsupialization** have low success rates.

[3] Plunging ranula. ***March 21***
[5] Plunging ranula. ***July 15***

- Deep or plunging ranula.

- When the intrabuccal ranula has a cervical prolongation, it is called deep or plunging ranula.

Causes

- The buccal ranula insinuates through the mylohyoid muscle to present as a submental swelling.
- Mucus may escape from a posterior sublingual gland and may flow over the posterior margin of the mylohyoid and down into the neck to form a plunging ranula.

Clinical Features

- **Dumb-bell shaped swelling** in the submandibular or submental region of the neck:
  - o Painless.
  - o Soft on palpation.
  - o Bidigital palpation helps elicit cross fluctuation.

Diagnosis

- Made on USG or MRI, but confirmed by aspirating thick yellow treacly fluid from the cyst.

Treatment

- **Excision of sublingual gland + aspiration of the saliva out of the sac.** The sac is formed of connective tissue, not epithelium, so it melts away once the leak of saliva is resolved.
- A cervical approach is contraindicated.

26

Thyroid and Parathyroid Glands

[3] Thyroglossal cyst. *Sept 21, Dec 16, Feb 23*

[5] Thyroglossal cyst. *July 15, Dec 13*

- It is the **most commonly encountered congenital cervical anomaly.**

Cause/Embryology

- The thyroid gland descends early in fetal life from the base of the tongue towards its position in the lower neck with the isthmus of the thyroid gland lying over the 2nd and 3rd tracheal rings.
- At the time of its descent, the hyoid bone has not been formed and the track of the descent of the thyroid gland is variable; passing in front, through or behind the eventual position of the hyoid body.
- Thyroglossal duct cysts **represent a persistence of this track** and may therefore be found anywhere in or adjacent to the midline from the tongue base to the thyroid isthmus.

Clinical Features

- Almost always arises in the midline, but, when they are adjacent to the thyroid cartilage, they may lie slightly to one side of the midline.
- Moves upwards on swallowing and with protrusion of the tongue.
- May become infected and rupture onto the skin of the neck, presenting as a discharging sinus.
- More common in children, but may also be seen in adults, even as late as 50 - 70 years.

Investigations

- USG neck.
- Thyroid scintigraphy.
- Both tests are used to confirm the presence of a thyroglossal cyst and the presence of a thyroid gland in the normal location.

Treatment

- **Sistrunk's operation:** Excision of the whole thyroglossal tract.
- It involves removal of hyoid bone and the suprahyoid tract through the tongue base to the vallecula at the site of the primitive foramen cecum, together with a core of tissue on either side.

[5] Lingual thyroid. *March 24*

- A lingual thyroid is a condition where the thyroid gland fails to descend to its normal position in the neck during fetal development and instead remains at the **base of the tongue.**

Embryology

- A lingual thyroid represents a **failure of the median thyroid anlage to descend normally.**
- It **may be the only thyroid tissue present.**

Clinical Features

- Asymptomatic/incidental finding.

- Swelling at posterior part of the tongue.
- **Obstructive symptoms:**
  - o Choking.
  - o Dysphagia.
  - o Airway obstruction.
- Hemorrhage.
- Difficulty in speaking.
- Many of these patients develop hypothyroidism.

Investigations

- **Thyroid function tests:** May show the presence of hypothyroidism.
- **USG of neck:** Is used to see whether thyroid tissue is present in the neck or not.
- **Radionuclide imaging:** Technetium Tc 99m pertechnetate (^{99m}Tc) is taken up by the thyroid gland and is therefore used to localise an ectopic (e.g., lingual) thyroid.
- **FNAC:** Used to confirm if the swelling at the base of tongue is thyroid tissue or not.

Treatment

A. Medical Treatment

- Administration of exogenous thyroid hormone to suppress thyroid-stimulating hormone (TSH).
- Radioactive iodine (RAI) ablation, followed by hormone replacement.

B. Surgery

- Surgical excision is rarely needed.
- **Indications:** Obstructive symptoms, hemorrhage.
- If required, it should be preceded by an evaluation of normal thyroid tissue in the neck to avoid inadvertently rendering the patient hypothyroid (in case lingual thyroid is the only thyroid tissue present).

[10] Discuss the aetiology, clinical features, investigations and treatment of primary thyrotoxicosis. *March 22*

- Primary hyperthyroidism is also called **Graves' disease** or **diffuse toxic goitre.**
- Graves' disease is a **diffuse vascular goitre which appears at the same time as hyperthyroidism**, is **autoimmune**, mostly occurs in **younger women** and is frequently **associated with eye signs.**

Aetiology

- It is an **autoimmune disease.**
- Strong **family history.**
- **Genetic factors:**
  - o **HLA haplotypes: HLA-B8, DR3.**
  - o CTLA-4 gene.
  - o **CD40** is a Graves' susceptibility gene.
- Associated with other autoimmune conditions such as type 1 diabetes mellitus, Addison's disease, pernicious anemia and myasthenia gravis.

Pathogenesis

Initiation or **triggers**, e.g., postpartum state, iodine excess, lithium therapy, bacterial and viral infections

↓

Sensitised T-helper lymphocytes stimulate B-lymphocytes

↓

Production of **autoantibodies directed against the thyroid hormone receptor**
TSI or thyroid stimulating immunoglobulins stimulate the TSH receptors (TSH-RAb)

↓

Whole of functioning thyroid tissue is involved, i.e., there is diffuse hypertrophy and hyperplasia

↓

Thyrocytes grow and synthesize excess thyroid hormones

↓

Primary thyrotoxicosis

Clinical Features

- Peak incidence is between 40 and 60 years of age.
- F : M = 5 : 1.
- The clinical manifestations of Graves' disease can be divided into those related to hyperthyroidism and those specific to Graves'.

A. Symptoms Related to Hyperthyroidism

- Heat intolerance.
- Increased sweating and thirst.
- Weight loss despite adequate calorie intake.
- Symptoms of increased adrenergic stimulation include palpitations, nervousness, fatigue, emotional lability, hyperkinesis and tremors.

- Increased frequency of bowel movements and diarrhea.
- Female patients often develop amenorrhea, decreased fertility and an increased incidence of miscarriages.
- Children experience rapid growth with early bone maturation.
- Older patients may present with cardiovascular complications such as atrial fibrillation and congestive heart failure.

B. Symptoms Specific to Graves' Disease

- **Graves' Ophthalmopathy:**
  - o **Von Graefe's lid lag sign:** Upper eyelid lags behind the eyeball as patient is asked to look downwards.
  - o **Dalrymple's revealing sign:** Spasm of upper eyelid revealing sclera above the corneo-scleral limbus.
  - o **Stellwag's staring sign:** Staring look and infrequent blinking of eyes.
  - o **Joffroy's wrinkling sign:** Absence of wrinkling on forehead when patient looks upwards with face inclined downwards.
  - o **Moebius sign:** Inability or failure to converge the eyeballs.
  - o **True infiltrative eye disease:** Periorbital edema, conjunctival swelling and congestion (chemosis), proptosis, limitation of upward and lateral gaze, keratitis, blindness due to optic nerve involvement.
- **Dermopathy:** Thickened skin in pretibial region and dorsum of foot.
- Bony involvement is rare and leads to sub-periosteal bone formation and swelling in the metacarpals, called thyroid acropachy.
- Gynecomastia in young men.
- Onycholysis or separation of finger nails from their beds.

On Examination

- Thyroid gland is **diffusely and symmetrically enlarged**, as evidenced by an enlarged pyramidal lobe.
- Overlying bruit or thrill over the thyroid gland.
- Loud venous hum in supraclavicular space.

GPE

- Tachycardia.
- Atrial fibrillation.
- Widening of pulse pressure.
- **Collapsing pulse:** Rapid fall off in transmitted pulse wave.
- Fine tremors.
- Muscle wasting.
- Proximal muscle group weakness with hyperactive tendon reflexes.

Investigations

1. **Thyroid Function Tests:**
   - Low TSH with or without an elevated free T4 or T3 level.
   - If eye signs are present, other tests are generally not needed.
2. **Iodine^{123} uptake and scan (Radioactive Iodine uptake and scan):**
   - An elevated uptake, with a diffusely enlarged gland, confirms the diagnosis of Graves' disease and helps to differentiate it from other causes of hyperthyroidism.
3. **Technetium scintigraphy:**
   - Using pertechnetate, which is trapped by the thyroid, but not organified.
   - Can be used to determine etiology instead of RAI.
4. **TSH-R or TSAb:**
   - Elevated TSH receptor or Thyroid Stimulating antibodies are diagnostic of Graves' disease.
5. **Anti Tg and anti TPO antibodies** are elevated but are not specific.
6. **CT or MRI scans of the orbits** are useful in evaluating Graves' ophthalmopathy.
7. **USG neck** allows assessment of the thyroid gland.

Treatment

- Non-specific measures are rest and sedation and in established thyrotoxicosis should be used only in conjunction with specific measures, i.e., the use of anti-thyroid drugs, surgery and radioiodine.

A. **Anti-Thyroid Drugs**

- Carbimazole, propylthiouracil are commonly used.
- **Used to restore the patient to a euthyroid state and to maintain this for a prolonged period in the hope that a permanent remission will occur**, i.e., that production of TSH-R Ab will diminish or cease.
- The overactive thyroid tissue is autonomous and recurrence of the hyperthyroidism is certain when the drug is discontinued.
- Therefore, these drugs are generally administered in preparation for surgery.

B. **Radioactive Iodine Therapy - I^{131}**

- Destroys thyroid cells and reduces the mass of functioning thyroid tissue to below a critical level.
- **Advantages:**
  - o No surgery.
  - o No prolonged drug therapy.
- **Disadvantages:**
  - o Isotope facilities must be available.
  - o Patient must be quarantined while radiation levels are high and avoid pregnancy and close physical contact, particularly with children.
  - o Eye signs may be aggravated.

C. **Surgery**

- Surgery cures by reducing the mass of overactive tissue by reducing the thyroid below a critical mass.
- **Extent of thyroidectomy performed is determined by the desired outcome** (risk of recurrence v/s euthyroidism) and surgeon experience.
- **Total or near-total thyroidectomy is the procedure of choice** for the surgical management of Graves' disease.
- Surgery may result in a reduction in TSH-R Ab.

[5] Secondary thyrotoxicosis. *June 13*

- Secondary thyrotoxicosis is also known as toxic nodular goitre.
- Secondary thyrotoxicosis is when **a simple nodular goitre is usually present for a long time before hyperthyroidism sets in.**
- It is very rarely associated with eye signs.

Aetiopathogenesis

- Usually **occurs in older individuals**, who often have a prior history of a non-toxic multinodular goitre.
- **Over several years, one or more thyroid nodules become overactive and the hyperthyroidism is due to autonomous thyroid tissue (called toxic adenoma).**
- In many cases of toxic nodular goitre, the **nodules are inactive, and it is the internodular thyroid tissue that is overactive.**

Clinical Features

- Occur in middle aged or elderly.
- Patient gives a history of a non-toxic/simple multi-nodular goitre.
- Presentation is insidious.
- Symptoms and signs of hyperthyroidism are similar to Graves' disease, but extrathyroidal manifestations are absent.
- **Cardiovascular system is involved:**
  - o Atrial fibrillation.
  - o Congestive heart failure.
- **Hyperthyroidism can also be precipitated by iodide containing drugs such as contrast media and the anti-arrhythmic agent amiodarone (Jod-Basedow phenomenon).**

Investigations

1. **Thyroid Function Tests:**
   - Low TSH with or without an elevated free T4 or T3 level.
2. **Iodine^{123} uptake:**
   - Shows multiple nodules with increased uptake and suppression of the remaining gland.
3. **USG neck:**
   - Allows assessment of the thyroid gland.

Treatment

1. **Anti-thyroid drugs:**
   - Carbimazole and propylthiouracil are commonly used.

- Hyperthyroidism must be adequately controlled before going for definitive treatment in the form of radioactive iodine or surgical resection.

2. **Surgery:**
   - Near total or total thyroidectomy is recommended to avoid recurrence and the consequent increased complication rates with repeat surgery.
3. **Radioactive Iodine – Iodine[131]**
   - **Indications:**
     - o Elderly patients who represent very poor operative risks.
     - o No airway compression from the goitre.
     - o Thyroid cancer is not a concern.
   - **Drawbacks:** Requires larger doses than in Graves' disease.

[10] 40-year-old lady presents with swelling in the front of the neck of 10 years duration, gradually increasing in size: ***CBME March 24***
A. List the differential diagnosis
B. Symptoms of hyperthyroidism
C. Complications of multinodular goitre
D. Investigations for multinodular goitre

DIFFERENTIAL DIAGNOSIS OF SWELLINGS WHICH MOVE WITH DEGLUTITION

- Swellings in the front of the neck which are fixed to the larynx or trachea move with deglutition:
  - o Thyroid swellings.
  - o Thyroglossal cysts.
  - o Subhyoid bursitis.
  - o Pre or para-tracheal lymph node enlargement.

DIFFERENTIAL DIAGNOSIS OF THYROID SWELLINGS

A. **Simple Goitre (Euthyroid)**
   a. **Diffuse hyperplastic:**
      - Physiological.
      - Pubertal.
      - Pregnancy.
   b. **Multinodular goitre.**
B. **Toxic Goitre**
   a. **Diffuse (Graves' disease).**
   b. **Multinodular goitre.**
   c. **Toxic adenoma.**
C. **Neoplastic**
   a. **Benign:**
      - Follicular adenoma.
   b. **Malignant:**
      - Papillary thyroid carcinoma.
      - Medullary thyroid carcinoma.
      - Follicular thyroid carcinoma.
      - Anaplastic carcinoma.
      - Lymphoma.
      - Secondaries.
D. **Inflammatory**
   a. **Autoimmune:**
      - Chronic lymphocytic thyroiditis.
      - Hashimoto's disease.
   b. **Granulomatous:**
      - de Quervain's thyroiditis.

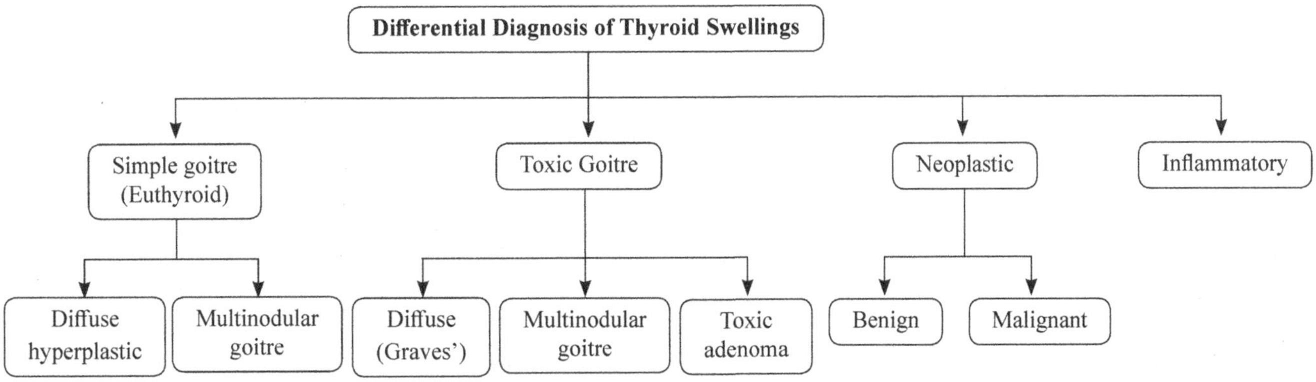

c. **Fibrosing:**
   - Riedel's thyroiditis.

d. **Infective:**
   - Acute (bacterial thyroiditis, viral thyroiditis, 'subacute thyroiditis').
   - Chronic (tuberculous, syphilitic).

e. **Others:**
   - Amyloid.

MULTINODULAR GOITRE

Aetiology

- **Simple goitre develops as a result of stimulation of the thyroid gland by TSH:**
  - o Due to increased secretion from a microadenoma in the anterior pituitary.
  - o In response to a chronically low level of circulating thyroid hormones.
- **Endemic Goitre:**
  - o Most important factor is dietary deficiency of iodine.
  - o Low iodide content in water and food, e.g., Himalayan region.
  - o Defective iodine absorption by intestines.
- **Sporadic Goitre:**
  - o Defective hormone synthesis (dyshormonogenesis) due to enzyme deficiencies.
  - o Genetic defect/family history.
- **Goitrogens:**
  - o Vegetables of brassica family (cabbage, kale, rape).
  - o **Drugs:** Para-aminosalicylic acid (PAS), anti-thyroid drugs.
  - o Iodides in large quantity (Wolff-Chaikoff effect).
- The heterogeneous structural and functional response in the thyroid resulting in characteristic nodularity may be due to the presence of clones of cells particularly sensitive to growth stimulation.

Natural History of Simple Goitre

- The stages in goitre formation are:

  a. Persistent growth stimulation causes **diffuse hyperplasia**; all lobules are composed of active follicles and iodine uptake is uniform. This is a diffuse hyperplastic goitre, which may persist but is reversible if stimulation ceases.

  b. Later, as a result of fluctuating stimulation, a **mixed pattern** develops with areas of **active** lobules **and** areas of **inactive lobules.**

  c. Active lobules become more vascular and hyperplastic until hemorrhage occurs, causing **central necrosis** and leaving only a **surrounding rind of active follicles.**

  d. **Necrotic lobules coalesce to form nodules** filled either with iodine-free colloid or a mass of new but inactive follicles.

  e, **Continual repetition** of this process **results in a nodular goitre**. Most nodules are inactive, and active follicles are present only in the internodular tissue.

Pathology

- Multinodular goitre is a **type of simple goitre.**
- As the name suggests, multiple nodules form a multinodular goitre.
- **Occasionally, only one macroscopic nodule is found**, but microscopic changes will be present throughout the gland; this is one form of a clinically solitary nodule.
- **Nodules may be colloid or cellular.**
- Cystic degeneration and hemorrhage are common, as is subsequent calcification.

Clinical Features

- Nodules **appear early in endemic goitre** (10-20 years) and **later** (20-30 years) **in sporadic goitre**, although the patient may be unaware till 40-60 years of age.
- F > M.
- Patient is euthyroid.
- Painless.
- Usual complaint is of cosmesis.
- **Compression Symptoms:**
  - o Trachea – dyspnoea.
  - o Esophagus – dysphagia.
  - o Recurrent laryngeal nerve – hoarseness of voice.

On Examination

- Nodules are palpable and often visible.
- Smooth.
- Usually firm in consistency.
- Non-tender.
- Moves with deglutition.
- Sometimes, it may be hard and irregular (due to calcification); in such cases it may simulate a carcinoma.
- A painful nodule, sudden appearance or rapid enlargement of a nodule raises suspicion of carcinoma but is usually due to hemorrhage into a simple nodule.

Complications

1. **Tracheal obstruction:**
   - Due to gross lateral displacement, or compression by retrosternal extension of the goitre.
   - Acute respiratory obstruction may be because of hemorrhage into a nodule impacted in the thoracic inlet.
2. **Secondary thyrotoxicosis:**
   - Transient episodes of mild hyperthyroidism are common.
3. **Carcinoma:**
   - An increased incidence of cancer (usually follicular) has been reported from endemic areas.
   - Dominant or rapidly growing nodules in longstanding goitres should always be subjected to FNAC.

Investigations

1. **Thyroid Function Tests:**
   - To exclude hyperthyroidism.
2. **Thyroid antibodies:**
   - Tested to differentiate from autoimmune thyroiditis.
3. **Ultrasonography:**
   - Gold standard assessment.
   - Gland substance as well as thyroid nodules can be assessed.
   - Number, size, shape, margins, vascularity, microcalcifications can be used to predict the risk of malignancy within a specific nodule.
4. **FNAC:**
   - Only required for a nodule within the goitre that demonstrates ultrasonographic features of concern.
   - It may or may not be the largest 'dominant' nodule.
   - Performed under ultrasound guidance to ensure that the correct nodule is sampled.
5. **CT scan of the chest and neck:**
   - To assess tracheal or oesophageal deviation or compression, if there are swallowing or breathing symptoms.
   - To assess a retrosternal goitre.

Prevention

- In endemic areas, goitre has been reduced by the introduction of **iodised salt.**

Treatment

- Most patients are asymptomatic and do not require operation.
- **Indications of surgery:**
  - o Features of **underlying malignancy.**
  - o For **pressure symptoms**, e.g., tracheal compression.
  - o For **cosmetic reasons.**
- Risks and benefits of surgery should be considered, as most patients are elderly and the goitre grows slowly.
- **Surgical options:**
  1. **Total thyroidectomy** with immediate and lifelong replacement of thyroxine.
  2. Some form of **partial resection**, e.g., subtotal thyroidectomy.
- Most surgeons favour **total thyroidectomy in** the setting of **bilateral disease.**

- If it is **asymmetrical** with one lobe more significantly involved than the other, particularly in older patients, **total lobectomy of the more affected side** is done.
- **Total lobectomy of more affected lobe + subtotal resection of c/l lobe (Dunhill procedure)** is also an option in asymmetrical disease.

[5] Retrosternal goitre. *Dec 12*

- A goitre which extends inferiorly, posterior to the sternum is called a retrosternal goitre.
- It may or may not extend into the mediastinum.

Aetiopathogenesis

- Most retrosternal goitres arise from the lower pole of a nodular goitre.
- If the neck is short and the pretracheal muscles are strong, as in men, the negative intrathoracic pressure tends to draw these nodules into the superior mediastinum.
- Very few retrosternal goitres arise from ectopic thyroid tissue.
- It can also arise from the slow growth of a multinodular gland down into the mediastinum.

Clinical Features

- Often asymptomatic and discovered incidentally.
- Dyspnea, cough and stridor (due to compression of trachea).
- Dysphagia (due to compression of esophagus).
- Engorgement of neck veins and superficial veins on the chest wall.
- In severe cases, there may be obstruction of the superior vena cava.
- Paralysis of recurrent laryngeal nerve.
- It may be malignant.
- It may be toxic.

Investigations

- **CT chest and CT neck:**
    - o Performed in the surgical position, i.e., arms down and neck extended.
- Thyroid Function Tests.

Treatment

- Elderly patients with incidentally detected retrosternal goitre can be observed.
- Treatment of choice is total thyroidectomy.
- **Indications for surgery are:**
    1. Significant airway compression.
    2. Symptomatic patients.
    3. Young patients in whom symptoms are likely to develop.
- Vast majority of retrosternal goitres can be removed transcervically (> 95%).
- **Indications of joint treatment with thoracic surgery:**
    - o Malignancy.
    - o Patients undergoing revision surgery.
    - o Goitres extending into posterior mediastinum.
    - o Diameter of goitre > diameter of thoracic inlet.
    - o Immobile and fixed gland.

[10] Classify thyroid neoplasms and describe in detail about papillary carcinoma of thyroid. *Dec 17*

CLASSIFICATION OF THYROID NEOPLASMS

A. Benign

- Follicular adenoma.

B. Malignant

1. **Primary:**
    a. Differentiated follicular epithelium:
        - o Follicular thyroid carcinoma.
        - o Papillary thyroid carcinoma.
    b. Poorly differentiated follicular epithelium:
        - o Anaplastic carcinoma.
    c. Parafollicular cells:
        - o Medullary thyroid carcinoma.
    d. Lymphoid cells.
        - o Lymphoma
2. **Secondary:**
    - Metastatic.
    - Local infiltration.

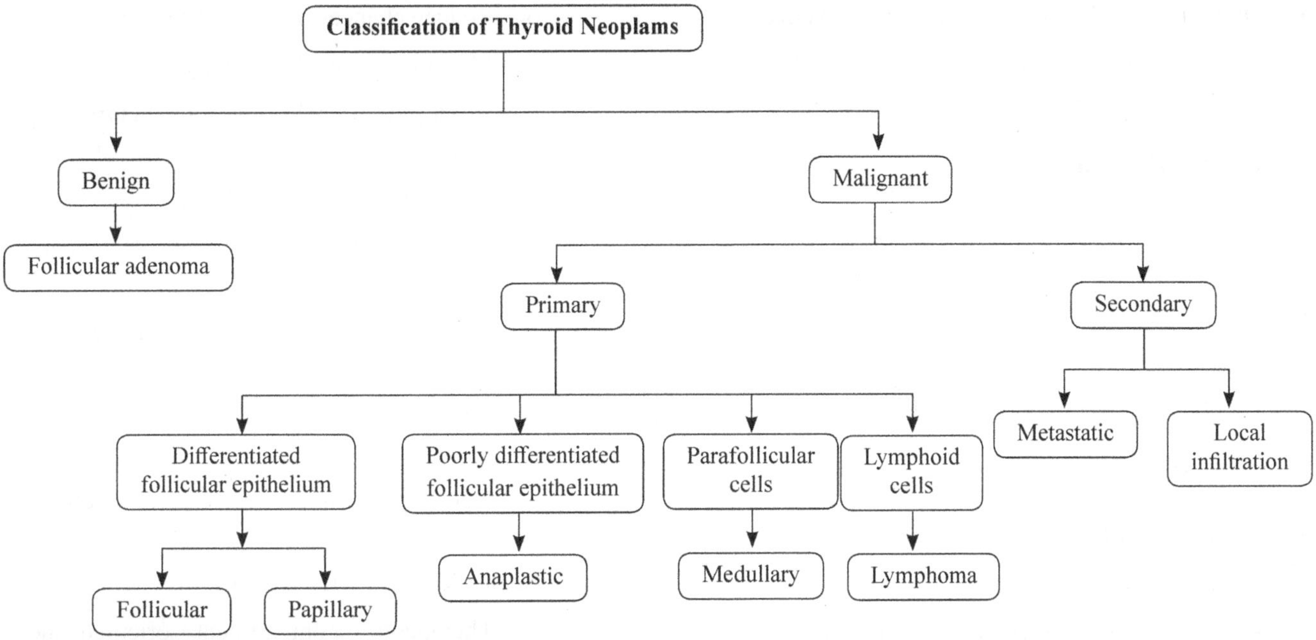

[10] Draw and illustrate the triangles of neck. Discuss the clinical features, presentation and management of Papillary Thyroid Carcinoma. ***June 14***

[5] Papillary carcinoma of thyroid. ***March 22***

[5] Enumerate clinical features and management of papillary thyroid carcinoma. ***CBME June 24***

PAPILLARY THYROID CARCINOMA

- It is the most common malignancy of the thyroid gland.
- Papillary thyroid carcinoma is differentiated cancer of the follicular epithelium of the thyroid gland.

Aetiology

- **Irradiation of the thyroid under 5 years of age:**
  - o It is the most common thyroid cancer in individuals exposed to external radiation.
- **Genetic basis:**
  - o ret/PTC3, ret/PTC1 oncogene.
- **Idiopathic:**
  - o Great majority of thyroid cancers have no known aetiological factor.

Clinical Features

- F > M = 2:1.
- 30-40 years.
- Incidence is increasing rapidly across the world due to increased rates of imaging, detecting previously occult disease.
- It is common in areas which are sufficient in iodine.
- Most common presenting symptom is a thyroid swelling (goitre).
- May also present with enlarged cervical lymph nodes.
- History of being exposed to radiation in childhood.
- Pain, often referred to the ear, suggests nerve involvement from infiltrating tumours.
- Recurrent laryngeal nerve paralysis suggests locally advanced disease.
- Spreads via lymph.
- Organs in which mets are seen : lungs > bone > liver > brain.
- Mets in the bone are osteolytic.
- But, distant mets are uncommon.
- Multiple foci may occur in the same lobe as the primary tumour or, less commonly, in both lobes. This is due to:
  - o Lymphatic spread in the rich intrathyroidal lymph plexus.
  - o Multicentric growth.
- It has a high rate of occult micro-mets.

On Examination

- Firm and irregular.

- Often indistinguishable from a benign swelling.
- Small papillary tumours may be impalpable, even when lymphatic mets are present.

High Risk Patients

- Older patients.
- Large tumours.
- Extrathyroidal extension.
- Distant mets.
- Cervical mets (particularly in lateral neck).

Investigations

1. **Ultrasound of the neck:**
   - Most accurate at assessment of thyroid swellings.
   - Gives information on the presence, size and number of thyroid nodules.
   - Can detect metastatic lymph nodes in the neck.
   - TIRADS (Thyroid Imaging Reporting and Data System) estimates the risk of malignancy.
2. **FNAC.**
3. **Radioiodine uptake scan:**
   - Indicated in thyrotoxic patients.
   - Used to assess the function of a nodule:
     - o Hot nodule - very rarely malignant.
     - o Cold nodule - has a higher chance of being malignant.
4. **CECT neck and chest:**
   - Its indications are:
     - o Patients with widespread nodal disease.
     - o Suspicion of locally invasive disease affecting the airway.
   - Accurately assesses visceral invasion.
   - Detects disease in mediastinum and thorax.

Treatment

A. Surgery

- **The aims of surgery are:**
  - o Remove macroscopic disease.
  - o Reduce chances of recurrence.
  - o Minimise surgical morbidity.

a. High risk patients with nodal or distant metastases:

- Total thyroidectomy is done.
- Total thyroidectomy also prepares the patient for radioactive iodine.

b. Low risk patients with single focus of disease limited to thyroid:

- Lobectomy is done.
- It has the advantage of protecting the c/l recurrent laryngeal nerve and parathyroid glands.

c. Neck metastases are present:

- Therapeutic compartment oriented neck dissection, i.e., central or lateral neck dissection, depending on site of involvement.

d. No neck mets:

- Elective central neck dissection.
- Recommended in patients who are considered at highest risk of having occult mets in the central neck (e.g., extrathyroid extension).
- Not recommended routinely in low risk patients.
- Elective lateral neck dissection has significant morbidity and despite there being high rates of occult mets in papillary thyroid carcinoma, it has been abandoned.

e. Incidentally detected papillary carcinoma:

- i.e., thyroid surgery was done for a different reason and papillary carcinoma was detected on HPE.
  - i. **Low risk patients:**
    - o Further surgery is unlikely to be beneficial.
    - o Active surveillance is therefore recommended.
  - ii. **High risk patients (younger patients with larger tumours):**
    - – Radioactive iodine may be recommended, in which case, completion thyroidectomy may be required.

B. Thyroxine

- After surgery, thyroid cells (both normal and malignant) are suppressed using high doses of thyroxine.
- **High risk patients:** Thyroxine is prescribed at levels that suppress TSH without making the patient biochemically hyperthyroid.
- **Low risk patients:** Thyroxine is prescribed at physiological levels.
- Side effects of long-term TSH suppression are cardiac arrhythmias and osteoporosis.

C. Radioactive Iodine (I^{131})

- It is rarely indicated in low risk cases.
- Used almost universally in high risk cases.
- It is given to deliver tumoricidal doses of radioactivity directly to thyroid tissue, both benign and malignant.
- Total thyroidectomy and neck dissection should be done first in order for any residual microscopic disease or distant metastases to receive an optimal dose.
- It is not an alternative to surgical resection for resectable disease.
- Thyroglobulin, which is a post-op tumour marker for papillary thyroid cancer, decreases after treatment with radio-iodine.

TRIANGLES OF NECK

- The neck is divided into anterior and posterior triangles by the sternocleidomastoid muscle.

Anterior Triangle

- Extends from the inferior border of the mandible to the sternum below:
- **Boundaries:**
  - o **Laterally:** Anterior border of sternocleidomastoid.
  - o **Superiorly:** Inferior border of mandible.
  - o **Medially:** Midline of neck.
- It is further subdivided into several smaller triangles as follows:

  a. **Submandibular triangle or digastric triangle:**
  - o Outlined by the inferior border of the mandible superiorly and, the anterior and posterior bellies of the digastric muscle inferiorly.

  b. **Submental triangle:**
  - o Outlined by the hyoid bone inferiorly, the anterior belly of the digastric muscle laterally and midline.

  c. **Muscular triangle:**
  - o Outlined by the hyoid bone superiorly, the superior belly of the omohyoid muscle and the anterior border of the sternocleidomastoid muscle laterally, and the midline.

  d. **Carotid triangle:**
  - o Outlined by the superior belly of the omohyoid muscle anteroinferiorly, the stylohyoid muscle and posterior belly of the digastric superiorly, and the anterior border of the sternocleidomastoid muscle posteriorly.

Posterior Triangle

- Extends backwards to the anterior border of the trapezius muscle and inferiorly to the clavicle.
- **Boundaries:** Posterior border of sternocleidomastoid muscle, anterior border of trapezius muscle and the middle one-third of the clavicle.

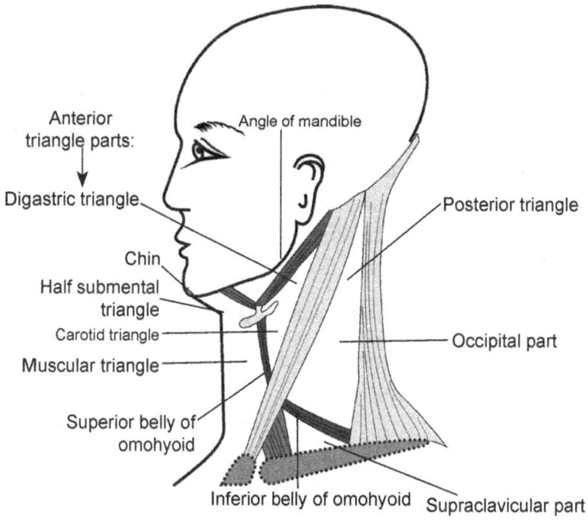

The triangles of neck. Note that the anterior and posterior triangles are subdivided by the digastric and inferior belly of omohyoid muscles respectively

Figure: Triangles of neck

[5] Complications of thyroidectomy. ***Dec 19***

[3] Mention the complications of thyroidectomy. ***Dec 13***

COMPLICATIONS OF THYROIDECTOMY

1. **Hemorrhage:**
   - It is the most common life-threatening complication of thyroidectomy

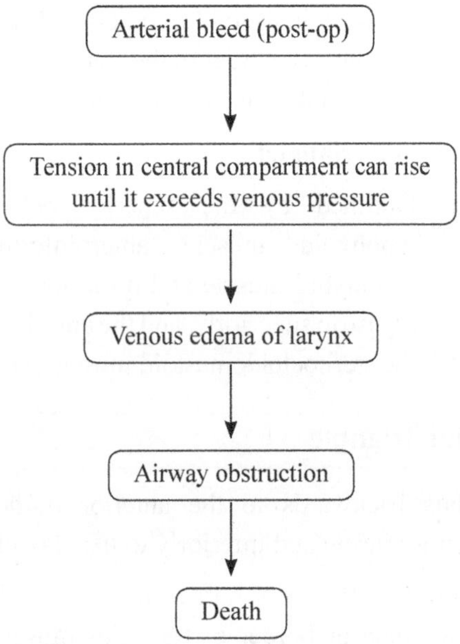

   - If hematoma develops post-op, treatment is as follows:
     - o Remove skin sutures bedside, in order to release some pressure.
     - o Shift patient to OT for wound exploration.
     - o Endotracheal intubation should be used to secure the airway while the hematoma is evacuated and the bleeding point is controlled.
2. **Recurrent laryngeal nerve injury:**
   - RLN innervates all the intrinsic muscles of larynx, except cricothyroid.
   - **Unilateral RLN injury:**
     - o Paralysis of i/l vocal cord.
     - o Vocal cord can lie in one of two positions:
       - **a. Paramedian:** Normal but weak voice.
       - **b. Abducted:** Hoarse voice and an ineffective cough.
   - **Bilateral RLN injury:**
     - o Airway obstruction:
       - ♦ **Treatment:** Emergency tracheostomy.
     - o Loss of voice:
       - ♦ **Treatment:** Speech therapy, medialization procedures.
   - **If both vocal cords come to lie in an abducted position:** Air movement can occur, but, patient has an ineffective cough. Such patients are at increased risk of repeated respiratory tract infections from aspiration.
3. **Injury to external branch of superior laryngeal nerve:**
   - Leads to loss of tension in the vocal cord with diminished power and range in the voice.
   - For most patients, changes are subtle and only demonstrable on formal voice assessment.
4. **Thyroid insufficiency:**
   - Thyroxine replacement is required following total thyroidectomy.
   - Supplementation may also be required in patients undergoing lobectomy.
5. **Parathyroid insufficiency:**
   - **Causes:**
     - o Removal of parathyroid glands.
     - o Infarction through damage to parathyroid end arteries.
   - Most cases present 2-5 days after surgery, with hypocalcemia.
     - o This complication is limited to total thyroidectomy, and is not seen in lobectomy, because when lobectomy is performed, the c/l parathyroid glands are sufficient to maintain calcium levels.
6. **Thyrotoxic crisis or thyroid storm.**
7. **Wound infection.**
8. **Hypertrophic or keloid scar.**
9. **Stitch granuloma.**

[5] Thyroid storm. ***June 19, Dec 17, Dec 14***

[3] Thyroid storm. ***June 14***

- It is an acute exacerbation of hyperthyroidism.

Causes/Precipitating Factors

1. Occurs if a thyrotoxic patient has been inadequately prepared for thyroidectomy.
2. Non thyroid surgery.
3. Abrupt cessation of antithyroid medications.
4. Infection.
5. Trauma in patients with untreated thyrotoxicosis.
6. Amiodarone administration.
7. Exposure to iodinated contrast agents.
8. Following radioactive iodine therapy.

Clinical Features

- Fever.
- CNS agitation or depression.
- Cardiovascular dysfunction.
- GI dysfunction.
- Hepatic failure.

Treatment

- Shift patient to ICU.
- IV fluids.
- Cooling the patient with ice packs.
- Non aspirin compounds are used to treat pyrexia.
- Oxygen administration.
- Diuretics for cardiac failure.
- Digoxin for uncontrolled atrial fibrillation.
- Sedation.
- Beta blockers (propranolol) are given to reduce peripheral T_4 to T_3 conversion and decrease the hyperthyroid symptoms.
- Lugol's iodine (orally) or sodium iodide (IV) decrease iodine uptake and thyroid hormone secretion.
- Propylthiouracil and carbimazole block the formation of new thyroid hormone and reduces peripheral conversion of T_4 to T_3.
- Corticosteroids prevent adrenal exhaustion and block hepatic thyroid hormone conversion.

[3] Tetany. *June 19, Dec 18*

- Tetany refers to a condition characterized by involuntary muscle contractions, often caused by hypocalcemia.

Causes

1. **Parathyroid tetany:**
   - Occurs **as a complication of total thyroidectomy** and is because of the following reasons:
     - o Inadvertent removal of parathyroid glands.
     - o Infarction through damage to the parathyroid end arteries.
   - May also occur **after surgery to the parathyroids themselves.**
2. Tetany in the newborn may occur within the first few days of life **in the child born of a mother with undiagnosed hypoparathyroidism**.

Clinical Features

- Symptoms usually appear on **POD-2 or POD-3.**
- First symptom is **mild circumoral or digital numbness** and paresthesia.
- **Carpopedal spasm**, i.e., painful cramps of hands and feet.
  - o **Accoucheur's hand or obstetrician's hand:** Extended fingers are flexed at their metacarpophalangeal joints, with the thumb strongly adducted.
  - o Toes are plantar flexed and the ankle joints extended.
- **Laryngeal spasm:** Pain and stridor.
- Cardiac arrhythmias.
- **Chvostek's sign:**
  - o Tapping/percussion over the branches of the facial nerve at the angle of the jaw will produce twitching at the corner of the mouth, the ala of the nose and the eyelids.
- **Trousseau's sign:**
  - o A sphygmomanometer cuff applied to the arm and inflated above the systolic blood pressure for 2 minutes will produce carpal spasm.

Investigations

- Total and ionized calcium levels.

- Serum magnesium levels.
- **ECG:** Prolonged QT interval, QRS complex change.

Treatment

A. Acute Symptomatic Hypocalcemia

- Emergency.
- IV + oral calcium.
- Vitamin D replacement.
- 10 ml of 10% calcium gluconate is administered slowly IV.
- Supplemental magnesium may also be required, because of the synergistic action of transporters for calcium and magnesium.

B. Mild Hypocalcemia

- Oral calcium and vitamin D supplementation.

[5] Enumerate clinical features and write a note on management of parathyroid adenoma. *CBME March 24*

- A parathyroid adenoma is a **benign tumour** of the parathyroid gland that **causes overproduction of parathyroid hormone (PTH)**, leading to hyperparathyroidism.
- It is **usually solitary**, i.e., affects one gland only.
- Multi-gland involvement is rare.

Aetiology

- **Majority** are **sporadic** in nature.
- **Familial disease:**
  - o Can occur in multiple endocrine neoplasia (**MEN**) **type 1 or type 2A.**
  - o As a familial cluster.

Pathogenesis

- Parathyroid adenoma secretes parathormone (PTH) and therefore **presents as primary hyperparathyroidism (PHPT).**
- PHPT is defined as **hypercalcemia in the presence of an unsuppressed and therefore relatively, or absolutely, elevated PTH level.**

Clinical Features

- 40 to 60 years.
- F : M = 3 : 1.
- **Typically identified incidentally** with an elevated total calcium or following routine DEXA scan.
- **Vague constitutional symptoms**, such as fatigue, muscle weakness, depression or some mild memory impairment on questioning.
- **Most common** clinical manifestation of symptomatic PHPT is **kidney stones.**
- Hypercalciuria.
- **Postmenopausal** women present with significant **osteopenia or osteoporosis** in the distal 1/3rd of radius with a minimal reduction in the lumbar spine.
- Pancreatitis.
- **Band keratopathy** is pathognomonic and is due to the **deposition of calcium phosphate crystals in the cornea.**
- Bone findings were typical findings but are rarely seen nowadays:
  - o **Osteitis fibrosa cystica or Brown tumours:** Subperiosteal bone resorption, which is most apparent along the radial aspect of the middle phalanx.
  - o Distal **tapering of the clavicles.**
  - o Classical **'salt and pepper'** erosions of the **skull.**
- Above findings led to the traditional mnemonic that PHPT patients presented with **'bones, stones, abdominal groans and psychiatric overtones'.**

Investigations

A. Lab Investigations

- PHPT is a biochemical diagnosis.
- Elevated PTH + elevated total or ionised calcium.
- Low serum phosphate.
- Normal creatinine levels.
- Normal vitamin D levels.
- 24-hour urinary excretion of calcium may be normal or elevated.
- Alkaline phosphatase may be elevated in patients in whom there is concomitant bone disease.

B. Localisation Studies

- Only when the disease has been confirmed biochemically, should localisation studies be undertaken.

a. **Non-Invasive:**
   - o Sestamibi scan:
     - ♦ Single-isotope dual-phase scan.
     - ♦ Dual-isotope subtraction imaging.
     - ♦ Single-photon emission computed tomography (SPECT).
   - o USG.
   - o 4D CT scan.
   - o PET-CT scan.
   - o MRI.

b. **Invasive:**
   - o USG or CT guided fine needle aspiration with concomitant PTH assays.
   - o Parathyroid angiography.
   - o Selective venous sampling for the PTH gradient.

Treatment

A. Surgery

- Mainstay of treatment is surgery.
- **Indications of surgery:**
  - o All symptomatic patients.
  - o Asymptomatic patients who have the following:

Measurement of serum calcium	0.25 mmol/L (1.0 mg/dL) above the upper limit of normal
Skeletal	• BMD by DEXA; T score -2.5 at lumbar spine, total hip, femoral neck or distal one-third of radius • Vertebral fracture
Renal	• Creatinine clearance <60 mL/min • 24-hour urinary calcium >10 mmol/dL (>400 mL/day) or increased risk of stone formation by risk analysis
Age	< 50 years

- Options of surgery are as follows:
  1. **Single adenoma:**
     - o Minimally invasive (focused) parathyroidectomy:
  2. **Discordant imaging or where imaging fails to identify any parathyroid abnormalities.**
     - o 3½ gland parathyroidectomy.
     - o 4 gland parathyroidectomy + autotransplantation in brachioradialis.
- Traditionally a bilateral cervical exploration was performed, but with improvements in localisation studies, minimally invasive approach is preferred.

[5] Multiple endocrine neoplasia. ***June 14***
[3] Types of MEN syndrome. ***June 13, Dec 12***
[3] Clinical manifestations of MEN-1. ***CBME March 24***
[3] Mention the components of MEN-1 and MEN-2 syndrome. ***CBME June 24***

MEN - 1	MEN - 2A	MEN - 2B
Also called Wermer's syndrome	Also called Sipple syndrome	
Autosomal dominant	Autosomal dominant	Autosomal dominant
Mutations occur in the MEN-1 gene (tumour suppression gene), which encodes the protein Menin	Mutations occur in codon 634 of RET proto-oncogene (cysteine codon)	Mutations occur in codon 918 of RET proto-oncogene (tyrosine kinase codon)
—	Medullary thyroid cancer is the first manifestation which can occur as early as 5-6 years	Medullary thyroid cancer occurs earlier than MEN-2A and is more aggressive
Parathyroid hyperplasia: • All 4 parathyroid glands are involved • Young onset (20-30 years) • Primary hyperparathyroidism is the earliest and most common manifestation • Most common symptom is nephrolithiasis	**Primary hyperparathyroidism is less common than MEN-1 and has a milder clinical course:** • Majority of patients will be asymptomatic • Mild elevations in serum calcium level • Asymmetrically enlarged parathyroid glands	—

Contd.

MEN - 1	MEN - 2A	MEN - 2B
Anterior pituitary adenomas: • **1st most common:** Prolactinomas (cause galactorrhea) • **2nd most common:** Non-functioning tumour	—	—
Pancreaticoduodenal endocrine tumours: Although most patients have multiple tumours, one hormone syndrome is usually dominant: • Gastrinomas/Zollinger Ellison syndrome is the most common • Insulinomas • **Non-functioning:** Secrete pancreatic polypeptide • VIPoma • Somatostatinoma • Glucagonoma	—	—
Adrenal tumours: • Non-functioning adenomas are most common • Adrenocortical carcinoma • Phaeochromocytoma	Unilateral or bilateral phaeochromocytomas are seen	Unilateral or bilateral phaeochromocytomas are seen
Foregut carcinoids: Neuroendocrine tumours of lung, bronchus, thymus, stomach, duodenum, small intestine	—	—
Other features: • Subcutaneous or visceral lipomas • Facial cutaneous angiofibromas • Collagenomas	**Other features:** • Cutaneous lichen amyloidosis • Hirschsprung's disease	**Other features:** • Facial and oral mucosal neuromas • Marfanoid habitus • Ganglioneuromatosis of GIT
Treatment: • Aim of surgical intervention is to obtain and maintain normocalcemia for the longest time possible. • Bilateral cervical exploration with at least a subtotal parathyroidectomy (removal of 3½ glands) and cervical thymectomy. • A total parathyroidectomy and forearm autotransplantation is an acceptable alternative. • Treatment of pituitary tumours is drugs >>> surgery.	**Treatment:** • Presence of a phaeochromocytoma should be excluded prior to surgical intervention. If present, unilateral or bilateral subtotal resection should be done. • Total thyroidectomy should be done. • **Parathyroids:** Resection of grossly enlarged glands, but with preservation of parathyroid tissue where possible.	**Treatment:** • Presence of a phaeochromocytoma should be excluded prior to surgical intervention. If present, unilateral or bilateral subtotal resection should be done. • Total thyroidectomy should be done.

MEN - 4

- It is an autosomal dominant syndrome.
- Due to an inactivating pathogenic variant in the CDKN1B gene.
- It comprises the same set of tumours as MEN-1, but it is a rarer cause of hereditary PHPT.
- Treatment is the same as MEN-1.

OTHER IMPORTANT TOPICS

TYPES OF THYROID SURGERY

- All thyroid operations can be assembled from three basic elements:
  1. Total lobectomy.
  2. Isthmusectomy.
  3. Subtotal lobectomy.
- **Total thyroidectomy** = 2 × total lobectomy + isthmusectomy.
- **Subtotal thyroidectomy** = 2 × subtotal lobectomy + isthmusectomy.
- **Near-total thryroidectomy** = total lobectomy + isthmusectomy + subtotal lobectomy.
- **Lobectomy** = total lobectomy + isthmusectomy.

THYROTOXICOSIS

- Hyperthyroidism results from an excess of circulating thyroid hormones.
- The term thyrotoxicosis is retained because hyperthyroidism is not responsible for all manifestations of the disease.

Clinical Types that are Relevant to a Surgeon

a. **Primary thyrotoxicosis:** Diffuse toxic goitre or Graves' disease.

b. **Secondary thyrotoxicosis:** Toxic nodular goitre.

c. Toxic nodule.

d. Hyperthyroidism due to rarer causes.

Causes of Hyperthyroidism

A. Increased Hormone Synthesis (Increased Radioactive Iodine Uptake)

- Grave's disease or diffuse toxic goitre.
- Toxic multinodular goitre.
- Toxic adenoma.
- **Drug induced:** Amiodarone, iodine.
- Thyroid cancer.
- Struma ovarii.
- Hydatidiform mole.
- TSH secreting pituitary adenoma.

B. Release of Pre-formed Hormone (Decreased Radioactive Iodine Uptake)

- **Thyroiditis:** Acute phase of Hashimoto's thyroiditis, subacute thyroiditis.
- Factitious or iatrogenic thyrotoxicosis.
- Hamburger thyrotoxicosis.

27

Adrenals

[MCQ] Conn's syndrome consists of: *CBME June 24*

A. Raised aldosterone level*

B. Decreased aldosterone level

C. Decreased thyroxine level

D. Raised PTH level

ADRENALDISORDER	ENZYME INVOLVED
Conn's syndrome or hyperaldosteronism	Increased plasma aldosterone
Cushing's syndrome	Excessive glucocorticoids
Congenital adrenal hyperplasia also known as adrenogenital syndrome	21-hydroxylase deficiency, decreased cortisol (glucocorticoid)
Addison's disease	Glucocorticoid and mineralocorticoid deficiency

OTHER IMPORTANT TOPICS

Classification of Adrenal Tumours

A. Functioning Tumours

a. Benign:

- o Aldosteronoma.
- o Cortisol-producing adenoma.
- o Sex steroid-producing adenoma.
- o Pheochromocytoma.

b. Malignant:

- o Adrenocortical cancer.
- o Malignant pheochromocytoma.

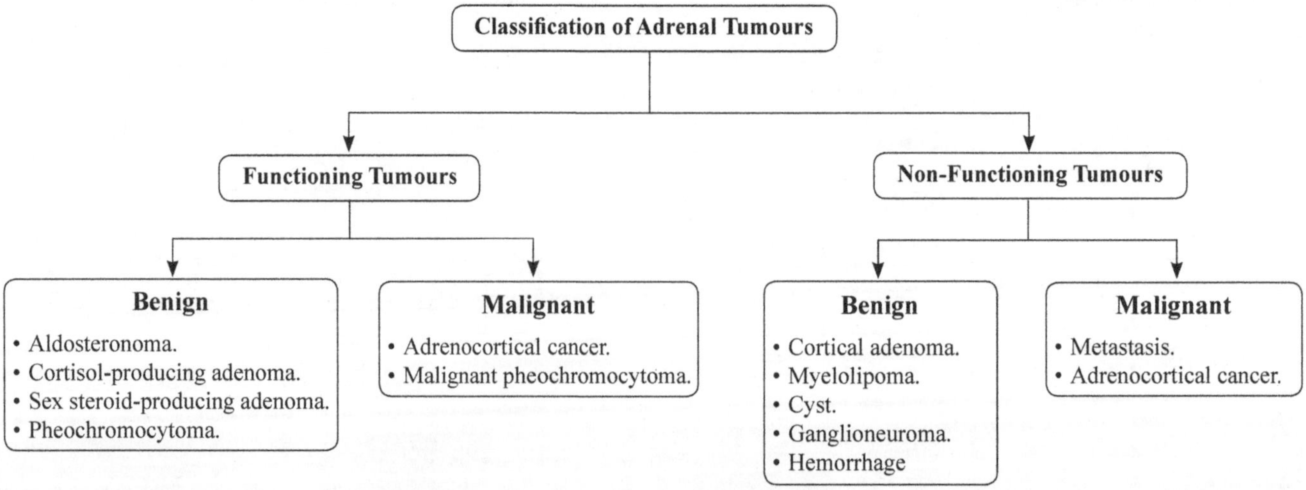

B. Non-Functioning Tumours

a. **Benign:**

- o Cortical adenoma.
- o Myelolipoma.
- o Cyst.
- o Ganglioneuroma.
- o Hemorrhage.

b. **Malignant:**

- o Metastasis.
- o Adrenocortical cancer.

INCIDENTALOMA

- **Definition:** An asymptomatic adrenal mass detected on imaging not performed for suspected adrenal disease is termed an incidentaloma.

Aetiology

- Includes benign and malignant tumours of the adrenal gland, cortex and medulla.
- Can also be of extra-adrenal origin.
- These tumours can be either non-functioning (silent) or functioning (secreting excess hormones).
- In patients with a history of malignant disease, metastatic disease is the most likely cause of adrenal masses, particularly when they are bilateral.
- In those without a clear history of malignant disease, 80% will turn out to be nonfunctioning cortical adenomas.

Incidence

- As the use of CT and MRI has become widespread, the incidence of incidentaloma has increased.
- Autopsy studies suggest a prevalence of clinically inapparent adrenal masses of the order of 2%, which increases with age.

Clinical Features

- By definition, patients with incidentalomas do not have clinically overt symptoms.
- Subtle abnormalities may be present.
- Weight gain.
- Skin atrophy.
- Facial fullness.
- Diabetes.
- Hypertension.
- Loss of normal diurnal variation in cortisol secretion.

Investigations

The following should be assessed in parallel:

A. Is the Tumour Benign or Malignant?

- Cushing's syndrome and virilising tumours are associated with higher rates of malignancy.
- The optimal way to determine malignancy is by means of a non-contrast CT scan and measurement of the density of the lesion by Hounsfield units (HU).
- Benign tumours are low density (≤10 HU).
- **In cases of uncertainty.**
  - o FDG-PET scan.
  - o MRI with chemical shift.
  - o Contrast CT and measurement of washout.
- **Radiological findings suspicious of malignancy are:**
  - o Diameter >40 mm.
  - o >10 HU density.
  - o Contrast-enhanced washout CT.
    - ♦ Relative <40%.
    - ♦ Absolute <60%.
  - o **MRI chemical shift:** No change in signal intensity on out-of-phase imaging.
  - o **FDG-PET:** Positive uptake.

B. Is the Tumour Functionally Active? This is determined by:

- Clinical assessment.
- 1 mg overnight dexamethasone suppression test.
- Measurement of plasma or urinary metanephrines.
- Plasma aldosterone-renin ratio (ARR).
- Sex hormones and steroid precursors.

Treatment

- All patients should be discussed in a multidisciplinary setting.
- The most important aspect of management is to distinguish the subset of adrenal masses that are likely

to have a clinical impact from the large proportion that are not.

A. Conservative

- Indications are:
  - o Small (<40 mm).
  - o Benign.
  - o Non-functioning tumours.
- Follow up CT/MRI at 6 months as tumours >30 mm have an increased risk of developing hyperfunction over time.

B. Surgery

- The treatment of choice for patients with unilateral tumours causing hormone excess is adrenalectomy.
- **Indications of adrenalectomy:**
  - o All tumours >40 mm in diameter.
  - o Tumours showing imaging characteristics of malignancy.
  - o Tumours showing significant growth.
- Open adrenalectomy is recommended for unilateral adrenal masses with radiological findings suspicious of malignancy.
- Laparoscopic adrenalectomy is recommended for unilateral adrenal masses with radiological findings suspicious of malignancy with a diameter <60 mm, but without evidence of local invasion.

PHAEOCHROMOCYTOMA

- **Definition:** Tumors that arise from the neuro-ectodermal tissue of the adrenal medulla are termed pheochromocytomas (PCC).
- Tumors that arise from the extra-adrenal para-sympathetic and sympathetic ganglia are termed paragangliomas (PGL).
- PCCs and PGLs are collectively abbreviated to PPGL.
- Phaeochromocytomas often are called the 10 percent tumour, because 10% are bilateral, 10% are malignant, 10% occur in children, 10% are extra-adrenal and 10% are familial.

Aetiology

- **Sporadic:** 75% of cases.
- Rest of the PCC occur as part of inherited endocrine tumor syndromes:

A. Hereditary PPGL syndromes.

- Associated with germline mutations

B. MEN-2.

C. von Hippel-Lindau disease:

- Patients with vHL develop PCC much more frequently than PGL.
- vHL tumors overproduce only noradrenaline.

D. Neurofibromatosis type 1:

- Can occur at any age with peak incidence between 30 and 50 years.
- No gender predilection.

Pathology

- 10% are malignant tumors. The differentiation between malignant and benign tumors is difficult, except when metastases are present.
- **Factors in favour of malignancy:**
  1. An increased PASS (pheochromocytoma of the adrenal gland scale score).
  2. High Ki-67.
  3. Vascular invasion.
  4. Breached capsule.
- PCC produce the following:
  1. Catecholamines – adrenaline and noradrenaline.
  2. Calcitonin.
  3. ACTH.
  4. VIP.
  5. PTHrP – Parathyroid hormone related protein.

Clinical Features

- Symptoms and signs are caused by catecholamine excess and are typically intermittent.
- Adrenal tumor + headache + palpitations + sweating is indicative of PCC.
- Paroxysms may be precipitated by physical training, induction of GA and drugs (contrast media, tricyclic anti-depressants, metoclopramide and opiates).
- Hypertension may occur continuously, be intermittent or absent. It is the most common symptom in PCC.
- Other symptoms – pallor, weight loss, hyperglycemia, nausea, psychological effects.
- A minority of patients may be asymptomatic.

Diagnosis

A. Biochemical

- Catecholamines are converted to metanephrines by the enzyme **catecholamine O-methyl transferase (COMT).**

Catecholamine O-methyl Transferase (COMT)

Catecholamines ————————→ *Metanephrines*

- This conversion happens within the tumor.
- Diagnosis is confirmed by:
  - o Elevated catecholamine metabolites (metanephrines) in plasma and/or
  - o Raised 24 hours urinary excretion of fractionated metanephrines.
  - o Measurement of plasma and urinary metanephrines is more sensitive than measurement of plasma and urinary catecholamines.
- If at least 1 of these substances are four times greater than the upper limit, it is 100% diagnostic.
- Plasma dopamine is regarded as a marker of tumour burden.

B. Radiological

- Once a biochemical diagnosis is established, imaging (CT or MRI) is done to:
  - o Determine tumour location.
  - o Assess its size and risk of malignancy.
  - o Tumours appear vascular and frequently possess cystic areas or central necrosis.
  - o Swiss cheese configuration is seen.
- MRI is preferred because contrast media used for CT scans can provoke paroxysms.
- Malignant phaeochromocytomas are diagnosed by the presence of local invasion or metastatic disease.
- If initial imaging is negative or reveals extra-adrenal disease, functional investigations are done:
  - o ^{123}I -MIBG (Meta Iodo Benzyl Guanidine)
  - o ^{111}In-octreotide scanning.
  - o 6- [^{18}F] fluoro dopamine PET scan.

Treatment

Medical management to control blood pressure followed by prompt surgical excision.

A. Pre-Operative Control of Blood Pressure

- An alpha-blocker (phenoxybenzamine) is used to block the effects of catecholamine excess and its consequences during surgery. It is given in increasing doses, till the patient reports symptomatic postural hypotension.
- Additional β-blockers are required if tachycardia or arrhythmias develop. But, this should not be introduced until the patient is α-blocked.
- **Other regimens:**
  1. α blockers (prazosin or doxazosin) ± β blockers.
  2. Using calcium channel blockers alone.
  3. Using the catecholamine synthesis blocker (metyrosine) in the setting of cardiac failure.

B. Intra-Op

- With adequate pre-operative blockade, anesthesia is as safe as in patients with a non-functioning adrenal tumor.
- In some patients, dramatic changes in heart rate and blood pressure may occur and requires sudden administration of pressor or vasodilator agents.
- A central venous catheter and invasive arterial monitoring are used.
- Special attention is required when the adrenal vein is ligated as a sudden drop in BP may occur.

C. Post-Operative Care

- Observed for 24 hours in ICU as hypovolemia and hypoglycemia may occur.
- Infusion of large volumes of fluid or administration of noradrenaline can be necessary to correct post-op hypotension in the presence of unopposed α blockade.
- Lifelong yearly biochemical tests should be performed to identify recurrent, metastatic or metachronous PCC.

D. Surgical Treatment

- Either by laparoscopic or open surgery.
- Laparoscopic surgery is now routinely done.
- **Indications of open approach:**

- o > 10 cm in size.
- o Radiological signs of malignancy are detected.

Treatment of Malignant Phaeochromocytoma

- Surgical excision is the only chance for cure.
- **If there is direct invasion:** Laparotomy and en bloc excision of involved adjacent organs offers the best chance of cure.
- **If mets are present:** Excision of primary tumor is still recommended to improve symptom control and improve the efficiency of adjuvant radiolabelled MIBG and octreotide therapy.

28

Breast

[3] Triple assessment. *March 22*

- It is a combined approach **used in the assessment of a patient presenting with breast lump, nipple discharge or other breast symptoms.**
- The predictive value and **diagnostic accuracy** of it is **99.99%.**
- It is a combination of the following **three** things:
  a. **Clinical assessment**
     - o History.
     - o Examination (inspection and palpation)
  b. **Radiological imaging**
     - o USG.
     - o Mammography.
  c. **Tissue sampling/Pathology**
     - o FNAC or fine needle aspiration cytology.
     - o Core biopsy.

[5] Benign breast diseases. *Dec 19*

- Benign breast disease is also known as **Aberrations of Normal Development and Involution (ANDI).**

Nomenclature

- The nomenclature of benign breast disease in the past has been confusing owing to the use of a variety of terms (fibrosis, adenosis, epitheliosis, fibroadenosis, fibrocystic disease) for clinical patterns of pain, nodularity, benign lumps and nipple discharge. However, such terms do not relate to clinical or histological features.
- Since **most benign disorders are derived from minor aberrations of the normal process of development, cyclical hormone related change and involution**, the concept of ANDI was developed to help in the better understanding and treatment of benign breast disease.

Aetiology

- The **breast is a dynamic structure** that undergoes alterations due to the **cyclical changes** in estrogen and progesterone in every menstrual cycle.
- These **hormones act as growth factors** on the epithelial and stromal cells of the **TDLU (Terminal Ductal Lobular Unit).**
- The pathogenesis of ANDI involves **disturbances in the breast physiology** extending from a perturbation of normality to well-defined disease processes.

Pathology

- This can be considered in **3 phases**:
  - o **Lobule development at 15-25 years.**
  - o **Cyclical changes at 15-50 years.**
  - o **Involution at 35-55 years.**
- Lobular proliferation leads to the development of fibroadenoma.
- Involution leads to cyst formation.

Clinical Features

- The **most common** manifestations of ANDI are **breast pain** and **benign nodularity.**

- Breast pain **usually follows the menstrual cycle,** appearing around day 14 and increasing in severity until day 28, when it becomes severe. This is **called cyclical pronounced mastalgia with premenstrual exacerbation.**
- **Nodularity or lumpiness** may be either localized or spread diffusely throughout the breast.
  - o It is often bilateral.
  - o It is most conspicuous in upper outer quadrant.
  - o The nodularity may be cyclical, appearing 1-2 weeks prior to menstruation and regressing with the onset of menses.
- A **discrete lump in the breast is commonly a fibroadenoma in the young and a cyst in the middle-aged.**

Investigations

- Triple assessment.
- USG/Mammography.
- Biopsy is done if there are suspicious features on imaging.

Treatment

- If triple assessment is normal, **reassurance** that the symptoms are not due to cancer helps the majority of women.
- **Mastalgia:**
  - o Type of pain, **cyclical or non-cyclical**, should be identified by recording a pain chart for 1 month.
  - o Wear **sports bra.**
  - o **Flaxseed** 30 g daily or oil of evening primrose.
  - o **Topical NSAID cream** (diclofenac or piroxicam).
  - o **Systemic drugs**: Tamoxifen, Danazol, Ormeloxifene.
  - o **Combination drugs:** LHRH agonist alone or with antiestrogen (tamoxifen or ormeloxifene).
- **Nodularity:**
  - o The **Cardiff-Lucknow nodularity scale**, that grades the nodularity on a scale of 0 to 4, provides an objective measurement of nodularity.
  - o If necessary, treatment with an **anti-estrogen such as tamoxifen or ormeloxifene** has been found to control nodularity within a few weeks.

[5] Fibroadenoma. *Dec 14*

- A fibroadenoma is the **most common cause of a breast lump in women aged 15-25 years.**
- It is a **benign** breast disease.
- It is considered to be a **part of ANDI**, i.e., Aberrations of Normal Development and Involution.

Aetiology

- Most benign disorders are derived from minor **aberrations of the normal process of development, cyclical hormone-related changes and involution.**
- This is because the breast is a dynamic structure that undergoes alterations due to the cyclical changes in estrogen and progesterone in every menstrual cycle.

Pathology

- It arises from **hyperplasia of a lobule.**
- Usually **grows to 2-3 cm in size.**
- Surrounded by a **well-defined capsule.**
- Although there are **2 microscopic variants**, both patterns are often seen in the same tumour and the distinction is unimportant.
  1. **Peri-canalicular**
     - o Normal duct structures are surrounded by a concentric overgrowth of connective tissue stroma.
  2. **Intra-canalicular**
     - o Stroma projects into the ducts to form elongated and distorted clefts.

Clinical features

- Solitary (most of the cases).
- Firm.
- Well defined.
- Lobulated.
- Extremely mobile lump (called mouse tumour).
- Usually painless.
- Usually grows 2-3 cm in size.

Investigations

- **USG breast:**
  - o Well-circumscribed, mobile, solid mass.

- **Biopsy/FNAC:**
  - o Not done routinely.
  - o A clinically typical fibroadenoma, confirmed on USG, may be treated conservatively without the need for a biopsy.
  - o A biopsy should be obtained if the patient is > 25 years or if there are atypical features on USG.

Treatment

1. **Surgical excision:**
   - Indications:
     - o Age > 30 years.
     - o Suspicious features on imaging, such as micro-lobulation.
     - o Atypia on histology.
     - o Size > 5 cm.
     - o Family history of breast cancer.
     - o Patient's preference.

B. **Drugs:**
   - Regression has been observed with anti-estrogen drugs such as Tamoxifen and Ormeloxifene.

GIANT FIBROADENOMAS

- Occasionally occur during puberty.
- > 5 cm in diameter.
- Often rapidly growing.
- Can be enucleated through a sub-mammary incision.

[5] Phyllodes tumour. *Dec 12*

[3] Phyllodes tumour. *Sept 21*

- Also known as cystosarcoma phyllodes.
- It is a **true mixed neoplasm comprising both epithelial and mesenchymal elements** and resembling a fibroadenoma.
- These tumours are **classified as benign, borderline or malignant.**

Clinical Features

- Usually occur in **women > 30 years**, but can appear in younger women.
- Present as a **large (sometimes massive)** tumour with an unevenly **bosselated surface.**
- Occasionally, the **overlying skin is ulcerated owing to pressure necrosis.**
- Despite their size, phyllodes tumours **remain mobile on the chest wall** and **rarely infiltrate the skin until late.**
- Usually **sharply demarcated** from the surrounding breast tissue, which is compressed and distorted.

Classification

- Phyllodes tumours are classified according to histological behaviour:
  - a. **Benign:** Mitotic rate < 4 per 10 hpf.
  - b. **Borderline:** 4-9.
  - c. **Malignant:** > 10.
- **Connective tissue composes the bulk** of these tumours, which have mixed gelatinous, solid and cystic areas.
- **Cystic areas represent sites of infarction and necrosis.**
- These gross alterations give the **cut tumour surface its classical leaf-like (phyllodes) appearance.**

Investigations

- Mammography.
- FNAC.
- Core needle biopsy.

Treatment

1. **Wide local excision** with a 2 cm margin along with the overlying skin and underlying pectoralis major muscle because of a high incidence of local recurrence.
2. **Mastectomy**: For massive tumours, recurrent tumours and those of the malignant type.
3. **Post-op radiotherapy** may be offered to women with **recurrent or malignant Phyllodes tumours**.
4. **Systemic chemotherapy** may be offered for **malignant phyllodes.**
5. **Axillary dissection is not recommended** because axillary lymph node mets rarely occur.

[5] Paget's disease of breast. *Dec 18*

- It is a unique type of **ductal carcinoma in situ arising in the nipple.**

Clinical Features

- It presents as a **chronic, eczematous eruption of the nipple.**
- The **nipple-areola complex slowly gets eroded and destroyed.**
- A **palpable mass may or may not be present** in the underlying breast.
- It **may become invasive** with **metastasis to the axillary lymph nodes.**

HPE

- Presence of **large, pale, vacuolated cells called Paget cells in the rete pegs of the epithelium.**

Differential Diagnosis

- Superficial spreading melanoma.

Investigations

- USG.
- Mammogram.
- FNAC.
- Core needle biopsy.

Treatment

A. Paget's Disease Without Associated Underlying Malignancy

- Central core excision + radiotherapy
- Central core excision means removing a cone of major milk ducts (lactiferous ducts) along with the nipple and areola complex down to the pectoralis major muscle.

B. Paget's Disease with Underlying Malignancy

- Mastectomy and evaluation of the axillary node status.

[3] Mondor's disease. ***Dec 13***

[MCQ] Mondor's disease is : ***CBME March 24***

A. Infection of scalp

B. Spontaneous thrombophlebitis of veins of leg

C. Spontaneous thrombophlebitis of veins of breast*

D. Infection of cheek

- **Definition:** It is thrombophlebitis of the superficial veins of the breast and anterior chest wall.

Aetiology

- The cause is **obscure** as there is no history of injury or infection.

Clinical features

- The **pathognomonic feature is a tender thrombosed subcutaneous cord**, usually attached to the skin.
- When the skin over the breast is stretched by raising the arm; **a narrow, shallow, subcutaneous groove alongside the cord** becomes apparent.
- Patient **may complain of pain.**

Differential Diagnosis

- Lymphatic permeation from an occult carcinoma of the breast.

Treatment

- The only treatment required is to **restrict arm movements.**
- The condition **usually subsides within a few months** without recurrence, complications or deformity.
- A course of **antibiotics (amoxicillin-clavulanic acid)** may be given to the patient.
- **Analgesics** for pain relief.

[5] TNM staging of breast cancer. ***July 15***

[3] TNM staging of breast cancer. ***Dec 14***

T_x : Primary tumour cannot be assessed.

T_0 : No evidence of primary tumour.

T_{is} : Ductal carcinoma in situ (DCIS).

T_1 : < 2 cm in greatest dimension.

T_2 : 2- 5 cm.

T_3 : > 5 cm.

T_{4a} : Invasion of chest wall.

T_{4b} : Skin involvement (ulceration, satellite nodules, peau d'orange).

T_{4c} : Both a and b are present.

T_{4d} : Inflammatory carcinoma.

N_x: Regional lymph nodes cannot be assessed.

N_0: No regional lymph node mets (by imaging or clinical examination).

N_1: Ipsilateral level I, II axillary lymph nodes.

N_2: Ipsilateral level I, II axillary lymph nodes that are clinically fixed or matted ***or*** ipsilateral internal mammary nodes in the absence of axillary lymph node mets.

N_3: Ipsilateral level III lymph nodes ± level I, II ***or*** ipsilateral internal mammary nodes with level I, II mets ***or*** mets in ipsilateral supraclavicular lymph nodes ± axillary or internal mammary lymph node involvement.

M_0: No clinical or radiographic evidence of distant mets.

M_1: Distant mets present.

[10] 40 years old female came with painless rapidly progressive lump in left breast for 4 months. On examination, 3 × 3 hard lump with peau d'orange appearance with 1 × 1 cm hard lump in level 1 axilla. Stage the condition. Write in detail risk factors, investigations and management of this patient. ***CBME June 24***

- The size of the lump is 3 × 3 cm, but there is peau d'orange appearance which makes it T_{4b}.
- A 1 × 1 cm hard lump in level 1 axilla makes it N_1.
- Metastases is not mentioned, which makes it M_0.
- Therefore, it is $T_{4b} N_1 M_0$.

[10] Discuss the differential diagnosis of carcinoma of breast. Describe the management of stage II breast cancer. ***March 22***

[10] Classify carcinoma breast. Discuss aetiology, clinical features and management of Ca breast - T2N0M0 in a 30 year old patient. ***Dec 16***

[5] Early breast cancer. ***Dec 13***

[10] Describe the aetiology, pathogenesis, clinical features, diagnosis and management of locally advanced breast carcinoma. ***Feb 23***

[10] 45 year old lady presents with a painless lump of 2 × 2 cm size to start within the right breast and has doubled the size in 6 months. ***CBME March 24***

A. What other history is needed?

B. What is your differential diagnosis?

C. How do you investigate?

D. Add a note on management of early breast cancer.

DIFFERENTIAL DIAGNOSIS OF BREAST LUMP

A. Benign

a. Non inflammatory:

- Fibroadenoma.
- Ductal papilloma.
- Phyllodes tumour.
- Hamartoma.
- Galactocele.
- Breast cyst.
- Hematoma.
- Traumatic fat necrosis.

b. Inflammatory:

- Breast abscess.
- Antibioma.
- Periductal mastitis (produces an evanescent mass).

B. Malignant

- Ca breast.
- Phyllodes tumour.

BREAST CANCER

- It is the **most common cancer in women.**

Risk Factors

- The events increasing the **estrogenic exposure** of the breast, **increase the risk** for cancer:
  - o Early menarche.
  - o Late menopause.
  - o Nulliparity.
  - o Late first pregnancy.
  - o Hormone replacement with high estrogen therapy.
- **Risk factors can be broadly divided into:**

A. Modifiable Risk Factors (those that can be modified by adopting a healthy diet and lifestyle)

- Obesity.
- Nulliparity.

- Breastfeeding is protective.
- Age at first childbirth > 35 years has high risk.
- Use of hormone replacement therapy increases risk.
- Smoking.
- Alcohol.
- History of radiation exposure.

B. Non-modifiable Risk Factors

- **Age:** Risk increases with age.
- **Sex:** F > M.
- **Ethnicity:** Whites, Parsis.
- Family history.
- **Genetic predisposition:** BRCA 1 and BRCA 2 mutations.
- Early menarche (< 12 years).
- Late menopause (> 55 years).
- **High risk breast lesions:**
  - o Proliferative conditions without atypia.
  - o Complex fibroadenoma.
  - o Papillomatosis.
  - o **Proliferative disease with atypia:** Atypical ductal and lobular hyperplasia.
  - o LCIS (lobular carcinoma in situ).

Pathology

- **Arises from:**
  - o **90%:** Milk ducts or lactiferous ducts, i.e., ductal carcinoma.
  - o **10%:** Lobules, i.e., lobular carcinoma.
- **In situ disease:**
  - o Remains confined to the epithelium of the duct or lobule with no breach in the basement membrane.
- **Invasive or infiltrative:**
  - o Infiltration of surrounding tissue through a breach in the basement membrane.
- Tumour may be well differentiated, moderately differentiated or poorly differentiated.
- **Lobular Carcinoma In Situ (LCIS) is a high risk benign lesion and not a cancer.**
- **Invasive carcinoma is usually of no special type (NST), which represents the most common variety of breast cancer.**

Modified Bloom-Richardson Scoring System

- For tumour grade.
- Includes the sum of individual scores for 3 variables:
  1. Percentage of tumour cells with **tubule formation.**
  2. **Nuclear pleomorphism.**
  3. Size and number of **mitoses**/HPF.
- Each is assigned from 1 to 3 points according to the degree of deviation from normal breast epithelium.

Grade	Total score
I	3-5
II	6-7
III	8-9

Classification

A. Histological

- Based on histology, breast cancer is classified as follows:

  1. In situ disease
  - o Ductal carcinoma in situ.

  2. Invasive or infiltrative
  - o No special type (most common).
  - o Ductal carcinoma.
  - o Lobular carcinoma.

  3. Rare histological variants
  - o Colloid or mucinous carcinoma.
  - o Medullary carcinoma.
  - o Tubular carcinoma.
  - o Papillary carcinoma.

B. Molecular

- The tumour cells may over-express estrogen receptors (ER positive), progesterone receptors (PR positive), human epidermal growth factor receptor 2/neu (HER 2/neu positive) and androgen receptors (AR positive).
- The degree of mitoses can be detected by the Ki – 67 mitotic index (proliferative index).

Classification	Hormone Receptor	HER 2/neu	Others
Luminal A	Positive (either or both ER/PR)	Negative	Ki-67 low
Luminal B	Positive (either or both ER/PR)	Negative	Ki-67 high
Basal type (triple negative)	Negative	Negative	Ki-67 usually high
HER 2/ neu enriched	Negative	Positive	Ki-67 high
Claudin low	Negative	Negative	Claudin low

Spread

- Breast cancer spreads by the following routes:

A. Local Spread

- tumour increases in size and **invades adjacent breast parenchyma.**
- **May involve:**
  - o **Skin:** Ulceration and satellite nodules.
  - o **Pectoralis major.**
  - o **Serratus anterior.**
  - o **Chest wall.**
- **Contraction of collagen leads to shortening of Cooper's ligament** pulling the skin inwards and giving rise to:
  - o Dimpling (single Cooper's ligament is shortened).
  - o Puckering or tethering (many Cooper's ligament are shortened).
  - o Nipple retraction.
- Tumour cells release a number of growth factors:
  - o FGF or Fibroblast Growth Factor.
  - o TGF-α and TGF-ß or Transforming Growth Factor.
  - o VEGF or Vascular Endothelial Growth Factor.
- FGF induces mitosis of adjacent fibrocytes, which convert to fibroblasts and lay down collagen (desmoplastic reaction).

B. Lymphatic Spread

- Occurs **mainly to axillary lymph nodes.**
- Tumours from inner half of breast may also spread to the **internal mammary nodes.**
- Involvement of the contralateral lymph nodes in the absence of a contralateral primary represents metastatic disease.

C. Hematogenous Spread

- Occurs to the **skeletal system:** Lumbar vertebrae > neck of femur > thoracic vertebrae > rib > skull.
- Bone mets is **generally osteolytic**, although osteosclerotic and mixed types may be seen.
- May also occur to the liver, lungs and brain.
- Extensive bone marrow replacement by tumour cells may result in release of immature blast cells in the peripheral blood, giving rise to '**leukoerythroblastic anemia**'.

Clinical Features

- The **most common presentation is a discrete lump** in the breast.
- **Most common tumour site is the upper outer quadrant** of the breast, because it has the highest number of lymphatics.
- Nipple retraction.
- Nipple discharge (blood or serous).
- **Skin changes:**
  - o Ulceration.
  - o **Peau d' orange:** It is a sign of locally advanced disease due to obstruction of cutaneous lymphatic drainage of the breast, by infiltration of either subdermal lymphatics or axillary lymph nodes by tumour cells.
- **Cancer en cuirasse** is due to extensive tumour infiltration of the skin of the breast, chest (in cases of post mastectomy recurrence), upper limb and abdomen.
- Swelling in the axilla due to lymphatic spread.
- **Metastatic symptoms:**
  - o Bony pain.
  - o Cough.
  - o Breathlessness.
  - o Haemoptysis.
  - o Headache.
  - o Visual disturbances.
  - o Neurological deficit.

- o Epileptic fits.
- o Abdominal distension (due to ascites).
- o Jaundice.
- o Anorexia.
- o Weakness.
- o Weight loss.
- o Hypercalcemia.

Investigations

- **Triple assessment:**
  - o Clinical (history and examination).
  - o Imaging (USG and mammography).
  - o Pathology (core biopsy).
- **USG of breast:**
  - o Primary imaging modality in young women (< 35 years) with dense breast tissue.
  - o Can distinguish cystic from solid lesions.
  - o Solid masses with an irregular shape and ill-defined margins are suspicious of malignancy and require biopsy.
- **USG of axilla:**
  - o Performed when cancer is diagnosed, with guided percutaneous biopsy of any suspicious lymph nodes.
- **Mammography:**
  - o Done as 1st line imaging investigation in women > 35 years old.
  - o May also be used as an initial screening tool for asymptomatic women.
  - o **Dose of radiation:** 0.1 cGy or 1 mGy per film.
  - o 2 views are taken:
    - ♦ Medio-lateral-oblique.
    - ♦ Craniocaudal.
  - o Features suggestive of cancers:
    - ♦ Irregular, spiculated mass.
    - ♦ Fine, pleomorphic microcalcifications.
    - ♦ Architectural distortion.
  - o Biopsy is required for definitive diagnosis, when malignancy is suspected on mammography.
- **MRI:**
  - o It is highly sensitive for breast pathology.
  - o **Indications:**
    - ♦ Women with dense breast or discordant or equivocal findings on mammogram/USG.
    - ♦ To distinguish scar from recurrence in women who have had previous Breast Conservation Therapy for cancer.
    - ♦ To assess multifocality and multicentricity.
  - o Women with BRCA gene or other genetic mutations or a strong family history.
  - o Women with breast implants.
  - o MRI guided biopsy may be performed for lesions not visible on USG or mammogram.
- **PET scan:**
  - o Used as a staging investigation in breast cancer, especially in patients who have symptoms/signs suggestive of mets.
  - o FDG[18] - PET scan is usually combined with CT scan which gives anatomical information along with detection of metabolically active tissue.
- **FNAC:**
  - o Fine Needle Aspiration Cytology.
  - o Is gradually being replaced by core needle biopsy.
- **Core needle biopsy:**
  - o Done under local anesthesia.
  - o Gives information on the histological type as well as the molecular subtype (ER, PR, Her-2-neu, Ki-67).
  - o If necessary, passage of biopsy needle can be guided by USG, mammogram or sometimes MRI.
  - o Needle tip should be used to take a sample from only the solid part of the mass, avoiding areas of cystic degeneration and blood vessels in and around the lesion.
  - o **Needle size:**
    - ♦ Breast tissues - 14G.
    - ♦ Axillary nodes - 18G.
- **Vacuum assisted biopsy:**
  - o 8G or 11G needles are used.
  - o This allows more extensive biopsies to be taken
  - o Useful in the management of microcalcifications and removal of benign lumps such as fibro-adenoma.

Treatment

- The treatment of breast cancer is **multimodal** and includes:
  - o Surgery.
  - o Systemic treatment (chemotherapy, targeted therapy, hormonal therapy).
  - o Radiotherapy.
- Treatment of breast cancer depends on the stage of the disease.

A. Early Breast Cancer (Stages 0,I,II)

- The mainstay of treatment of early breast cancer is **surgery.**
- The aim of surgery is to **remove all disease in the breast and axilla with negative margins**. There should be no tumour cells on the cut edge of the tumour for invasive cancer.
- However, in patients with DCIS, a minimum of 2 mm is considered a safe margin.
- There are various surgical options:
  - o Mastectomy.
  - o Modified radical mastectomy.
  - o Skin and nipple sparing mastectomy.
  - o Breast Conservation Surgery.
  - o Wide Local Excision.
  - o Oncoplasty.

Mastectomy

- Removal of the entire breast tissue including the skin over the tumour, the nipple areola complex and the axillary tail.
- **Indications:**
  - o Large tumour (in relation to the size of the breast).
  - o Multicentric disease.
  - o Diffuse microcalcification on a mammogram indicative of DCIS.
  - o BRCA positive cancers.
  - o Local recurrence following BCS.
  - o The patient's preference.

Modified Radical Mastectomy

- Mastectomy + axillary lymph node dissection.
- Level I and II nodes are routinely removed.
- Level III axillary dissection is reserved for patients who have enlarged level I and II lymph nodes.
- **Indications:**
  - o Staging.
  - o Local disease control in patients with axillary lymph node positive tumours
  - o Patients with > 3 sentinel lymph nodes that are positive for macrometastasis.

Skin and Nipple Sparing Mastectomy

- **Indications :**
  - o DCIS.
  - o tumour is > 1 cm away from skin and > 2 cm away from nipple.
- Breast can then be reconstructed using autologous tissue flaps/fat or a silicone breast implant.

Breast Conservation Surgery (BCS)

- Removing the tumour along with a 1 cm margin of normal breast tissue.
- Patients with involved margins should have a revision of margins called a cavity shave.
- **All patients with BCS receive radiotherapy.** BCS together with radiotherapy is called breast conservation therapy (BCT).

  BCS + RT = BCT
- Contraindications of BCS:
  - o Multicentric tumour.
  - o Diffuse microcalcifications on a mammogram.
  - o Large tumour to breast ratio.
  - o Two times positive surgical margins after re-excision.
  - o History of previous breast or chest wall irradiation.
  - o SLE or other collagen vascular disease (these patients have a high risk of a radiation reaction).
  - o Ankylosing spondylitis.
  - o Severe orthopnoea (as the patient cannot lie on the radiation table).

Wide Local Excision

- WLE of upto 20% of the breast volume can be achieved by excision of the tumour with adequate margins and closure of the defect by approximation of the breast tissue with absorbable sutures.

Oncoplasty

- Volume loss > 20% or an unfavourable breast-to-tumour ratio requires an oncoplastic procedure.
- Oncoplasty is defined as a tumour excision with wide margins followed by repair of the defect by local rearrangement/ replacement of the breast tissue and the nipple areola complex to maintain shape and symmetry.
- This may be achieved by:
  - o Volume displacement (level 1).
  - o Volume replacement (level 2) using a distant or local flap.

Level 1 Oncoplasty or Volume Displacement

- Volume displacement technique involves a dual plane mobilisation of the breast parenchyma, i.e., the dermoglandular plane and the plane between breast parenchyma and pectoralis muscle, to close the defect created after wide local excision.

Level 2 Oncoplasty or Volume Replacement

- More complex procedures that involve skin excision and glandular mobilization to allow major volume resection, usually > 20% of breast volume.
- Although the mainstay of treatment of early breast cancer is surgery, neoadjuvant chemotherapy is indicated in select cases of early breast cancer:
  - o To downsize the tumour to facilitate BCS.
  - o Her-2/neu positive tumours.
  - o Triple negative breast cancer.
  - o Premenopausal women (age < 50 years).
  - o Patients with axillary node mets.

B. Locally Advanced Breast Cancer (Stage III A, III B)

- The treatment of LABC is neo-adjuvant systemic therapy, followed by surgery, followed by adjuvant therapy (radiotherapy and/or chemotherapy)

Neo-Adjuvant Systemic Therapy

- Consists of chemotherapy, targeted therapy or hormonal therapy prior to surgery.
- **Aims:**
  - o To downsize the disease.
  - o To know the in vivo response of the tumour to therapy.

1. Neo-adjuvant targeted therapy

- Administered for HER-2/ neu positive tumours > 5 mm in diameter.
- **Drugs:** Trastuzumab, Pertuzumab.

2. Neo-adjuvant hormonal therapy

- Given to elderly or frail women with ER and/ or PR positive status, who are deemed unfit to receive systemic chemotherapy.
- **Drugs:**
  - o **Selective Estrogen Receptor Modulator:** Tamoxifen (used in pre-menopausal women).
  - o **Aromatase inhibitors:** Anastrozole, Letrozole, exemestane (used in post-menopausal women).
- Takes longer (around 3-6 months) for the response to be seen.

3. Neo-Adjuvant chemo therapy

- The indications for NACT are as follows:
  - o **Locally Advanced Breast Cancer T3, T4/ N2, N3 disease:** To downsize the tumour.
  - o **Select cases of early breast cancer:**
    - ♦ To downsize the tumour to facilitate breast conservation surgery (BCS).
    - ♦ HER2/neu-positive tumours.
    - ♦ Triple-negative breast cancer (TNBC).
    - ♦ Premenopausal women (age <50 years).
    - ♦ Patients with axillary node metastasis.
- The patient is assessed 3 weeks after the 2nd cycle of NACT:
  - a. For patients with complete response and partial response, the entire chemotherapy regimen may be delivered prior to surgery.
  - b. For patients showing stable or progressive disease, the patient should undergo surgery and be given 2nd line chemotherapy after surgery.

Surgery

- Following NACT, patients should be offered the option of mastectomy or BCS, if suitable.
- Patients with initial skin or chest wall involvement and those with inflammatory carcinoma should undergo MRM.

Adjuvant Radiotherapy

- It decreases the risk of locoregional and systemic recurrence and improves survival.
- **Indications of radiotherapy after mastectomy:**
  - o Tumour size > 5 cm.
  - o Skin or chest wall involvement.
  - o Lymphovascular invasion.
  - o Axillary lymph node positive for mets.

Adjuvant Chemotherapy

- The purpose is to control putative micromets, delay relapse and prolong survival
- The following regimens are used:
  1. **CMF:** Cyclophosphamide, Methotrexate, 5-Fluoro Uracil
  2. **Anthracycline based regimens:**
     - ♦ CAF - Cyclophosphamide, Adriamycin/ Doxorubicin, 5-Fluoro Uracil
     - ♦ CEF - Cyclophosphamide, Epirubicin, 5 -Fluoro Uracil
  3. **Taxane based regimens:** Docetaxel, Paclitaxel
- Indications of adjuvant chemotherapy are:
  - o All invasive carcinomas > 1 cm in diameter.
  - o Presence of lymphovascular invasion.
  - o High grade.
  - o Her-2/neu positive.
  - o Triple negative breast cancer.
  - o Node positive tumours.

C. Metastatic Carcinoma of Breast (Stage IV)

- **Aims:**
  - o Palliating symptoms.
  - o Improving quality of life.
  - o Prevention of potentially disabling complications.
  - o Attempt to prolong life.
- Endocrine therapy for ER/PR positive tumours is preferred for patients with bony mets and limited visceral mets.
- Systemic chemotherapy is preferred for patients with hormone receptor-negative cancers, hormone refractory mets and patients with visceral crisis.
- **Bony mets:**
  - o Palliative radiotherapy to lesions in weight bearing areas (e.g., vertebra, femur).
  - o Palliative radiotherapy to painful bony deposits.
  - o Bisphosphonates.
- Symptomatic pleural effusions are palliated by intercostal chest drainage and pleurodesis.
- Surgical resection of metastatic lesions may be indicated in solitary visceral metastasis in patients with good performance status and favourable tumour biology.

[3] Tamoxifen. *March 21*

- It is a SERM, i.e., Selective Estrogen Receptor Modulator.

Mechanism of Action

- It acts by competing with the circulating estrogens for binding to the cytoplasmic estrogen receptors (ER).
- It is a non-steroidal anti-estrogen.
- It causes cell death of ER positive and ER negative cells.
- The response rates are high in ER positive breast carcinomas, but some ER negative tumours also respond.

Uses

- Used as hormonal treatment for breast cancer.
- **Early cases:** Used as adjuvant therapy.
- **Advanced cases:** Used in the form of palliative treatment.
- Used in the treatment of primary as well as metastatic breast cancer in premenopausal women.
- Primary prophylaxis of breast cancer in high risk women.
- Reduces recurrence rates in i/l and c/l breast.
- Treatment of mastalgia, if pain score is > 3 on a VAS of 0-10.

Side Effects

- Hot flashes.
- Nausea, vomiting.
- Higher incidence of DVT.
- Higher incidence of endometrial cancer.

[3] BRCA. *March 24*

- BRCA is short for **BR**east **CA**ncer gene.
- These genes produce proteins that help repair damaged DNA.
- **There are two BRCA genes:** BRCA1 and BRCA2.
- **BRCA1 (17q):**
  - o Situated on long arm of chromosome 17.
  - o Associated with a 50–85% lifetime risk of developing breast cancer.
  - o 40% risk of ovarian cancer.
  - o Breast cancers in *BRCA1* are mostly triple negative breast cancer.
- **BRCA2 (13q):**
  - o Situated on long arm of chromosome 13.
  - o Associated with an up to 50–60% lifetime risk of breast cancer.
  - o 20% risk of ovarian cancer.
  - o Also associated with cancer of the prostate, colon, gallbladder, bile duct, stomach and pancreas.
- BRCA mutation is more common in males with breast cancer.
- Women with a BRCA mutation may be offered a bilateral risk-reducing mastectomy with immediate breast reconstruction, as it reduces the risk of breast cancer by 90%.
- Chemoprophylaxis with tamoxifen or anastrozole may reduce the risk to 50%.
- Premenopausal women may be offered bilateral salpingo-oophorectomy after they have completed their family at around 35–40 years of age.

[5] Gynecomastia. *March 22*
[3] Gynaecomastia. *Oct 20*

- **Definition:** Gynaecomastia refers to an enlarged breast in the male.

Causes

1. **Physiological:**
   - **Occurs during 3 phases of life:** Neonatal period, adolescence and senescence.
   - Common to each of these phases is an excess of circulating estrogens in relation to circulating testosterone.
2. **Pathological:**
   - The pathophysiologic mechanisms that may initiate gynaecomastia are:

   a. **Estrogen excess states:**
   - o Increase in the secretion of estradiol by the testes or by non-testicular tumors, e.g. Leydig cell tumors, Sertoli cell tumors, choriocarcinoma, seminoma, adrenal cortical neoplasms, lung carcinoma.
   - o Nutritional alterations such as protein and fat deprivation.
   - o Endocrine disorders such as hyper/hypothyroidism
   - o Hepatic disease, e.g., non-alcoholic and alcoholic cirrhosis

   b. **Androgen deficiency states:**
   - o Primary testicular failure:
     - ♦ Klinefelter's syndrome (47 XXY).
   - o Secondary testicular failure:
     - ♦ Trauma.
     - ♦ Orchitis.
     - ♦ Cryptorchidism.
     - ♦ Bilateral testicular atrophy (seen with leprosy).

   c. **Pharmacologic causes:**
   - o **Drugs with estrogenic activity:** E.g., digitalis, estrogens, anabolic steroids, marijuana.
   - o **Drugs that enhance estrogen synthesis:** E.g., human chorionic gonadotropin.
   - o Drugs that inhibit the action or synthesis of testosterone: E.g., cimetidine, ketoconazole, phenytoin, spironolactone.

- o **Others:** E.g., reserpine, theophylline, verapamil.

d. **Idiopathic.**

Clinical Features

- During puberty, the condition is often unilateral.
- Senescent gynaecomastia is bilateral.
- In the non-obese male, breast tissue measuring at least 2 cm in diameter must be present to diagnose gynaecomastia.

Investigations

- Mammography.
- USG.
- Serum estrogen, testosterone.

Treatment

- Reassurance.
- **Surgery:**
  - o Local excision.
  - o Liposuction.
  - o Subcutaneous mastectomy.

OTHER IMPORTANT TOPICS

BREAST ABSCESS

- **Definition:** A breast abscess is a collection of pus in the breast tissue.

Causes

- Lactational (puerperal) mastitis.
- **Non-lactational mastitis:**
  - o Periductal mastitis.
  - o Idiopathic granulomatous mastitis.
  - o Tubercular mastitis.

Pathogenesis

- Lactational mastitis is more common.
- Most cases are caused by *Staph aureus.*
- Hospital acquired cases may be due to MRSA.
- **May be bacterial or non-bacterial:**

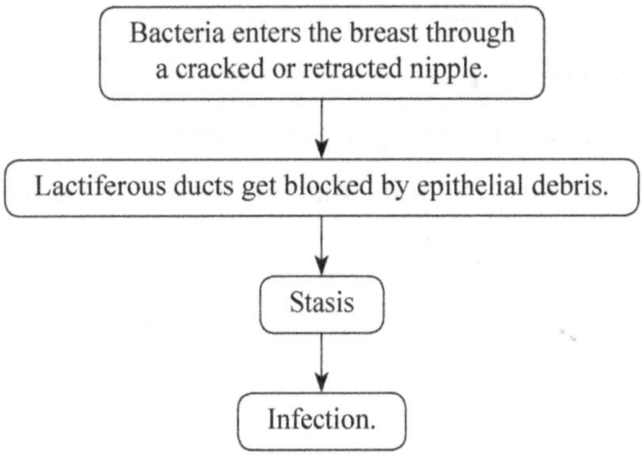

- Breast abscess formation is most commonly seen at 2 stages during lactation:
  1. In the first month after the first childbirth, owing to inexperience or inappropriate and inadequate breastfeeding.
  2. At weaning, due to trauma to the nipple by the baby's teeth.

Clinical Features

- Breast abscess is preceded by cellulitis.
- An abscess presents as a fluctuant lump (fluctuation may be absent in a deep-seated abscess).
- Pain.
- **Signs of inflammation:** Redness, swelling, tenderness.
- Fever.
- Malaise.
- Difficulty in feeding.
- Axillary nodes are enlarged and tender.

Investigations

- USG shows the presence of liquefaction necrosis.
- Pus should be sent for C/S.

Treatment

A. During Cellulitis Stage

- **Antibiotics:** Cloxacillin, flucloxacillin or erythromycin.
- Breastfeeding from both breasts should be encouraged 2-hourly, followed by emptying of the breast.
- Supportive bra.

- Cold compression.
- Analgesics.

B. Presence of Pus

- USG guided aspiration/drainage.

C. Abscesses > 3 cm in Diameter or Those Containing > 30 ml Pus

- A vacuum suction catheter is inserted under ultrasound guidance to drain the pus.
- Patient should be reviewed on alternate days and any residual collection should be aspirated.
- Catheter is irrigated with cold normal saline until complete resolution.

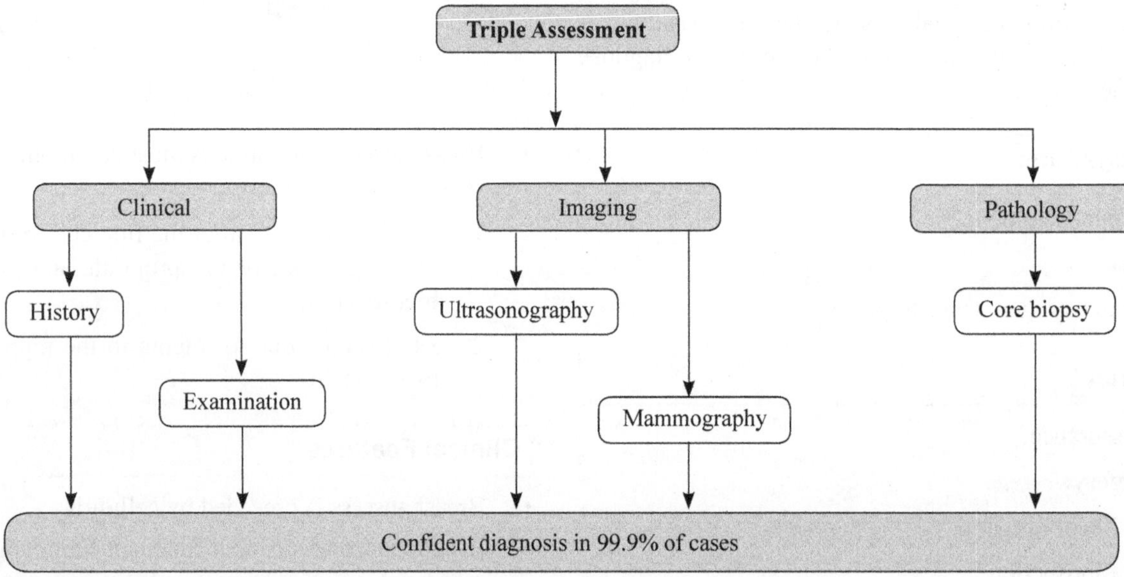

Figure: Triple assessment

29

Arteries

PERIPHERAL VASCULAR DISEASE OR THROMBOANGIITIS OBLITERANS (TAO) OR BUERGER'S DISEASE

[10] 40 years man presented with pain in the right calf while walking for the last 6 months. He also noticed change in colour of the 2nd toe of right foot. ***CBME March 24***

A. What is the probable diagnosis?

B. What other history would you like to take?

C. Relevant investigations to be done?

D. Add a note on management of thromboangiitis obliterans.

[10] Discuss the aetiology, clinical features and management of thromboangiitis obliterans. ***August 22, March 21, June 13***

[10] Enumerate causes of peripheral vascular disease. Discuss clinical features, investigations and management of a case of Buerger's disease. ***Oct 20***

[10] Discuss the investigation and principles of management of ischemic limb. ***Dec 19***

[10] What are the causes of leg ulcer? Write in detail about thromboangiitis obliterans. ***Dec 18***

[10] A 50 year old hypertensive male patient presents to the clinic with claudication pain over the right thigh with gangrene of right 4th and 5th toe. Discuss in detail the management of this particular patient. ***June 16***

[10] Describe the aetiology, clinical features, investigations and management of thromboangiitis obliterans. ***Dec 13***

[10] Describe the aetiopathogenesis, clinical features, investigations and principles of management of arterial occlusive disease. ***March 24***

[5] Buerger's disease. ***Dec 15***

[3] Intermittent claudication. ***March 22, Dec 12***

[3] Doppler scan. ***June 16***

[5] Digital Subtraction Angiography. ***June 14***

[3] Ankle - Brachial Pressure Index. ***Feb 23***

[3] Duplex scan. ***July 23***

- Thromboangiitis obliterans (TAO) is also known as peripheral vascular disease (PVD) or Buerger's disease.
- TAO is characterized by the following:
  1. Chronic occlusive disease of small and medium sized arteries of the limb.
  2. Thrombophlebitis of superficial or deep veins.
  3. Raynaud's syndrome.
- Usually one or two of the three manifestations are present, and occasionally all three.
- There may also be involvement of the neighboring nerve.
- Thrombophlebitis of superficial veins may be migratory.

Aetiology of TAO

- Cigarette smoking.
- Young males.
- Although TAO occurs almost exclusively in young male smokers, it occurs rarely, even in female smokers.

Aetiology of Peripheral Arterial Disease

- There has been a dramatic rise in peripheral arterial disease, which is thought to be due to an increase in the underlying risk factors:
  1. Population ageing (i.e., increased longevity).
  2. Diabetes mellitus.
  3. Hypertension.
  4. Obesity.
  5. Smoking.

Pathology of TAO

- Inflammatory changes in the walls of arteries and veins, leading to thrombosis.

Clinical Features of Chronic Arterial Stenosis or Occlusion in the Leg

1. **Intermittent Claudication:**
   - Occurs as a result of anaerobic muscle metabolism due to accumulation of excessive P substances in the muscle, which are not absorbed properly due to inadequate blood supply.
   - Classically described as debilitating cramp-like pain felt in the muscles that is:
     - o Brought on by walking.
     - o Not present on taking the first step (unlike osteoarthritis).
     - o Relieved by rest in both the standing and sitting positions, usually within 5 minutes (unlike nerve compression from a lumbar intervertebral disc prolapse or osteoarthritis of the spine or spinal stenosis, which are typically relieved only when resting in the sitting position for > 5 minutes).
   - The distance that a patient is able to walk without stopping is called claudication distance and varies only slightly from day to day.
   - Claudication distance is decreased by:
     1. Increasing the work demands and hence the oxygen requirements of the muscles affected, e.g. walking uphill, increasing the speed of walking and/or carrying heavy weights.
     2. By general health conditions that reduce the oxygen delivery capacity of the arterial system, e.g., anemia or cardiorespiratory disease.
   - The muscle group affected by claudication is classically one anatomical level below the level of arterial disease.
   - Claudication is usually felt in the posterior calf as the superficial femoral artery is the most commonly affected artery.
   - Aortoiliac disease may cause buttock claudication. **Leriche syndrome**: Buttock claudication + sexual impotence which is secondary to arterial insufficiency.
   - **Boyd's grading/classification of claudication pain:**
     - o **Grade 1:** Patient complains of pain; however, if the patient continues to walk, the metabolites increase the muscle blood flow and may sweep away the substance P produced by exercise and pain disappears.
     - o **Grade 2:** Pain continues and the patient can still walk with some effort.
     - o **Grade 3:** Pain compels the patient to take rest.
     - o **Grade 4:** Pain on rest.
2. **Rest pain:**
   - As the disease progresses, the claudication distance decreases and perfusion to the leg may be so severely compromised that anaerobic metabolism occurs even at rest.
   - Typically affects foot and/or calf.
   - Pain is exacerbated by lying down or elevation of the foot because of the loss of gravitational effects on the perfusion pressure in the foot.
   - Pain is worse at night and may be lessened by hanging the foot out of bed or by sleeping in a chair (restoring the effects of gravity).
3. **Ulceration and gangrene:**
   - Seen in severe arterial insufficiency.

- Present as painful erosions between the toes or as shallow, non-healing ulcers on the dorsum of the feet, shins and especially around malleoli.
- **Dry gangrene:** Blackened mummified tissues.
- **Wet gangrene:** Dry gangrene + supra-added infection.
- **Chronic limb-threatening ischemia (CLTI):** Patients with ischemic rest pain ± tissue loss (ulceration/gangrene). Management consists of urgent vascular assessment/revascularization to prevent major amputation.

4. **Temperature:**
   - A chronically ischemic limb tends to equilibrate with the temperature of its surroundings and may feel quite warm under the bed clothes.
5. **Sensation and movement:**
   - Does not produce paralysis and sensation is usually intact.
6. **Colour:**
   - Colour changes with:
     - o Elevation – foot pallor.
     - o Dependency – red/purple colour.
   - This is called dependent rubor or the sunset foot sign.
7. **Capillary refill time:**
   - Normal is 2-3 seconds.
   - In severe ischemia, it may be prolonged to 10 seconds.
8. **Arterial pulsations are diminished or absent**
9. **Arterial bruit:**
   - Heard on auscultation.
   - Suggests a stenosis.

Investigations

- The aims of investigations are:
  1. To confirm the presence and severity of peripheral arterial disease.
  2. To identify the anatomical location of disease.
  3. To assess the suitability of the patient for intervention.

A. General Investigations

- Since arterial disease is often a multisystem disease process, the following investigations need to be done:
  - o Total blood count.
  - o Blood glucose.
  - o Lipid profile.
  - o Renal function tests – urea, creatinine, electrolytes.
  - o ECG.
  - o 2D-ECHO.
  - o Exercise testing.
  - o Arterial blood gases (ABG).
  - o Pulmonary function tests.

B. Specific Investigations

1. **Doppler ultrasound blood flow detection**
   - Principle/mechanism:
     - o The doppler probe transmits a continuous wave ultrasound signal at an artery and a receiver within the probe itself, picks up the reflected beam.
     - o Change in frequency in the reflected beam compared with that of the transmitted beam is due to the doppler shift, which results from the reflection of the beam by moving blood cells.
     - o Any frequency change is converted into an audio signal, that is typically pulsatile.
   - Doppler USG can be used with a sphygmomanometer to assess systolic blood pressure in small vessels. This is possible even when the arterial pulse cannot be palpated.
   - Normal artery: Triphasic signal.
   - Diseased artery: Biphasic or monophasic signal.
   - Although the presence of a doppler signal indicates moving blood, it does not necessarily indicate that the blood flow is sufficient to maintain limb viability and prevent limbs loss.

- **Ankle Brachial Pressure Index (ABPI or ABI)**
  - o Can be measured bedside.
  - o It is the ratio of systolic pressure at the ankle to that in the i/l arm, i.e., highest pressure in the dorsalis pedis, posterior tibial or peroneal artery : highest brachial systolic pressure.
  - o Normal value = 0.9 – 1.4.

- o Arterial obstruction/claudication (i.e. hemodynamically significant arterial lesion) is < 0.9
- o Chronic limb threatening ischemia (CLTI) is < 0.4
- o Media sclerosis and calcification of arterial wall is > 1.4
- o These values are merely a guide and normal values may be present with intermittent claudication.
- o Retesting after exercise, to the onset of pain can be useful.
- o A drop in the resting ABI of > 20% after exercise is indicative of flow-limiting arterial disease.

- **Toe brachial pressure index (TBI):**
  - o TBI + ABI is a more reliable diagnostic tool for the detection of significant large vessel steno-occlusive disease in patients with diabetes mellitus.
  - o This is because toes (digital arteries) are rarely affected by sclerosis.
  - o TBI <0.6 suggests a significant arterial lesion that may have been overlooked if ABI was used in isolation.

2. **Duplex doppler USG:**
   - Non-invasive technique.
   - Uses B-mode ultrasound to provide an image of vessels.
     - o Image is created because of the varying ability of different tissues to reflect the ultrasound beam.
     - o A second ultrasound beam is then used to insonate the imaged vessel and the doppler shift obtained is analyzed.
     - o Colour coding allows detailed visualization of blood flow, turbulence, etc.
   - Different colours indicate changes in direction and velocity of flow with areas of high flow usually indicating a stenosis.
   - **Advantages:**
     - o As accurate as angiography in experienced hands.
     - o Cost-effective.
     - o Safe.
   - **Limitations:**
     - o Aortoiliac segment can be difficult to visualize because of bowel gas or obesity.
     - o Subjective, i.e., based on operator experience.
     - o Calcification of vessels limits the ability to accurately assess the severity of steno-occlusive disease.
   - When duplex ultrasound is inadequate, DSA (Digital Subtraction Angiography) or CT angiography are used.

3. **DSA or Digital Subtraction percutaneous Angiography**
   - **Principle:**
     - o Common femoral artery is accessed percutaneously using the Seldinger technique.
     - o Radio-opaque dye is injected into the arterial tree.
     - o Images obtained are digitalized and the extraneous background (bone, soft tissues, etc) is removed to provide clearer images.
   - **Advantages:**
     - o Provides dynamic arterial flow information.
     - o Can be combined with a definitive endovascular intervention when indicated.
   - **Disadvantages:**
     - o Expensive.
     - o Usage should be limited to patients in whom an intervention is anticipated.
     - o **Complications:** Bleeding, hematoma, false aneurysm formation, thrombosis, arterial dissection, distal embolization, renal dysfunction, allergic reaction.

4. **CT angiography:**
   - It is a minimally invasive alternative to DSA.
   - **Uses:**
     - o When Doppler ultrasound is not possible (intra-thoracic arteries) or produces poor images (aortoiliac segment).
     - o When planning revascularization procedures.
   - **Drawbacks:**
     - o Exposure to ionizing radiation.
     - o Use of iodinated contrast.

- o Interactions between contrast and certain diabetic drugs such as metformin.

5. **MR angiography:**
   - Non-invasive.
   - **Advantages:**
     - o No ionizing radiation.
     - o No iodinated contrast.
     - o Useful in diabetics who have calcified crural vessel disease, which is difficult to assess using Duplex Doppler ultrasound or CT angiography.
     - o MR angiography has the ability to differentiate contrast from vessel wall calcification.
   - **Disadvantages:**
     - o Contraindicated in patients with claustrophobia or certain metallic implants, e.g., pacemakers.
     - o Uses Gadolinium as contrast agent and patients with renal dysfunction are at risk of gadolinium induced nephrogenic systemic fibrosis.

Management of Arterial Stenosis or Occlusion

A. General

- **Aims of treating claudication:**
  1. Prevention of major cardiovascular morbidity through risk factor modification.
  2. Symptom relief/improvement.
- Stop smoking; this arrests, but does not reverse the disease.
- Control diabetes mellitus.
- Control of hypertension.
- Control of hyperlipidemia.
- Weight loss in obese patients.
- A structured exercise program of at least 2 hours of exercise per week for 3 months.

B. Non-Surgical Management

a. Drugs:

- Statins should be prescribed even when the lipid profile is normal, as it may stabilize atherosclerotic plaques and protect against cardiac death.
- **Antiplatelet drugs:** Clopidogrel 75 mg/day or aspirin 75 mg/day.
- Vasodilators were used earlier; they are unlikely to provide any benefit.
- For patients with rest pain or tissue necrosis, intervention is usually required to prevent major amputation.

b. Percutaneous transluminal angioplasty:

- **Indications:** Claudication, rest pain or tissue necrosis.
- **Procedure:**
  - o Done under LA.
  - o Following percutaneous femoral artery puncture, a guidewire is inserted and negotiated through the stenosis or occlusion under fluoroscopic control.
  - o A balloon catheter is positioned within the lesion over the guidewire and inflated at high pressure for 30 seconds.
  - o Satisfactory dilation is confirmed by performing an angiogram.
- **Use:** It is very successful in dilating the iliac and femoropopliteal segments, but results below the knee are less successful.
- **Subintimal angioplasty:**
  - o Used to treat long occlusions.
  - o Guidewire crosses the lesion in the subintimal space (in the arterial wall) and a new lumen is created by inflation of the balloon.
- **Complications:** Failure, hematoma, bleeding, thrombosis, distal embolization.
- These complications may impact on the surgeon's ability to perform a subsequent open surgical revascularization procedure.

c. Stenting:

- If the vessel fails to stay adequately dilated (often caused by elastic recoil of the artery), it may be possible to hold the lumen open using a metallic stent.
- Stent is introduced on a balloon catheter and expanded by balloon inflation.
- A self-expanding stent may also be used.

C. **Surgery**

- The indication for surgery is patients with severe symptoms (chronic limb threatening ischemia or lifestyle limiting claudication) where angioplasty has failed or is not possible.
- **Treatment depends on the level of the block:**
  1. **Aortoiliac occlusion:**
     - o Aorto-bifemoral bypass using a Dacron graft is generally used. However, in unfit patients, axillo-bifemoral bypass is an alternative.
  2. **If only one iliac system is occluded:**
     - o Ilio-femoral or femoro-femoral crossover graft is used.
  3. **Superficial femoral artery disease:**
     - o Femoro-popliteal bypass.
     - o Autologous Great Saphenous Vein when used as conduit gives best results.
     - o Alternatives to GSV: Lesser Saphenous Vein, arm veins. If no vein is available, prosthetic PTFE (poly tetra fluoro ethylene) graft may be used.
     - o Many surgeons construct the lower anastomosis using a small collar of vein (Miller cuff or St Mary's boot) between the PTFE and the recipient artery, which may improve patency.
  4. **Isolated common femoral artery or profunda disease:**
     - o End-arterectomy and patch (vein or prosthetic) or a short bypass in the groin.
  5. **If occlusion extends beyond the popliteal artery into the tibial (crural) vessels:**
     - o Femoro-distal bypass.
     - o If limb salvage is not possible, amputation is done; and the level of amputation is determined by the level of the block.

GANGRENE

[10] Discuss aetiology, clinical features and management of thromboangiitis obliterans. Add a note on gangrene. ***June 17***

- **Definition:** Gangrene refers to the death of macroscopic portions of tissue, which turns black because of the breakdown of hemoglobin and the formation of iron sulphide.

Sites Affected

- It usually affects the most distal part of a limb, the appendix, a loop of small intestine, and sometimes organs such as the gallbladder, the pancreas or the testis.

Types of Gangrene According to Cause

1. **Secondary to arterial obstruction from disease:**
   - Thrombosis of an atherosclerotic artery.
   - Embolus from the heart in atrial fibrillation or after coronary thrombosis.
   - Arteritis with neuropathy in diabetes.
   - Buerger's disease.
   - Arterial shutdown in Raynaud's disease.
   - Ergotism.
   - **Intra-arterial injections:** Thiopentone, cytotoxic substances.
2. **Infective:**
   - Boils and carbuncles, gas gangrene, Fournier's gangrene.
3. **Traumatic:**
   - **Direct:** Crushes, pressure sores and the constriction groove of strangulated bowel.
   - **Indirect:** Due to injury of vessels at some distance from the site of gangrene, e.g., pressure on the popliteal artery by the lower end of a fractured femur.
4. **Physical:**
   - Burns, scalds, frostbite, chemicals, irradiation and electricity.
5. **Venous gangrene.**

Clinical Features

- **Absence of:**
  - o Arterial pulsation.
  - o Venous return.
  - o Capillary response to pressure (colour return).
  - o Sensation.
  - o Warmth.
  - o Function.
- Colour of the part changes through a variety of shades according to circumstances (pallor, dusky,

grey, mottled, purple) until finally taking on the characteristic dark brown, greenish-black or black appearance, which is due to the disintegration of hemoglobin and the formation of iron sulphide.

Types

1. Dry gangrene.
2. Moist/wet gangrene.

DRY GANGRENE	WET GANGRENE
Occurs when the tissues are desiccated by gradual slowing of the bloodstream.	Occurs when venous + arterial obstruction are present.
Typically occurs as a result of atherosclerosis.	Infection and putrefaction are always present.
Affected part becomes: • Dry. • Wrinkled. • Discolored/black.	Affected part becomes: • Swollen. • Discolored. • Epidermis may be raised in blebs. • Crepitus is present.
If the blood supply of the proximal tissues is adequate, the line of demarcation (between normal tissue and the gangrenous part) appears and separation begins to take place neatly and with the minimum of infection (separation by aseptic ulceration).	There is more infection, and suppuration extends into the neighboring living tissue, thus causing the final line of demarcation to be higher than in dry gangrene (separation by septic ulceration).

Investigations

- Arterial doppler.
- Venous doppler.
- CT angiogram.
- MR angiogram.

Treatment

- The principles of Rx are as follows:
  - **A. Limb saving attitude** is needed in most cases of symptomatic gangrene affecting hands and feet.
    - o How much of a limb or digit can be salvaged depends on the blood supply proximal to the gangrene.
  - **B. Poor circulation should be improved by surgical revascularization,** which enables a more conservative debridement or distal amputation.
  - **C. Major limb amputation** may be required in the presence of life-threatening sepsis, when the blood supply cannot be improved or in patients whose limb is non-functional because of contractures, stroke, etc.
    - o Cardiac failure, atrial fibrillation and anemia are treated in order to improve the tissue oxygenation.

DIABETIC FOOT

[3] Diabetic foot. ***Dec 16***

- Diabetic foot is a complication of diabetes that occurs when high blood sugar levels damage nerves and blood vessels in the feet.

Cause

- Diabetic foot is usually caused by a combination of 3 factors:
  1. Ischemia secondary to macrovascular disease and microvascular dysfunction.
  2. Peripheral sensorimotor neuropathy, which leads to trophic skin changes.
  3. Immunosuppression caused by an excess of sugar in the tissues, which predisposes to infection.

Aetiopathogenesis

- Macrovascular disease is atherosclerotic and typically affects the crural vessels with relative sparing of the pedal vessels.
- Increased microcirculatory shunting causes micro-vascular dysfunction.
- Sensory neuropathy (classically in a stocking distribution) renders the patients at high risk of soft tissue injury and its subsequent neglect.
- Neuropathy may extend to the joints of the foot and ankle, resulting in loss of nociceptive and proprioceptive protective reflexes and a repeated cycle of joint injury and bony destruction.

Motor involvement
↓
Imbalance between flexor and extensor muscle groups of the foot
↓
Altered foot biomechanics and abnormal pressure loading
↓
Thick callosities develop on the sole of foot

- Ischemia and neuropathy act synergistically to increase the risk of diabetic foot ulceration and reduce its subsequent healing potential.
- Superadded infection due to poor wound care can spread rapidly and proximally in subfascial planes, leading to fulminant foot sepsis, gangrene and death.

Clinical Features

- History of longstanding and/or uncontrolled diabetes.
- There is usually history of trivial trauma such as a thorn prick, which may go unnoticed due to loss of sensation.
- Thick callosities develop on the sole of the foot which are followed by ulceration.
- Abscess and cellulitis of foot.
- There is change of colour and temperature where gangrene is impending.
- Both dry and wet gangrene are seen.
- Charcot's arthropathy.

Investigations

- C/S swab from wound.
- X-Ray foot: To rule out osteomyelitis.
- HbA1c.
- CBC.
- Doppler ultrasound.
- Duplex.

Treatment

- Control of diabetes.
- **Treatment depends on the degree of arterial involvement:**
  - o Gangrene is treated by liberal debridement of dead tissue.
  - o Any pus should be drained.
  - o Antibiotics.
- Angioplasty for macrovascular disease.
- Primary amputation should be considered for patients who present with life-threatening systemic upset.

RAYNAUD'S DISEASE AND RAYNAUD'S SYNDROME

[3] Raynaud's disease. *Dec 19*

RAYNAUD'S DISEASE

- Idiopathic condition.
- Usually occurs in young women.
- Affects hands more than the feet.

Aetiopathogenesis

- There is abnormal sensitivity in the arteriolar response to cold.
- **Raynaud's phenomenon:**
  - o Arterioles constrict and the digits (usually the fingers) turn white and become incapable of fine movements
  - o Capillaries then dilate and fill with slowly flowing deoxygenated blood, resulting in the digits becoming swollen and dusky.
  - o As the attack passes off, the arterioles relax, oxygenated blood returns into the dilated capillaries and the digits become red.
- Thus, the condition is recognized by the characteristic sequence of blanching, dusky cyanosis and red engorgement, often accompanied by pain.

Clinical Features

- F > M.
- Usually occurs in young women.
- Affects hands more than feet.
- Superficial necrosis is seen but is very uncommon.

Treatment

- Protection from cold (wear gloves).
- Avoidance of pulp and nail bed infection.
- Calcium channel blockers, e.g., nifedipine.
- Electrically heated gloves are useful in winter.

- Sympathectomy was used in the past, but is now obsolete as it is ineffective and its effects are short-lived.

RAYNAUD'S SYNDROME

- It is the peripheral arterial manifestation of a collagen disease such as systemic lupus erythematosus or rheumatoid arthritis.

Clinical Features

- Same as for Raynaud's disease, but they may be much more aggressive.
- May also follow the use of vibrating tools in industry, called 'vibration white finger'.
- When secondary to collagen disease, it leads frequently to necrosis of digits and multiple amputations.

Treatment

- Directed primarily at the underlying condition.
- Nifedipine, i.e., calcium channel blockers.
- Steroids.
- Vasospastic antagonists.
- Patients with vibration white finger should avoid vibrating tools.
- Protection from cold (gloves).
- Avoidance of pulp and nail bed infection.
- Sympathectomy yields disappointing results and is not recommended.

THORACIC OUTLET SYNDROME

[3] Adson's test. ***March 21***

Thoracic Outlet Syndrome

- Thoracic Outlet Syndrome refers to compression of the subclavian vessels and nerves of the brachial plexus in the region of the thoracic inlet.

Aetiology and Pathogenesis

- The subclavian vessels and the brachial plexus can be compressed at various locations as they pass between the thoracic inlet and the upper extremity. From medial to lateral, these anatomic regions are as follows:

1. Interscalene triangle.
2. Costoclavicular space.
3. Subcoracoid area.

Causes

- Cervical rib.
- Bony degenerative cervical spine changes.
- Physical trauma.
- Anatomical defects.
- Tumours.
- Poor posture.

Clinical Features

- Most commonly seen in middle aged women.
- Symptoms vary depending on the anatomic structure that is compressed.
- The most common structure to be compressed is nerves.
- **Symptoms due to nerve compression:**
  - o Numbness.
  - o Tingling.
  - o Weakness.
  - o Pain in the arm, hand or fingers.
  - o Muscle atrophy.
  - o Impaired sensation and coordination.
  - o Difficulty with hand movements.
- **Symptoms due to subclavian artery compression:**
  - o Fatigue
  - o Weakness.
  - o Coldness.
  - o Upper extremity claudication.
  - o Thrombosis.
  - o Paresthesia.
  - o Thrombosis with distal embolisation can cause Raynaud's phenomenon.
- **Symptoms due to venous compression:**
  - o Edema.
  - o Venous distension.
  - o Collateral formation.

- Cyanosis of affected limb.
- Effort thrombosis (called Paget-Schroetter syndrome).

Clinical Maneuvers

- These are evocative tests performed to elicit symptoms in patients suspected of having Thoracic Outlet Syndrome:

1. **Adson or Scalene test:**
    - The patient inspires maximally and holds their breath while the neck is fully extended and the head is turned towards the affected side.
    - This maneuver narrows the space between the scalenus anterior and medius, resulting in compression of the subclavian artery and the brachial plexus.
    - Decrease or loss of i/l radial pulse suggests compression.
2. **Halsted's costoclavicular test:**
    - The patient is instructed to place their shoulders in a military position, i.e., drawn backwards and downwards.
    - This narrows the costoclavicular space between the first rib and clavicle, causing neurovascular compression.
    - Reproduction of neurologic symptoms or decrease or loss of i/l radial pulse suggests compression.
3. **Wright's hyperabduction test:**
    - The patient's arm is hyperabducted to 180°.
    - This causes the neurovascular structures to be compressed in the subcoracoid region by the pectoralis tendon, the head of the humerus, or the coracoid process.
    - Decrease or loss of i/l radial pulse suggests compression.
4. **Roos test:**
    - The patient abducts the involved arm 90° with external rotation of the shoulder.
    - Maintaining this body position, the patient is asked to open and close their hands rapidly for 3 minutes.
    - This reproduces symptoms.

Investigations

- Chest X-ray.
- Cervical spine X-ray.
- CT scan.
- MRI.
- Doppler studies.
- **Vascular imaging:**
    - Conventional angiography/venography.
    - CT angiography.

Treatment

- Physiotherapy.
- Repetitive upper extremity mechanical work and muscular trauma are avoided.
- **Surgery:**
    - Aim is to release the narrowing/pressure point at the thoracic outlet.
    - **Options are:**
        1. Detachment of the anterior and middle scalene muscles from the first rib.
        2. Resection of first rib.
        3. Release of the pectoralis minor muscle from its insertion on the coracoid process.
        4. Neurolysis of dense fibrosis along the brachial plexus.

30

Veins

VARICOSE VEINS

[10] Describe the symptoms, signs, investigations and treatment of varicose veins. ***Sept 21***

[10] Discuss the clinical features, presentation and management of varicose veins. ***June 19***

[10] Define varicose veins. Discuss pathophysiology, clinical features and management of varicose veins. ***Dec 14***

[5] Complications of varicose veins. ***Dec 16***

[3] Mention complications of varicose veins. ***June 17, Dec 13***

- **Definition:** A dilated, elongated and tortuous vein is called a varicose vein.

Aetiology

- F > M.
- **Age:** Chances of varicose veins increases with age.
- **Obesity and height:** Increasing BMI is associated with a higher prevalence of varicose veins.
- Pregnancy increases the risk of varicose veins.
- Family history.
- Occupation and lifestyle factors:
  - o Contrary to conventional medical belief, there is inconclusive evidence regarding increased prevalence of varicose veins in smokers, in patients who suffer constipation and in those with occupations that involve prolonged standing.

Types

- Varicose veins can be classified as:
  - **A. Primary**
    - o Result from intrinsic abnormalities of venous wall.
  - **B. Secondary**
    - o Associated with deep and/or superficial venous insufficiency.

Pathophysiology

- The direction of blood flow in normal conditions is as follows:

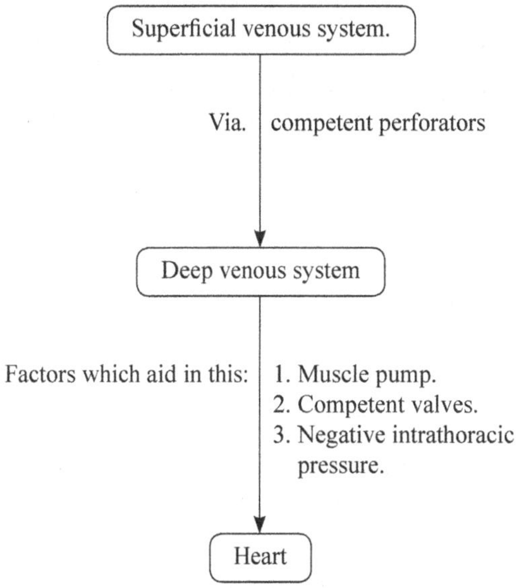

  - o If this mechanism breaks down, the blood becomes stagnated in the superficial veins and thus becomes distended and tortuous to become varicose veins.

- **The underlying factor of varicose veins is venous hypertension.**
- Venous hypertension leads to vein wall damage. This venous damage goes on to reduce the function of the affected veins, worsening the venous hypertension in a vicious cycle.

Clinical Features

- The most common symptom of varicose veins is pain.
  - o Patients describe aching, heaviness, throbbing, burning or bursting over affected areas and sometimes over the whole limb.
  - o Such symptoms typically increase throughout the day or with prolonged standing.
  - o Some patients may suffer from cramp in the calf shortly after retiring to bed.
  - o Symptoms are relieved by elevation or compression hosiery.
- Swelling of the ankle towards evening.
- Patients may present with no other symptom except dilated and tortuous veins of the leg.
- **Clinical features due to complications of varicose veins:**
  - o Skin over varicosities may itch.
  - o Skin may be thickened and/or pigmented.
  - o Eczema of affected skin.
  - o Venous ulceration.
  - o Symptoms can be very severe and interfere with the day-to-day activities of the patient.

On Examination

- Tortuous, dilated, subcutaneous vein is clinically obvious.
- The distribution of varicosities may indicate which superficial axis is defective:
  - o Medial thigh and calf varicosities suggest Great Saphenous Vein (GSV) incompetence.
  - o Posterolateral calf varicosities are suggestive of Short Saphenous Vein (SSV) incompetence.
  - o Anterolateral thigh and calf varicosities may indicate isolated incompetence of Anterior Accessory of Great Saphenous Vein (AAGSV).
- **Saphena Varix:**
  - o Large, dilated veins around the sapheno-femoral junction (SFJ) may present as a (usually painless) lump.
  - o Increases on standing.
  - o Decreases on lying down.
  - o Gentle palpation over the varix during coughing may elicit an impulse and it may be mistaken for a groin hernia.
- Skin over medial part of lower surface of leg should be inspected to exclude edema, pigmentation, eczema or ulceration.
- Lipodermatosclerosis may be present over medial surface of lower leg.

Complications

1. **Thrombophlebitis of superficial veins**
   - Veins become red and feel like tender cords in the subcutaneous tissue.
2. **Pigmentation**
   - Particularly seen in lower part of leg.
   - Brownish to blackish pigmentation, due to hemosiderin deposits from breakdown of RBCs which have leaked out of the veins.
3. **Eczema or chronic dermatitis**
   - Due to extravasation and breaking down of RBCs in the lower part of the leg, the skin may itch.
4. **Ankle flare**
   - In case of varicosity of GSV, small veins from the sole of the foot and ankle which drain into GSV become dilated and this gives rise to swelling of the ankle, called ankle flare.
5. **Venous ulcer**
   - Mostly found on or near the medial malleolus.
6. **Hemorrhage**
   - Hemorrhage from ruptured varicose veins may follow minor trauma.
   - It can be profuse.
7. **Periostitis**
   - Occurs in long-standing cases, particularly if a

venous ulcer is formed over the medial surface of the tibia.

8. **Calcification**
   - Occasionally seen in the walls of the veins which are varicosed for many years.

9. **Equinus deformity of foot**
   - May result from long-standing varicosity.
   - It is due to the bad practice of the patient of walking on the toes for relief of pain due to varicosity. After some years, the Achilles tendon may be shortened and leads to such deformity.

10. **Lipodermatosclerosis**
    - It is a condition where there is skin thickening, fibrosis and pigmentation.
    - The cause is related to increased venous pressure during ambulation.
    - Progression to an ulcer is common.

11. **Champagne bottle leg**
    - The constriction from lipodermatosclerosis causes an inverted champagne bottle appearance of the leg.

Investigations

- Tourniquet tests, hand held Doppler and varicography have been abandoned.
  1. **Duplex ultrasound scanning:**
     - o Should be done for all patients with varicose veins prior to any intervention.
     - o High frequency linear array transducer of 7.5-13 MHz is used to obtain good quality images.
     - o B-mode settings are used.
     - o Pulsed wave spectral or colour Doppler settings should be optimised for the low flow velocities encountered within veins.
     - o Antegrade venous flow towards heart shows as blue colour.
     - o Reverse venous flow shows as red colour.
     - o Visible venous flow can be augmented by a calf squeeze.
     - o The aim of duplex is to establish the following:
       - ♦ Presence of reflux in the deep and superficial venous system.
       - ♦ The exact distribution and extent of reflux in the superficial venous system, including affected junctions (sapheno-femoral and saphenopopliteal junction) and perforators.
       - ♦ Presence of obstruction in the deep venous system.
       - ♦ Suitability of incompetent superficial veins for the different treatment options available (based upon diameter, extent, tortuosity, saphena varix).
       - ♦ Presence of thrombus within the superficial veins.
       - ♦ An indication of a pelvic source of reflux or obstruction.
     - o Superficial veins should be examined with patient in standing position.
     - o Scan commences in the groin and proceeds distally.
     - o **Mickey Mouse sign:** Great Saphenous Vein and Common Femoral Vein lying medial to Common Femoral Artery.
  2. **Pelvic and iliac veins may be investigated using transabdominal or transvaginal duplex scan.**
  3. **Magnetic Resonance (MR) venography.**
  4. **Contrast venography.**
  5. **Intravenous ultrasound (IV US).**

Treatment

- The various options for treatment are:

  A. **Compression stockings.**

  B. **Endothermal ablation:**
     1. Endovenous Laser Ablation (EVLA).
     2. Radio Frequency Ablation (RFA).

  C. **Non-endothermal, non-tumescent ablation:**
     1. USG guided foam sclerotherapy.
     2. Catheter directed sclerotherapy and mechanicochemical ablation.
     3. Endovenous glue.

D. Open surgery–Junction ligation and stripping.

E. Adjunctive surgical techniques:

1. Phlebectomy.
2. Perforator ligation.
3. SEPS or Subfascial Endoscopic Perforator Surgery.

A. Compression Hosiery/Stockings

- **Mechanism of action:** Graduated external pressure improves deep venous return and reduces venous pressures.
- May be knee length or thigh length.
- It improves varicose vein symptoms.
- It is classified according to the pressure it exerts (British classification):
  - o Class I: 14-17 mm Hg.
  - o Class II: 18-24 mm Hg.
  - o Class III: 25-35 mm Hg.

B. Endothermal Ablation

- It is now the gold standard treatment and has replaced surgical ligation and stripping.
- Performed as an OPD procedure under local anesthetic.
- Treats only junctional and truncal incompetence.
- Varicosities can be managed concomitantly or sequentially by either phlebectomy or sclerotherapy.
- **Procedure:**
  - o A treatment device is inserted into the incompetent axial vein percutaneously.
  - o Tumescent local anesthetic solution is injected around the vein.
  - o The treatment device then produces thermal energy that destroys the structure of the vein, resulting in permanent occlusion.
  - o **2 types of technologies are used:**
    1. Endo Venous Laser Ablation (EVLA).
    2. Radio Frequency Ablation (RFA).

Endo Venous Laser Ablation (EVLA)

- This procedure is very good for the treatment of any vein that will allow the passage of a guide - wire.
- Laser energy is used to generate the thermal energy.

Radio Frequency Ablation (RFA)

- Uses the same treatment principles as EVLA, but an electromagnetic current is used to create the thermal energy.
- The most popular device is the ClosureFast Device.

C. Non-Endothermal, Non-Tumescent Ablation

1. USG guided foam sclerotherapy

- Sclerosing agent is injected directly into the superficial veins.
- Most commonly used sclerosant is sodium tetradecyl sulphate.
- Sclerosant has detergent action and causes cellular death and initiates an inflammatory response, aiming to result in thrombosis, fibrosis and obliteration (sclerosis).
- Blood deactivates the action of the sclerosant. The use of foam increases the effective volume of the agent, maximizing endothelial contact and displacing any blood that deactivates it.
- Tessari method is the most widely used method of preparing the foam sclerosant.

2. Catheter directed sclerotherapy and mechano-chemical ablation

- The efficacy of sclerotherapy relies on endothelial contact with fresh, undiluted sclerosant.
- Some have therefore experimented with catheter-delivered sclerotherapy rather than trying to milk the sclerosant down the vein lumen.

3. Endovenous glue

- Endoluminal application of cyanoacrylate adhesive.

D. Open Surgery

- The role of open surgery as a primary treatment of a refluxing superficial axis has been considerably reduced with the development of the minimally invasive techniques.
- **Principle:**
  - o The principles of open surgery, i.e., ligation and stripping is to fully dissect the point of junctional incompetence and to remove the refluxing axial vein and dilated tributaries.

- **Procedures done:**
  1. For Great Saphenous Vein varicosity:
     - o Saphenofemoral junction ligation and GSV stripping, called Trendelenburg's procedure.
  2. For Short Saphenous Vein varicosity:
     - o Saphenopopliteal junction ligation and SSV stripping.
- The operation is usually performed under GA but locoregional anesthesia can also be used.
- Flush ligation is done, as it prevents recurrence.

E. Adjunctive Surgical Techniques

1. Phlebectomy

- Usually performed through small stab incisions using small mosquito forceps and/or phlebectomy hooks.
- **Indications:**
  - o May be performed following Trendelenburg's procedure, i.e., in the same sitting.
  - o As a sole treatment in patients with isolated tributary incompetence.

2. Perforator Ligation

- **Indications:**
  - o In venous ulcers, as it promotes their healing.
  - o **In uncomplicated varicose veins:** Perforators may be ligated through a small, duplex-guided incision.

3. SEPS or Subfascial Endoscopic Perforator Surgery

- Preferred in patients with skin changes.

[3] CEAP classification. ***March 24***

- CEAP (<u>C</u>linical–a<u>E</u>tiology–<u>A</u>natomy–<u>P</u>athophysiology) is a descriptive classification used for chronic venous disorders and is widely utilised.

Clinical Classification

- C0: No signs of venous disease.
- C1: Telangiectasia or reticular veins.
- C2: Varicose veins.
- C3: Oedema.
- C4a: Pigmentation or eczema.
- C4b: Lipodermatosclerosis (LDS) or atrophie blanche.
- C4c: Corona phlebectatica.
- C5: Healed venous ulcer.
- C6: Active venous ulcer.

  Clinical classification can be further characterised as **symptomatic (s), asymptomatic (a) or recurrent** following previous successful treatment or healing **(r)**, e.g., C2a, C2s, C6r.

Aetiological Classification

- Ec: Congenital.
- Ep: Primary.
- Es: Secondary (post-thrombotic).
- En: No venous cause identifed.

Anatomical Classification

- As: Superficial veins.
- Ap: Perforator veins.
- Ad: Deep veins.
- An: No venous location identified.

Pathophysiological Classification

- Pr: Reflux.
- Po: Obstruction.
- Pr,o: Reflux and obstruction.
- Pn: No venous pathophysiology identifiable.

VENOUS OR VARICOSE ULCER

[5] Venous ulcer. ***Dec 19***

[10] What is venous ulcer? Describe in detail aetiology, pathology, clinical features and management of varicose veins in the lower limb. ***Dec 17***

[3] Varicose ulcer. ***Dec 15***

[MCQ] Following are features of venous ulcer except: ***CBME March 24***

A. Sloping edge

B. Occurs at pressure sites*

C. Venous hypertension

D. Surrounding skin pigmentation

[5] Etiopathogenesis and management of venous ulcer. ***CBME June 24***

- Venous ulcer is the most common cause of chronic lower limb ulcers.
- Some patients with venous leg ulcers have concomitant arterial occlusive disease. This is called a mixed ulcer.

Pathophysiology

- The exact pathophysiology of ulcer development has not been established.
- **At present, ambulatory venous hypertension is the only accepted underlying cause of venous ulceration. This theory also explains why venous ulcers are never seen in the upper limb.**
- Venous hypertension may be the result of primary valve incompetence of the saphenous veins, incompetence of the perforating veins or incompetence or obstruction of the deep veins.

Clinical Features

- Characteristically develop in the **gaiter region**:
  - o This is located circumferentially around the lower leg from approximately mid-calf to just below the medial and lateral malleoli.
  - o This is the region where many of the Cockett perforators join the posterior tibial vein to the surface vein.
  - o Majority of the ulcers develop on the medial side of the calf.
- Ulcers often develop in response to **minor trauma.**
- Many patients notice some **itching before the ulcers develop** (this is probably because of mast cell degranulation).
- **Venous ulcers are sometimes accompanied by varicose veins, where it is called a varicose ulcer.**

On Examination

- Venous ulcer is usually vertically oval in shape.
- Sloping edge.
- Floor contains granulation tissue covered by a variable amount of slough and exudate.
- Almost all venous ulcers have surrounding haemosiderosis (seen as pigmentation).
- The more chronic ulcers develop lipodermatosclerosis with associated fibrosis of the subcutaneous tissue.
- LDS manifests as thickening, pigmentation, inflammation and induration of the calf skin.
- The pigmentation comes from haemosiderin and melanin.
- Multiple ulcers are sometimes present which are in different stages of healing.

Investigations

- **Duplex scan**
  - o To assess status of deep veins, superficial veins and perforators.
- **Biopsy**
  - o Done to rule out malignancy.
  - o This is because a Marjolin's ulcer can develop in a chronic longstanding venous ulcer.
- All patients should have their peripheral pulses palpated and, if there is any doubt, their arterial doppler pressures should be measured.
- Sensation and proprioception should be assessed to exclude neuropathy, especially in diabetics.
- CBC.
- FBS, PPBS, HbA1c.
- ESR.
- CRP.

Treatment

- The cause of a venous leg ulcer is venous hypertension and the keystone of management is to decrease this hypertension using:
  1. Venous ablation.
  2. Compression therapy.

A. Superficial Venous Ablation or Surgery

- In patients with venous leg ulcers, treatment of superficial venous incompetence accelerates healing and reduces recurrence.

B. Compression Therapy

- Compression therapy is applied over the primary dressing for the venous ulcer.
- The most clinical and cost-effective compression regimes are two-layer compression hosiery or four layer compression bandaging.
- Four layer dressing includes:

1. Orthopedic wool

- o Distributes the pressure and reduces

undue pressure on sensitive areas susceptible to pressure damage.

- o Also helps to absorb excess exudate that escapes the primary dressing.

2. **Cotton crepe**
   - o Smoothens the wool and holds it in place.
3. **Elastic bandage**
   - o First compressive layer.
   - o Contributes about 1/3rd of the interface pressure.
4. **Cohesive bandage**
   - o Second compressive layer.
   - o Increases stiffness.
   - o Adds 2/3 of the interface pressure.

C. Other Treatments

- Pentoxifylline increases microvascular perfusion and this augments ulcer healing.
- Horse chestnut seed extract improves symptoms and reduces leg volume in chronic venous hypertension.
- Biological dressings, including fetal keratinocytes and collagen meshes.
- Split skin grafting.
- Ulcer excision + SSG.

VENOUS THROMBOEMBOLISM

[10] Discuss the aetiology, clinical features and management of Deep Vein Thrombosis of lower limb. ***Dec 13***

[5] Deep vein thrombosis. ***August 22, March 20***

[3] Deep Vein Thrombosis. ***March 24***

DEEP VEIN THROMBOSIS

- Autopsy studies suggest that **venous thromboembolism is the most common direct cause of death in surgical patients**.
- Venous thrombosis is the formation of a semisolid coagulum within the venous system and may occur in:
  - o **Superficial system:** Superficial vein thrombosis or thrombophlebitis.
  - o **Deep system:** Deep vein thrombosis.

Aetiology

- The 3 factors of **Virchow's triad** are:
  1. Contact of blood with an abnormal surface (e.g., endothelial damage).
  2. Abnormal flow (e.g., stasis).
  3. Abnormal blood (e.g., thrombophilia).
- Any of these factors result in thrombus formation.

Risk Factors

A. Patient Factors

- Age.
- Obesity.
- Varicose veins.
- Immobility.
- Pregnancy.
- Puerperium.
- High dose estrogen therapy.
- Previous deep vein thrombosis or pulmonary embolism.
- Thrombophilia.
  - o **Congenital causes:**
    - ♦ Deficiency of anti-thrombin III, protein C or protein S.
    - ♦ Antiphospholipid antibody or Lupus anticoagulant.
    - ♦ Factor V Leiden gene defect or activated protein C resistance.
    - ♦ Dysfibrinogenemias.
  - o **Acquired causes:**
    - ♦ Antiphospholipid antibody or lupus anticoagulant.

B. Disease or Surgical Procedure

- Trauma or surgery, especially of pelvis, hip and lower limb.
- Malignancy, especially pelvic and abdominal metastatic.
- Heart failure.

- Recent myocardial infarction.
- Paralysis of lower limb(s).
- Infection.
- Inflammatory bowel disease.
- Nephrotic syndrome.
- Polycythemia.
- Paraproteinemia.
- Paroxysmal nocturnal hemoglobinuria antibody or lupus anticoagulant.
- Behcet's disease.
- Homocystinemia.

Pathology

- The thrombus **commences as a platelet aggregate**.
- Subsequently, **fibrin and RBCs form a mesh** until the lumen of the vein wall occludes.
- The thrombus then **progresses as a propagated loose red fibrin clot containing many RBCs.**
- This may extend up to the next large venous branch and it is **possible for the clot to break off and embolise to the lung as a pulmonary embolus.**
- The clot **lodges in the pulmonary arteries.**
- This may totally **occlude perfusion to all or part of one or both lungs.**

Clinical Features

- The most common presentation of a DVT is **pain and swelling, especially in the calf.**
- Occlusion of a length of the deep femoral vein will cause **painful congestion** and **oedema** of the leg.
- **Phlegmasia cerulea dolens or blue leg:**
  - o It is due to extensive DVT of the major axial deep venous channels of the lower extremity with relative sparing of collateral veins.
  - o Characterised by pain and pitting edema with associated cyanosis.
- **Phlegmasia alba dolens or white leg:**
  - o When the thrombosis extends to the collateral veins, massive fluid sequestration and more significant oedema ensue.
  - o The affected extremity is extremely painful and oedematous and pale secondary to arterial insufficiency from dramatically elevated below lower knee compartment pressures.
- Both blue and white leg can be complicated by **venous gangrene** and the need for amputation.
- Unilateral > Bilateral.
- Some patients have no symptoms of thrombosis and **may first present with signs of a pulmonary embolus.**
  - o Pleuritic chest pain.
  - o Hemoptysis.
  - o Shortness of breath.
- A **low grade pyrexia** may be present, especially in a patient who is having repeated pulmonary embolus.

On Examination

- Clinical examination for DVT is unreliable.
- Mild pitting edema of the ankle.
- Dilated surface veins.
- Stiff calf.
- Tenderness over the course of the deep veins.
- **Homan's sign:**
  - o Resistance (not pain) of the calf muscles to forcible dorsiflexion of the foot.
  - o Unreliable.
  - o May cause embolism.
- **Moses' sign or Bancroft's sign:**
  - o Seen in thrombosis of posterior tibial veins.
  - o It is considered positive if pain is elicited when the calf muscle is compressed forwards against the tibia, but not when the calf muscle is compressed from side to side.
- If a patient has pulmonary emboli which causes right heart strain, the following signs may be present:
  - o Cyanosis.
  - o Dyspnoea.
  - o Raised neck veins.
  - o Fixed split second heart sound.
  - o Pleural rub.

Differential Diagnosis of DVT

- Ruptured Baker's cyst.
- Calf muscle hematoma.
- Ruptured plantaris muscle.
- Thrombosed popliteal aneurysm.
- Arterial ischemia.

Differential Diagnosis of a Pulmonary Embolism

- Myocardial infarction.
- Pleurisy.
- Pneumonia.
- Aortic dissection.

Investigations

- **Venous duplex ultrasound:**
  - o Can detect thrombosis throughout the deep or superficial venous system.
- **Compression ultrasound:**
  - o Involves applying pressure with the USG probe over the common femoral and popliteal veins.
  - o Normally, veins will compress tightly shut.
  - o In the presence of DVT, they will not fully compress.
- **Ascending venography:**
  - o Thrombus is seen as a filling defect.
  - o Rarely required nowadays unless thrombolysis is being considered.
- **MR venography.**
- **CT pulmonary angiogram:**
  - o Diagnoses pulmonary embolism, which is seen as filling defects in the pulmonary arteries.
- **Pulmonary angiography:**
  - o Rarely required unless thrombolysis is being considered.
- **Modified Wells' score is used as a guide to predict DVT:**
  - o **Low probability:** -2 to 0.
  - o **Moderate probability:** 1-2.
  - o **High probability:** > 2.

Variable	Score
Lower limb trauma or surgery or immobilisation in a plaster cast	1
Bedridden for >3 days or surgery in last 4 weeks	1
Tenderness along the line of femoral or popliteal veins	1
Entire limb swollen	1
Calf >3 cm larger circumference than the other side	
10 cm below the tibial tuberosity	1
Pitting oedema	1
Dilated collateral superficial veins (not varicose veins)	1
Previous DVT	1
Malignancy (including treatment up to 6 months ago)	1
Intravenous drug abuse	3
Alternative diagnosis more likely than DVT	-2

Prophylaxis

A. Mechanical Methods

- Graduated elastic compression stockings.
- External pneumatic compression.

B. Pharmacological Methods

- More effective than mechanical methods, although they carry an increased risk of bleeding.
- **Low Molecular Weight Heparin (LMWH)**
  - o Given subcutaneously.
  - o OD dose.
  - o Lower risk of bleeding complications.
  - o Contraindicated in patients with renal impairment.
- **Low-dose unfractionated heparin**
  - o Can be used in patients with renal impairment.

Treatment of Pulmonary Embolus

- Most pulmonary emboli can be treated by anti-coagulation and observation.
- If patient has severe right heart strain and shortness of breath:
  - o Thrombolysis.
  - o Radiologically guided catheter embolectomy.

Treatment of DVT

- These are:
    - o Rapid anticoagulation (with parenteral drugs) to reduce the risk of pulmonary embolism.
    - o Maintenance of anticoagulation with oral drugs.
    - o Inferior Vena Cava filters.
    - o Endovascular surgery.

Rapid Anticoagulation to Reduce the Risk of Pulmonary Embolism

- Rapidly anticoagulate the patient with a 'treatment dose' of subcutaneous LMWH.
- **If patient has renal impairment:** Give intravenous unfractionated heparin.
- Patients who have a sensitivity towards heparinoids, such as those with heparin induced thrombocytopenia, should be commenced on another anticoagulant:
    - o Fondaparinux (Indirect factor Xa inhibitor).
    - o Bivalirudin (Direct thrombin inhibitor).

Maintenance of Anticoagulation

- After rapid anticoagulation via IV or SC route, patient is started on oral anticoagulation for at least 3 months (or longer depending upon the persistence of risk factors or in recurrent cases).
- New or novel anticoagulants are used:
    - o **Direct inhibitors of factor Xa:** Rivaroxaban, Apixaban.
    - o **Direct thrombin inhibitors:** Dabigatran.
- Novel anticoagulants are as effective as Vitamin K antagonists (warfarin) in preventing recurrent symptomatic venous thromboembolism but are associated with less major bleeding complications.

Inferior Vena Cava Filters

- Patients who cannot be safely anticoagulated (usually because of bleeding risks) should be considered for a temporary IVC filter, until either they are safe to be anticoagulated or the risk of embolisation has subsided and the filter may be retrieved.

Endovascular Surgery

- **Aims:**
    - o To restore patency.
    - o To reduce the risk of chronic post-thrombotic syndrome.
- **Procedures done:**
    - o Thrombus removal.
    - o Lysis.
    - o Stenting techniques.

OTHER IMPORTANT TOPICS

PULMONARY EMBOLISM

- It is an important condition within surgery, and autopsy studies suggest that it is the most common direct cause of death in surgical patients.

Risk Factors for Pulmonary Embolism

A. Patient Factors

- o Age.
- o Obesity.
- o Immobility.
- o Pregnancy, Puerperium.
- o High-dose oestrogen therapy.
- o Thrombophilia.

B. Disease or Surgical Procedure

- Trauma (fracture) or surgery, especially of pelvis, hip and lower limb.
- Malignancy, especially pelvic and abdominal metastatic.
- Heart failure.
- Recent myocardial infarction.
- Paralysis of lower limb(s).
- Paroxysmal nocturnal hemoglobinuria antibody or lupus anticoagulant.
- Homocystinemia.

Aetiopathogenesis

- **The most important factor is a hospital admission** for treatment of a medical or surgical condition.
- While called **pulmonary,** this is a **disorder of the clotting system more than a primary insult to the lung parenchyma.**

- Thrombus **can arise from DVT in the legs/pelvis, venae cavae or the right atrium.**
- The **clot breaks off and embolises to the lungs.**
- It passes through the large veins of the limb and vena cava, through the right heart and **lodges in the pulmonary arteries.**
- This **may totally occlude perfusion to all or part of one or both lungs.**
- Its primary pathophysiology is to **increase pulmonary vascular resistance and ultimately, right heart failure.**
- Can cause significant dead space physiology with resultant **hypoxia**.

Clinical Features

- Can present in the early postoperative period.
- This results in a **clinical spectrum from tachycardia and pain, through respiratory failure (despite adequate ventilation) to cardiovascular collapse and death.**
- Signs and symptoms depend on the size of the embolus.
- Dyspnoea.
- Shortness of breath results from chronic pulmonary hypertension.
- Cough.
- Hemoptysis.
- Pleuritic chest pain.
- Sudden cardiovascular collapse.
- A **low-grade pyrexia** may be present, especially in a patient who is having repeated pulmonary embolus.
- **The two-level Wells Pulmonary Embolism score can be used to determine its probability**:
  - o **Unlikely:** < 4.
  - o **Suggestive of PE:** > 4.

Variable	Score
Clinical signs and symptoms of DVT (minimum of leg swelling and pain on palpation of deep veins)	3
Alternative diagnosis less likely than Pulmonary Embolism	3
Heart rate >100 bpm	1.5
Immobilisation >3 days or surgery within past 4 weeks	1.5
Previous DVT or PE	1.5
Hemoptysis	1
Malignancy (treatment or palliation within past 6 months)	1

On Examination

- Cyanosis.
- Raised neck veins.
- A fixed split 2nd heart sound.
- Pleural rub.

Differential Diagnosis

- Myocardial infarction.
- Pleurisy.
- Pneumonia.
- Aortic dissection.

Investigations

- ECG.
- **Venous duplex ultrasound** is performed to look for thrombosis in the venous system.
- **CT pulmonary angiography** is the gold standard to definitively diagnose pulmonary embolism. It demonstrates the presence of filling defects in the pulmonary arteries.
- **Transesophageal ECHO** can be rapidly used to evaluate for presence of right ventricular dilatation/failure and "right heart strain".

Prevention

- Prevention is the best weapon.
- Early ambulation.
- Intermittent pneumatic compression.
- Prophylactic anticoagulation in at risk populations.

Treatment

A. Supportive Measures

- Shift to ICU.
- Oxygen therapy.
- Analgesia.

B. Massive Pulmonary Embolism with Cardiovascular Collapse

- Resuscitation.
- Patient may need inotropes.
- Thrombolysis or radiologically guided catheter embolectomy can be considered in patients with severe right heart strain and shortness of breath.

C. Anticoagulation

- After initial resuscitation, the patient will need anticoagulation, initially parenteral anticoagulation followed by long-term oral anticoagulation.
- Rapidly anticoagulate patients with **a treatment dose of subcutaneous Low Molecular Weight Heparin (LMWH).**
- Patients with renal impairment should be given IV unfractionated heparin.
- Patients with sensitivity to heparinoids, e.g., heparin-induced thrombocytopenia, should be given another anticoagulant, such as fondaparinux or bivalirudin.
- After this, patient should be given oral anticoagulation for at least 3 months.
- This prevents clot propagation.
- Oral anticoagulation using **'novel' anticoagulants,** such as rivaroxaban, apixaban or dabigatran, is as effective as warfarin but are associated with less bleeding complications.

D. Vena Cava Filter

- An inferior vena cava filter may be needed if anticoagulation is not possible or if the patient has an embolism while anticoagulated, e.g., **Greenfield filter.**

31

Lymphatics

[5] Cystic hygroma. *March 21*

[3] Enumerate clinical features of cystic hygroma. *CBME March 24*

- It is a **congenital condition** characterized by a **fluid filled sac or cyst that forms most commonly in the neck region.**
- It is **filled with clear lymph** and **lined by a single layer of squamous epithelium.**

Embryology

- About the 6th week of embryonic life, the **primitive lymph sacs** develop in the mesoblast stage, the principal pair being situated **in the neck, between the jugular and subclavian veins**, called jugular lymph sacs.
- **Sequestration** of a portion of a jugular lymph sac, from the lymphatic system **causes cystic hygroma**.

Clinical Features

- Usually presents in the **neonate** or in **early infancy**.
- It may occasionally present at birth and be so large as to **obstruct labour**.
- Swelling usually occurs in the **neck** and **may involve the face, submandibular region, tongue and floor of the mouth.**
- **Less common sites:** Cheek, axilla, groin, mediastinum.
- **May be bilateral**.
- **Soft** in consistency.
- Partially **compressible.**
- Visibly **increases in size when the child coughs or cries.**
- It is **brilliantly transilluminant.**
- May become infected.
- The behaviour of cystic hygromas during infancy is unpredictable. Sometimes, the cyst expands rapidly and occasionally respiratory difficulty ensues.

Investigations

- **MRI:** Diagnoses the cystic hygroma and also shows its relationship to surrounding structures.

Treatment

- If it causes **respiratory difficulty**, it requires immediate **aspiration** and **occasionally, a tracheostomy**.
- **Definitive treatment is complete excision of the cyst at an early stage.**
- Injection of a **sclerosant** may reduce the size of the cyst. However, they are commonly multi-cystic and so, may not resolve completely.

[3] Lymphadenitis. *August 22*

- Due to acute inflammation of the drainage area, the regional **lymph nodes become acutely inflamed** and the condition is known as acute lymphadenitis.
- Affected lymph nodes become **enlarged, painful** and tender.

- **Overlying skin becomes warm and red with brawny oedema.**
- There is a varying degree of **pyrexia.**
- Due to **periadenitis**, which may be present in all the severe forms, the **lymph nodes may be matted together**.
- Cause is generally infectious:
  - o Bacterial.
  - o Viral.
  - o Parasitic.
- **Investigations:** FNAC may be required in case of doubt.
- **Treatment:**
  - o Antibiotics.
  - o Treatment of the underlying cause.

[3] Secondary lymphedema. *June 19*

- **Definition:** Lymphedema may be defined as abnormal limb swelling caused by the accumulation of increased amounts of high protein interstitial fluid due to defective lymphatic drainage in the presence of (near) normal net capillary filtration.
- Secondary lymphedema or acquired lymphedema is lymphedema in which there is a **clear underlying cause.**

Causes

1. **Trauma and tissue damage**
   - Lymph node excision, radiotherapy.
2. **Malignant disease**
   - Lymph node mets, infiltrative carcinoma, lymphoma.
3. **Venous disease**
   - Chronic venous insufficiency, venous ulceration .
4. **Infection**
   - Cellulitis, lymphadenitis, filariasis.
5. **Inflammation**
   - Rheumatoid arthritis, dermatitis.
6. **Endocrine disease**
   - Pretibial myxedema.
7. **Immobility and dependency.**

Clinical Features

- They are the same for primary and secondary lymphedema.
- **Characteristically involves the foot:**
  - o **Contour of ankle is lost** because of infilling of submalleolar depressions.
  - o **Buffalo hump** forms on dorsum of foot.
  - o **Toes appear square** because of confinement of footwear.
- **Stemmer's sign:** Skin on dorsum of toes cannot be pinched because of subcutaneous fibrosis.
- Usually **spreads proximally to knee level** and less commonly affects the whole leg.
- **Advanced disease:**
  - o Chronic eczema.
  - o Fungal infection of skin (dermatophytosis) and nail (onychomycosis).
  - o Fissuring.
  - o Verrucae and papillae (warts).
- In the initial stages, lymphedema pits and decreases on lying down. As it progresses, edema becomes non-pitting and is associated with irreversible skin changes.

Grading

- Brunner's grade is used to clinically grade lymphedema.

Grade	Clinical features
Subclinical (latent)	There is excess interstitial fluid and histological abnormalities in lymphatics and lymph nodes, but no clinically apparent lymphedema
I	Edema pits on pressure and swelling largely or completely disappears on elevation and bed rest
II	Edema does not pit and does not significantly reduce upon elevation, positive Stemmer's sign
III	Edema is associated with irreversible skin changes, i.e., fibrosis, papillae

Investigations

- Lymphangiography.
- Isotope lymphoscintigraphy.

- CT.
- MRI.
- USG.
- Lymphofluoroscopy.

Treatment

- **Relief of pain:** NSAIDs, opioids, etc.
- Skin care.
- Manual lymphatic drainage.
- Multi-layer lymphedema bandaging.
- Exercise.
- Surgery.

[5] Surgeries for filarial leg. ***June 14***

SURGERIES FOR LYMPHEDEMA

- Only a small minority of patients with lymphedema benefit from surgery.
- Operations for lymphedema fall into 3 categories:

A. Bypass Procedures

- **Indications:**
  - o Proximal ilioinguinal lymphatic obstruction with normal distal lymphatic channels.
- **Methods:**
  - o Omental pedicle.
  - o Gillies skin bridge.
  - o Neilubowicz anastomosis of lymph nodes to veins.
  - o Kinmonth's ileal mucosal patch.
  - o Direct microsurgical lymphaticovenular anastomosis.

B. Liposuction

- Used in the treatment of chronic lymphedema in patients with non-pitting edema.

C. Limb Reduction Procedures

1. **Sistrunk**
   - A wedge of skin and subcutaneous tissue is excised and the wound is closed primarily.
   - Most commonly carried out to reduce the girth of the limb.
2. **Homans**
   - Involves raising skin flaps to allow the excision of a wedge of skin and a larger volume of subcutaneous tissue down to the deep fascia.
   - It is the most satisfactory operation for the calf.
   - It is contraindicated in the presence of venous obstruction or active malignancy.
3. **Thompson**
   - It is a modification of the Homans' procedure aimed to create new lymphatic connections between the superficial and deep systems.
   - Buried dermal flap is used.
4. **Charles**
   - Excision of all of the skin and subcutaneous tissues down to the deep fascia, with coverage using split skin grafts.

[5] Chyluria. ***July 18***

- **Definition:** Chyluria is the presence of chyle in the urine.
- Intestinal lymph is also called chyle and it transports cholesterol, long chain fatty acids, triglycerides and the fat soluble vitamins directly to the circulation bypassing the liver.

Causes

1. Filariasis (most common cause).
2. Ascariasis.
3. Malaria.
4. Tuberculosis.
5. Trauma to the lymphatic system.
6. Iatrogenic (surgery).
7. Malignancies affecting the lymph nodes.

Pathogenesis

- There is an abnormal connection (fistula) between the lymphatic system and the urinary system.
- This allows leakage of chyle into the urine.

Clinical Features

- Painless passage of milky white urine.

- Increases after a fatty meal.
- Chyle may clot leading to renal colic.
- Hypoproteinemia.

Investigations

- IV urography.
- Lymphangiography.

These can demonstrate the lymphourinary fistula.

Treatment

- Low fat and high protein diet.
- Increased oral fluids to prevent clot colic.
- Laparotomy and ligation of dilated lymphatics.
- To sclerose the lymphatics either directly or via instrumentation of the bladder, ureter and renal pelvis.

[5] Hodgkin's lymphoma. *Dec 16*

- Also known as Hodgkin's disease.
- **Definition:** It is a group of malignant conditions that are characterized by the **presence of Reed-Sternberg cells** on histology.
- They **arise from germinal center B-cells.**

Aetiology

- Exact cause is unknown, but several factors are thought to be contributory.
- Epstein-Barr virus infection.
- Genetic factors.
- Family history.
- **Immunosuppression:** AIDS, organ transplants.
- **Environmental factors:** Pesticides, industrial chemicals.

Clinical Features

- M > F.
- **Bimodal age distribution:**
  - o **1st peak:** 20-40 years.
  - o **2nd peak:** 50 years.
- **Asymptomatic lymphadenopathy:**
  - o **Most common:** Cervical lymph nodes are involved.
  - o **Less common:** Other groups (axiliary, inguinal).
- **Constitutional symptoms:**
  - o Night sweats.
  - o Weight loss.
  - o Pruritus.
  - o Fatigue.
  - o Fever and chills.
  - o Loss of appetite.
- Some people c/o pain in affected lymph nodes after consuming alcohol.
- Pressure effects such as superior vena cava obstruction from enlarged mediastinal lymph nodes.
- Bone pain, particularly in the back, indicates vertebral collapse secondary to bone mets.
- Anemia and pancytopenia develop with dissemination bony mets.
- Skin deposits in advanced cases.
- Jaundice due to excessive hemolysis of red cells or diffuse liver involvement.
- **On examination lymph nodes are:**
  - o Discrete.
  - o Non-tender.
  - o Rubbery in consistency.
  - o Lymph nodes become matted as the disease advances.
  - o Splenomegaly.
  - o Hepatomegaly.

Spread

- Hodgkin lymphomas arise in a single lymph node or chain of lymph nodes and typically spread in a step-wise fashion to anatomically contiguous nodes.

Classification

According to the WHO/REAL classification:

A. Classical Hodgkin's lymphoma

1. Nodular sclerosis.
2. Mixed cellularity.
3. Lymphocyte depletion.
4. Lymphocyte rich.

B. Nodular Hodgkin's Lymphoma

1. Lymphocyte predominant.

WHO/REAL classification

- **Classical HodgKin's Lymphoma**
  1. Nodular sclerosis
  2. Mixed cellularity
  3. Lymphocyte depletion
  4. Lymphocyte rich
- **Nodular HodgKin's Lymphoma**
  1. Lymphocyte predominant

Staging

- **Ann Arbor staging with Cotswold modifications:**
  - I. Disease in a single lymphatic site.
  - II. Disease in ≥ 2 lymphatic sites on the same side of the diaphragm.
  - III. Disease on both sides of the diaphragm and includes splenic involvement.
  - IV. Disease with additional non-contiguous extra-lymphatic implication with or without associated lymphatic involvement.

Subscripts

E - Added to I, II or III and indicates single or contiguous extralymphatic spread.

S - Splenic involvement.

A - Constitutional symptoms are absent.

B - Constitutional symptoms are present.

Investigations

- ^{18}F-FDG PET/CT scan.
- CT with IV contrast.
- Incision or excision biopsy.

Treatment

- **Early stages: Radiation + chemotherapy.**
- **Advanced stages: Chemotherapy ± radiation.**
- Two regimens of chemotherapy are used:

1. **ABVD**
   - Adriamycin (doxorubicin), bleomycin, vinblastine, dacarbazine.
2. **BEACOPP**
   - Bleomycin, etoposide, doxorubicin, cyclophosphamide, vincristine, procarbazine, prednisone.
   - **Monoclonal antibodies:** Rituximab, obinutuzumab.

[5] Non-Hodgkin's lymphoma. ***July 23***

- It is a group of malignant tumours of lymphoid tissues which are derived from **germinal centre B cells.**
- Unlike Hodgkin's lymphomas, **Reed-Sternberg cells are absent** in non-Hodgkin lymphomas.

Classification

- Non-Hodgkin's lymphomas are classified into 27 distinct pathological subtypes, as per the **WHO/ REAL classification.**
- Common subtypes are:
  1. Diffuse large B-cell lymphoma.
  2. Follicular lymphoma.
  3. Mantle cell lymphoma.
  4. Marginal zone lymphoma.

Aetiology

- The exact course is not understood, but several risk factors are known:
  - o **Infections:** Epstein-Barr virus, H pylori.
  - o **Autoimmune diseases:** Rheumatoid arthritis, Sjogren's syndrome.
  - o **Immunosuppression:** AIDS, organ transplant.
  - o Family history.
  - o **Environmental factors:** Pesticides, industrial chemicals.

Clinical Features

- It usually manifests as painless lymphadenopathy.
- Multiple peripheral nodes are involved (more frequently involved when compared to Hodgkin's lymphoma).
- Mesenteric nodes and Waldeyer's ring are commonly involved.
- Extranodal involvement is common.

- Splenomegaly may be seen.
- It spreads in a non-contiguous manner.
- **Constitutional symptoms:**
  - o Night sweats.
  - o Weight loss.
  - o Pruritus.
  - o Fatigue.
  - o Fever and chills.
  - o Loss of appetite.

Staging

- Ann Arbor staging with Cotswold modifications (same as Hodgkin's lymphoma).

Investigations

1. **^{18}F-FDG PET/CT scan**
   - Stages the malignancy.
   - Helps with targeting FDG-avid lymph node with biopsy.
2. **Biopsy**
   - Incision or excision biopsy is gold standard for diagnosis.
   - Obtained before initiation of steroids, as steroids lyse lymphoid tissue and might obscure the diagnosis.

Treatment

1. **Chemotherapy**
   - **Combination regimens:** ABVD, BEACOPP.
   - **ABVD:** Adriamycin (Doxorubicin), Bleomycin, Vinblastine, Dacarbazine.
   - **BEACOPP:** Bleomycin, Etoposide, Adriamycin (Doxorubicin), Cyclophosphamide, Vincristine (Oncovin), Procarbazine, Prednisone.
2. **Monoclonal antibodies**
   - Rituximab, Obinutuzumab.
3. **Chimeric antigen receptor (CAR) T-cell therapy.**
4. **Radiation.**

OTHER IMPORTANT TOPICS

PRIMARY LYMPHEDEMA

- Primary lymphedema is that in which the **cause is unknown** (or at least uncertain and unproven).

Aetiology

- It is thought to be caused by **'congenital lymphatic dysplasia,'** which is an inherited abnormality of the lymphatic system.
- It is possible that **many sporadic cases** of primary lymphedema occur in the presence of a (near-) normal lymphatic system and are actually **examples of secondary lymphedema for which the triggering events have gone unrecognised.**
- More common in the legs than the arms because of gravity, bipedal posture and the fact that the lymphatic system of the leg is less well developed.

Types

- It is usually further subdivided on the basis of the presence of family history, age of onset and lymphangiographic findings:
  1. **Congenital**
     - o Onset < 2 years old.
     - o Can be sporadic.
     - o Can also be familial (Nonne–Milroy's disease)
  2. **Praecox**
     - o Onset 2–35 years old.
     - o Sporadic.
     - o Familial (Letessier–Meige's disease).
  3. **Tarda**
     - o Onset > 35 years old.
     - o Clinical features, Investigations and Treatment of secondary lymphedema are the same as primary lymphedema.

MALIGNANCIES ASSOCIATED WITH LYMPHEDEMA

- Lymphangiosarcoma (Stewart–Treves' syndrome).
- Kaposi's sarcoma (human immunodeficiency virus).
- Squamous cell carcinoma.
- Liposarcoma.
- Malignant melanoma.
- Malignant fibrous histiocytoma.
- Basal cell carcinoma.
- Lymphoma.

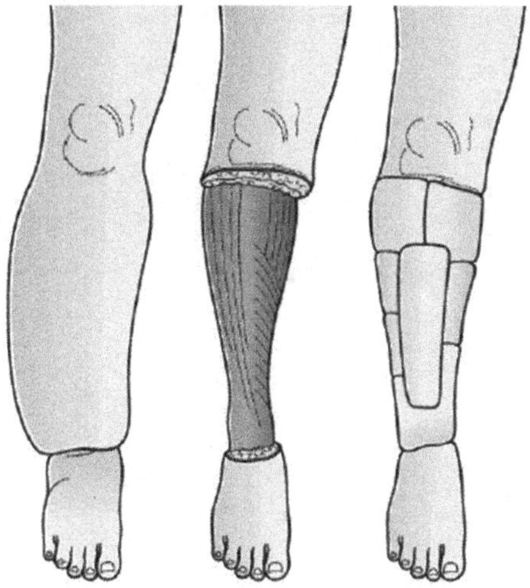

The Charles procedure involves circumferential excision of lymphedematous tissue down to, and including, the deep fascia followed by split-skin grafting. This procedure gives a very poor cosmetic result but does allow the surgeon to remove very large amounts of tissue and is particularly useful in patients with severe skin changes.

Figure 1: Charles procedure

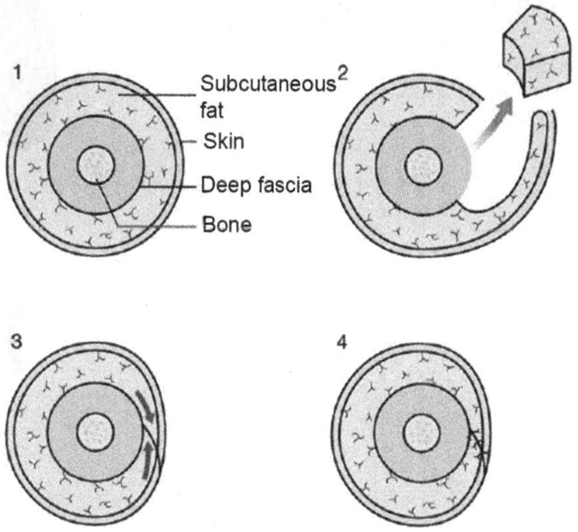

A cross-sectional representation of Thompson's reduction operation; red arrows illustrate the buried dermal flap sutured to deep fasica.

Figure 2: Thompson procedure

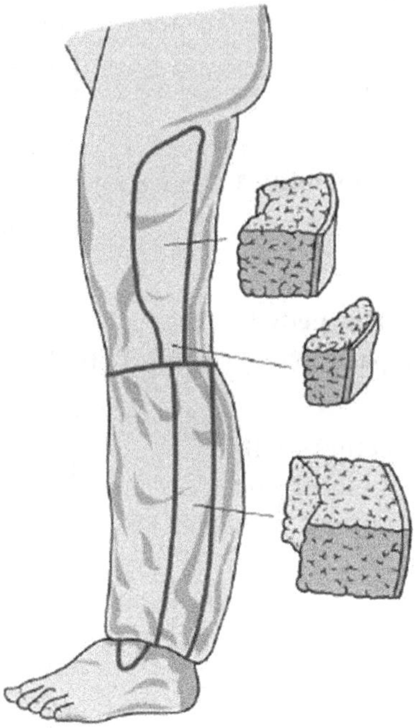

Homans' procedure involves raising skin flaps to allow the excision of a wedge of skin and a larger volume of subcutaneous tissue down to the deep fascia. Surgery to the medial and lateral aspects of the leg must be separated by at least 5 months to avoid skin flap necrosis.

Figure 3: Homans procedure

32

Liver

[5]	Surgical lobes of liver. ***June 17***
[3]	Surgical segments of liver. ***June 16***

- Historically, the liver was divided into left and right lobes by the obvious external landmark of the falciform ligament. This was anatomically incorrect in relation to the blood supply of the liver.

Segmental/Functional Anatomy

- The concept of segmental anatomy **facilitates anatomical liver resection.**
- The liver is composed of **8 segments.**
- Each segment is supplied by its **own portal pedicle (triad)** which contains: **Portal vein + hepatic artery + bile duct.**
- **The 8 segments are grouped into 4 sectors, with each sector containing 2 segments (except for medial sector of left hemilever which contains only one segment).**
- Sectors are separated by **scissurae**.
- Since there are 4 sectors, there are 3 scissurae.
- The scissurae **contain the main hepatic veins:** Right hepatic vein, middle hepatic vein and left hepatic vein.
- The **4 sectors are grouped into 2 hemilivers:** Right hemiliver and left hemiliver, with each hemiliver containing 2 sectors.

A. Right Hemiliver or Right Liver.

- Contains 4 segments grouped into 2 sectors.
  - o **Anterior sector:** Segments V and VIII.
  - **Posterior sector:** Segments VI and VII.
- The anterior and posterior sectors are separated by the right scissura which contains the right hepatic vein.
- The right hemiliver is **supplied by the right hepatic artery and the right branch of the portal vein and biliary drainage is via the right hepatic duct.**
- Between the right hemiliver and the left hemiliver is the **main scissura**. This **contains middle hepatic vein**. The main scissura is **also known as Cantlie's line** (between the gallbladder fossa and the middle hepatic vein).

B. Left Hemiliver or Left Liver

- **Contains 3 segments, grouped into 2 sectors:**
  1. **Lateral sector:** Segments III and IV.
  2. **Medial sector:** Segment II.
- The lateral and medial sectors are separated by the **left scissura** which **contains the left hepatic vein**.
- The left hemiliver is **supplied by the left hepatic artery and the left branch of the portal vein and biliary drainage is via the left hepatic duct.**

C. Caudate Lobe/Segment I

- It is the **dorsal portion of the liver.**
- The vascular supply and biliary drainage to the caudate lobe comes from **both the left and right pedicles.**

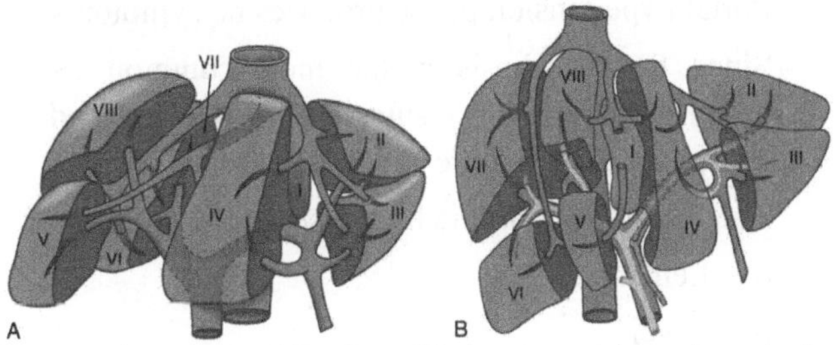

Segmental anatomy of the liver. (A) As seen at laparotomy in the anatomic position. (B) In the ex vivo position (From Blumgart LH, Hann. LE. Surgical and radiologic anatomy of the liver and biliary tract. In: Blumgart LH, Fong Y, eds. *Surgery of the Liver and Biliary Tract*. London: WB Saunders;2000: 3-34.)

Figure 1: Surgical segments of liver

[3] Signs of liver cell failure. ***Dec 18***

- **The features of chronic liver disease are as follows:**
  - o Lethargy.
  - o Fever.
  - o Jaundice.
  - o Scratch marks.
  - o Protein catabolism (wasting).
  - o Coagulopathy (bruising).
  - o Cardiac manifestation because of hyperdynamic circulation.
  - o **Cutaneous:** Spider naevi, palmar erythema.
  - o Loss of body hair.
  - o Parotid enlargement.
  - o Testicular atrophy.
  - o Gynecomastia.
  - o Dupuytren's contracture.
  - o Asterixis or flapping tremors.
  - o Clubbing.
  - o Purpura.
  - o Pigmented ulcers.
- When chronic liver disease becomes decompensated, patients present with following symptoms, leading to a diagnosis of portal hypertension:
  1. Hepatic encephalopathy.
  2. Ascites.
  3. **Collateral vessels:**
     - o Variceal bleeding from esophageal & gastric varices, i.e., hematemesis.
     - o **Caput medusa:** It is a cutaneous manifestation and consists of dilated, enlarged, superficial veins radiating from the umbilicus.
  4. Splenomegaly and hypersplenism
     - o Manifests as thrombocytopenia, leucocytopenia, erythrocytopenia.

[10] Describe the aetiology, clinical features and management of portal hypertension. ***June 16***

[5] Clinical features and management of portal hypertension. ***Dec 19***

[5] Management of portal hypertension. ***June 19***

[5] Esophageal varices. ***June 19***

[5] Caput medusae. ***July 18***

PORTAL HYPERTENSION

- **Definition:** Portal hypertension is defined by a portal pressure gradient, (i.e., difference in pressure between the portal vein and the hepatic veins), greater than 5 mm Hg.
- However, higher pressures (8-10 mm Hg) are typically required to begin stimulating the development of portosystemic collateralization.

Causes

- The most common cause of portal hypertension is liver cirrhosis.

A. Prehepatic

- Portal vein thrombosis
- Extrahepatic portal vein obstruction (EPVO) or cavernous transformation of portal vein
- Splenic vein thrombosis
- Arteriovenous fistula

B. Intrahepatic

- Liver cirrhosis (it has multiple etiologies)
- Congenital hepatic fibrosis
- Veno-occlusive disease
- Noncirrhotic portal fibrosis
- Schistosomiasis
- Nodular regenerative hyperplasia

C. Posthepatic

- Budd-Chiari syndrome (hepatic vein or inferior vena cava obstruction)
- Constrictive pericarditis

Pathophysiology

- Portal hypertension **usually occurs because of increased portal venous resistance** that is pre-hepatic, intrahepatic or posthepatic in location.
- Several **factors** contribute to this:
  - o Increased passive resistance secondary to **fibrosis and regenerative nodules.**
  - o **Increased hepatic vascular resistance because of active vasoconstriction** (by noradrenaline, endothelin and other humoral vasoconstrictors).
  - o **Increased portal venous inflow** secondary to a hyperdynamic systemic circulation and splanchnic hyperemia.
- Portal hypertension stimulates the development of **portosystemic collateralization.**
- **Collateral vessels usually develop where the portal and systemic venous circulations are in close apposition.**
- Sites of development of collateral vessels, i.e., portosystemic anastomoses:
  1. **Esophagogastric junction**
     - o Esophagogastric varices is the most important site of portosystemic anastomoses clinically.
     - o It is the collateral network through the coronary and short gastric veins to the azygos vein.
  2. **Periumbilical region (called caput medusae)**
     - o It is a cutaneous manifestation, with visible collateral veins radiating from the umbilicus.
     - o Named after Medusa, who in Greek mythology had her fine hair turned into snakes.
  3. **Retroperitoneal collateral vessels.**
  4. **Hemorrhoidal venous plexus.**

Clinical Features

- Portal hypertension is **most commonly due to liver cirrhosis.**
- It is common in clinical practice and represents a significant clinical challenge. Patients have often been ill for long periods, repeatedly presenting as emergencies.
- Portal hypertension per se produces no symptoms.
- Since liver cirrhosis is the most common cause, portal hypertension **occurs on a background of compensated Chronic Liver Disease.**
- The features of chronic liver disease are as follows:
  - o Lethargy.
  - o Fever.
  - o Jaundice.
  - o Scratch marks.
  - o Protein catabolism (wasting).
  - o Coagulopathy (bruising).
  - o Cardiac manifestation because of hyperdynamic circulation.
  - o **Cutaneous:** Spider naevi, palmar erythema.
  - o Loss of body hair.
  - o Parotid enlargement.
  - o Testicular atrophy.
  - o Gynecomastia.
  - o Dupuytren's contracture.
  - o Asterixis or flapping tremors.
  - o Clubbing.
  - o Purpura.
  - o Pigmented ulcers.
- When chronic liver disease becomes decompensated, patients present with following symptoms, leading to a diagnosis of portal hypertension:
  1. Hepatic encephalopathy.
  2. Ascites.
  3. Collaterals:
     - Variceal bleeding from esophageal and gastric varices, i.e., hematemesis.
     - **Caput medusa:** It is a cutaneous manifestation and consists of dilated, enlarged, superficial veins radiating from the umbilicus.
  4. **Splenomegaly and hypersplenism:**
     - Manifests as thrombocytopenia, leucocytopenia, erythrocytopenia.

Investigations

- The key aspects of assessing a patient with suspected chronic liver disease or complications of portal hypertension are the following:

1. Diagnosis of the underlying liver disease.
2. Estimation of functional hepatic reserve.
3. Definition of portal venous anatomy and hepatic hemodynamic evaluation.
4. Identification of the site of upper GI hemorrhage, if present.

- Estimation of functional hepatic reserve is useful in determining whether definitive (e.g., hepatic transplantation) or palliative (e.g., endoscopic variceal ligation or a shunt procedure) treatment is indicated.

A. Liver Function Tests

Child Pugh Score

Factor	Number of Points		
	1	2	3
Bilirubin (mg/dl)	< 2	2-3	>3
Albumin (g/dl)	> 3.5	2.8-3.5	<2.8
Prothrombin Time (increased seconds)	1-3	4-6	>6
Ascites	None	Slight	Moderate
Encephalopathy	None	Minimal	Advanced

- It is a quantitative score of liver function.
- It is the most commonly used scoring system.
- It is used for cirrhotic patients who require liver surgery.
- **Class A:** 5-6 points.
- **Class B:** 7-9 points.
- **Class C:** 10-15 points.
- This score correlates with mortality and survival rates after hepatectomy.
- Class B and C patients have higher perioperative mortality after any partial hepatectomy than class A patients, who can generally withstand a major hepatectomy.

B. Measurement of Pressure

- The best evidence for portal hypertension is by directly measuring the hepatic vein wedge pressure, i.e., the difference in pressure between the portal vein and the hepatic veins.
- This gradient is best estimated by transfemoral-hepatic vein catheterization with a balloon tip catheter.
- Portal hypertension is when pressure > 5 mm Hg.
- Pressure at which portosystemic collateralization starts to develop: 8-10 mm Hg.

C. Detection of Varices

- **CT scan of abdomen:**
  - o Detects intra-abdominal varices, especially retroperitoneal.
  - o **Can visualize the rest of the abdomen:** Ascites, splenomegaly, liver span.
- **Upper GI endoscopy**
  - o It is both diagnostic as well as therapeutic.
  - o Investigation of choice for diagnosis of esophageal and/or gastric varices.

Treatment

- The treatment of portal hypertension revolves around the treatment of bleeding from esophagogastric varices.
  - o Responsible for 1/3rd deaths in all patients with cirrhosis.
  - o 50 % deaths are due to uncontrolled bleeding.
  - o Risk of death is mainly related to the underlying hepatic functional reserve.

A. General Measures

- Airway.
- IV access with 2 large bore IV lines.
- IV fluids.
- Matching and cross matching of blood.
- Blood and products transfusion.
- Correct coagulopathy (with vitamin K).

B. Pharmacotherapy

- Reduces variceal blood flow, which in turn reduces variceal pressure.
- Should be initiated at the onset of variceal bleeding.
- **Splanchnic vasoconstrictors:** Terlipressin, vasopressin, octreotide, somatostatin.
- Prophylactic antibiotics.

C. Endoscopy

- Endoscopic intervention is the mainstay of treatment for control of acute variceal bleeding.
- **Options are:**
  1. Band ligation.
  2. Sclerotherapy.

D. Balloon Tamponade

- It is effective for massive or refractory variceal bleeding, but is only recommended as a 'bridge' to definitive treatment.
- If the rate of blood loss prohibits endoscopic evaluation, balloon tamponade is used to provide temporary hemostasis:
  1. Sengstaken - Blakemore tube.
  2. Minnesota tube.
- **Complications:** Esophageal pressure necrosis

E. TIPSS (Transjugular Intrahepatic Portosystemic Shunt)

- It has become the preferred treatment for acute variceal bleeding when pharmacotherapy and endoscopic treatment fail.
- It is a radiological procedure and has replaced the surgical portocaval shunt.
- **Method:**
  - o A TIPSS is inserted under local anesthetic, analgesia and sedation using fluoroscopic guidance and USG.
  - o Via the internal jugular vein, SVC and hepatic vein, a guidewire is inserted through the hepatic parenchyma into a branch of the portal vein.
  - o The tract is dilated and a metallic stent is then inserted and expanded, forming a porto-venous channel.
  - o A satisfactory drop in portal venous pressure is usually associated with good control of the variceal hemorrhage .
- **Complications of TIPSS:**
  1. Perforation of liver capsule, with potentially fatal intraperitoneal hemorrhage.
  2. TIPSS occlusion.
  3. Post-TIPSS encephalopathy.
- Contraindication: Portal vein occlusion.

F. Surgical Shunts

- Rarely performed, because of their high morbidity and mortality.
- **Indication:** Failure of medical management in non-cirrhotic patients with extrahepatic portal vein occlusion.
- Effectively prevent rebleeding by reducing portal pressure.
- **Types:**
  1. Selective.
  2. Non-selective.
  3. Partial.

G. Liver Transplantation

- It is the only therapy that treats portal hypertension and the underlying liver disease.

H. Recurrent or Refractory Variceal Bleeding:

- **Sugiura procedure:** Splenectomy + esophago-gastric devascularization.

[3] Liver function tests. *June 14*

- It helps recognize the presence of hepatic disease and gives clues about the cause of that disease.

A. Bilirubin

- o Total Bilirubin = Direct (conjugated bilirubin) + indirect (unconjugated bilirubin).
- o Increased levels may be associated with:
  - ♦ Increased hemoglobin breakdown.
  - ♦ Hepatocellular dysfunction resulting in impaired bilirubin transport and excretion or mechanical biliary obstruction.

B. Alkaline Phosphatase (ALP)

- o Elevated with cholestatic liver disease or biliary obstruction.

C. Gamma Glutamyl Transpeptidase (GGT)

- o Marker of alcohol intake.

D. Aspartate Transaminase (AST)/SGOT and Alanine Transaminase (ALT)/SGPT

- o Raised levels usually reflect acute hepatocellular damage.

E. Total Protein, Albumin, Globulin

F. Prothrombin Time/International Normalised Ratio (PT/INR)

- o The synthetic functions of the liver are indicated by the ability to synthesize proteins (albumin levels) and clotting factors (PT).
- o The standard method of monitoring liver function in patients with chronic liver disease is serial measurement of bilirubin, albumin and Prothrombin Time.

[10] Describe the aetiopathogenesis, clinical features and management of amoebic liver abscess. ***July 23***

[10] Discuss the aetiology, clinical features, investigations and management of amoebic liver abscess. ***June 13***

[3] Amoebic liver abscess. ***March 22, Oct 20***

- It is caused by the organism ***Entamoeba histolytica.***

Pathogenesis

- **Causative organism**: *Entamoeba histolytica.*
- **Mode of infection**: Faeco-oral route.
- **Risk factors:**
  - o Substandard hygiene and sanitation.
  - o Populations from poorer socio-economic status are more vulnerable.
- **Majority** of the people remain **asymptomatic carriers.**
- Right liver > left liver.

Life Cycle

Pathogenesis of Amoebic Liver Abscess

Organism **enters the gut through food or water** contaminated with the cyst

↓

In the small bowel, the **cysts hatch and a large number of trophozoites are released**

↓

Carried to the colon

↓

Flask shaped ulcers form in the submucosa

↓

Contd.

Trophozoites multiply, ultimately forming cysts

↓

Cysts

↓

Enter the portal circulation | Excreted in the faeces

↓ (Enter the portal circulation)

Get trapped in the interlobular veins of the liver

↓

Multiply in the portal triads

↓

Focal infarction of hepatocytes

↓

Trophozoites produce proteolytic enzymes

↓

Areas of necrosis eventually **coalesce** to form the **abscess cavity**

- Abscess cavity contains chocolate-coloured, odourless, **anchovy sauce -** like fluid that is a mixture of necrotic liver tissue and blood.
- There may be **secondary infection** of the abscess, which causes the pus to smell.
- **Chronic infection** of the large bowel may result in a **granulomatous lesion** along the large bowel, most commonly seen **in the cecum, called an ameboma.**

Clinical Features

- Younger adults.
- M > F.
- History of insidious onset of non-specific symptoms, such as abdominal pain, anorexia, fever, night sweats, malaise, cough and weight loss.
- These symptoms gradually progress to more specific symptoms.
- Pain in the RUQ and right shoulder tip.
- Hiccoughs.
- Non-productive cough.

- Past history of bloody diarrhea.
- History of travel to an endemic area.

On Examination

- Patient looks toxic.
- Anemic.
- Upper abdominal rigidity.
- Tender hepatomegaly, often with tender and bulging intercostal spaces and overlying skin edema.
- In chronic cases, a mass in the RIF may be an ameboma.
- Pleural effusion.
- Basal pneumonitis.
- Jaundice.
- Ascites.
- Rarely, the patient may present as an emergency owing to the effects of rupture of an abscess into the peritoneal, pleural or pericardial cavity.

Investigations

A. Blood

- Anemia.
- Leukocytosis.
- **Raised inflammatory markers:** ESR, CRP.
- Hypoalbuminemia.
- **LFT is deranged:**
  - o Elevated alkaline phosphatase.
- Serological tests are more specific:
  - o Majority of patients show antibodies in the serum which are detected by ELISA.
  - o Other tests such as Indirect Hemagglutination Assay (IHA).
  - o Detection of parasite by antigen detection or DNA PCR.

B. Colonoscopy

- While amebiasis may affect the entire colon, it has a predilection for the cecum and ascending colon.
- Flask shaped ulcers.
- Discrete exudate-covered areas of ulceration with normal areas in between.
- Biopsy can also be taken.

C. Imaging

USG

- Seen as a hypoechoic or anechoic lesion with ill-defined borders.
- Internal echoes suggest necrotic material or debris.
- Investigation is very accurate and is used for aspiration, which is both diagnostic and therapeutic.

CT Scan

- Helpful when there is doubt about the diagnosis on USG.
- Diagnoses the lesion.
- May also show a raised right hemidiaphragm, a pleural effusion and evidence of pneumonitis.

Treatment

A. Medical Treatment

- Very effective.
- Should be the first choice in the elective situation.
- Metronidazole and tinidazole are the effective drugs.
- After treatment with metronidazole and tinidazole; diloxanide furoate, a luminal amebicide that is not effective against hepatic infestation, is used for 10 days to destroy any intestinal amebae.

B. Percutaneous Aspiration/Drainage

- Done under USG guidance or CT guidance.
- Aspiration is carried out when imminent rupture of an abscess is expected, especially when involving the left lobe.
- Pigtail catheter drainage may be considered in those patients who are not responding to IV metronidazole in the first 48-72 hours to improve antibiotic penetration.
- The threshold for draining a left liver lobe abscess should be low, as it has a propensity to rupture into either the peritoneal, pleural or pericardial cavity.

C. Surgery

- Open surgery, i.e., laparotomy is indicated only for complications (e.g., rupture into pleural, peritoneal or pericardial cavities).
- Drainage + lavage.

[10] Describe the aetiopathogenesis, clinical features, diagnosis and management of hydatid cyst of liver. ***Feb 23***

[5] Hydatid cyst of liver. ***Sept 21, June 17, Dec 12***

[3] Hydatid disease. ***June 14***

- Hydatid disease or echinococcosis is a **zoonosis** that **occurs primarily in sheep grazing areas** of the world, but is **common worldwide because the dog is the definitive host.**

Aetiopathogenesis

- **Causative organism:** *Echinococcus granulosus,* commonly called the **dog tapeworm** is the most common.
- **Others:** E multilocularis, E ligartus.
- **Definitive host: Dog.**
- **Intermediate hosts: Humans, sheep and cattle.**
- **Mode of infection:**
  - o Humans commonly contract the disease from dogs by direct contact.
- There is no human to human transmission.
- Humans may also eat salads on which ova have been deposited.
- Sheep and cattle are infected by eating contaminated grass.
- Dogs become infected by eating offal of infested sheep and cattle:
  - o The adult tapeworm resides in the ileum of dogs. It expels eggs (*via* the dog's feces) which are deposited on grass, vegetables, etc. Cattle, sheep or human beings ingest these eggs. Close contact with an infected dog causes contamination by the oral route.
  - o The eggs enter the human GIT. Humans are an end stage to the parasite. In the human duodenum, it releases an oncosphere containing hooklets that penetrate the mucosa, allowing access to the bloodstream.
  - o In the blood, the oncosphere reaches the liver through a radical of the portal vein, where it develops its larval stage, called the hydatid cyst.
  - o The **right lobe is commonly affected.**

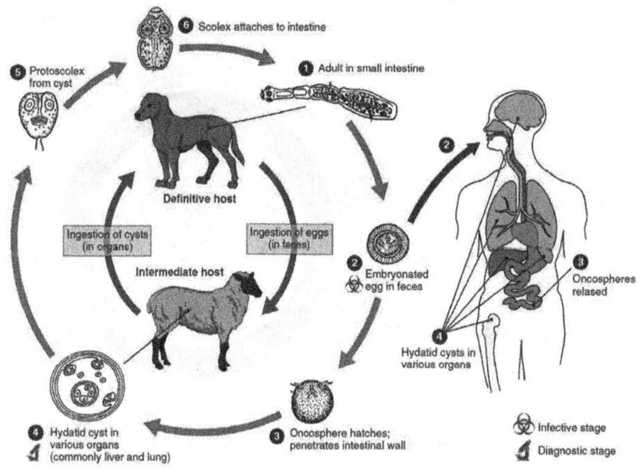

Figure 2: Life cycle of *Echinococcus granulosus*

Pathology

A hydatid cyst consists of 3 layers:

1. **Outer layer - pericyst or pseudocyst (adventitia)**
   - Consists of fibrous tissue.
   - It is the result of reaction of the liver to the parasite, i.e., it is derived from compressed host organ liver.
   - It blends intimately with the liver, from which it is inseparable.
2. **Intermediate layer - ectocyst (laminated membrane)**
   - It is formed of the parasite itself.
   - It is elastic and contains the hydatid fluid.
   - It closely resembles a water filled balloon.
   - Unless bacterial infection has occurred, it peels readily from the adventitia.
   - Hydatid fluid is crystal-clear and may contain hooklets and scolices.
   - It is non-infective.
3. **Inner layer - endocyst (germinal membrane)**
   - It is the only living part of a hydatid cyst and is infective.
   - It contains viable parasites that can separate, forming daughter cysts.
   - Brood capsules within the hydatid cyst develop from the germinal membrane (epithelium). These are small, intracystic cellular masses in which future worm heads develop into scolices.

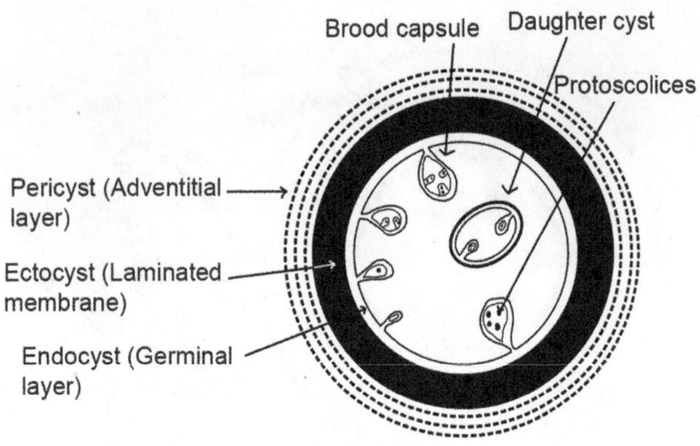

Figure 3: Structure of hydatid cyst

Clinical Features

- Most common organ affected is liver.
  - o 2nd most common organ affected is the lung.
  - o But, the parasite can colonise virtually every organ in the body.
- Common in sheep farmers, people who handle dogs.
- For a long time, patient remains asymptomatic.
- Gradually enlarging painful mass in the RUQ, which arises from the liver.
- Swelling causes pressure effects, therefore, a hepatic lesion causes dull pain from stretching of the liver capsule.
- **Course of the disease:**
  1. **Occasionally, the parasite dies**. The fluid is absorbed, and all that remains is an encapsulated, laminated, bile-stained membrane.

     In long standing cases, the walls of the cyst may calcify.
  2. **Usually, the cyst enlarges gradually and becomes manifest by its size.**

     Sometimes, sessile cysts float in the peritoneal cavity, or they may be confused with mesenteric, pancreatic or renal cysts.
  3. **Complications arise:**

     a. **Jaundice**
       - o Due to pressure of cysts on the bile ducts or due to the presence of daughter cysts within the bile ducts.

     b. **Rupture**
       - o Into the biliary tree.
       - o **Into the peritoneum:** Anaphylaxis, diffuse peritonitis, urticaria.
       - o Into the pleural cavity.

     c. **Suppuration, i.e., secondary infection.**

Investigations

- Raised eosinophil count.
- **Serological tests:** ELISA, immunoelectrophoresis.
- **USG:**
  - o Initial investigation of choice.
  - o May show abnormality in the gallbladder and bile ducts.
- **CT scan:**
  - o Best imaging technique.
  - o Diagnostic feature is a space occupying lesion with a smooth outline with septa.
- **MRCP.**
- The intradermal Casoni's test is now obsolete.

Treatment

- Ideally managed in a tertiary unit by a multidisciplinary team of a surgeon, physician and interventional radiologist.
- **Asymptomatic and inactive cysts are left alone:** Its size is monitored by USG.
- **Active cysts should first be treated by a full course of albendazole. Praziquantel is also used.**
- Surgical options available are:
  1. **PAIR**
     - o Puncture, Aspiration, Injection, Reaspiration.
     - o After puncture and aspiration of contents, a scolicidal agent is injected into the cyst, e.g., hypertonic saline (15-20%), ethanol (75-95%) or povidone iodine (5-10%).
     - o After injection, contents are re-aspirated.
     - o Before PAIR is done, it must be ensured that the hydatid cyst does not communicate with the biliary tree.
     - o If scolicidal agent is accidentally injected into the biliary tree, it may cause sclerosing cholangitis.
     - o Can be done by open surgery or laparoscopically.

2. **Pericystectomy with omentoplasty**
   - o Done especially if the lesion is in a peripheral part of the liver.
3. **Hepatic segmentectomy**
   - o Done especially if the lesion is in a peripheral part of the liver.
4. **Laparoscopic marsupialisation (deroofing) of the cyst**
   - o Removal of the cyst containing the endocyst along with the daughter cysts.

[3] Hemangioma of liver. *June 19*

- It is the **most common benign tumour** of the liver.

Pathology

- Consist of an abnormal plexus of vessels.
- **Enlargement is by ectasia** rather than by neoplasia.
- Usually solitary.
- Usually < 5 cm in diameter.
- Those > 5 cm are called giant hemangiomas.
- Occur with equal incidence in the right and left hemilivers.

HPE

- Endothelium-lined, blood filled spaces separated by thin fibrous septa.

Clinical Features

- Usually asymptomatic and found incidentally on imaging studies.
- Large compressive masses may cause vague upper abdominal symptoms.
- Sometimes, symptoms which are ascribed to liver hemangiomas are usually due to some other cause.
- Rapid expansion or acute thrombosis can occasionally cause symptoms.
- Spontaneous rupture is very rare.
- **Kasabach-Merritt syndrome:**
  - o Associated with giant hemangiomas.
  - o Thrombocytopenia.
  - o Consumptive coagulopathy.

Investigations

- **USG is diagnostic.**
- **CT scan with delayed contrast enhancement:**
  - o Done in cases of diagnostic uncertainty.
  - o Shows the characteristic appearance of slow contrast enhancement owing to small vessel uptake.
- **MRI.**
- **Isotope-labelled RBC scans** are an accurate test, but are rarely necessary.
- Percutaneous biopsy is not recommended.

Treatment

- Diagnosis is usually **incidental** and therefore **requires no treatment.**
- **Indications of surgical resection:**
  - o Symptomatic patients.
  - o Diagnostic uncertainty.
- The **preferred approach to resection is enucleation with arterial inflow control.**
- Anatomic resections may be necessary in some cases.

[5] Secondaries in liver. *July 18, Dec 17, Dec 16, Dec 15, July 23*

- The **most common malignant tumors of the liver are metastatic lesions**.

Pathology

- The liver is a common site of metastases from gastrointestinal tumours, presumably **because of dissemination through the portal venous system**.
- **Tumours which commonly metastasize to liver:**
  - o Cancers of GIT and pancreatobiliary system.
  - o Genitourinary system (renal, prostate).
  - o Neuroendocrine system.
  - o Breast.
  - o Eye (melanoma).
  - o Skin (melanoma).
  - o Soft tissue (retroperitoneal sarcoma).
  - o Gynecologic system (ovarian, endometrial, cervical).

- **Metastatic adenocarcinoma to the liver of unknown primary is often a primary intrahepatic cholangiocarcinoma.**

Survival

- The **most relevant metastatic tumour of the liver (secondaries) to the surgeon is colorectal cancer** because of the well documented potential for long-term survival after complete resection.
- Tumours other than colorectal cancer which manifest as isolated or limited hepatic metastases can also be resected for potential long-term survival, but data on these are less convincing than for colorectal cancer.

Presentation of Patients with Liver Mets

- Symptoms and signs of advanced malignant disease indicate poor prognosis:
  - o Pain.
  - o Ascites.
  - o Jaundice.
  - o Weight loss.
  - o Palpable mass.

Investigations of Patients with Primary Colorectal Cancer with Liver Mets

- Serial physical examinations.
- CT/ MRI.
- LFT:
  - o Mild elevations in LFT results are common in metastatic colorectal cancer to the liver, but are not effective as a screening tool.
  - o The levels most commonly elevated are those of ALP, GGT and lactate dehydrogenase.
- CEA.
- Colonoscopy.
- Staging laparoscopy.

Treatment

- **Synchronous colon and liver resection** may be done.
- **Liver first approach** is a newer approach.
- Usually, liver mets are treated **after treating the primary:**

1. **Surgical resection**
   - o An R0 resection with a negative surgical margin of 1 cm is considered the gold standard.
2. **Surgical resection + chemotherapy**
   - o R1 resection ($\geq$ 1 mm margin microscopically negative).
   - o **Drugs:** 5-Fluorouracil, folinic acid, oxaliplatin, monoclonal antibodies against:
     - ♦ VEGFR – Vascular endothelial growth factor receptor.
     - ♦ EGFR – Epidermal growth factor receptor.
3. **Loco-regional therapies**
   - Embolization.
   - Percutaneous ablation.
   - Hepatic artery infusion chemotherapy.
   - Internal radiation.

[3] Budd-Chiari syndrome. *August 22, Dec 19*

- **Definition:** It is a **collective term for conditions that impede hepatic venous outflow at any level from the small hepatic veins to the junction of the IVC with the right atrium.** Cardiac and pericardial diseases and sinusoidal obstruction syndrome are excluded from this definition.

Causes

- Hypercoagulable states: Antithrombin 3, protein C or protein S deficiency.
- Extrinsic compression.
- Congenital or acquired IVC webs (rare).

Pathophysiology and Clinical Features

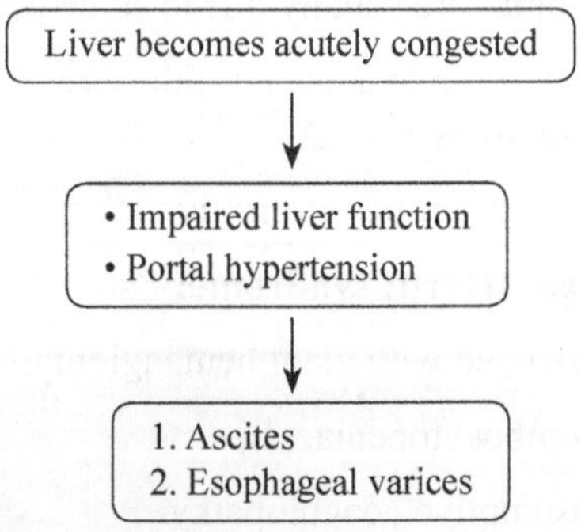

- Mainly affects young women.
- **Classic triad: Abdominal pain + ascites + hepatomegaly.**
- Fulminant hepatic failure may result from acute thrombosis.
- If chronic, the liver progresses to established cirrhosis.

Investigations

- **Colour and pulsed doppler ultrasonography.**
- **CT scan:**
  - o Demonstrates a large, congested liver or cirrhosis.
  - o Gross enlargement of the caudate lobe. This is because it is preserved and hypertrophies, as it drains directly to the SVC.

Treatment

- Depends on the stage of disease at presentation and the specific findings in each patient:
  1. **Fulminant liver failure, established cirrhosis and complications of portal hypertension:**
     - o Liver transplantation.
  2. **If liver parenchyma is relatively normal:**
     - o Transjugular Intrahepatic Portosystemic Shunt or a side-to-side portocaval shunt.
     - o IVC compression is relieved by the insertion of a retrohepatic expandable metallic stent.
- Patients with secondaries in liver usually require lifelong anticoagulation.

OTHER IMPORTANT TOPICS

PYOGENIC LIVER ABSCESS

Aetiology/Route of Spread

- Biliary tract pathology (most common source).
- Portal spread from GIT (diverticulitis and appendicitis).
- Contiguous spread from subphrenic or intra-abdominal collections.
- Bacteremia secondary to trauma or infected cysts.
- Necrotic tumours following chemotherapy.

Risk Factors

- Elderly.
- Diabetes.
- Immunosuppressed.
- Cirrhosis of liver.
- Chronic renal failure.

Causative Organisms

- Usually polymicrobial.
- **Most common organisms:** *Klebsiella, E coli, Streptococcus milleri.*

Pathogenesis

- **Mostly affects the right hemiliver**, probably because of preferential laminar blood flow to the right side.
- Liver is **exposed to loads of bacteria from the portal vein** on a regular basis and usually clears this bacterial load without any problems.
- Hepatic abscess occurs when an **inoculum of bacteria, regardless of route of exposure, exceeds the liver's ability to clear it.**
- **Biliary obstruction results in bile stasis** with the potential for subsequent bacterial colonisation, infection and ascension into the liver.
- Any **systemic infection** (e.g., endocarditis, pneumonia, osteomyelitis) can result in bacteremia and infection of the liver through the hepatic artery.

Clinical Features

- Age > 50 years.
- Slightly more common in males.
- Classic description is of fever, jaundice and right upper quadrant pain, with tenderness on palpation.
- Chills.
- Anorexia.
- Constitutional symptoms: Malaise, vomiting.
- Rupture of abscess may cause peritonitis.

Investigations

1. **USG**
   - Round or oval area that is less echogenic than the surrounding liver.

2. **CECT**
   - Multiloculated cystic mass.
   - Air-fluid level.
   - Rim enhancement.
   - Can detect small abscesses.
3. **Blood tests**
   - Increased WBC count.
   - Deranged LFT:
     - o ALP is mildly elevated.
     - o SGOT and SGPT are increased.
     - o Mild elevations of PT and INR.
     - o Total bilirubin may be elevated.

Treatment

A. **Antibiotics**
- Penicillin + aminoglycoside + metronidazole.
- Cephalosporin + metronidazole.

B. **CT Guided Percutaneous Drainage**
- Pig-tail catheterisation is better than simple aspiration.

C. **Open Surgical Drainage**
- **Indications are:**
  - o Failure of percutaneous drainage.
  - o Patients who require surgical treatment of the primary pathologic process.

HEPATOCELLULAR CARCINOMA

- HCC is a malignant tumour arising from hepatocytes.
- It is the most common primary liver cancer.
- It is the leading cause of death in patients with cirrhosis.

Aetiology

- Wide geographical variation reflects the incidence of aetiological factors.
- Chronic hepatitis B virus (HBV) infection:
  - o HBV infection precedes the development of HCC.
  - o Sequence of HBV infection to cirrhosis to HCC is seen.
  - o HBV vaccination programmes reduce the incidence in high-risk areas.
- Hepatitis C virus (HCV) increases the risk of HCC by promoting end-stage liver disease.
- Aflatoxin contamination of rice in some parts of the world is probably responsible for seasonal variations.
- Lifetime alcohol exposure remains an intractable risk factor.
- Obesity.
- Diabetes mellitus.

Clinical Features

- M: F = 3 : 1.
- Age: 50-60 years.
- RUQ abdominal pain that sometimes radiates to the right shoulder.
- Weight loss.
- Palpable mass.
- In countries endemic for HBV, presentation at a younger age is common and probably related to childhood infection.
- Tends to manifest at a later stage.
- Nonspecific symptoms of advanced malignancy: Anorexia, nausea, lethargy, weight loss.
- Hepatic decompensation in a patient with known mild cirrhosis or even in patients with unrecognized cirrhosis.
- Can rarely manifest as a rupture, with the sudden onset of abdominal pain followed by hypovolemic shock secondary to intraperitoneal bleeding.
- Other rare presentations:
  - o Hepatic vein occlusion (Budd-Chiari syndrome).
  - o Obstructive jaundice.
  - o Hemobilia.
  - o Fever of unknown origin.
- **Paraneoplastic syndrome:** Usually hypercalcemia, hypoglycemia and erythrocytosis.

Investigations

A. **Imaging**
- **Aims:**
  - o Pre-op assessment.

- Accurate tumour staging.
- To determine technical and oncological resectability.
- Exclude metastatic disease.

- USG is used for screening and early detection but definitive diagnosis and treatment planning rely on CT or MRI.
- **Triple-phase CT chest/abdomen/pelvis:**
  - Arterial enhancement followed by washout in the delayed phase is seen.
- MRI of liver.
- Liver-specific contrast agents improve sensitivity and specificity.

B. Tumour Markers

- **Alpha-Fetoprotein:**
  - Cut off value is 400 ng/ml.
  - Not specific to HCC and can be elevated with intrahepatic cholangiocarcinoma and colorectal metastases.
  - Used as an adjunctive test in patients with liver masses.
  - Particularly useful in monitoring treated patients for recurrence after normalization of levels.

Staging

- Barcelona Clinic Liver Group (BCLC) is the most commonly used.
- Patients with HCC usually have underlying liver cirrhosis and the Child Turcott Pugh score is used to assess it.

Treatment

1. Surgical resection

- It is a compromise as it requires resection of the tumour, while preserving sufficient functional parenchyma.
- HCC spreads within the liver by direct invasion of portal and hepatic venous systems.
- Anatomical resections that include removal of the entire venous drainage of a tumour, including occult micrometastases, is the optimal approach.

2. Liver transplantation

- It is an attractive option as it definitely treats the tumour as well as the underlying cirrhosis, and the donor liver provides functioning parenchyma.

3. Ablation

- Ethanol injection.
- Acetic acid injection.
- Thermal ablation (cryotherapy, radiofrequency ablation, microwave ablation).

4. Transarterial

- Embolisation.
- Chemoembolisation.

5. Radiotherapy

- Combination transarterial and ablative: External beam radiation.

6. Systemic

- Chemotherapy.
- Hormonal.
- Immunotherapy.

33

Gallbladder and Biliary Tree

[10] Describe aetiopathogenesis of biliary calculi. Write about clinical features and management of biliary stones. *June 17*

[5] Aetiopathology of gallstones. *August 22*

[5] Gallstones. *June 19, Dec 16, Dec 15*

[5] Management of cholelithiasis. *Dec 18, Dec 17*

[5] Types of gallstone. *Feb 13*

[3] List the complications of gallstones. *July 15, Dec 14*

GALLSTONES

- Gallstones are the most common biliary pathology.

Type of Stones

- USA, Europe: 80% are cholesterol or mixed stones.
- Parts of Asia: 80% are pigment stones.
- Gallstones can be divided into 3 main types:

A. Cholesterol Stones

- Consist almost entirely of cholesterol.
- Often solitary (cholesterol solitaire).

B. Mixed Stones

- Cholesterol is the major component.
- **Other components:** Calcium salts, bile acids, bile pigments and phospholipids.
- Usually multiple.
- They are often faceted.

C. Pigment Stones (Black/Brown)

- Contains < 30% cholesterol.
- Patients with cirrhosis have a higher incidence of pigment stones.

Black Stones

- Insoluble bilirubin pigment polymer + calcium phosphate + calcium bicarbonate + cholesterol.
- Associated with hemolysis, e.g., Hereditary spherocytosis, sickle cell anemia.

Brown Stones

- Calcium bilirubinate + calcium palmitate + calcium stearate + cholesterol.
- More common in bile ducts.
- Related to bile stasis and infection
- Associated with the presence of foreign bodies within the bile ducts, such as stents or parasites (*Clonorchis sinensis* and *Ascaris lumbricoides*).

Aetiopathogenesis

Four major factors explain most gallstone formation:

1. **Supersaturation of secreted bile.**
2. **Concentration of bile in the gallbladder.**
   - Cholesterol is insoluble in water and is secreted in phospholipid vesicles.
   - Whether cholesterol remains in solution or not, depends on the type and relative concentrations of phospholipids and bile acids in the bile.

- **Lithogenic bile means:**
  a. **When bile is supersaturated with cholesterol, i.e., cholesterol secretion increases:**
     - o Age.
     - o Sex.
     - o Genetics.
     - o Obesity.
     - o High calorie diet.
     - o Drugs (oral contraceptives).

  b. **Bile acid concentrations are low, i.e., depleted bile acid pool:**
     - o Ileal disease.
     - o Ileal resection.
     - o Bowel transit time.
     - o Fecal enteric flora.
     - o Deoxycholate.
     - o Cholestyramine.
- In lithogenic bile, unstable unilamellar phospholipid vesicles form and cholesterol crystals nucleate.

3. **Crystal nucleation:**
   - Nucleation of cholesterol monohydrate crystals from multi-lamellar vesicles is a crucial step in gallstone formation.
4. **Gallbladder dysmotility:**
   - Impaired GB function, i.e., abnormal emptying, absorption, excretion may aid the aggregation of nucleated cholesterol crystals.

Clinical Features

- Gallstones are asymptomatic in the majority of cases (> 80%).
- Approx. 1-2% will develop symptoms requiring surgery.
- Increased incidental detection during imaging for other symptoms.
- Gallstones become symptomatic when they obstruct a visceral structure such as a cystic duct.
- RUQ or epigastric pain.
- Pain may be described as colicky.
- The typical biliary 'colic' more often is dull, continuous and severe, lasting for several minutes or even hours. There is associated nausea and vomiting.
- Frequently, pain starts during the night and wakes the patient.
- Minor episodes may occur intermittently during the day.
- In the majority of cases, the process is limited by the stone slipping back into the body of the GB.
- Associated symptoms have a questionable relation to gallstones.
- Dyspepsia.
- Flatulence.
- Food intolerance, particularly to fats.
- Alteration in bowel frequency.

Effects and Complications of Gallstones

- Biliary colic.
- Acute cholecystitis.
- Chronic cholecystitis.
- Empyema of the GB.
- Mucocele of the GB.
- Perforation of the GB.
- Biliary obstruction (jaundice).
- Acute cholangitis.
- Acute pancreatitis.
- Intestinal obstruction (gallstone ileus).

Investigations

A. Liver Function Tests

- Raised alkaline phosphatase is indicative of stones in the biliary tree.

B. USG

- Transabdominal USG is the initial imaging modality of choice.
- **Advantages of USG:** It is accurate, readily available, inexpensive and quick to perform.
- **Disadvantages:** It is operator dependent and may be compromised by excessive body fat and bowel gas.
- **Information provided by USG:**
  - o Size of GB.
  - o Thickness of GB wall.
  - o Presence of stone or polyps.

- o Can diagnose acute calculous cholecystitis.
- o Size of CBD.
- o Presence of stones within extrahepatic biliary tree.

- Wall acoustic shadow is seen in cholelithiasis.

C. MRCP

- Magnetic Resonance CholangioPancreatography.
- Provides excellent images of the gallbladder and biliary system (gives information on anatomy and stones).
- Advantages: It is not operator dependent.
- Indicated if alkaline phosphatase is raised.

Treatment

- For patients with **symptomatic gallstones, cholecystectomy is the treatment of choice** (if there are no medical contraindications).
- **Asymptomatic gallstones do not need intervention.**
- However, **prophylactic cholecystectomy may be performed for asymptomatic gallstones in the following:**
  - o > 3 cm gallstones.
  - o Choledocholithiasis.
  - o Chronic hemolytic conditions (sickle cell disease, hereditary spherocytosis).
  - o Gallbladder polyps > 1 cm in diameter.
  - o Suspicion/risk of malignancy (anomalous pancreatic ductal drainage/long common channel of bile and pancreatic ducts).
  - o Calcification of the wall (porcelain gallbladder).
  - o Some ethnic groups or subjects living in areas with a high prevalence of GB cancer associated with gallstones, e.g., North India.
  - o Transplant patients (during transplantation).
  - o Bariatric surgery.
  - o In diabetic patients with gallstones, one should have lower threshold for cholecystectomy: Considering higher rate of gangrene.
- Cholecystectomy can be performed via the open or the laparoscopic route.
- Laparoscopic cholecystectomy is the most preferred option and is one of the most common surgeries done.

[10] Classify gallstones. Discuss aetiopathogenesis and management of acute calculous cholecystitis. ***March 22***

[10] Discuss the aetiology of gallstones. Describe the clinical features, investigations and management of acute calculous cholecystitis. ***Dec 13***

[5] Acute cholecystitis. ***June 16***

[3] Murphy's sign. ***March 21***

ACUTE CALCULOUS CHOLECYSTITIS

- Acute calculous cholecystitis is the inflammation of the gallbladder, as a result of blockage of the cystic duct by a stone.

Aetiopathogenesis

- Acute calculous cholecystitis is because of **blockage of the cystic duct by a stone.**
- **In chronic calculous cholecystitis or biliary colic, the blockage is temporary and repetitive; while in acute calculous cholecystitis the blockage does not resolve, leading to inflammation with edema and subserosal hemorrhage.**
- Obstruction is followed by **infection of the stagnant pool of bile.**
- Without resolution of the obstruction, the **gallbladder will progress to ischemia and necrosis.**
- Eventually, **empyema develops** and acute cholecystitis becomes **acute gangrenous cholecystitis.**
- When acute gangrenous cholecystitis gets complicated by infection with a **gas forming organism** it is called **acute emphysematous cholecystitis.**
- **If gallbladder wall perforates, localized peritonitis develops.**
- Occasionally, **complete obstruction of the cystic duct** leads to reabsorption of bile salts by the gallbladder epithelium and secretion of uninfected mucus, resulting in a **mucocele** of the GB.

Clinical Features

- The development of acute calculous cholecystitis is marked by fever.
- Right upper quadrant pain or pain in the epigastrium.

On Examination

- Tenderness and guarding in the RUQ.
- **Murphy's sign:**
  - o Seen in acute cholecystitis.
  - o Elicited by asking the patient to breathe in, whilst gently palpating the gallbladder area (right subcostal).
  - o Patient will experience pain and 'catch their breath' just before the zenith of inspiration, i.e., there is voluntary cessation of inspiration.
  - o It suggests inflammation of the visceral and parietal peritoneal surfaces.
  - o It can also be elicited during USG.
  - o Sometimes, a mass may become palpable as the omentum walls off an inflamed gallbladder.

Investigations

A. USG

- The following features are seen in acute calculous cholecystitis on USG:
  - o Presence of stone(s) in the gallbladder.
  - o Thickening of the GB wall (> 3 mm).
  - o Presence of pericholecystic fluid.
  - o Direct tenderness when the probe is pushed against the GB (ultrasonographic murphy's sign).

B. HIDA Scan (Hepatic Imino Diacetic Acid Scan)

- Can be used in atypical cases to demonstrate obstruction of the cystic duct, which definitively diagnoses acute cholecystitis.
- Imino diacetic acid is injected intravenously. It reaches the liver where it is processed and secreted with bile, thus allowing identification of bile flow.
- The failure to fill the gallbladder 2 hours after injection demonstrates obstruction of the cystic duct, as seen in acute cholecystitis.

C. CT Scan

- May show similar findings to USG, but is less sensitive.
- Can diagnose the presence of complications such as perforation.

D. MRCP

- Should be performed to exclude choledocholithiasis (if LFT is deranged and alkaline phosphate is raised).

E. Blood Tests

- CBC: Leukocytosis.
- Increased cRP.
- LFT.

Tokyo Consensus Guidelines

It is the diagnostic criteria for acute cholecystitis.

A. Local Signs of Inflammation, etc.

- Murphy's sign.
- RUQ pain/tenderness/mass.

B. Systemic Signs of Inflammation, etc.

- Fever.
- Elevated CRP.
- Elevated WBC count.

C. Imaging Findings

- **Suspected diagnosis:** 1 item in A + 1 item in B.
- **Definite diagnosis:** 1 item in A + 1 item in B + 1 item in C.

Treatment

A. Conservative Treatment

- Non-operative treatment is based on 4 components:
  1. NPO and IV fluids till pain resolves.
  2. IV analgesics.
  3. IV antibiotics: Broad spectrum antibiotics effective against Gram-negative aerobes, e.g., Cefazolin, cefuroxime, ciprofloxacin.
  4. Subsequent management: When the temperature, pulse and other physical signs show that the inflammation is subsiding, oral fluids are reinstated, followed by a regular diet.

B. Surgical

1. Cholecystectomy

- Whether open or laparoscopic, it is the treatment of choice for acute cholecystitis.
- The timing of surgery in acute cholecystitis remains controversial.

- Early laparoscopic cholecystectomy, undertaken by an experienced surgeon with excellent operating facilities within 5-7 days of the onset of the attack is safe and shortens total hospital stay.
- Nevertheless, the conversion rate in laparoscopic cholecystectomy is higher in acute than in elective surgery.

2. **Interval cholecystectomy**
   - If early operation is not indicated, one should wait for approx. 6 weeks for the inflammation to subside before operating.
3. **Subtotal/partial cholecystectomy**
   - The GB is transected at the infundibulum.
   - Cauterization of the remaining mucosa.
   - It is done when Calot's is frozen.
   - This is acceptable as it avoids injury to the CBD.
4. **Percutaneously placed cholecystostomy tube**
   - Done under local anesthesia with some sedation.
   - Done under USG guidance.
   - Acts as a temporizing measure by draining the infected bile.
   - Indicated in patients with a prohibitively high operative risk.
   - It results in improvement in symptoms and physiology, allowing a delayed cholecystectomy 3-6 months after medical optimization.

[10] Describe the aetiology, clinical features and management of obstructive jaundice. ***June 14***

[5] Obstructive jaundice. ***Dec 19***

[5] Clinical features and investigations of obstructive jaundice. ***June 13***

Definitions

- **Medical jaundice:** Source of hyperbilirubinemia is from hemoglobin breakdown through the process of conjugation.
- **Surgical/obstructive jaundice:** Hyperbilirubinemia occurs from a blockage of excretion.

Causes

- Choledocholithiasis or CBD stones.
- Biliary strictures.
- Cholangiocarcinoma.
- Choledochal cyst.
- Biliary atresia.
- Carcinoma head of pancreas.
- Serous cystic neoplasm of pancreas.
- Intraductal papillary mucinous neoplasm.
- Hepatocellular carcinoma (rare).

Clinical Features

- These depend on the cause of the obstructive jaundice. However, there are a few **common clinical features:**
  - o Darkening of urine.
  - o Scleral icterus.
  - o Pruritus.
- **Choledocholithiasis** causing obstructive jaundice:
  - o It is more likely to be painful because the onset of obstruction is acute, causing rapid distension of the bile duct and activation of pain fibres.
  - o Pain is usually colicky in nature.
  - o Clay-coloured stools.
  - o Cholangitis is ascending infection of CBD, secondary to obstruction and increased intraluminal pressure. They present with RUQ pain, fever and jaundice – known as Charcot's triad; which may progress to septic shock with mental status changes and hypotension – called Reynold's pentad, which has 100% mortality, if not treated promptly.
- The presentation of **cholangiocarcinoma** depends on the origin and manifestations of biliary obstruction at that site:
  - o Painless jaundice.
  - o Steatorrhea.
  - o Ash-coloured or silver-grey stools due to sloughing of tumour.
- **Choledochal cyst**
  - o Infants typically present with obstructive jaundice and an abdominal mass.

- **Biliary strictures**
  - o History of hepatobiliary surgery.
  - o Cholangitis, jaundice
- **Biliary atresia**
  - o Infants present shortly after birth with jaundice, pale stools and dark urine.
  - o Advanced disease presents with failure to thrive, hepatomegaly and ascites from liver cirrhosis.
- **Pancreatic ductal adenocarcinoma**
  - o Ca pancreas involving head or periampullary region causes jaundice.
  - o Although painless jaundice has frequently been described, a significant number of patients present with pain in addition to jaundice, typically arising in the epigastrium and radiating to the back.
  - o Weight loss.
- Serous cystic neoplasms have a predilection for the head of the pancreas and may thus present with obstructive jaundice.

Investigations

A. Liver Function Tests

- Hyperbilirubinemia.
- Increased alkaline phosphatase.
- Other markers of hepatic synthetic function, such as prothrombin time and albumin level, are generally unaffected until later in the disease or when the biliary obstruction is long-standing.
- Tumour markers such as CEA and CA 19-9 are unreliable for diagnosis of cholangiocarcinoma, but if elevated, may be useful post-operatively in the surveillance of recurrence.

B. USG

- Evaluates most of the biliary tree.
- Can separate patients with medical jaundice from surgical jaundice.
- It is the study of choice for the initial evaluation of jaundice or symptoms of biliary disease.
- Can sometimes identify the cause of obstructive jaundice showing CBD stones or even cholangiocarcinoma.
- May show intrahepatic biliary ductal dilation.

C. CT Scan

- Provides anatomic delineation.
- Can be used to identify the cause and site of biliary obstruction.
- It is the investigation of choice for retroperitoneal organs such as the pancreas.

D. MRCP

- Provides superior anatomic definition of the intrahepatic and extrahepatic biliary tree and pancreas.
- Extremely useful in planning resection of biliary or pancreatic neoplasms.

E. ERCP

- Diagnostic and therapeutic.
- Useful in taking bile cytology and brushings for diagnosis of cholangiocarcinoma.

F. Cholangiography

- Useful in biliary strictures

G. Endoscopic Ultrasound

- Useful in evaluating lesions of the pancreatic head.

Treatment

Depends on the underlying cause:

A. Choledocholithiasis

- ERCP is used to perform CBD clearance and also for the placement of stent in CBD.
- If stones are too big to be cleared by ERCP, choledochoduodenostomy or choledochojejunostomy is done.
- Cholecystectomy (Lap/open) is also done in choledocholithiasis.

B. Choledochal Cyst

- Radical excision of the cyst + reconstruction of the biliary tract using a Roux-en-Y loop of jejunum is the treatment of choice (hepaticojejunostomy).

C. Biliary Stricture

- Re-establishing biliary enteric communication.

D. Cholangiocarcinoma

- Resection of the lesion with negative margins, liver transplantation .
- ERCP with metallic stenting.

E. Biliary Atresia

- Kasai procedure, i.e., Hepaticojejunostomy.

F. Ca Head of Pancreas

- Whipple's procedure.

[3] Gallstone ileus. ***Dec 18***

- It is a rare complication of cholelithiasis, which occurs as a result of **impaction of one or more gallstones within the gastrointestinal tract.**

Aetiopathogenesis

- An episode of acute cholecystitis leads to erosion of inflamed tissues, resulting in a **cholecysto intestinal fistula.**
- A majority of **small gallstones pass through the intestines spontaneously**.
- However, **gallstones of size 2-5 cm get impacted, usually in the terminal ileum or at the ileocecal valve** owing to the relatively narrow lumen and less active peristalsis here.
- Impacted stones may lead to **necrosis and perforation** followed by **peritonitis.**
- Less common locations include the stomach and the **duodenum (Bouveret's syndrome)**.

Clinical Features

- More common in elderly and in women.
- Acute, intermittent or chronic episodes of partial or complete gastrointestinal obstruction.
- On examination, signs of obstruction are seen:
  - o Dehydration.
  - o Abdominal distension.
  - o Tenderness.
  - o High pitched bowel sounds.

Investigations

- **X-ray abdomen:**
  1. Partial or complete intestinal obstruction.
  2. Pneumobilia or contrast material in the biliary tree.
  3. Ectopic calcified gallstone:
     - o These 3 together constitute **Rigler's triad.**
     - o A change in the position of such a gallstone on serial films (called tumbling sign).
- **CT abdomen:**
  - Superior to plain X-rays and USG.
  - Shows an abnormal gallbladder with air, an air fluid level or fluid accumulation with an irregular wall.

Treatment

- Management of intestinal obstruction.
- **Enterolithotomy** is the most common surgical procedure performed.
- A **cholecystoenteric fistula should not be resected unless the patient is stable** or there are residual gallstones that may cause infection or recurrent ileus.
- The fistula is resected in a separate sitting when the patient stabilizes.

[3] Enumerate components of Charcot's triad. ***CBME March 24***

[3] Components of Charcot's triad. ***CBME June 24***

[3] Charcot's triad and its significance. ***August 22, Dec 15***

[3] Charcot's triad. ***June 19, Dec 18, July 23***

- Charcot's triad has 3 components:
  1. Clinical jaundice.
  2. Fever.
  3. Pain in the right upper quadrant.
- **Importance:** Charcot's triad is important as it **helps diagnose ascending cholangitis**, which is a potentially **life threatening emergency** associated with infection of the biliary tree.
- Charcot's triad **may progress to septic shock with mental status changes and hypotension, called Reynold's pentad** which has a mortality of 100% without prompt treatment.

[3] Courvoisier's rule. ***July 18, Dec 17, March 24***

[3] What is Courvoisier's rule? Mention the exceptions. ***Dec 12***

- Courvoisier's law states that: **'In obstruction of the CBD due to stone, distension of the gallbladder rarely occurs, as the organ usually is already**

shriveled. In obstruction from other causes, distension is common'.

- So, most patients with jaundice due to stone have a fibrotic, non-distended gallbladder, whilst those with malignant obstruction have a distended and palpable gallbladder.
- Another factor is that malignant obstruction is often complete, whereas stone obstruction may not be so complete as to cause distension.
- **Exceptions** to Courvoisier's law:
  1. **Double impaction** of stones, i.e., One in the cystic duct and the other in the CBD.
  2. **Oriental cholangiohepatitis.**
  3. **A pancreatic calculus obstructing the ampulla of Vater.**
  4. **Mucocele** of gallbladder due to a stone in the cystic duct.

[5] Choledochal cyst. ***March 22, Oct 20, Dec 16, Dec 15***

[3] Types of choledochal cyst. ***July 18***

- **Definition:** Choledochal cysts are **congenital dilatations of the intra and/or extrahepatic biliary system**.
- Rare disorder.
- **Now called biliary malformations rather than cysts.**

Aetiopathogenesis

- Pathogenesis is **unclear.**
- Although classified as a single disease, there are **multiple theories** for aetiology, but the **most accepted is the anomalous pancreatobiliary junction theory.**
- More common in Asian populations.
- Considered to be a **premalignant** condition.

Types

I: Fusiform dilation involving only the extrahepatic biliary tree.

II: Saccular diverticulum off the CBD which may be mistaken for an accessory gallbladder.

III: Appears as a cystic dilation of the intramural CBD (i.e., within the wall of the duodenum). This is also called choledochocele.

IV:

a: Multiple cysts involving the intrahepatic and extrahepatic biliary tree.

b: Multiple cysts limited to the extrahepatic biliary tree.

V: Cystic dilatation of only the intrahepatic ducts, also called **Caroli disease.**

Type I choledochal cyst is the most common form.

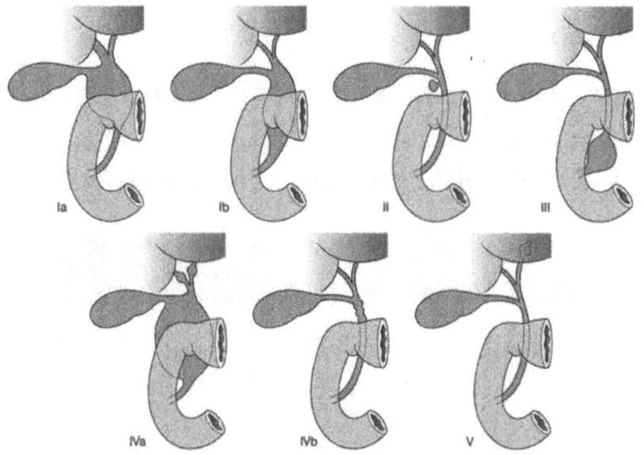

Classification of choledochal cysts. Type Ia and Ib (80-90%): diffuse cystic dilatation; note the extension into the intrapancreatic portion in type Ib. Type II (3%): diverticulum of the common bile duct. Type III (5%): diverticulum within the intrapancreatic portion. Type IV (10%): extension into the liver; type IVa: fusiform dilatation of the entire extrahepatic bile duct with extension into the intrahepatic ducts; type IVb: multiple cystic dilatations involving only the extrahepatic bile duct. Type V: cystic dilatation only of the intrahepatic ducts.

Figure: Types of choledochal cyst

Clinical Features

- They are sometimes diagnosed in infancy, however, they can present in adulthood.
- Jaundice is the most common symptom.
- Fever.
- RUQ pain.
- Rarely, a RUQ mass is palpable.
- Non-specific problems: Weight loss, nausea, vomiting.
- They are considered pre-malignant conditions and have an increased risk of developing cholangiocarcinoma.
- Pancreatitis is sometimes seen in adults.
- Rarely, a long-standing malformation can cause liver injury and even cirrhosis.

Investigations

- **USG:** Confirms the presence of an abnormal cyst.
- **MRCP:** Reveals the anatomy in detail, in particular the relationship between the lower end of the bile duct and the pancreatic duct.

- **CT:** Delineates the extent of intra or extrahepatic dilatation.

Treatment

- **Radical excision of the cyst + reconstruction of the biliary tract using a Roux-en-Y loop of jejunum** is the treatment of choice (**Hepaticojejunostomy**).
- Complete resection is important because of an **association with** the later development of **cholangiocarcinoma.**
- **Type III** needs **endoscopic management with sphincterotomy**. It should be accompanied by **biopsy of the cyst epithelium to exclude dysplasia**.

[5] Calot's triangle. *June 14*

- Calot's triangle, also called the hepatobiliary triangle was initially described by Calot as the space bordered by:
  1. Inferiorly/laterally – cystic duct.
  2. Medially – common hepatic duct.
  3. Superiorly – cystic artery.
- This has been modified in contemporary literature as the area bounded by:
  a. Superiorly – inferior surface of the liver.
  b. Laterally – cystic duct and the medial border of the gallbladder.
  c. Medially – common hepatic duct.
- It is also known as the hepatocystic triangle.

Importance

- It is an important surgical landmark as the cystic artery usually can be found within its boundaries.
- The cystic lymph node often lies superficial to the cystic artery and acts as a landmark to locate this artery in difficult cases.
- During laparoscopic cholecystectomy, it helps surgeons identify the cystic artery and cystic duct.
- Dissection of the Calot's is important to achieve Critical View of Safety which is essential for safe laparoscopic cholecystectomy.

[3] Indications of CBD exploration. *Dec 17, Dec 15*

- Common bile duct exploration is indicated when there's a need to directly visualize and address issues within the bile duct that cannot be adequately managed through less invasive means such as ERCP:
  1. Presence of common bile duct stones not amenable to endoscopic removal.
  2. Suspected or confirmed bile duct strictures or obstructions causing jaundice, cholangitis, or pancreatitis.
  3. Failed ERCP attempts to clear the bile duct.
  4. Suspicion of bile duct injury during cholecystectomy or other abdominal surgeries.
  5. Evaluation and management of bile duct tumors or other pathology affecting bile duct drainage.

[3] Saint's triad. *June 14*

- Saint's triad consists of 3 conditions which may coexist:
  1. Gallstones.
  2. Diverticulosis of the colon.
  3. Hiatus hernia.
- It is important to find out which lesion is the cause of the patient's dyspeptic symptoms.

OTHER IMPORTANT TOPICS

CA GALL BLADDER

- It is an aggressive malignant disease and carries an extremely poor prognosis.

Aetiology

- Extremely variable by geographical region and racial-ethnic groups, common in parts of North India.
- Association with pre-existing gallstone disease (gallstones > 3 cm), implying that chronic inflammation may play a role.
- Calcification of the gallbladder wall (porcelain gallbladder).
- Chronic infection, e.g., Typhoid carriers.
- Primary sclerosing cholangitis, especially with concomitant inflammatory bowel disease.
- Abnormal pancreatic biliary junction.

- Gallbladder polyps: The risk of malignant transformation increases with increasing size of the polyp.

Pathology

- Majority (90%) of tumours are adenocarcinomas.
- Squamous carcinomas may arise from areas of mucosal squamous metaplasia.
- Tumour most commonly is nodular and infiltrative, with thickening of the gallbladder wall, often extending to the whole gallbladder.
- 90% originate in the fundus or body of the gallbladder.

Spread

- Direct extension into the liver.
- Seeding of the peritoneal cavity.
- Involvement of the perihilar lymphatics and neural plexuses.

Clinical Features

- F > M.
- Age: 60-80 years.
- No specific presenting symptoms, therefore, presentation with late-stage disease is common.
- May be asymptomatic.
- Symptoms, if present, are usually indistinguishable from those of benign gallbladder disease such as biliary colic or cholecystitis, particularly in older patients.
- Jaundice and anorexia are late features.
- Palpable mass is a late sign.
- Weight loss.
- Other common symptoms: Chronic epigastric pain, early satiety and a sense of fullness.

Investigations

- Laboratory findings are generally non-specific but may be consistent with biliary obstruction:
  - o Anaemia.
  - o Leukocytosis.
  - o Mild elevation in transaminases.
- **Tumour markers:**
  - o Serum CA19-9.
  - o Carcinoembryonic antigen.
- **USG** is used to make the pre-op diagnosis.
- **CT thorax, abdomen and pelvis** is used to confirm the diagnosis.
- **MRI/MRCP** is also used to confirm the diagnosis.
- **Percutaneous biopsy:**
  - o Under radiological guidance.
  - o May be considered to obtain tissue for pathological examination, but only in unresectable disease prior to palliative treatment.
- **Diagnostic laparoscopy:**
  - o Useful in staging the disease.
  - o Can detect peritoneal or liver metastases, which would preclude further surgical resection.
- **PET scan** has a role in detecting metastatic disease.

Treatment

A. Pre-op Diagnosis

- Majority of patients have advanced disease at presentation and are not candidates for surgical therapy.
- Staging laparoscopy is mandatory prior to formal laparotomy to detect occult metastases not picked up on imaging.
- Radical en bloc resection includes the gallbladder, wedge hepatectomy (2 cm of liver in the gallbladder bed or segments IVb and V if there is concomitant liver infiltration) or extended hepatectomy and bile duct resection if the bile duct is involved or the cystic duct margin is positive on intraoperative frozen section.
- Regional lymphadenectomy (paracholedochal portal, along the right hepatic artery and retroduodenal nodes) should be considered.
- Aim is to remove the tumour entirely and achieve negative histopathological margins.

B. Incidental Gallbladder Cancer

- Diagnosed following HPE of gallbladder after it has been removed for presumed benign disease.
- In these cases, the need for further surgery is determined by the stage of disease:

a. **For early-stage disease confined to the mucosa of the gallbladder with a negative cystic duct margin and no evidence of recurrence on imaging.**
   - o No further treatment is indicated.

b. **For transmural disease:**
   - o A radical en bloc resection of the gallbladder fossa and surrounding wedge of liver along with the regional lymph nodes.
   - o If the initial procedure was performed laparoscopically, the surgeon should examine the laparoscopic port sites.
   - o Routine resection of port sites is no longer recommended.
   - o Finding of disease at the port sites is a sign of generalised peritoneal disease and carries a very poor prognosis.
   - o Adjuvant oral chemotherapy: Capecitabine ± gemcitabine/oxaliplatin.

C. Advanced Disease

- Non-operative approach.
- Palliative therapy.
- Obstructive jaundice is relieved by endoscopic and/or percutaneous methods.

34

Pancreas

[3] Annular pancreas. *August 22*

- It is a **congenital anomaly** of the pancreas.

Cause

- It is the result of **failure of complete rotation of the ventral pancreatic bud** during development.
- A **ring of pancreatic tissue surrounds the second or third part of the duodenum.**

Clinical Features

- Most often seen in **association with congenital duodenal stenosis** or atresia.
- More prevalent in children with **Down syndrome.**
- Duodenal obstruction typically causes **vomiting in the neonate.**
- Vomiting can be **bile stained if the duodenal obstruction is below the ampulla of Vater.**
- It may be a cause of **acute pancreatitis** in later life.

On Examination

- Peristaltic waves may be seen.
- Upper abdominal distension may be seen.

Investigations

- **Plain abdominal X-ray** shows the **'double bubble'** sign of the interrupted gastroduodenal shadow produced by the rigid ring of pancreatic tissue.
- **CECT.**

Treatment

- **The usual treatment is bypass: Duodenoduodenostomy** or **duodenojejunostomy**, if it is causing duodenal obstruction.
- **If it is a cause of pancreatitis, resection of the head of the pancreas** should be considered.

[10] Describe aetiology, pathology, clinical features and management of acute pancreatitis. *Sept 21*
[10] Describe the clinical features, investigations and management of acute pancreatitis. *Dec 14*
[3] Write causes of acute pancreatitis. *Dec 12*
[3] Ranson's score. *Oct 20, June 17, Dec 15*
[3] Ranson's criteria. *Dec 17, July 23*

ACUTE PANCREATITIS

- Acute pancreatitis is an **acute inflammation of the pancreatic parenchyma**, which presents as an **emergency**.
- **Definition:** Acute pancreatitis is defined as an acute condition presenting with:
  - o Abdominal pain.
  - o A three-fold or greater rise in the serum levels of the pancreatic enzymes amylase or lipase **and/or.**
  - o Characteristic findings of pancreatic inflammation on CECT.

Aetiology

- **Gallstones or biliary calculi is the most common cause of acute pancreatitis.**
- **Alcoholism is the 2nd most common cause** of acute pancreatitis.
- Post ERCP.
- Abdominal trauma.
- Following biliary, upper gastrointestinal or cardio-thoracic surgery.
- Ampullary tumours.
- Drugs (corticosteroids, azathioprine, asparaginase, valproic acid, thiazides, estrogens).
- Hyperparathyroidism.
- Hypercalcemia.
- Hypertriglyceridemia.
- Pancreas divisum.
- Sphincter of Oddi dysfunction.
- Autoimmune pancreatitis.
- Hereditary pancreatitis.
- Viral infections (mumps, coxsackie B).
- Malnutrition.
- Scorpion bite.
- Idiopathic.

Pathogenesis

- The underlying mechanism of all causes of acute pancreatitis is as follows:

Injury to acinar cells →impaired secretion of zymogen granules

Or

Damage to ductal epithelium → delayed enzymatic secretion

↓

Premature activation of pancreatic enzymes within the pancreas

↓

Autodigestion, i.e., Acute pancreatitis

Pathophysiology of Acute Pancreatitis

Cellular injury has been initiated

↓

Inflammatory process

↓ (two branches)

1. Pancreatic edema
2. Pancreatic hemorrhage

↓

Pancreatic necrosis

Inflammatory mediators are released into the circulation (IL-1, IL-6, TNF-α)

↓

SIRS

↓

MODS

↓

Death

Systemic Complications of Acute Pancreatitis

- Hemodynamic instability.
- Bacteremia (due to translocation of gut flora).
- Acute respiratory distress syndrome.
- Pleural effusions.
- GI hemorrhage.
- Renal failure/acute kidney injury.
- Disseminated intravascular coagulation.

Phases of Acute Pancreatitis

Acute pancreatitis has 2 phases:

A. Early Phase

- Usually lasts a week.
- Caused by the intense inflammatory cascade triggered by pancreatic inflammation.
- Characterised by SIRS, MODS which are the cause of death in early phase.

B. Late Phase

- Typically seen in those who suffer a severe attack.
- Can last from weeks to months.

- Characterized by persistent systemic signs of inflammation and/or local complications, particularly fluid collections and peri-pancreatic sepsis.
- In the late phase, deaths are often due to septic complications.

Clinical Features

- **Pain is the cardinal symptom**
  - o Characteristically develops quickly and reaches maximum intensity within minutes.
  - o Persists for hours or even days.
  - o Frequently severe, constant and refractory to the usual doses of analgesics.
  - o Usually experienced first in the epigastrium but may be localized to either upper quadrant or felt diffusely.
  - o Radiates to the back.
  - o Some patients may gain relief by sitting or leaning forwards.
- **Nausea, repeated vomiting and retching**
  - o Retching may persist despite the stomach being kept empty by nasogastric aspiration.
- **Hiccoughs.**

On Examination

- Appearance may be that of a patient who is well, or at the other extreme, one who is gravely ill with profound shock, toxicity and confusion.
- Bleeding into the fascial planes can produce bluish discolouration of:
  - o **Flanks: Grey Turner's sign.**
  - o **Umbilicus: Cullen's sign.**
- Tachypnea.
- Tachycardia.
- Hypotension.
- Body temperature is often normal or even subnormal, but frequently rises as inflammation develops.
- Mild icterus can be caused by biliary obstruction in gallstone pancreatitis.
- Acute swinging pyrexia suggests cholangitis.
- Subcutaneous fat necrosis may produce small, red, tender nodules on the skin of the legs.
- P/A
  - o Distension due to ileus.
  - o Ascites with shifting dullness.
  - o A mass may develop in the epigastrium owing to inflammation.
  - o Guarding in upper abdomen.
- Pleural effusion.
- Patient may be confused and exhibit the signs of metabolic derangement together with hypoxemia.

Investigations

Blood Tests

A. Serum Amylase

- A serum amylase level three times above normal is indicative of acute pancreatitis.

B. Serum Lipase

- More sensitive and specific than amylase.

Imaging

A. X-rays of Chest and Abdomen

- Not diagnostic of acute pancreatitis but are useful in the differential diagnosis.
- **Non-specific findings:**
  - o **Sentinel loop**–Generalised or local ileus.
  - o **Colon cut off sign.**
  - o **Renal halo sign.**
  - o Occasionally, calcified gallstones or pancreatic calcifications may be seen.
  - o CXR may show a pleural effusion, and in severe cases, a diffuse alveolar interstitial shadowing may suggest Acute Respiratory Distress Syndrome.

B. USG

- Does not establish a diagnosis of acute pancreatitis.
- Detects gallstones as a potential cause.
- Rules out acute cholecystitis as a differential diagnosis.

- Determines whether the CBD is dilated or not.
- Should therefore be performed within 24 hours in all patients.

C. CECT Abdomen and Pelvis

- CECT is the imaging **investigation of choice.**
- It is indicated in the following situations:
  - o Diagnostic uncertainty.
  - o In patients with severe acute pancreatitis, to distinguish interstitial from necrotizing pancreatitis.
  - o Severity of pancreatitis detected on CT may be staged according to the Balthazar criteria.
  - o In patients with organ failure, signs of sepsis or progressive clinical deterioration.
  - o When a localized complication is suspected, such as a fluid collection, pseudocyst or a pseudoaneurysm.

D. Cross-sectional MRI

- Yields similar information to that obtained by CT.

E. MRCP

- Detects stones in the CBD.
- Directly assesses the pancreatic parenchyma.

F. ERCP

- Diagnostic as well as therapeutic.
- Allows the identification and removal of stones in the CBD in gallstone pancreatitis.

Assessment of Severity

- It is important to identify those patients who will develop severe pancreatitis as they require aggressive early management and transfer to a specialist unit.
- Various prognostic scoring systems have been used, all aimed at predicting persistent organ failure.
- Severity stratification assessments should be performed in patients at 24 hours, 48 hours and 7 days after admission.
- Scoring systems specific for acute pancreatitis:
  - o Ranson score.
  - o Glasgow score.
- Several other scoring systems that are used in ICUs can also be applied:
  - o APACHE.
  - o SAPS.
  - o SOFA.
  - o MODS.
  - o Modified Marshall score.
- Regardless of the scoring system used, persisting organ failure indicates a severe attack.

Ranson Score

- It is a scoring system which is specific for acute pancreatitis.
- A score of ≥ 3 at 48 hours indicates a severe attack.

ALCOHOLIC OR OTHER CAUSE	BILIARY CAUSE
On admission	**On admission**
Age > 55 yrs	Age > 70 yrs
WBCs > 16,000/µl	WBCs > 18,000/µl
Blood glucose > 200 mg/dl	Blood glucose > 220 mg/dl
LDH > 350 U/l	LDH > 250 U/l
AST > 250 U/l	AST > 250 U/l
At 48 hours	**At 48 hours**
Drop in hematocrit > 10%	Drop in hematocrit > 10%
BUN increase > 5 mg/dl	BUN increase > 2 mg/dl
Calcium < 8 mg/dl	Calcium < 8 mg/dl
PaO_2 < 60 mm Hg	PaO_2 < 60 mm Hg
Base deficit > 4 mEq/l	Base deficit > 5 mEq/l
Fluid loss > 6 litres	Fluid loss > 4 litres

Treatment

A. Treatment of Mild Attack of Pancreatitis

- IV fluids.
- Frequent but non-invasive observation.
- A brief period of NPO may be sensible in a patient who is nauseated and in pain *but* early oral feeds is recommended.
- Antibiotics are not indicated.
- Analgesics.
- Anti-emetics.
- CT scan is unnecessary, unless there is evidence of deterioration.

B. Treatment of Severe Acute Pancreatitis

- Admission to HDU/ICU.
- Invasive monitoring of vital signs, central venous pressure, urine output, arterial blood gases.

- Analgesia.
- Aggressive fluid resuscitation, **RL is fluid of choice.**
- Supplemental oxygen.
- Frequent monitoring of hematological and biochemical parameters (including LFT, RFT, INR, serum calcium, blood glucose).
- Nasogastric drainage (only initially):
  - o Not essential.
  - o May be of value in patients with vomiting.
  - o External nutrition, i.e., Feeding via a nasogastric tube.
- Antibiotics:
  - o Prophylactic IV antibiotics may be used to prevent local and other septic complications.
  - o IV cefuroxime or IV imipinem or IV ciprofloxacin + IV metronidazole.
  - o Antibiotics should be given promptly if there is evidence of cholangitis or concomitant respiratory or urinary infection.
- CECT is essential if there is organ failure, clinical deterioration or signs of sepsis.
- ERCP within 72 hours for severe gallstone pancreatitis or signs of cholangitis.
- Supportive therapy for organ failure if it develops (inotropes, ventilatory support, hemofiltration etc).
- If nutritional support is required, consider enteral (nasogastric) feeding.

[5] Write the surgical management of chronic calcific pancreatitis. ***CBME June 24***

CHRONIC PANCREATITIS

- **Definition:** Chronic pancreatitis is a progressive inflammatory disease in which there is irreversible destruction of pancreatic tissue.

Aetiopathogenesis

1. **High alcohol consumption**
   - It is the most common cause of chronic pancreatitis.
2. **Genetic factors**
   - Normally, if trypsinogen becomes prematurely activated within the pancreas, it is inhibited by ***SPINK1*** and destroyed. Mutations in the *SPINK1* gene, therefore cause chronic pancreatitis.
   - Mutations in the ***CFTR* gene.**
3. **Metabolic factors**
   - Hyperlipidemia.
   - Hypercalcemia.
4. **Pancreatic duct obstruction**
   - Stricture formation after trauma.
   - After acute pancreatitis.
   - Occlusion of the duct by pancreatic cancer.
5. **Congenital abnormalities**
   - Pancreas divisum.
   - Annular pancreas.
   - Predispose to chronic pancreatitis if associated with papillary stenosis.
6. **Hereditary pancreatitis**
   - Autosomal dominant.
   - Gain-of function mutation in the cationic trypsinogen gene (*PRSS1*) on chromosome 7, leads to production of a degradation-resistant form of trypsin.
7. **Cystic fibrosis.**
8. **Infantile malnutrition.**
9. **Tropical pancreatitis.**
10. **Autoimmune pancreatitis.**
11. **Idiopathic:**
    - Has been subdivided into early-onset and late-onset forms.

Pathology

- At the onset of the disease when symptoms have developed, the pancreas may appear normal.
- Later, the pancreas enlarges and becomes hard as a result of fibrosis.
- The ducts become distorted and dilated with areas of both stricture formation and ectasia.
- Calcified stones weighing from a few milligrams to 200 mg may form within the ducts.

- The ducts may become occluded with a gelatinous proteinaceous fluid and debris and inflammatory cysts may form.

HPE

- Lesions affect the lobules.
- Ductular metaplasia.
- Atrophy of acini.
- Hyperplasia of duct epithelium.
- Interlobular fibrosis.

Clinical Features

- More common in South India.
- M > F = 4:1.
- Mean age of onset is about 40 years.
- Pain is the outstanding symptom in the majority of patients:
  - o The site of pain depends on the part of pancreas affected.
  - o If the disease is mainly in the head of the pancreas, then epigastric and right subcostal pain is common.
  - o If it is limited to the left side of the pancreas, left subcostal and back pain are the presenting symptoms.
  - o In some patients, the pain is more diffuse.
  - o Radiation to the shoulder can occur.
  - o The pain is often dull and gnawing.
  - o Severe flare-ups of pain, due to acute attacks may be superimposed on a background of chronic pancreatitis.
  - o The pain prevents sleep.
  - o Pain forces the patient to take leave from work.
  - o Recurrent pain may sometimes be the only clinical symptom.
- Nausea is common during attacks and vomiting may occur.
- Weight loss is common because the patient does not feel like eating.
- Analgesic use and abuse are frequent.
- Loss of exocrine function leads to steatorrhoea.
- Loss of endocrine function may lead to development of diabetes.
- Infection is not infrequent, possibly related to the diabetes mellitus.

Complications/Sequelae

- Hereditary pancreatitis and pancreatitis occurring at a young age predispose the patient to developing **pancreatic cancer**, particularly if the patient smokes tobacco.
- **All the complications of acute pancreatitis can occur with chronic pancreatitis.**

Investigations

A. Serum Amylase

- Rises only in the early stages of the disease.

B. Pancreatic Function Tests

- Confirm the presence of pancreatic insufficiency or that more than 70% of the gland has been destroyed.

C. Abdominal X-rays

- Pancreatic calcifications may be seen on abdominal radiographs.

D. CT/MRI

- Shows the outline of the gland and the main area of damage.
- Possibilities for surgical correction can be determined.
- Calcification is seen very well on CT but not on MRI.
- A normal-looking pancreas on CT or MRI does not rule out chronic pancreatitis.

E. MRCP

- Will identify the presence of biliary obstruction.
- Shows the state of the pancreatic duct.
- Use of intravenous secretin during the study may demonstrate a pancreatic duct stricture which is not apparent on standard MRCP.

F. ERCP

- ERCP is the most accurate way of elucidating the anatomy of the duct.
- In conjunction with the whole organ morphology, it can help determine the type of operation required, if operative intervention is indicated.

G. USG

- Sonographic findings characteristic of chronic pancreatitis include:
  - o Presence of stones.
  - o Visible side branches.
  - o Cysts.
  - o Lobularity.
  - o An irregular main pancreatic duct.
  - o Hyperechoic foci and strands.
  - o Dilatation of the main pancreatic duct.
  - o Hyperechoic margins of the main pancreatic duct.
- The presence of ≥ 4 of these features is highly suggestive of chronic pancreatitis.

Treatment

A. Medical Measures

- Most patients can be managed with medical measures.
- Stop alcohol consumption.
- Stop smoking.
- **Pain management:**
  - o Eliminate obstructive factors (duodenum, bile duct, pancreatic duct).
  - o Escalate analgesia in a stepwise fashion.
  - o For intractable pain, consider CT/EUS-guided coeliac axis block.
- Diet should be low in fat, and high in protein and carbohydrates.
- Pancreatic enzyme supplementation with meals.
- Correct malabsorption of the fat-soluble vitamins and vitamin B_{12}.
- Micronutrient therapy with methionine, vitamins C and E, selenium.
- Medium-chain triglycerides are given to patients with severe fat malabsorption, as they are directly absorbed by the small intestine without the need for digestion.
- Reducing gastric secretions may help.
- Treat diabetes mellitus.

B. Intervention

- Intervention can be endoscopic, radiological or surgical.
- **Indications:**
  - o To relieve obstruction of the pancreatic duct, bile duct or the duodenum.
  - o In dealing with complications (e.g., pseudocyst, abscess, fistula, ascites or variceal hemorrhage).
  - o Decompressing an obstructed pancreatic duct can provide pain relief in some patients (the assumption is that ductal hypertension causes the pain).

C. Endoscopic Intervention

- Endoscopic pancreatic sphincterotomy might be beneficial in patients with papillary stenosis + high sphincter pressure and pancreatic ductal pressure.
- Placement of a stent across the stricture. The stent should not be left for more than 4–6 weeks as it gets blocked. Those who get pain relief may benefit from a surgical bypass.
- Pancreatic duct stones may be extracted at ERCP; this may sometimes be combined with extracorporeal shock wave lithotripsy.
- Pseudocysts may be drained internally under endoscopic ultrasound guidance.

D. Radiological Intervention

- Percutaneous or transgastric drainage of pseudocysts under ultrasound or CT guidance may be performed.

E. Surgery

- **Indications for surgery:**
  - o Conservative treatments fail to alleviate symptoms.
  - o Complications such as pancreatic pseudocysts.
  - o Persistent pain.
  - o Obstructive jaundice.
- **Goals of surgery:**
  - o To overcome obstruction.
  - o To remove mass lesions.
  - o Pain relief.

- o Prevent complications.
- o Preserve pancreatic function as much as possible.

Surgical Options Available

- **Mass in the head of the pancreas:**
  - o Pancreatoduodenectomy or Whipple's procedure.
  - o Duodenum-preserving resection of the pancreatic head or Beger procedure.
- **If the duct is markedly dilated:**
  - o Longitudinal pancreaticojejunostomy or Frey procedure.
- **Disease limited to the tail of the pancreas:**
  - o Distal pancreatectomy.
- **Patients with intractable pain and diffuse disease:**
  - o Total pancreatectomy with autologous islet cell transplantation.

Whipple's Procedure

- Involves removal of the pancreatic head, duodenum, proximal jejunum, gallbladder and distal common bile duct.
- Reconstruction is performed by connecting the remaining pancreas to the stomach or jejunum and connecting the remaining bile duct to the jejunum.

Distal Pancreatectomy

- Indicated when the pancreatic body and tail are primarily affected by calcifications or when there are localized complications such as pseudocysts.
- Removal of the pancreatic tail and sometimes the body, sparing the pancreatic head.

Total Pancreatectomy with Autologous Islet Cell Transplantation

- Considered in selected cases where severe pain persists despite other surgical interventions.
- Involves removal of the diseased part of the pancreas (usually the head or body/tail) while isolating and preserving pancreatic islet cells.
- These cells are then processed in a lab and transplanted back into the patient's liver via the portal vein, where they can restore insulin production and reduce the risk of diabetes mellitus post-surgery.

Frey Procedure

- Specifically designed for patients with chronic pancreatitis affecting the pancreatic head, with pain as the predominant symptom.
- Involves a partial pancreatic head resection along with longitudinal pancreaticojejunostomy.
- This procedure aims to decompress the pancreatic duct and alleviate pain while preserving pancreatic function.

Puestow Procedure (Lateral Pancreaticojejunostomy)

- Used for patients with diffuse pancreatic ductal obstruction causing pain and/or pseudocysts.
- Involves longitudinal opening of the pancreas along its length and anastomosis of the pancreatic duct to a loop of jejunum.
- This procedure aims to relieve obstruction and pain by allowing pancreatic secretions to drain more freely into the intestine.

[5] Enumerate the clinical features and management of pancreatic pseudocyst. ***CBME March 24***

[5] Pseudocyst of pancreas. ***March 22, March 21, Oct 20, Dec 18, Dec 16, June 16, July 15, Dec 14***

PSEUDOCYST OF PANCREAS

- **Definition:** Pseudocyst of pancreas is a complication of acute pancreatitis that is a collection of amylase-rich fluid enclosed in a well-defined wall of fibrous or granulation tissue.

Aetiopathogenesis

- Typically arise following an attack of mild acute pancreatitis.
- Lie outside the pancreas.
- Represents an acute peri-pancreatic fluid collection that has not resolved and matured.
- Formation of a pseudocyst requires $\geq$ 4 weeks from the onset of acute pancreatitis.
- More than half have a communication with the main pancreatic duct.

- Pseudocysts are often single but are occasionally multiple.
- The term pseudocyst is often used more loosely to include sterile walled off necrosis that has failed to resolve or a collection that has developed in the context of chronic pancreatitis or after pancreatic trauma.

Clinical Features

- **Epigastric swelling:**
  - o Appears during the conservative treatment.
  - o Or in traumatic cases, during or after convalescence for an injury that did not require laparotomy.
- Sometimes, patient may give a history of an episode of acute pancreatitis.
- Persistent pain.
- Early satiety.
- Nausea.
- Weight loss.
- There is a swelling, sometimes as large as a melon, placed centrally above the umbilicus.
- Swelling is fixed.
- It may be so tense that fluctuation cannot be elicited.
- Transmitted pulsation from the abdominal aorta is very noticeable.

Complications

1. **Infection:**
   - Abscess.
   - Systemic sepsis.
2. **Rupture:**
   - a. **Into the gut**
     - GI bleeding.
     - Internal fistula.
   - b. **Into the peritoneum**
     - Peritonitis.
3. **Enlargement:**
   - a. **Pressure effects**
     - Obstructive jaundice from biliary compression.
     - Bowel obstruction.
   - b. **Pain.**
4. **Erosion into a vessel:**
   - Hemorrhage into the cyst.
   - Hemoperitoneum.

Investigations

- **Barium meal:**
  - o Shows projection of the pseudocyst into hollow viscera, especially the stomach.
- CT scan.
- **MRCP:**
  - o Demonstrates communication of the cyst with the pancreatic duct system.
  - o Ductal anomalies can be seen.
- **EUS + FNA of cyst fluid:**
  - o Endoscopic ultrasound + fine needle aspiration of cyst fluid.
  - o Cyst fluid should be sent for the following:
    - a. **CEA (CarcinoEmbryonic Antigen)**
      - ♦ Pseudocyst has low CEA levels.
      - ♦ Levels > 400 ng/ml indicates a mucinous neoplasm.
    - b. **Amylase levels**
      - ♦ Pseudocyst usually has high amylase levels.
    - c. **Cytology**
      - ♦ Typically reveals inflammatory cells in pseudocyst fluid.

Treatment

- Pseudocysts usually resolve spontaneously, but complications can develop.
- **Indications for therapeutic intervention:**
  - o Symptomatic patients.
  - o If complications develop.
  - o Distinction has to be made between a pseudocyst and a tumour.
  - o Pseudocysts that are less likely to resolve spontaneously:

- ♦ Thick walled.
- ♦ Large (> 6 cm in diameter).
- ♦ Have lasted for a long time (> 12 weeks).
- ♦ Have arisen in the context of chronic pancreatitis.

- There are 3 possible approaches to draining a pseudocyst:
  1. Percutaneous.
  2. Endoscopic.
  3. Surgical.

Percutaneous

- A percutaneous transgastric cystogastrostomy can be performed under imaging guidance.
- A double pig tailed drain is placed with one end in the cyst cavity and the other end in the gastric lumen.
- Percutaneous drainage to the exterior should not be done.

Endoscopic

- Usually involves puncture of the cyst through the stomach or duodenal wall under endoscopic ultrasound guidance.
- Placement of a tube drain with one end in the cyst cavity and the other end in the gastric lumen.
- Sometimes, ERCP and placement of a pancreatic stent across the ampulla may help to drain a pseudocyst that is in communication with the duct.

Surgical

- Involves internally draining the cyst into:
  - o **Stomach:** Cystogastrostomy.
  - o **Jejunum:** Cystojejunostomy.

[5] ERCP. ***March 24***
[3] ERCP. ***Sept 21***
[3] Indications for ERCP. ***July 18, CBME June 24***

ERCP

- Endoscopic Retrograde CholangioPancreatography.

Method

- Performed using a side-viewing fibreoptic duodenoscope.
- Ampulla of Vater is intubated.
- Water soluble contrast is injected into the biliary and pancreatic ducts.
- An X-ray is then taken, which displays the anatomy radiologically.
- This provides excellent images of the ductal anatomy.
- A plain radiograph can sometimes be taken before contrast studies to delineate calcification.

Indications and Uses

ERCP is both diagnostic as well as therapeutic.

A. Diagnostic

- Diagnosis of pancreatic ductal adenocarcinoma.
- Diagnosis of cholangiocarcinoma.
- Bile or pancreatic fluid and brushings from duct strictures can yield cells that confirm the suspected diagnosis of carcinoma, i.e., brush cytology.
- In carcinoma pancreas, the main pancreatic duct may be narrowed or completely obstructed at the site of the tumour, or the distal bile duct may be narrowed. Concurrent narrowing of both ducts result in the so called double duct sign.
- Changes seen in chronic pancreatitis include:
  - o Presence of pancreatic duct strictures.
  - o Dilation of main pancreatic duct with stones.
- Can identify choledocholithiasis.

B. Therapeutic

- Can relieve obstruction in case of malignant strictures.
- Placement of biliary stents in cholangiocarcinoma.
- Placement of pancreatic stents in pancreatic ductal adenocarcinoma.
- CBD stones can be removed and stent placed in CBD.
- Pancreatic duct stones can be removed and stent placed in main pancreatic duct.

[3] Serum amylase. *March 21*

- Measurement of serum amylase is the most widely used test of pancreatic damage.
- It rises within a few hours of pancreatic damage and declines over the next 4-8 days.
- A markedly elevated serum amylase level is highly suspicious but not diagnostic of acute pancreatitis.
- Causes of raised severe amylase level:
  - o Acute pancreatitis.
  - o Upper GI perforation.
  - o Mesenteric infarction.
  - o Torsion of an intra-abdominal viscus.
  - o Retroperitoneal hematoma.
  - o Ectopic pregnancy.
  - o Macroamylasemia.
  - o Renal failure.
  - o Salivary gland inflammation.

[5] Insulinoma. *Dec 12*

- It is the **most common type of pancreatic neuro-endocrine tumour**.
- **Definition:** It is an insulin producing tumour of the pancreas.

Aetiology

- Unknown.

Pathology

- Equally scattered throughout the pancreas.
- Tumours are graded according to the WHO-NET criteria.

Grade	Mitoses/10 High Power Fields	Ki-67 Index
I	< 2	< 3
II	2-20	3-20
III (well differentiated with high proliferative index)	> 20	> 20
NEC (poorly differentiated neuro-endocrine carcinoma)	> 20	> 20

- Tumours < 2 cm without signs of invasion are considered benign.
- > 90% are both benign and solitary.
- 10% are associated with MEN 1.

Clinical Features

- Have been diagnosed in all age groups (highest 30-60 years).
- F > M.
- **Whipple's triad:**
  1. Symptoms induced by fasting.
  2. There is hypoglycemia at the time of symptoms (< 45 mg/dl).
  3. Symptoms are relieved by the administration of glucose.
- Patients typically develop sporadic symptoms of neuroglycopenia, i.e., shortage of glucose in the brain resulting in neuronal dysfunction and death if left untreated.
  - o Classically, these manifest while fasting or during exercise.
  - o Some may develop symptoms postprandially.
  - o Some patients develop loss of consciousness and coma.
- The release of catecholamines produces symptoms such as sweating, weakness, hunger, tremor, nausea, anxiety and palpitations.
- Sometimes, patients may have been investigated for epilepsy or drug abuse, before the correct diagnosis is established.
- Weight gain.

Diagnosis

1. **72-hour monitored fast**
   - Gold standard.
   - Looks for documented endogenous hyperinsulinism in association with symptoms and signs of low plasma glucose (< 54 mg/dl) and high C-peptide.
2. **Prolonged oral glucose tolerance test**
   - Is done if the 72-hour monitored fast test is negative and the suspicion of insulinoma is high.

3. **CT or MRI**
    - Performed after a positive fast test.
    - In the majority of cases, insulinomas are visualized.
4. **Endoscopic ultrasound**
    - Done if insulinoma is not visualized.
    - Has a very high positive detection rate.
5. **Visceral angiography with arterial stimulation venous sampling**
    - Reserved for negative EUS studies or when more than one lesion has been identified.
6. **Scintigraphy with radiolabeled glucagon-like peptide 1.**

Treatment

A. **Surgery**
- Laparoscopic enucleation of the tumour is the treatment of choice as most insulinomas are small, sporadic and solitary.
- **Contraindications to enucleation:**
    - o Close proximity to the main pancreatic duct.
    - o Larger tumours.
- Post-op blood sugar levels begin to rise in most patients within the first few hours after removal of the tumour.

B. **Medical**
- All patients undergoing surgery should be treated with **diazoxide**, which suppresses insulin secretion by direct action on the beta cells.
- Patients are given frequent small meals to avoid hypoglycemia.
- For patients with unresectable or metastatic disease, **SomatoStatin Analogues (SSA) and everolimus** are effective in controlling hypoglycemia.

B. **Other Options:**
- Chemotherapy.
- Peptide receptor radionuclide therapy (PRRT).
- Chemoembolization.

[3] Inverted 3 sign. *Dec 17*

- Frostberg inverted 3 sign is a radiological sign seen on barium meal.
- There is effacement and distortion of the mucosal pattern on the medial wall of D2 (second part of duodenum) due to focal mass and local edema.

Causes

1. Carcinoma of the head of the pancreas is most common.
2. Duodenal carcinoma.
3. Pancreatitis.

OTHER IMPORTANT TOPICS

ACUTE NECROTIZING PANCREATITIS

- Also known as pancreatic necrosis.
- **Definition:** It is the presence of nonviable pancreatic parenchyma or peripancreatic fat and can manifest as a focal area or diffuse involvement of the gland.

Pathogenesis

- Pancreatic necrosis is typically associated with lysis of peripancreatic fat. This may lead to an ***acute necrotic collection*** **(ANC).**
- This is typically an intra- or extra-pancreatic collection containing fluid and necrotic material, with no definable wall.
- Gradually, **over a period of over 4 weeks**, this may develop a well-defined inflammatory capsule and evolve into ***walled-of necrosis*** **(WON).**
- Collections associated with necrotising pancreatitis are sterile to begin with but often **become subsequently infected**, probably because of **translocation of gut bacteria (*Escherichia coli, Klebsiella, Enterococcus*).**
- The **risk** is directly related to the **amount of necrosis.**
- Infected necrosis is associated with a mortality rate of up to 50%.

Clinical Features

- Acute necrotic collection occurs in a background of acute pancreatitis.
- The main complication of acute necrotic collection is infection.
- Infected necrotic collection should be suspected in patients with prolonged fever, elevated white blood cell count, or progressive clinical deterioration.

- It should also be suspected if the patient develops sepsis, SIRS, and/or organ failure later in the course of the disease (>7 days after the onset of acute pancreatitis).

Investigations

1. **CT with IV contrast**
   - Absence of parenchymal enhancement or low attenuation.
   - Evidence of air within the pancreatic necrosis.
2. **Aspiration of fluid**
   - Done percutaneously with a fine needle, under CT or USG guidance.
   - Used to determine if it has become infected or not.
   - Purulent aspirate means that it is infected.
   - Aspirate should be sent for microbiological assessment and C/S.

Treatment

A. Sterile Necrotic Material

- Conservative management.
- Should not be drained or interfered with, as it resolves on its own.

B. Infected Fluid

- If it is infected, it should be drained.
  - **a. Internal drainage**
    - o Internal drainage into the stomach under endoscopic ultrasound guidance should be considered first.
    - o A plastic or covered metal stent can be used to create a communication between the collection and the gastric lumen.
    - o The stent may be left in situ for weeks if necessary, and may need to be changed if blocked.
  - **b. Percutaneous drainage**
    - o Should be considered if internal drainage is not possible.
    - o The tube drain inserted should have the *widest* bore possible.
    - o Antibiotics as per C/S report.
    - o The fluid can be quite viscous with particulate matter, and the drain may need regular flushing with full aseptic precautions.
  - **c. Pancreatic necrosectomy**
    - o Should be considered if sepsis worsens despite conservative measures.
    - o Challenging operation with high morbidity and mortality.
    - o Laparoscopic approach can be considered if expertise is available.
    - o Thorough debridement of the dead tissue around the pancreas is carried out.
    - o A feeding jejunostomy may be a useful adjunct to the procedure.
    - o If gallstones are the precipitating factor of the pancreatitis, a cholecystectomy should be included.
    - o Once a necrosectomy has been completed, further necrotic tissue may form. There are several possible ways of dealing with this:
      1. **Closed continuous lavage.**
      2. **Closed drainage.**
      3. **Open packing.**
      4. **Closure and relaparotomy.**

C. Supportive Management

- ICU care.
- **IV antibiotics:** Carbapenems are the drugs of choice.
- **Nutritional support is essential:** Parenteral and nasojejunal approaches are more popular than nasogastric feeding.

AUTOIMMUNE PANCREATITIS

- Autoimmune pancreatitis has been described relatively recently.
- **Features include:**
  - o Diffuse enlargement of the pancreas.
  - o Diffuse and irregular narrowing of the main pancreatic duct.
- It may occur in association with other autoimmune diseases, as a multisystem disorder, or may affect the pancreas alone.

- There may be changes in the biliary tree (autoimmune cholangiopathy) as well, which may be confused with neoplasia.
- Autoantibodies may be present and levels of the immunoglobulin subtype IgG4 are elevated.
- Steroids can be given as treatment.

TROPICAL PANCREATITIS

- It is a form of idiopathic pancreatitis.
- Has been described in resource-poor countries in Asia, Africa and Central America.
- **Possible mechanisms:**
  - o Malnutrition.
  - o Ingestion of cyanogenic glycosides in cassava.
  - o Exposure to hydrocarbons released by kerosene or paraffin lamps.
- Begins at a young age.
- Associated with a high incidence of diabetes mellitus and stone formation.

REVERSE FIGURE 3 SIGN

- Also called E sign.
- Seen on barium swallows.
- **Cause:** Coarctation of the aorta.
- It is formed by prestenotic dilatation of the ascending aorta, indentation of the coarctation site (or, 'tuck') and post-stenotic dilatation of the descending aorta.

35

Spleen

[5] Functions of spleen. *Dec 18*

The spleen has the following functions:

1. **Immune function**
   - The spleen contains:
     - o 70% of total T-lymphocytes.
     - o 10-15% of total B-lymphocytes.
   - Processes foreign antigens.
   - It is the major site for the specific IgM production.
   - **Synthesises non-specific opsonins:** Properdin and tuftsin (these bind to the specific receptors on the surface of macrophages and leukocytes, stimulating their phagocytic, bactericidal and tumoricidal activity).
2. **Filter function**
   - Spleen removes old platelets and RBCs. This process takes place in the sinuses and the splenic cords.
   - The red pulp of the spleen removes bacteria and in particular, pneumococci.
3. **Reservoir function**
   - Spleen contains 8% of the red cell mass.
   - An enlarged spleen may contain a much larger proportion of the blood volume.
   - Massive splenic enlargement will be associated with a larger proportion of blood volume in the spleen, leading to pancytopenia, which can be corrected by splenectomy.
4. **Cytopoiesis, i.e., hematopoietic function**
   - From the 4th month of intrauterine life, some degree of hematopoiesis occurs in the fetal spleen.
   - Stimulation of the white pulp may occur following antigenic challenge.
   - This results in the proliferation of T and B cells and macrophages.
5. **Pitting**
   - Particulate inclusions within RBCs such as Howell Jolly and Heinz bodies are removed and the repaired RBCs are returned to the circulation. This process is called pitting.

[5] Hypersplenism. *June 17*

- Hypersplenism is an indefinite clinical syndrome that is characterized by:
  - o Splenic enlargement, i.e., **splenomegaly.**
  - o **Cytopenias:** Any combination of anemia, leukopenia, or thrombocytopenia.
  - o **Compensatory bone marrow hyperplasia.**
  - o **Improvement after splenectomy.**

Causes

- Portal hypertension.
- **Blood disorders:**
  - o Acute leukemia, chronic leukemia.
  - o Idiopathic thrombocytopenic purpura.

- Hereditary spherocytosis.
- Autoimmune hemolytic anemia.
- Thalassemia.
- Sickle cell disease.

- **Malignancies:**
  - Hodgkin's lymphoma.
  - Non-Hodgkin's lymphoma.
  - Other lymphomas.
- **Metabolic disorders:**
  - Gaucher's disease.
  - Felty syndrome.

Clinical Features

- **Splenomegaly, defined as weight of > 175 g:**
  - **Normal:** 90-150 g.
  - **Massive:** > 1 kg.
- **Mechanical symptoms:**
  - Pain.
  - Early satiety.
- **Cytopenias:**
  - **Anemia:** Requires frequent transfusions, which can lead to iron overload.
  - **Leucopenia:** Frequent infections.
  - **Thrombocytopenias:** Problems with coagulation, bleeding.

Treatment

- **Splenectomy:** Open or laparoscopic or robotic.
- When the spleen is the sole site of the disease or a major contributor to the underlying pathophysiology, splenectomy is performed with curative intent.
- In most conditions, it is performed for effective palliation of symptoms and complications in patients refractory to medical management.

[5] Rupture of spleen. *June 19*

Causes

- **Blunt direct injury** to LUQ of abdomen.
- **Iatrogenic injury:** During a surgical procedure, particularly in the LUQ, when adhesions are present.
- Occasionally, a fall without direct trauma to the trunk can rupture the spleen, especially if it is diseased or enlarged, e.g., infectious mononucleosis, malaria.

Clinical Features

Cases of ruptured spleen may be divided into 3 groups:

1. Patient **succumbs rapidly**, never recovering from the initial shock.
2. **Initial shock with recovery from shock:**
   - This is the **usual type** seen in surgical practice.
   - After the initial shock has passed off, there are signs which point to **intra-abdominal bleeding:**

     a. **General signs:**
     - General signs of internal hemorrhage are variable.
     - Increasing pallor, a rising pulse rate, sighing respiration and restlessness.

     b. **Local signs:**
     - Abdominal **guarding:** Most pronounced in left upper quadrant.
     - Local **bruising and tenderness** in left upper quadrant.
     - **Abdominal distension** is due to the irritative effect of the intraperitoneal blood which produces peritonism and ileus.
     - **Kehr sign:**
       - **Pain** referred to **left shoulder**.
       - **Hyperesthesia** may be present in this area.
       - Can often be demonstrated 15 minutes after elevation of the foot of the bed.
       - It is due to **blood in contact with** the undersurface of the **diaphragm**.
       - Pain is mediated through afferent fibres in the **phrenic nerve.**
     - **Ballance sign:**
       - There is a **dull note in both flanks**, but on the right side it can be made to shift, whereas on the left it is constant.
       - The interpretation is that there is blood in the peritoneal cavity, but the

blood in the neighbourhood of the lacerated spleen has coagulated.

- o **DRE:**
  - ♦ Tenderness and sometimes a soft swelling, due to blood or clot in the rectovesical pouch.

3. **The delayed type of case:**
   - After the initial signs have passed off, the symptoms of a serious intra-abdominal catastrophe are postponed for a variable period.
   - Cause of the **delayed hemorrhage** is local vasoconstriction with or without the formation of blood clot which seals the tear.
   - Causes of the hemorrhage are those of reactionary or secondary hemorrhage.

Investigations

- **CECT scan:**
  - o It is the most important investigation for assessment of abdominal trauma in a **hemodynamically stable** patient.

Treatment

- Vigorous resuscitation.
- **Hemodynamically unstable patient:**
  - o **Splenectomy should be performed for severe grades of injury** where control of bleeding takes precedence over measures to salvage the spleen.
- **Hemodynamically stable patients:**
  - o **Splenic angiography with embolization of actively bleeding vessels.**

[3] Splenic abscess. *Dec 19*

- It is an **unusual but potentially life-threatening illness** if not promptly identified and treated.

Causes

- May arise from an **infected splenic embolus.**
- Associated with typhoid and paratyphoid fever.
- Osteomyelitis.
- Otitis media.
- Puerperal sepsis.
- May be associated with pancreatic necrosis.
- Any intra-abdominal infection.

Clinical Features

- Symptoms are non-specific.
- Vague abdominal pain.
- Fever.
- Peritonitis (due to rupture of splenic abscess).
- Pleuritic chest pain.

Investigations

- CT is the preferred method for diagnosis.
- USG can also be used.

Treatment

- Treatment involves that of the underlying cause, and:
  1. **Percutaneous drainage** of the splenic abscess under radiologist guidance.
  2. **Splenectomy** is indicated when interventional radiology is not available.

[3] Mention indications for splenectomy. *Dec 12*

The common indications for splenectomy are:

A. Trauma

- Accidental.
- Iatrogenic, i.e., during a surgical procedure, e.g., during mobilisation of the esophagus, stomach, distal pancreas or splenic flexure of the colon.

B. Oncological

- Part of en bloc resection with the stomach as of a radical gastrectomy or, with the pancreas as part of a distal or total pancreatectomy.

C. Hematological

- To treat anemia or thrombocytopenia in:
  - o Hereditary spherocytosis.
- ITP or idiopathic thrombocytopenic purpura:
  - o Hypersplenism.

D. Portal Hypertension

- In association with shunt or variceal surgery for portal hypertension.

[5] Indications and complications of splenectomy. *Sept 21*

[5] Complications of splenectomy. *June 16*

[3] Enumerate complications of splenectomy. *CBME March 24*

The complications of splenectomy can be divided into:

A. Short-term Complications

- Hemorrhage.
- Left basal atelectasis.
- Pleural effusion.
- Gastric perforation, gastric fistula.
- Hematemesis.
- Gastric dilation.
- Pancreatitis.
- Localized pancreatic abscess.
- Pancreatic fistula.
- Post-op thrombocytosis.
- Increased risk of DVT and pulmonary embolism.

B. Long-term Complications

- OPSI or opportunist post splenectomy infection.
- Sepsis due to *Capnocytophaga canimorsus* may result from dog, cat or other animal bites.

[3] OPSI. *June 14*

- It stands for opportunist post splenectomy infection.
- It is the **most common fatal late complication** of splenectomy.

Cause

- It is caused by polysaccharide **encapsulated organisms:**
  1. *Streptococcus pneumoniae.*
  2. *Neisseria meningitidis.*
  3. *Hemophilus influenzae.*
- *Escherichia coli* can also cause post splenectomy septicaemia.

Patients Who Have Increased Risk of OPSI

1. Young patients.
2. Splenectomised patients treated with chemoradiotherapy.
3. Patients who have undergone splenectomy for thalassemia, sickle cell disease, autoimmune anemia, autoimmune thrombocytopenia, lymphoma.
4. Immunosuppression.

Clinical Features

- **May occur at any time after splenectomy:**
  - o Most infections occur > 2 years after splenectomy.
  - o The risk of overwhelming sepsis is greatest within the first 2-3 years after splenectomy.
- Usually **begins with flu like symptoms**: Fever, rigor, chills, sore throat, malaise, myalgias.
- Patient may also complain of diarrhea and vomiting.
- These symptoms **quickly progress to fulminant infection** with the development of hypotension, respiratory distress, DIC, coma, MODS and death.
- **Survivors often have multiple sequelae:**
  - o Peripheral gangrene requiring amputation.
  - o Deafness.
  - o Meningitis.
  - o Mastoid osteomyelitis.
  - o Bacterial endocarditis.
  - o Cardiac valvular destruction.

Prevention

A. Vaccination

- **Timing of vaccination:**
  - o **Elective splenectomy: The ideal time is 10-12 weeks before surgery *or* at least 14 days before surgery.**
  - o **Emergency splenectomy: Vaccines should be given 14 days after splenectomy or upon discharge, whichever comes first.**
- **Vaccines given are:**
  - o **Pneumococcus:** Repeated every 5 years.
  - o **Meningococcus C:** Repeated every 5 years.
  - o **Hemophilus influenza type B:** Repeated every 10 years.
- **Others:** Annual seasonal influenza, MMR, varicella, DPT.

B. Antibiotic Prophylaxis

- Benefit from the use of prophylactic antibiotics remains **controversial.**
- Depends on the age at which splenectomy was done:
  - i. **< 5 years:** Daily dose of penicillin until the age of 10 years.
  - ii. **> 5 years:** Daily dose of penicillin until the age of 16 years.
  - iii. **Adults:** Use of prophylactic antibiotics is less well defined.
- **Oral prophylaxis:** Penicillin, erythromycin, amoxicillin or co-amoxiclav.

C. Prompt Treatment of Symptoms

- Same antibiotics as used for prophylaxis.
- **If patient is allergic to penicillin and cephalosporins:** Chloramphenicol.

D. Patient Should Be Educated to Recognise Symptoms of Infection.

OTHER IMPORTANT TOPICS

IDIOPATHIC THROMBOCYTOPENIC PURPURA

- Also known as immune and autoimmune thrombocytopenic purpura.
- It is the most common hematologic indication for splenectomy.

Pathogenesis

- Characterized by a low platelet count (< 1,00,000/µL) despite normal bone marrow and the absence of other causes of thrombocytopenia.
- Results from autoantibodies to specific platelet membrane glycoproteins (antiplatelet IgG autoantibodies) that are responsible for platelet destruction within the reticuloendothelial system by macrophages and cytotoxic T cells.
- Also, there is dysfunction of megakaryocytes with low levels of thrombopoietin.
- There are two distinct clinical types:
  1. An acute condition in children.
  2. A chronic condition in adults.
- Acute ITP often follows an acute infection and usually resolves spontaneously.
- Chronic ITP persists longer than 6 months without a specific cause being identified.

Causes

- **Primary ITP:**
  - o There is no clear aetiology.
- **Secondary ITP:**
  - o Drug induced (heparin, quinine, sulphonamides).
  - o Infections (e.g., Hep C, HIV, Epstein-Barr virus).
  - o Rheumatologic conditions.

Clinical Features

- Adult form normally affects females between the ages of 15 and 50 years.
- Childhood form is distributed equally between males and females and commonly presents before the age of 5 years.
- Can be associated with other conditions:
  - o Systemic lupus erythematosus.
  - o Chronic lymphatic leukaemia.
  - o Hodgkin's disease.
- Purpuric patches (ecchymoses) occur on the skin and mucous membranes.
- Petechial hemorrhages in the skin following trauma or pressure.
- Spontaneous bleeding from mucous membranes (e.g., epistaxis).
- Menorrhagia in women.
- Prolonged bleeding of minor wounds.
- Hemorrhage from the urinary and gastrointestinal tracts and hemarthrosis are rare.
- Intracranial hemorrhage is also uncommon, but it is the most common cause of death.
- Presence of cutaneous ecchymoses and a positive tourniquet test.
- The spleen is palpable in < 10% of patients and gross splenic enlargement should raise suspicion of an alternative diagnosis.

Investigations

- Coagulation studies are normal and a bleeding time is not helpful in diagnosis.
- Platelet count in the peripheral blood film is reduced (usually <60 × 10^9/L).
- Bone marrow aspiration reveals plenty of platelet-producing megakaryocytes.

Treatment

- The course of the disease differs in children and adults.
- It usually regresses spontaneously in pediatric cases.

A. Medical Therapy

- Short courses of corticosteroids in both adults and children are usually followed by recovery.
- Steroid therapy should not be prolonged.

B. Surgery

- Splenectomy is usually recommended for refractory or relapsing ITP.
- 2/3rd of patients will be cured by surgical intervention and 15% will improve, but no benefit will be seen in the rest.
- The response to steroids predicts a good response to splenectomy if the disease relapses.
- Laparoscopic splenectomy is rapidly becoming the mainstay of treatment since the size of the spleen is usually normal or slightly enlarged and the spleen is not friable.
- It is important to identify and remove splenunculi as they have the potential to enlarge with time and lead to recurrence of symptoms.
- In the acute setting, blood transfusion or transfusion with platelets before surgery may be necessary, although these are generally withheld until the splenic vessels have been controlled.

SPLENUNCULI

- Splenunculi are single or multiple accessory spleens.
- Found in approximately 10–30% of the population.

Location

- Most common is near the hilum of the spleen.
- Gastrosplenic ligament.
- Tail of pancreas.
- Splenocolic ligament.
- Left transverse mesocolon.
- Greater omentum along the greater curvature of the stomach.
- Mesentery.
- Left mesocolon.
- Left ovary.
- Pouch of Douglas.
- Left testis.

Significance

- Failure to identify and remove these at the time of splenectomy may give rise to **persistent disease.**
- A **technetium 99m (99mTc)-labelled red blood cell scan** can be used to help localize accessory spleens if complete splenectomy is mandatory, e.g., immune thrombocytopenic purpura (ITP).

36

Abdominal Wall, Umbilicus and Hernia

[3] Classification of hernia. *Dec 15*

European Hernia Society (EHS) Classification for Groin Hernias

- The EHS classification is used to classify inguinal (and femoral) hernias.
- Primary or recurrent (P or R).
- Lateral, medial or femoral (L: Indirect, M: Direct, F: Femoral).
- Width or defect size in fingerbreadths (assumed to be 1.5 cm), with three sizes:
  - o $\leq$ 1 fingerbreadths ($\leq$ 1.5 cm).
  - o 2-3 fingerbreadths (1.5 – 4.5 cm).
  - o > 3 fingerbreadths (> 4.5 cm).
- A primary indirect inguinal hernia with a 3 cm defect size would be PL2.

Classification of Primary Abdominal Wall Hernias

A. Groin

- Inguinal:
  - o Indirect.
  - o Direct.
  - o Combined.
- Femoral.

B. Anterior

- Umbilical.
- Epigastric.
- Spigelian.

C. Pelvic

- Obturator.
- Sciatic.
- Perineal.

D. Posterior

- Lumbar:
  - o Superior triangle.
  - o Inferior triangle.

Types of Hernia by Complexity

- **Occult:** Not detectable clinically.
- **Reducible:** A swelling that appears and disappears.
- **Irreducible:** A swelling that cannot be replaced in the abdomen and is at risk of complications.
- **Incarcerated:** Irreducible, trapped, risk of strangulation.
- **Strangulated:** Acutely painful swelling with tissue ischemia; requires emergency surgery.
- **Obstruction:** Contents of the hernia (usually bowel) are in obstruction, i.e., no peristalsis is happening.

INGUINAL HERNIA

[10] Discuss aetiopathology, management and complications of inguinal hernia in a 60 year old male. *Dec 16*

[10] Discuss clinical features and management of indirect inguinal hernia. ***July 23***

[5] Inguinal hernia. ***August 22***

[5] Write clinical features and management of inguinal hernia. ***CBME March 24***

[5] Differential diagnosis of groin swelling. ***March 24***

[3] Complications of inguinal hernia. ***March 21, Dec 18, Dec 17, June 17, July 15***

[3] Complications of hernia. ***June 16***

[MCQ] Surgery for inguinal hernia includes all except: ***CBME March 24***

A. Lichtenstein repair
B. Stoppa repair
C. Desarda repair
D. Mc Evedy repair*

- Inguinal hernia is the most common hernia.
- **Most common hernia in males:** Inguinal hernia.
- **Most common hernia in females:** Inguinal hernia.

Surgical Anatomy

- **Superficial inguinal ring:** Triangular aperture in the aponeurosis of the external oblique, and lies 1.25 cm above and lateral to the pubic tubercle. It is bound by a superomedial and an inferolateral crus joined by criss-cross intercrural fibres.
- **Deep inguinal ring:** U-shaped opening in the transversalis fascia 1.25 cm above the midpoint of the inguinal ligament. The transversalis fascia is the fascial envelope of the abdomen and the competency of the DIR depends upon the integrity of this fascia.
- **Inguinal canal:**
  - o 3.75 cm long.
  - o Oblique, directed downwards and medially from the deep to the superficial inguinal ring.
  - o **Boundaries of inguinal canal:**
    - ♦ Anterior: External oblique aponeurosis.
    - ♦ Posterior: Fascia transversalis.
    - ♦ Roof/superiorly: Conjoint tendon.
    - ♦ Floor/inferiorly: Inguinal ligament.

Types of Inguinal Hernia

There are 2 broad types – Direct and Indirect.

A. Indirect Inguinal Hernia (Lateral)

- Enters the inguinal canal via the DIR, travels down the canal on the outer side of the spermatic cord (lateral and anterior), and may or may not enter the scrotum.

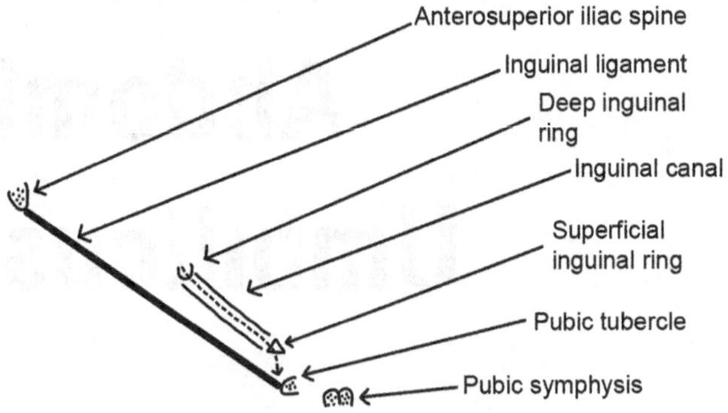

Figure 1: Pathway of indirect inguinal hernia

- There are **3 types** of indirect inguinal hernia:
  1. **Bubonocele:** Hernia is limited to the inguinal canal.
  2. **Funicular:** Hernia lies just above the epididymis. The contents of the sac can be felt separately from the testis, which lies below the hernia.
  3. **Complete (scrotal):** Hernia descends the full length of the scrotum. The testis appears to lie within the lower part of the hernia.

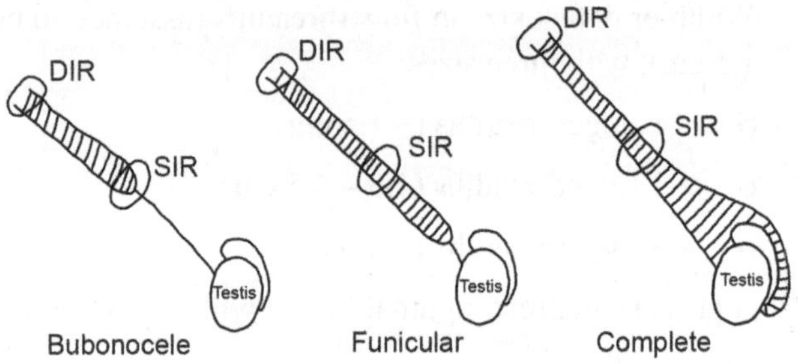

Figure 2: Types of indirect inguinal hernia

B. Direct Inguinal Hernia (Medial)

- Comes out directly through the posterior wall of the inguinal canal.
- The area it comes out through is called the **Hesselbach's triangle**. Its boundaries are:
  - o **Laterally:** Inferior epigastric vessels.
  - o **Medially:** Lateral edge of rectus abdominis muscle.
  - o **Below:** Inguinal ligament (iliopubic tract).

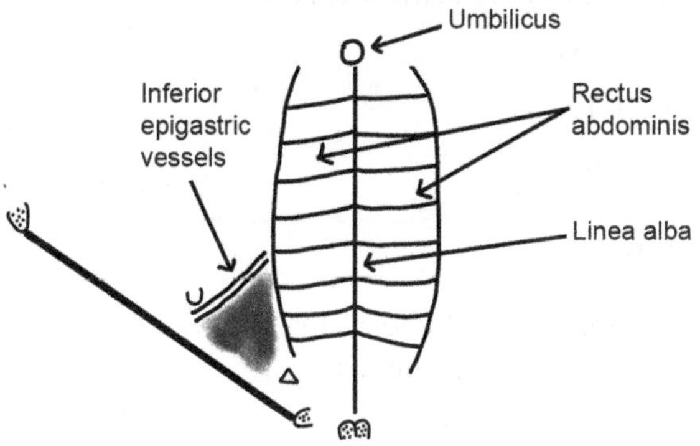

Figure 3: Hesselbach's triangle (shaded)

Aetiology

1. **Anatomical weakness:**
   - Areas of natural weakness due to absence of muscle.
   - Natural defects that allow structures to enter or leave the abdomen.
   - Injury, e.g., surgical scar, trauma.
2. **Developmental failures:**
   - Failure of normal development may lead to congenital hernias, e.g., indirect inguinal hernia arising through failure of processus vaginalis to close.
3. The risk of inguinal hernia is related to the anatomical shape of the pelvis and is **greater in patients with a wider and shorter pelvis.**
4. **Weakness of collagen:**
   - Genetic.
   - Smoking.
5. **Weakness due to ageing and pregnancy.**
6. **Primary neurological and muscle disease.**
7. **Increased intra-abdominal pressure:** Lifting heavy weights, obesity, chronic cough (COPD), constipation, BPH.

Composition of a Hernia

A hernia consists of 3 parts:

1. **Sac:**
   - Diverticulum of peritoneum consisting of mouth, neck, body and fundus.
   - Diameter of neck is important, because narrow neck predisposes to strangulation.
2. **Coverings of sac:**
   - Derived from the layers of the abdominal wall through which the sac passes.
3. **Contents of sac:**
   - Fluid, omentum and intestine.

Clinical Features

- M > F.
- Complains of **pain in the groin** or pain referred to the testicle when he is performing heavy work or on strenuous exercise.
- **Swelling in the region of the groin** in large hernias:
  - o There is a sensation of weight.
  - o Dragging on the mesentery may produce epigastric pain.

On Examination

- **Cough impulse:** Is both seen on inspection and felt during palpation.
- Neck of indirect hernia is lateral to inferior epigastric vessels.
- Direct hernia is medial to inferior epigastric vessels.
- **Saddle bag or pantaloon type:** Has both direct and indirect components.
- Neck of inguinal hernia is above and medial to the pubic tubercle.
- Digital control of internal ring helps in distinguishing between an indirect and a direct inguinal hernia.

Complications of Inguinal Hernia

1. **Irreducible hernia:**
   - When the **contents cannot be returned to the abdomen** and there is no evidence of other complications.
   - It is brought about by adhesions between the sac and its contents or from overcrowding within the sac.
   - Any degree of **irreducibility predisposes to strangulation.**
2. **Obstructed hernia:**
   - This is an irreducible hernia **containing intestine which is obstructed from within or from**

without; but there is no interference to the blood supply to the bowel.

- Symptoms are less severe and the onset more gradual than in strangulation.
- Often, the **obstruction culminates in strangulation.**

3. **Strangulated hernia:**
   - A hernia becomes strangulated when the **blood supply of its contents is seriously impaired**, rendering gangrene imminent.
   - Gangrene may occur as early as 5-6 hours after the onset of the first symptoms of strangulation.
4. **Incarcerated hernia:**
   - Irreducible, trapped and at risk for strangulation.
5. **Perforation of hernia contents.**
6. **Peritonitis.**

Differential Diagnosis of Inguinal Hernia/Groin Swelling

- **Males:**
  - o Vaginal hydrocele.
  - o Encysted hydrocele of the cord.
  - o Spermatocele.
  - o Incompletely descended testis in the inguinal canal.
  - o Lipoma of the cord.
- **Females:**
  - o Hydrocele of the canal of Nuck.
- **Common to both:**
  - o Femoral hernia.
  - o Enlarged inguinal lymph nodes.
  - o Saphena varix.
  - o Femoral artery aneurysm.
  - o Psoas abscess.
  - o Rupture of adductor longus with hematoma.

Investigations

- Inguinal hernia is a clinical diagnosis.
- **In case of diagnostic difficulties:**
  - o USG.
  - o CT scan.
  - o MRI.

Treatment

- The treatment of choice for uncomplicated inguinal hernia is **mesh hernioplasty.**
- **Indications of surgery:**
  - o It is **recommended to perform surgery when the patient presents with hernia**. This is because the hernia might become complicated in future.
- **Indications of conservative management:**
  - o It is safe to recommend no active treatment in cases of early asymptomatic direct hernia, particularly in **elderly patients** who do not wish for surgical intervention.
  - o But the patient should be warned to seek early advice if the hernia increases in size or becomes symptomatic.
- Irrespective of the approach, the **principle of hernia surgery** remains the same:
  - o **Reduction of contents.**
  - o **Closure of the fascial defect.**
  - o **Strengthening of the closure with mesh.**

The options for inguinal hernia surgery are:

A. **Open Approach**

   a. **Herniotomy**
      - Indicated in children who have indirect inguinal hernia.
      - The sac is excised and closed.

   b. **Open suture repair**
      - Bassini.
      - Shouldice.
      - Desarda.
      - Maloney darn.

   c. **Open flat mesh repair**
      - Lichtenstein's tension free mesh hernioplasty.
      - This is the operation of choice for inguinal hernias.

   d. **Open complex mesh repair**
      - It is not recommended any more.

- **Methods:**
  1. Mesh plugs.
  2. Hernia systems.

e. **Open preperitoneal repair**
  1. Indicated for bilateral hernias.
  2. Stoppa Rives repair.

B. Laparoscopic/Robot Assisted Repair

- **Indications:**
  1. Recurrence after open approach.
  2. Bilateral hernias.
  3. Any hernia in a female.
- **Laparoscopic surgical options**
  1. TEP or Total Extra Peritoneal.
  2. TAPP or Trans Abdominal Pre Peritoneal.

STRANGULATED INGUINAL HERNIA

[10] Discuss complications of inguinal hernia. Add a note on diagnosis and treatment of strangulated inguinal hernia. ***Dec 14***

[5] Strangulated inguinal hernia. ***Dec 12***

- **Definition:** A hernia becomes strangulated when the **blood supply of its contents is seriously impaired, rendering gangrene imminent**.
- **A femoral hernia is more likely to strangulate** because of the narrowness of the neck of the sac and its rigid walls.

Pathology

- The intestine is obstructed + blood supply is constricted.

At first, only venous return is impeded
↓
Wall of intestine becomes congested and bright red
↓
Congestion further increases
↓
Intestine becomes purple in colour
↓

Contd.

Intestinal pressure increases
↓
Strangulated loop becomes distended, often to twice its diameter
↓
Arterial supply becomes more and more impaired
↓
Walls of intestine lose their tone
↓
Intestine becomes flabby and friable
↓
1. Migration of bacteria through intestinal wall
2. Intestine becomes gangrenous
3. Mesentery involved by strangulation also becomes gangrenous
↓
Perforation of wall of intestine
↓
Peritonitis

- **Constricting agent:**
  - o Neck of the sac.
  - o Superficial inguinal ring.
  - o Adhesions within the sac.
- **Contents: Usually small intestine is involved in the strangulation**. The next frequent content to be strangulated is omentum. Sometimes, both are strangulated.

Clinical Features

- Femoral hernia > inguinal hernia (indirect > direct).
- **Sudden pain:**
  - o **At first situated over the hernia.**
  - o Followed by generalized abdominal pain.
  - o Pain is paroxysmal in character.
- Frequent episodes of **vomiting.**
- Patient may say that the **hernia has recently become larger.**
- History of hernia becoming irreducible.

On Examination

- Hernia is tense.
- Extremely tender.
- Irreducible.
- No expansile impulse on coughing.
- Unless the strangulation is relieved by operation, the paroxysms of pain continue until peristaltic contractions cease with the onset of **gangrene** when paralytic ileus (often the result of **peritonitis**) and **endotoxic shock** develop.

Investigations

- Strangulated hernia is a clinical diagnosis and does not require any investigations.
- If there is any doubt about diagnosis:
  - o USG.
  - o CT scan.
  - o MRI.

Treatment

- **Time is critical** in the presence of ischemic bowel.
- Principles of surgery are the same as in an elective setting.
- Open or laparoscopic surgery is possible (Hernia repair ± mesh).
- Mesh is generally not recommended.
- However, unless there is significant infection/ contamination, use of synthetic mesh is acceptable as long as the operation is covered by appropriate antibiotics.
- Some patients (20%) may require bowel resection which necessitates conversion to a midline laparotomy.
- If bowel looks ischemic, it should be wrapped in a warm saline mop and observed for viability after few minutes.

SLIDING INGUINAL HERNIA

[5] Sliding inguinal hernia. *March 22*

- Also known as Hernia-en-glissade.
- **Definition:** A sliding hernia is a hernia where the posterior wall of the **sac** is not **formed** of peritoneum alone, but by the **sigmoid colon and its mesentery in the left, the caecum on the right and, sometimes, on either side by a portion of the bladder.**

Aetiology

- **Same as inguinal hernia:**
  - o Anatomical weakness.
  - o Developmental failures.
  - o Genetic weakness of collagen.
  - o Sharp and blunt trauma.
  - o Weakness due to ageing and pregnancy.
  - o Primary neurological and muscle diseases.

Pathology

- Sliding hernia **occurs as a result of slipping of the posterior parietal peritoneum on the underlying retroperitoneal structures.**

Clinical Features

- Occurs almost exclusively in males.
- Left > right.
- Bilateral sliding hernias are very rare.
- **Age:** Almost always > 40 years, incidence increases with age.
- There are no clinical findings that are pathognomonic of a sliding hernia, but it **should be suspected in every large globular inguinal hernia descending well into the scrotum.**
- **Left side:** Contains sigmoid colon and its mesentery.
- **Right side:** Caecum.
- Urinary bladder may be present on the left or right.
- It is an intra-op diagnosis.

Investigations

- USG.
- CT scan.
- MRI.

Treatment

- The primary danger associated with a sliding hernia is the failure to recognize the visceral component of the hernia sac. This increases chances of intra-op injury to the bowel or bladder.
- To **prevent injury to the urinary bladder**, if any hernia is suspected to be a sliding hernia pre-

operatively, it should be catheterized using a **Foley's catheter**.

- The sliding hernia contents are reduced into the peritoneal cavity, and any excess hernia sac is ligated and divided.
- After reduction of the hernia, any of the techniques which are used for an inguinal hernia can be applied.
- The treatment of choice for an uncomplicated sliding hernia is **Lichtenstein's tension free mesh hernioplasty**.

FEMORAL HERNIA

[10] Enumerate groin hernia. Write about management of femoral hernia. ***Oct 20***

[5] Femoral hernia. ***June 19, July 18, July 23***

[3] Boundaries of femoral canal. ***June 16***

- A femoral hernia occurs through the femoral canal.
- It is important, because of all hernias it is the **most liable to become strangulated due to the narrowness of the neck of the sac and the rigidity of the femoral ring.**
- It is less common than inguinal hernia.

Surgical Anatomy of the Femoral Canal

- The femoral canal occupies the most medial compartment of the femoral sheath.
- It extends from the femoral ring above to the saphenous opening below.
- **Contents:**
  - o Fat.
  - o Lymphatic vessels.
  - o Lymph node of Cloquet.
- **Boundaries:**
  - o **Anteriorly:** Inguinal ligament.
  - o **Posteriorly:** Astley Cooper's iliopectineal ligament, the pubic bone and the fascia over the pectineus muscle.
  - o **Medially:** By the concave knife-like edge of Gimbernat's lacunar ligament. This is a strong curved ligament with a sharp unyielding edge that impedes reduction of a femoral hernia.
  - o **Laterally:** By a thin septum separating it from the femoral vein.
  - o It is closed above by the septum crurale which is a condensation of extraperitoneal tissue and below by the cribriform fascia.

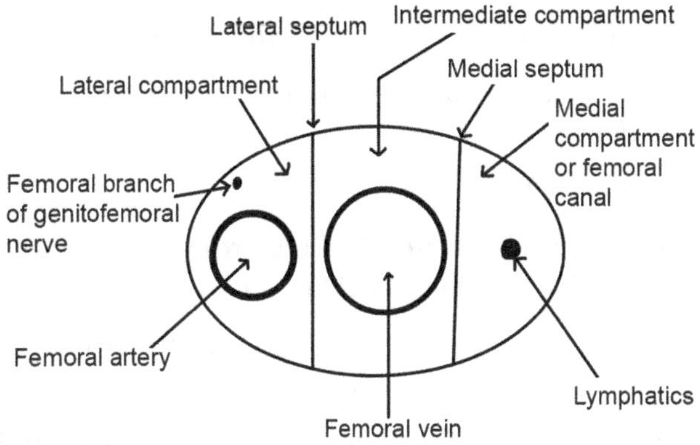

Figure 4: Cross-section of femoral sheath

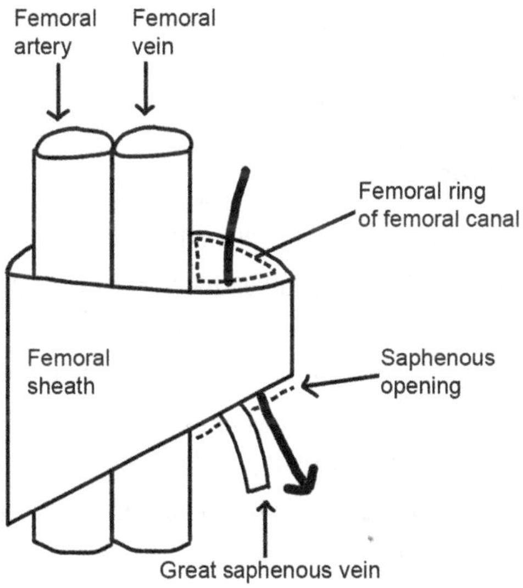

Figure 5: Pathway of femoral hernia

Aetiology

- The **female pelvis has a different shape** from the male, **increasing the size of the femoral canal and the risk of hernia**.
- In old age, the femoral defect enlarges further.
- Femoral hernia is therefore commonly seen in thin, elderly women:
  - o Anatomical weakness.
  - o Developmental failures.
  - o Genetic weakness of collagen.

- o Sharp and blunt trauma.
- o Weakness due to ageing and pregnancy.
- o Primary neurological and muscle diseases.

Clinical Features

- Femoral hernia are **more common in women**.
- It is rare before puberty and the **incidence increases with age**.
- Right > left.
- **Symptoms of a femoral hernia are less pronounced than those of an inguinal hernia.**
- A small femoral hernia may be unnoticed or ignored for years, until perhaps the day it strangulates.
- **Has a high tendency to become irreducible and strangulate**. 50% present as an emergency with very high risk of strangulation.
- Adherence of greater omentum sometimes causes a **dragging pain**.
- Rarely, a large sac is present.

On Examination

- Below and lateral to the pubic tubercle.
- Lies in the **upper leg** rather than in the lower abdomen.
- Inadequate exposure of this area during routine examination leads to failure to detect the hernia.
- Hernia often **rapidly becomes irreducible** and loses any cough impulse owing to the tightness of the neck.
- May only be 1-2 cm in size and can easily be mistaken for a lymph node.
- As it increases in size, it is reflected superiorly and becomes difficult to distinguish from a direct inguinal hernia.

Differential Diagnosis

- Inguinal hernia.
- Lymph node.
- Saphena varix.
- Femoral artery aneurysm.
- Psoas abscess.
- Rupture of adductor longus with hematoma.

Investigations

- In routine cases, no specific investigations are required.
- In cases of uncertainty:
  - o USG.
  - o CT scan.
  - o X-ray shows bowel obstruction in patients coming to the emergency (in complicated hernia).
- All patients with unexplained small bowel obstruction should undergo careful examination for a femoral hernia.

Treatment

- There is no alternative to surgery for femoral hernia.
- These cases should be treated with urgency.
- There are various options:

1. **Lockwood's low approach**
   - o Simplest operation.
   - o Suitable only when there is no risk of bowel resection.
   - o Transverse incision is made over the hernia.
   - o Some surgeons place a mesh plug into the hernia defect for further reinforcement.
2. **Lotheissen's inguinal approach**
   - o Initial incision is identical to that of inguinal hernioplasty.
   - o Flat mesh may be placed over the defect in the extraperitoneal plane.
3. **Mc Evedy's high approach**
   - o Complex operation.
   - o Ideal in the emergency situation where the risk of bowel strangulation is high.
   - o Transverse incision just above the inguinal canal, centered on the lateral border of the rectus muscle.
4. **Laparoscopic approaches**
   - o TAPP (Trans Abdominal Pre Peritoneal).
   - o TEP (Total Extra Peritoneal).
   - o Ideal for reducible femoral hernias presenting electively.

- o Laparoscopic approach is recommended in women.

INCISIONAL HERNIA

[3] Incisional hernia. *Oct 20*

- **Definition:** Incisional hernia is a hernia which **arises through a defect in the musculofascial layers of the abdominal wall at the site of a post-operative scar.** Therefore, they may appear anywhere where a laparotomy has been made.

Incidence

Laparotomy incisions >>> laparoscopic port site incisions.

Aetiology

Factors predisposing to an incisional hernia are as follows:

A. Patient Factors

- Genetic collagen disorders.
- Obesity.
- General poor healing due to malnutrition, immune suppression or steroid therapy.
- Chronic cough.
- Cancer.

B. Wound Factors

- Poor quality tissues.
- Wound tension.
- Wound infection.

C. Surgical Factors

- Inappropriate suture material.
- Poor closure technique.

Clinical Features

- Commonly appear as a **localized swelling involving part of a surgical scar** but may present as a diffuse bulging of the whole length of the incision.
- There may also be several discrete hernias along the length of the incision.
- Even with apparently singular hernias, unsuspected defects are frequently found at operation.
- Tend to increase steadily in size with time.
- Overlying skin may become thin and atrophic.
- Local trauma and microvascular damage to skin may lead to ulceration.
- **Episodes of intestinal obstruction** are common because there are usually coexisting internal adhesions.
- **Strangulation is less frequent** because most incisional hernias are shallow and wide necked.
- As with any hernia type, strangulation is most likely when the fibrous defect is small and the sac is large.

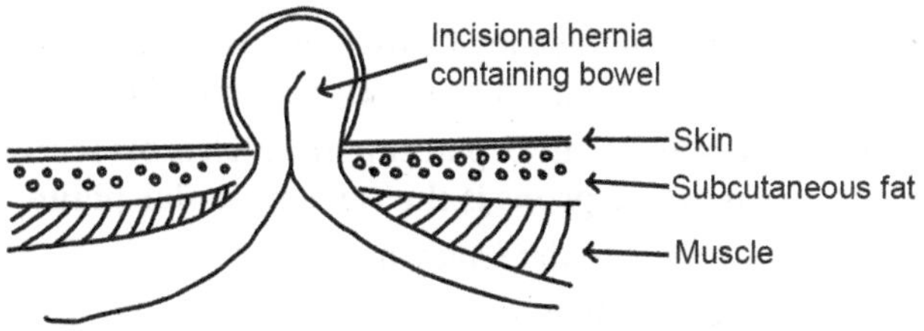

Figure 6: Incisional hernia

Investigations

- Incisional hernia is a clinical diagnosis and does not usually require any investigations.
- In case of uncertainty, complications or to plan surgery, the following are done:
  - o USG.
  - o CT scan.
  - o MRI.

Treatment

- Asymptomatic patients may not require treatment.
- Abdominal binder/belt often provides symptomatic relief and may prevent the hernia from increasing in size.
- Many patients with an incisional hernia have other comorbidities and discussion around the balance of benefits and risks of surgery is important.
- Patients should be optimized/prehabilitated before surgery:
  - o Weight loss if patient is obese.
  - o Stop smoking.
  - o Fitness improvement.
  - o Core strength exercising.

Surgical Options

- Irrespective of the technique used, the principles of surgery are the same:
  1. The repair should cover the whole length of the previous incision.
  2. Approximation of the musculofascial layers should be done with minimal tension.
  3. Prosthetic mesh should be used to reduce the risk of recurrence. **Mesh is contraindicated in a contaminated field.**

A. Open Repair
  - Mesh should ideally be used unless there is gross contamination, where mesh is contraindicated.
  - **The plane of mesh placement which is preferred by most surgeons is the retromuscular plane.**
  - **Simplest repair:** Onlay mesh.

B. Laparoscopic Repair
  - IPOM or intraperitoneal onlay mesh is most commonly used.

Features Which Can Prevent Incisional Hernias

- Ensuring healthy wound edges.
- Minimal wound tension.
- Good surgical technique.
- Small-stitch, small-bite technique.
- Optimal ratio of suture length to wound length is 4:1 (Jenkin's rule).

UMBILICAL HERNIA

[5] Umbilical hernia. ***June 16, July 15***

[3] Surgical management of umbilical hernia. ***CBME June 24***

- **Definition**: Any hernia in the immediate vicinity of the umbilicus is called an umbilical hernia.

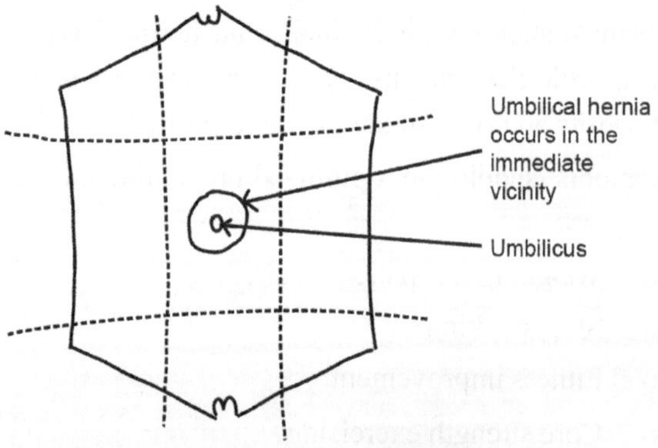

Figure 7: Umbilical hernia

Surgical Anatomy

- The umbilical defect is present at birth, but closes as the stump of the umbilical cord heals, usually within a week of birth.
- This process may be delayed, leading to the development of herniation in the neonatal period.
- The **umbilical ring may also stretch and reopen in adult life.**
- In adults, the **defects** can be not only through the umbilicus but also in the **median raphe (linea alba)** immediately adjacent to the true umbilicus, (**supraumbilical > infraumbilical**). These were earlier called paraumbilical hernias.
- However, under current guidelines, any hernia in the immediate vicinity of the umbilicus can now be called umbilical.

Aetiology

- Conditions that cause **stretching and thinning of the midline raphe (linea alba)**, predispose to reopening of the umbilical defect.
- Pregnancy.
- Obesity.
- Liver disease with cirrhosis and ascites.

Clinical Features

- It is commonly seen in:
  - o **Overweight men** with a thinned and attenuated midline raphe.
  - o **Postpartum women** with a weakened abdominal wall.
- F > M.
- Complains of pain due to tissue tension or symptoms of intermittent bowel obstruction.
- In large hernias:
  - o Overlying skin may become very thin.
  - o Overlying skin irritation and ulceration may be seen.
- Contents:
  - o Small umbilical hernias – extraperitoneal fat or omentum.
  - o Large hernias – small or large bowel.

- **Because the hernia neck is relatively narrow in relation to the size of the sac, they are prone to become irreducible, obstructed and strangulated.**

On Examination

- The bulge of the hernia is typically slightly to one side of the umbilical depression, creating a **crescent shaped appearance of the umbilicus**.

Investigations

- It is a clinical diagnosis.
- In the presence of uncertainty/complications:
    - o USG.
    - o CT scan.
    - o MRI.

Treatment

- As a result of the high risk of strangulation, surgery should be advised in cases where the hernia contains bowel.
- Small hernias may be left alone if they are asymptomatic, but they may enlarge and require surgery at a later date.
- Surgery may be performed via open technique or laparoscopically.

A. Open Umbilical Hernia Repair

- The choice of surgery depends on defect size:
    - a. Defect < 1 cm.
        - o Simple suture repair.
        - o Darn suture.
    - b. Defect 1-2 cm.
        - o Mayo's waistcoat over trousers repair.
    - c. Defect > 2 cm.
        - o Mesh hernioplasty.
        - o Mesh can be placed onlay, inlay or sublay.

B. Laparoscopic Approach

- IPOM or Intraperitoneal Onlay Mesh.

OTHER HERNIA

[3] Richter's hernia. *Dec 19*

- It is a rare variety of groin hernia.
- **Definition:** A Richter's hernia is one where **only a portion of the circumference of the bowel wall enters the hernia**.
- It is an intra-op finding/diagnosis.

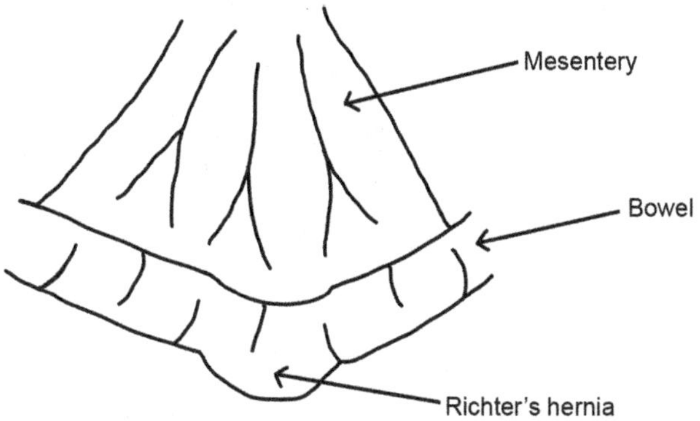

Figure 8: Richter's hernia

Clinical Features

- It may be small.
- May be difficult or even impossible to detect clinically.
- Has **high risk of strangulation.**
- Bowel obstruction may or may not be present.
- Bowel wall may become necrotic and perforate, with life threatening peritonitis.
- Femoral hernia may present in this way, often with diagnostic delay and high risk to the patient.

Treatment

- Hernioplasty (if there is no risk of infection).
- Herniorrhaphy (if there is risk of infection).
- Resection and anastomosis (if bowel is not viable).

[3] Maydl's hernia. *Dec 18*

- Also known as hernia-en-W or retrograde strangulation.
- It is an intra-op finding/diagnosis.
- It is a rare variety of inguinal hernia.

Description

- **2 loops of bowel remain in the sac.**
- **Connecting loop remains in the abdomen** and often becomes strangulated.

- The loops of intestine **look like a W.**

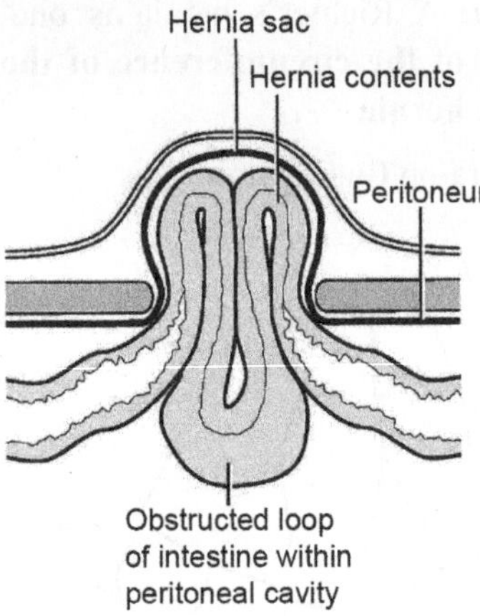

Figure 9: Maydl's hernia

Clinical Features

- The **connecting loop within the abdomen is the first to get strangulated:**
  - o Tenderness is elicited above the inguinal ligament.
  - o Intestinal obstruction is present.
  - o Generalised peritonitis may set in early, as the strangulated loop is inside the abdomen.
- The **fallacy of this condition is that even on opening the sac, the coils of intestine look normal.**
- Only on traction of these loops, one can find the strangulated loop inside abdomen.

[3] Littre's hernia. ***Dec 18, June 13***

- The finding of a **Meckel's diverticulum in an inguinal or femoral hernia is called Littre's hernia.**
- It is an intra-op finding/diagnosis.
- When found in the course of an abdominal surgery, a Meckel's diverticulum can safely be left alone, if it has a wide mouth and is not thickened.
- When there is doubt, it can be resected.

ABDOMINAL WALL

[3] Mention various types of abdominal incisions. ***June 17, Dec 16***

- Access to the abdominal cavity can be achieved in many ways.
- Exposure required (by the abdominal incision) will depend on:
  - o The surgical pathology anticipated.
  - o Procedure performed.
  - o Expertise of surgeon.
- Surgical exposure of abdomen can be achieved in the following ways:

A. Open Surgical Exposure

a. Intraperitoneal access:
- Longitudinal.
- Transverse.
- Oblique.
- Pelvic.

b. Retroperitoneal access:
- Flank incision.

c. Multicompartment access:
- Thoracoabdominal incisions.

B. Laparoscopic Exposure
- Multiport.
- Single port.
- Hand-assisted laparoscopy.

Examples

- **Subcostal:** For access to liver, gallbladder and biliary tree.
- Paramedian.
- **Transverse:** Preferred in children.
- **Periumbilical:** Camera port in laparoscopy.
- **McBurney's:** For appendicectomy.

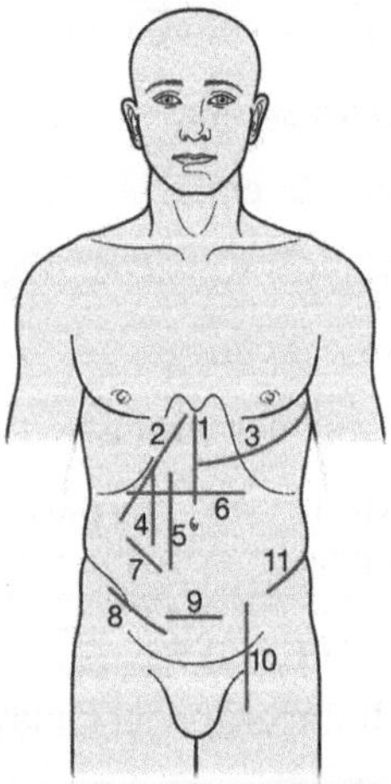

1. Midline 2. Kocher's 3. Thoracoabdominal 4. Rectus split 5. Paramedian 6. Transverse 7. McBurney's gridiron 8. Inguinal 9. Pfannenstiel 10. McEvedy 11. Rutherford Morison

Figure 10: Abdominal incisions

- **Pfannenstiel:** For access to uterus, ovaries and fallopian tubes.
- **Chevron incision:** Hepatopancreatobiliary incision.
- **Midline incision:** Exploratory laparotomy.
- **Inguinal incision:** Groin hernias.

[5] Desmoid tumour. *Dec 15, Dec 15 (Asked in both papers)*

[3] Desmoid tumour. *Sept 21, Oct 20*

- Also known as fibromatosis, aggressive fibromatosis or desmoid type fibromatosis.
- These are uncommon **mesenchymal neoplasms that are locally aggressive but lack metastatic potential.**

Aetiology

- **Associated with syndromes:**
  - FAP or familial adenomatous polyposis (germline mutations of APC gene).
  - Gardner syndrome.
  - Turcot syndrome.
- Sporadic desmoid tumours are most commonly associated with somatic mutations of the **CTNNB1 gene.**
- May be a result of **repeated trauma.**
- Associated with **pregnancy and oral contraceptive use.**
- Surgical history is an important risk factor.

Pathology

- Considered by some pathologists to be a hamartoma.
- Some believe it to be a fibroma.
- Express beta - catenin.

HPE

- Contain plasmodial cell masses resembling giant cells.
- Undergo central myxomatous change.

Clinical Features

- More common in women.
- Typically present as a **firm, non-painful, non-tender mass** in the abdominal wall.
- **Other sites:** Shoulder, hips, limbs, mesentery or pelvis.
- **Infiltrate surrounding structures and spread along tissue planes and muscles.**

Investigations

- **MRI** is the preferred modality for diagnosis, local staging and follow-up.
- **Core needle biopsy.**

Treatment

- Treatment of choice is surgical excision with a wide margin (to prevent recurrence) + reconstruction.
- Radiation is used as adjuvant therapy.
- Adjuvant chemotherapy, anti-hormonal therapies, NSAIDs.

UMBILICUS

[3] Sister Mary Joseph's nodule. *Sept 21*

- A **secondary malignant mass at the umbilicus** is called a Sister Mary Joseph's nodule.
- If tumour presents at the umbilicus, it is most probably **due to spread from the internal organs along internal ligaments**, e.g., from the liver along the falciform ligament.
- The primary neoplasm is often situated in the **stomach, pancreas, colon or ovary**, but a metastasis from the **breast**, probably transmitted along the lymphatics of the round ligament of the liver, is sometimes located here.
- It is described as a **red papular lesion** in the umbilicus.
- It is always a late manifestation of the disease, i.e., **advanced malignancy**.
- There is **little (if any) role for surgery** at this stage.

OTHER IMPORTANT TOPICS

BURST ABDOMEN

- Also known as abdominal dehiscence.

- **Definition:** Abdominal wound dehiscence describes partial or total disruption of the surgical wound, which can be superficial (skin and subcutaneous fat) or deep (fascial), with or without extrusion of abdominal viscera (evisceration).

Pathogenesis

- Burst abdomen is usually seen between the 6th and 9th day of operation, i.e., during the inflammatory phase of healing when wound strength is dependent on the suture material and holding capacity of the knot.
- The fascial layer provides most of the strength and anchor for abdominal incisions.
- Dehiscence can be caused by technical failure if the suture material breaks, knots become undone, or if the suture material cuts through the suture holding tissues.
- Over time (during the fibrotic phase), the intrinsic strength of the wound increases, and the integrity of wound is less dependent on the suture and suture technique.

Causes

A. Patient Factors

- Obesity.
- Jaundice.
- Malignancy.
- Hypoproteinemia.
- Anemia.
- Diabetes.
- Uremia.
- Immunosuppression.
- Sepsis/infected cases.
- Steroid use.
- Cough, vomiting and distension in the early post-op period.

B. Technical Factors

- Upper midline > transverse.
- Suture length:Wound length > 4:1 is recommended for proper fascial closure.
- Faulty suture placement (too close to the fascial edge, too far apart or under too much tension).

Clinical Features

- A serosanguineous (pink) discharge from the wound is the most pathognomonic sign of impending wound disruption. It signifies that intraperitoneal contents are lying extraperitoneally.
- Patient gives a history of 'felt something give way'.
- If skin sutures have been removed, omentum or coils of intestine may be forced through the wound and will be found lying on the skin.
- Symptoms and signs of intestinal obstruction may be present.

Investigations

- It is a clinical diagnosis and does not require any investigations.

Treatment

A. Emergency Surgery

- Done to replace the bowel, relieve any obstruction and resuture the wound.
- Protruding coils of intestine and omentum are washed gently with saline solution and returned to the abdominal cavity.
- **Tension suturing is done:** All layers are approximated by through and through sutures of monofilament nylon, which may be passed through a soft rubber or plastic tube collar.
- Abdominal wall may be supported by strips of adhesive plaster encircling the anterior 2/3rd of the circumference of the trunk.

B. Care While Awaiting Surgery

- Cover the wound with a sterile towel.
- Analgesics.
- IV fluids.
- Empty the stomach with a nasogastric tube.

EPIGASTRIC HERNIA

- **Definition:** Epigastric hernias arise through the midline raphe (linea alba) anywhere between the xiphoid process and the umbilicus.

Pathogenesis

- They begin with a transverse split in the midline

raphe so the defect is elliptical and usually < 1 cm in diameter.

- The hernia commonly contains only extra-peritoneal fat, which gradually enlarges, spreading in the subcutaneous plane to resemble the shape of a mushroom.
- When very large, they may contain a peritoneal sac but rarely any bowel.
- > 1 hernia may be present.
- The most common cause of recurrence is failure to identify a second defect at the time of original repair.

Clinical Features

- Patients are often fit, healthy men, but they are also seen in older, overweight men and women especially after multiple pregnancies.
- **Symptomless:** A small hernia is better felt than seen and may be discovered only in the course of routine abdominal palpation.
- Can be very painful even when the swelling is small due to the fatty contents becoming strangulated.
- It may be locally tender.
- It is unlikely to be reducible because of the narrow neck.
- A cough impulse may or may not be felt.

Investigations

- USG or soft tissue scan.
- CT scan.
- MRI.

Treatment

Surgery is the mainstay of treatment.

A. Primary Repair

- Repair usually consists of excision of the incarcerated preperitoneal tissue and simple closure of the fascial defect.

B. Mesh Repair

- Sometimes, the defects can be large and may contain omentum or other intra-abdominal viscera, and may require mesh repair.
- Mesh is ideally placed in the retro-rectus plane.

CONGENITAL INGUINAL HERNIA

- A congenital inguinal hernia is present since birth.

Aetiopathogenesis

- Prematurity.
- Low birth weight.
- M > F = 6 : 1.
- Right > left.
- It is usually due to a congenital weakness of the abdominal musculature.
- Persistence of processus vaginalis:
  - This causes indirect complete inguinal hernia.
  - It is a sort of pre-formed sac through which the contents herniate.
- Patent canal of Nuck in females.

Clinical Features

- Presents as an intermittent bulge in the groin extending to the scrotum or labia, often exacerbated by crying or straining.
- Most reduce on lying down or with gentle manipulation.
- A thickened cord in boys, or round ligament in girls, may be all that is palpable.
- May contain omentum, intestine, appendix (Amyand's) or a Meckel's diverticulum (Littre's).
- An ovary can prolapse and twist in a girl, requiring emergency exploration.

Treatment

- Reducible inguinal hernias are repaired electively.
- Complicated hernias are repaired on an emergency basis.
- Herniotomy is usually done, i.e., sac is opened, contents reduced and redundant sac excised.
- Mesh is not placed in children.

37

Peritoneum, Omentum and Mesentery

MESENTERIC CYST

[5]	Mesenteric cyst. *June 16, Feb 23, July 23*
[3]	Mesenteric cyst. *June 19*
[3]	Types of mesenteric cyst. *Dec 18, July 15, Dec 14, July 23*
[3]	Chylolymphatic cyst. *Feb 23*

- Cysts **may occur in any region of the mesentery.** They are **most often observed in the mesentery adjoining the small intestine (60%) or the colon.**

Types

1. Chylolymphatic.
2. Enterogenous.
3. Traumatic.
4. Hydatid.

Clinical Features

- Occurs most commonly in adults with a mean age of 45 years.
- But, 1/3rd of cases occur in children < 15 years.
- F > M.
- Rare.
- The **most common presentation is of a painless abdominal swelling** with characteristic physical signs:
    - o **Fluctuant swelling near the umbilicus.**
    - o Swelling moves freely in a plane at right angles to the attachment of the mesentery **(Tillaux's sign).**

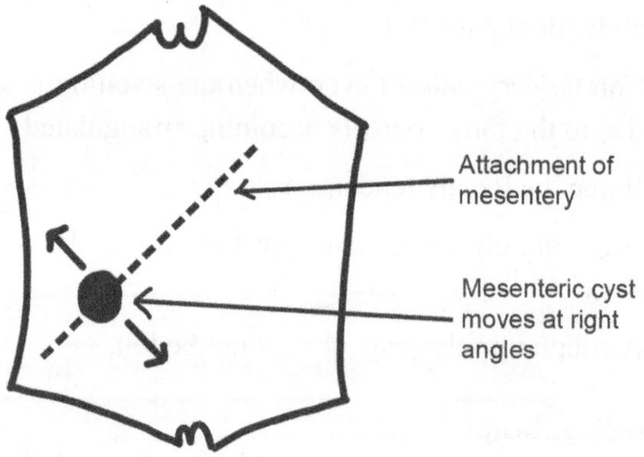

Figure 1: Movement of mesenteric cyst

- o There is a **zone of resonance around the cyst.**
- **Recurrent attacks of abdomen pain with or without vomiting** (pain resulting from recurring temporary impaction of a food bolus in a segment of bowel narrowed by the cyst or possibly from torsion of the mesentery).
- Acute **abdominal catastrophe**, due to:
    - o **Torsion** of that portion of the mesentery containing the cyst.
    - o **Rupture** of the cyst, often as a result of a comparatively trivial accident.
    - o **Hemorrhage** into the cyst.
    - o **Infection.**

Investigations

- USG.
- CT scan.

Treatment

- The treatment depends on the type of cyst:
  1. A **chylolymphatic cyst** has a blood supply that is independent from that of the adjacent intestine and, thus, **enucleation is possible without the need for resection of the gut**.
  2. The muscle in the wall of an **enterogenous cyst** and the bowel with which it is in contact have a common blood supply; therefore, removal of the cyst always entails **resection of the related portion of intestine**.

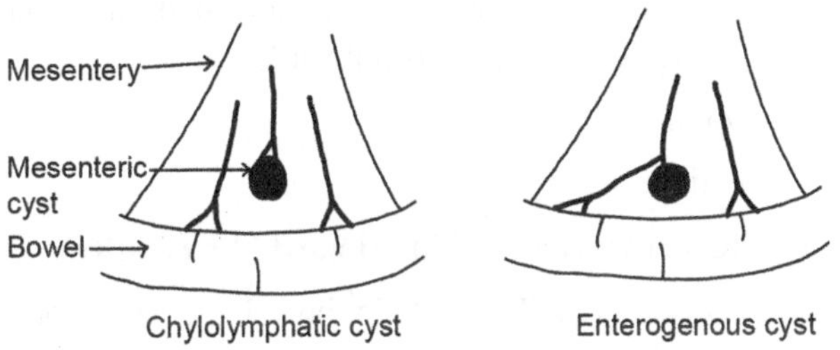

Figure 2: Types of mesenteric cyst

CHYLOLYMPHATIC CYST

- This is the most common variety.

Aetiopathology

- **Arises in congenitally misplaced lymphatic** tissue that has no efferent communication with the lymphatic system.
- **Most common in ileum.**
- Cyst is **thin walled**, composed of connective tissue **lined by flat endothelium.**
- Occasionally, the cyst attains a large size.
- Unilocular > multilocular.
- Almost always **solitary.**
- **Has a blood supply that is independent from that of the adjacent intestine.**

Treatment

- Enucleation of cyst.

ENTEROGENOUS CYST

- Also known as enteric duplication cyst.

Aetiopathogenesis

- **Causes:**
  1. Derived from a **diverticulum** of the mesenteric border of the intestine **that has become sequestrated** from the intestinal canal during embryonic life.
  2. **Duplication** of the intestine.
- Has a **thicker wall than a chylolymphatic cyst** and is lined by mucous membrane, which is sometimes ciliated.
- **Content is mucinous** and either colourless or yellowish brown as a result of past hemorrhage.
- Muscle in the wall of an enterogenous cyst and the bowel with which it is in contact have a common blood supply.

Treatment

- Removal of the cyst always entails resection of the related portion of intestine.

PERITONITIS

[5] Acute peritonitis. ***March 24***

[5] Management of peritonitis. ***Dec 19***

[3] Mention the clinical features of peritonitis. ***Dec 12***

[MCQ] Features of peritonitis include all except: ***CBME March 24***

A. Abdominal pain that increases on movement

B. Fever

C. Guarding

D. Increased bowel sounds*

- Peritonitis is inflammation of the peritoneum.

Types

- According to the primary underlying pathology, peritonitis can be of **2 types:**

1. **Localised or diffuse:**
   - o Clinically, this is the most useful categorisation of peritonitis.
2. **Acute or chronic.**

Causes of Peritoneal Inflammation

a. **Bacterial**
   - Gastrointestinal and non-gastrointestinal.

b. **Chemical**
   - Bile, barium.

c. **Allergies**
   - Starch peritonitis.

d. **Traumatic**
   - Operative handling.

e. **Ischemia**
   - Strangulated bowel, vascular occlusion.

f. **Miscellaneous**
   - Familial Mediterranean fever.

Paths to Peritoneal Infection

a. **GI perforation**
   - Perforated ulcer, appendicitis, diverticulum.

b. **Transmural translocation (without any perforation)**
   - Pancreatitis, ischemic bowel, primary bacterial peritonitis.

c. **Exogenous contamination**
   - Drains, open surgery, trauma, peritoneal dialysis.

d. **Female genital tract infection**
   - Pelvic inflammatory disease.

e. **Hematogenous spread (rare)**
   - Septicemia.

Clinical Features

Localised Peritonitis

- Bound intimately with the causative lesion, and the initial symptoms and signs are those of that lesion.
- Temperature increases.
- Pulse rate increases.
- As pain increases, there is associated **vomiting.**
- **Guarding and rigidity** of the abdominal wall over the area which is involved, with a positive release sign, e.g.:
  - o Subphrenic peritonitis–Shoulder tip pain.
  - o Pelvic peritonitis–PR/PV tenderness.
- **Course/natural history:**
  - o Resolves.
  - o Becomes an abscess.
  - o Becomes diffuse.

Diffuse or Generalised Peritonitis

A. **Initial Phase**
   - Patient complains of severe pain, which is:
     - o Made worse by moving or breathing.
     - o First experienced at the site of the original lesion and spreads outwards.
   - Vomiting.
   - Patient lies still.
   - Tenderness and rigidity **(board like rigidity).**
   - As **paralytic ileus** sets in, bowel sounds become absent.
   - Pulse rate increases.
   - Temperature changes are variable and can even be subnormal.

B. **Intermediate Phase**
   - In this phase, one of 3 things happen:
     1. Peritonitis may resolve.
     2. Condition may localise, producing one or more abscesses, with overlying swelling and tenderness.
     3. Patient may deteriorate and go into the terminal phase.

C. **Terminal Phase**
   - Abdomen becomes silent.
   - Distension of abdomen.
   - Circulatory failure with cold, clammy extremities and thready or irregular pulse.
   - **Hippocratic facies:**
     - o Sunken eyes.
     - o Dry tongue.
     - o Drawn and anxious face.

- SIRS.
- MODS.

Investigations

- The aim is to diagnose the underlying cause and guide treatment.
- **CT Scan:**
  - o **Investigation of choice**, as the whole abdomen can be visualised.
- **Erect CXR:**
  - o Air under diaphragm, i.e., pneumoperitoneum is seen.
- **Abdominal X-ray:** Both erect and supine.
- **Lateral Decubitus X-ray:**
  - o Done if patient is particularly unwell and unable to stand.
  - o Serves the same purpose as an erect X-ray (provided the patient has been appropriately positioned for long enough for the gas to rise within the peritoneal cavity).
- **USG:**
  - o Lacks specificity except in the case of tubo-ovarian pathology.
- Lab biomarkers will support a diagnosis of acute inflammation, but are rarely diagnostically specific.
- Diagnostic laparoscopy may be required if the above investigations are inconclusive.

Treatment

- **General care of patient:**
  - o Correction of fluid and electrolyte imbalance.
  - o Insertion of nasogastric drainage tube and urinary catheter.
  - o Broad spectrum antibiotics.
  - o Analgesia.
  - o Vital system support/shift to ICU.

A. Localised Peritonitis

- **Aims of treatment:**
  - o To treat the underlying cause.
  - o To lavage or dilute residual contamination.

B. Diffuse or Generalised Peritonitis

- **'Source control'** by removal or exclusion of cause, e.g., perforation repair if hollow viscus perforation is the cause of peritonitis.
- Peritoneal lavage ± drainage.
- **Surgical treatment of cause** when appropriate.

OTHERS

[5] Subdiaphragmatic abscess. *Sept 21, June 17*

- Also known as subphrenic abscess.

Causes

a. **Surgical operations:**
- Operations on stomach, pancreas, intestines, splenectomy.

b. **Abdominal trauma:**
- Hematoma, bile accumulation.

c. **Purulent processes:**
- Pancreatitis, liver abscess, pleural empyema.

Clinical Features

- Symptoms and signs are frequently unspecific.
- Remember the aphorism, '**pus somewhere, pus nowhere else, pus under diaphragm**'.
- **Common history:** When some infective focus in the abdominal cavity has been dealt with, the condition of the patient improves temporarily, but after an interval of a few days or weeks, symptoms of toxemia reappear.
- Condition of the patient deteriorates steadily and rapidly.
- Swelling.
- Wasting.
- Anorexia.
- Epigastric fullness and pain.
- Shoulder tip pain, i.e., pain in shoulder on affected side, because of irritation of sensory fibres in the phrenic nerve.
- Persistent hiccups.
- Swinging pyrexia.

On Examination

- Tenderness, rigidity.
- Palpable swelling.
- Sometimes, the liver is displaced downwards, but more often it is fixed by adhesions.
- **Chest:** Collapse of lung, basal effusion or empyema.

Investigations

- CT abdomen is the investigation of choice.
- X-ray abdomen.
- CXR.

Treatment

A. General Care

- Correction of fluid and electrolyte imbalance.
- Insertion of nasogastric drainage tube and urinary catheter.
- Broad spectrum antibiotics.
- Analgesia.
- Vital system support.

B. Surgical Treatment of Cause When Appropriate

- **'Source control'** by removal or exclusion of the cause.
- Peritoneal lavage ± drainage.

[5] Pseudomyxoma peritonei. *June 13*
[3] Pseudomyxoma peritonei. *Dec 19*

- **Definition:** It is a rare condition typified by **progressive peritoneal tumour deposits, mucinous ascites, omental cake and ovarian involvement** in females.

Aetiology

1. The vast majority of cases arise as a result of **perforation of a mucinous appendiceal tumour**.
   - Risk varies according to:
     - o Tumour subtype.
     - o Mode of presentation.
   - **Risk is highest with mucinous adenocarcinoma of appendix.**
2. Rupture of pseudomucinous cyst of ovary.

Pathology

- Abdomen is filled with a **yellow jelly**, large quantities of which are often **encysted.**

Clinical Features

- F > M.
- Progressive and massive abdominal distension.
- Anorexia.
- Symptoms of bowel dysfunction.
- It is invariably fatal without intervention.

Investigations

- High resolution CT scan of the abdomen and pelvis with oral and IV contrast.
- Full length colonoscopy should be performed to exclude a primary colorectal cancer.
- **Diagnostic Laparoscopy:**
  - o Provides additional staging information by allowing direct visualisation.
  - o Also facilitates tissue diagnosis.
  - o Ideally, **should be performed at a centre where subsequent CRS (cytoreductive surgery) would be undertaken.**

Treatment

Patient should be referred to a specialist centre with multidisciplinary expertise.

A. Cytoreductive Surgery + Hyperthermic Intra-Peritoneal Chemotherapy (HIPEC)

- It is the treatment of choice.
- This approach **combines multiple peritonectomy procedures with multivisceral resections** as required to achieve a complete surgical clearance of the tumor (i.e., complete cytoreduction) + **HIPEC (typically mitomycin C or oxaliplatin)** to eradicate presumed residual microscopic disease.
- The combined operation can take > 10 hours and may require total abdominopelvic peritonectomy, greater and lesser omentectomy, bilateral salpingo-oophorectomy, hysterectomy, cholecystectomy, splenectomy, partial gastrectomy, colectomy and anterior resection of rectum.

B. Systemic Chemotherapy

- It is indicated in:
  1. Patients with **high grade or invasive unresectable disease**. In such patients, systemic chemo is first line treatment.
  2. Adjuvant chemotherapy in patients with high grade tumour.
- Chemotherapy is not considered in patients with low grade tumour.

OTHER IMPORTANT TOPICS

PELVIC ABSCESS

- The pelvis is the most common site of intraperitoneal abscess.

Aetiopathogenesis

- The vermiform appendix is often pelvic in position.
- Fallopian tubes are frequent sites of infection.
- Can also occur as a sequel to any case of diffuse peritonitis.
- After anastomotic leakage following colorectal surgery.
- Pus can accumulate in the pelvis without serious constitutional disturbance, and may attain considerable size before being recognised.

Clinical Features

- Abdominal/pelvic pain.
- Complains of lower back pain or a pressure sensation in the pelvis (can be quite severe in intensity).
- Diarrhoea and passage of mucus in the stools, which is due to local irritation of the rectum by the collection in the pelvis.
- Passage of mucus, occurring for the first time in a patient who has, or is recovering from, peritonitis, is pathognomonic of pelvic abscess.
- The abscess may discharge into the anal canal as the pelvic collection points through an anastomotic leak (the point of least resistance).
- Malaise, lethargy, failure to recover from surgery as expected.
- Anorexia and weight loss.
- Sweats ± rigors.
- Nausea and vomiting.
- Complains of fever ± swinging pyrexia.

On Examination

- Rectal or vaginal examination can be extremely uncomfortable for the patient.
- Tenderness on per rectal or per vaginal examination.
- Bogginess on DRE.
- Bulging of the anterior rectal wall, which becomes softly cystic, as the abscess ripens.
- Tachycardia.

Investigations

- If any uncertainty exists, the presence of pus should be confirmed by ultrasonography or CT scanning.
- Transrectal or transvaginal ultrasound can be done to look for a collection in the pelvis.

Treatment

- **Drainage of the abscess:**
  - o Can be drained transanally or transgluteally.
  - o In women it can be drained transvaginally, through the posterior fornix.
  - o Transintestinal drainage is no longer done because of the high incidence of complications such as fistulae.
- **Laparotomy** may sometimes be indicated.

38

Esophagus

[5] Enumerate clinical features and add a note on management of achalasia cardia. ***CBME March 24***

[5] Achalasia cardia. ***August 22, Dec 17, June 17, June 16, Dec 15, Dec 14***

[3] Achalasia cardia. ***Sept 21***

- The term achalasia means failure to relax.
- There is **failure of relaxation of lower esophageal sphincter.**
- It is a **motility disorder** of the esophagus which **affects both the body and LES.**

Aetiopathology

Loss of inhibitory ganglion cells in the Auerbach's myenteric plexus

↓

Mismatch in excitatory and inhibitory activity of the LES

↓

1. Failure of LES relaxation
2. Absent peristalsis

↓

Esophagus dilates and contractions disappear

↓

Contd.

Esophagus empties mainly by the hydrostatic pressure of its contents, which is almost always incomplete

↓

Residual food and fluid in the esophagus

↓

Esophagus becomes progressively more tortuous and dilated, called megaesophagus

↓

Fermentation of food residues

↓

Retention esophagitis

↓

Increased risk of carcinoma esophagus

Causes

- Virus induced autoimmune effect.
- **Chagas disease**, due to the parasite *Trypanosoma cruzi.*
- **Allgrove syndrome = adrenal insufficiency + alacrima + achalasia.**

Clinical Features

- 30-60 years of age.

- Dysphagia to both solids and liquids.
- Regurgitation.
- Heartburn.
- Chest pain/odynophagia.
- Patients often present late and, having had relatively mild symptoms, remain untreated for many years.
- Weight loss.
- Due to significant stasis of food residue in the dilated esophagus:
  - o Aspiration related respiratory symptoms.
  - o Pneumonia.
  - o Retained food undergoes fermentation, which results in halitosis.
  - o Patients may report regurgitating food that they have ingested before.
- **Eckardt score** helps assess the severity of symptoms and monitors the treatment outcome.

Investigations

- **Barium swallow**
  - o Birds beak appearance.
  - o Sigmoidal shaped esophagus.
  - o Dilated esophagus with distal narrowing.
- **X-ray abdomen**
  - o Gastric air shadow/air fluid level seen in normal people may be absent.
  - o Timed barium esophagogram.
  - o Quantifies the height of the retained contrast at a specific time after ingestion.
  - o Determines severity of disease.
- **Endoscopy**
  - o Frothy saliva pooling in esophagus.
  - o Presence of food residue.
  - o Dilated and tortuous esophagus.
  - o High resolution manometry.
  - o Gold standard test for diagnosis.
  - o Distinguishes achalasia from other motility disorders of esophagus.

Treatment

- **Goal:** Symptom palliation only, since there is no therapy to reverse the neuronal degeneration.
- Therapies target the LES, aiming to reduce its contractility by drugs or by destroying the muscle fibers using endoscopic or surgical methods.

A. Drugs

- Limited role.
- Calcium channel blockers, nitrates, 5' –phosphodiesterase inhibitors.
- Reserved for patients who are poor candidates for endoscopic or surgical treatments.

B. Botulinum Toxin

- It is a potent presynaptic inhibitor of acetylcholine release from nerve endings.
- Injected endoscopically into LES.
- Repeated injections are required.
- Indicated in elderly patients with comorbidities.

C. Pneumatic Dilatation

- Involves stretching the LES with a non-compliant balloon to disrupt the sphincter muscle and render it less competent.
- Serial pneumatic dilatation is required.
- Has a risk of perforation.

D. Heller's Myotomy

- Involves cutting the muscles of the lower esophagus and gastric cardia.
- Anterior myotomy is typically done.
- Transabdominal and transthoracic approaches are advocated. Currently, the standard procedure is a laparoscopic approach.
- Usually combined with a partial fundoplication (anterior Dor or posterior Toupet) which offsets the underlying risk of GERD.

E. Per Oral Endoscopic Myotomy (POEM)

- It involves creation of a long esophageal myotomy using a flexible GI endoscope.
- After incising the esophageal mucosa, a tunnel is created in the esophageal wall, circular muscle is divided to a point distal to the LES and the esophageal mucosal opening is closed with clips.
- If done properly, it is as effective as laparoscopic Heller's myotomy.

F. Esophagectomy

- Reserved only for the treatment of patients with end-stage achalasia with a sigmoid or megaesophagus that is not responding to other methods.

[5] Tracheoesophageal fistula. *March 22, june 13*

- Congenital esophageal atresia or tracheoesophageal fistula is an important condition because its recognition within 48 hours of birth and subsequent surgical correction, is the only hope of survival.
- Oesophageal atresia is a congenital condition of oesophageal discontinuity that results in proximal oesophageal obstruction.
- A tracheoesophageal fistula is an abnormal fistulous communication between the esophagus and trachea.

Types

- There are 5 types:
  - o **Type A:** Both the proximal and the distal esophageal pouches are blind.
  - o **Type B:** The proximal esophageal pouch is connected to the trachea and the distal esophageal pouch is blind.
  - o **Type C:** The proximal esophageal pouch is blind and the distal esophageal pouch is connected to the trachea. This is the most common type.
  - o **Type D:** Both the proximal and distal esophageal pouch are separately connected to the trachea.
  - o **Type E:** The proximal and distal esophageal pouch are in continuity. There is a fistula between the trachea and the esophagus. This is the only type where the proximal and distal esophageal pouch are in continuity.

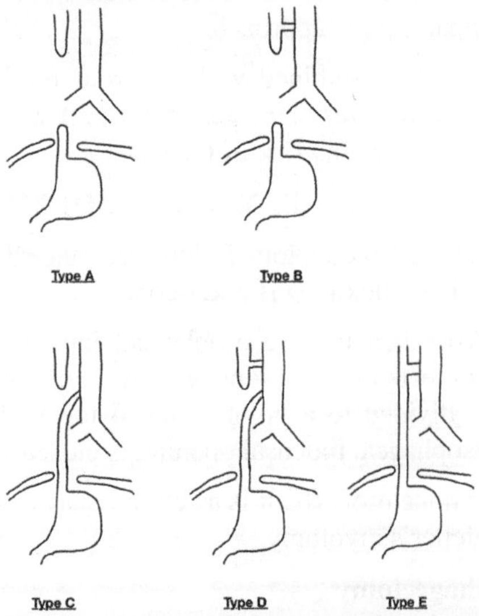

Figure 1: Types of tracheo-esophageal fistula

Clinical Features

- M > F
- When detected **antenatal or before birth:**
  - o When the esophagus ends blindly, amniotic fluid cannot be swallowed and polyhydramnios results.
  - o In type A, the stomach may be small or difficult to detect antenatally and is often wrongly referred to as absent.
- **Postnatal presentation:**
  - o The newborn baby regurgitates all its first, and subsequent feeds.
  - o Saliva pours, almost continuously, from its mouth (drooling). This is the classic symptom, as it is not seen in any other condition.
  - o Attacks of coughing and cyanosis occur on feeding.
  - o Type E presents with recurrent chest infections or coughing after feeds.

Investigations

- A nasogastric tube coiled in the upper esophageal pouch on a CXR suggests the diagnosis.
- Type E is diagnosed with the help of a contrast swallow.

Treatment

- A nasal or oral sump Replogle tube is placed to drain saliva and prevent aspiration.
- Positive airway pressure is avoided as air passing through the fistula causes gastric distension, compromised ventilation and risks perforation.
- If pressure support is needed, perhaps because of respiratory distress syndrome, prompt fistula ligation is needed.
- **Types A and B**
  - o Typically have a long gap and may require esophageal replacement. Colonic or jejunal interposition or gastric transposition is done some months after a cervical esophagostomy and a gastrostomy.
  - o In many cases, the ends can be brought together by progressive traction and delayed anastomosis.

- **Types C and D**
  - o Fistula is divided through a right thoracotomy or thoracoscopically.
  - o If the neonate is stable and the gap is favourable, an anastomosis is fashioned over a trans-anastomotic tube, which facilitates early feeding.
  - o If a primary anastomosis is not possible, a delayed anastomosis is done after a few weeks of growth.
- **Type E**
  - o Usually found in the neck on a contrast swallow.
  - o Repaired in the neck itself.

[3] Mention the causes of reflux esophagitis. ***June 16***

CAUSES OF REFLUX ESOPHAGITIS

- Hiatus hernia.
- Obesity.
- Overeating.
- Declining infection rates of *Helicobacter pylori.*
- Ineffective esophageal motility.
- Pregnancy.
- Alcohol.
- Smoking.
- Spicy or fatty foods.
- Chocolate.
- Coffee.

[3] GERD. ***June 17, July 23***

GASTROESOPHAGEAL REFLUX DISEASE

- **Definition:** A condition that develops when the reflux of stomach contents causes troublesome symptoms and/or complications.

Aetiopathology

- GERD can be explained by the interaction between:
  1. **Reflux barrier** (consists of the crural diaphragm and the LES).
  2. **Pressure difference between the thoracic and abdominal cavity.**
- Physiological relaxation of the LES in response to stretching of the gastric fundus, particularly after a meal to allow venting of swallowed air is termed **transient LES relaxations (tLESR).**
- GERD increases by the following:
  - o Increased number of tLESR.
  - o More compliant LES.
  - o Delay in acid refluxate clearance from the esophagus as a result of defective esophageal motility.

Causes/Predisposing Factors

- Hiatus hernia.
- Obesity.
- Overeating.
- Declining infection rates of *H. pylori.*
- Defective esophageal motility.
- Pregnancy.
- Alcohol.
- Smoking.
- Spicy or fatty foods, chocolate, coffee.

Clinical Features

- **Esophageal symptoms:**
  - o Heartburn (burning sensation behind the sternum).
  - o Regurgitation or water brash (perception of the flow of refluxed gastric contents into the mouth or hypopharynx).
  - o Dysphagia.
  - o Chest pain/epigastric pain.
  - o Dyspepsia.
  - o Nausea.
  - o Bloating.
  - o Belching.
- **Extraesophageal symptoms:**
  - o Chronic cough.
  - o Asthma.
  - o Laryngitis.
  - o Dental caries.
- Heartburn, regurgitation and dysphagia are typical symptoms.
- Symptoms are often provoked by food, particularly after a full meal with increased intragastric pressure or food that delays gastric emptying (e.g., oily, spicy

food).

- Refluxate causes an unpleasant taste, which is acidic or bitter.
- Intensive exercise may sometimes induce GERD.
- Some patients may complain of nocturnal symptoms especially when lying supine.

Investigations

- **Ambulatory 24 hours pH monitoring** is the gold standard test to diagnose GERD.
- **De Meester** score is used.
- **High Resolution Manometry** is used to exclude other disorders.
- **Endoscopy:**
  - o **Los Angeles grading** is used to grade severity.
- **Barium esophagram.**

Treatment

A. Lifestyle Modification

- **Healthy diet**
  - o Avoid overeating.
  - o Avoid dietary items that provoke symptoms (e.g., soda, alcohol, tea or coffee).
  - o Early dinner.
- Avoid lying down after meals.
- Elevation of the head end of the bed.
- Stop smoking.
- Lose weight.

B. Medical Management

- Antacids.
- **H_2 receptor antagonists:** Ranitidine.
- **Proton pump inhibitors:** Pantoprazole, omeprazole.
- **Prokinetics:** Metoclopramide, domperidone.
- PCABs or Potassium Competitive Acid Blockers.
- **Other treatment modulators:** Tricyclic antidepressants, SSRIs.

C, Surgical Management

- **Indications for surgery:**
  - o Incomplete symptom control with medical management.
  - o Intolerance or unwillingness to comply with long-term medical therapy.
  - o Regurgitation despite medication.
  - o Presence of a large hiatus hernia.
  - o Complications arising from GERD.
  - o Extraesophageal symptoms.
- **Anti-reflux surgery:**
  - o **Complete:** Nissen's fundoplication.
  - o **Partial:**
    - ♦ Anterior: Dor, Watson.
    - ♦ Posterior: Toupet.

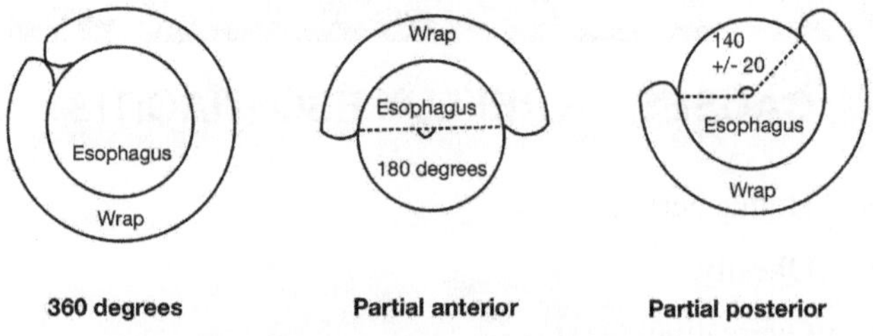

Figure 2: Types of fundoplication

[3] Hiatus hernia. ***June 19***
[5] Hiatus hernia. ***June 13***

- **Definition:** Hiatus hernia is a condition in which the abdominal contents migrate through the hiatal opening of the diaphragm into the mediastinum.

Types

There are four types of hiatus hernia:

1. Type I or sliding hiatal hernia

- Most common type.
- GEJ migrates cephalad into the posterior mediastinum.

2. Type II or rolling hiatal hernia

- Gastric fundus herniates into the mediastinum through the hiatal defect.
- GEJ remains in its normal intra-abdominal position.

3. Type III or mixed hiatal hernia

- It is a combination of 1 and 2, i.e., both the GEJ and fundus are located in the mediastinum.

4. **Type IV**
   - When abdominal viscera other than the stomach herniates (e.g., colon, spleen, pancreas or small bowel) cephalad to the esophageal hiatus and into the mediastinum.
   - Hiatal hernia types 2, 3 and 4 are also referred to as paraesophageal hernia.

Pathophysiology

- The **2 events** that facilitate the formation of hiatus hernia are:
  1. **Widening of diaphragmatic crura** at the esophageal hiatus.
  2. **Stretching of the phrenoesophageal membrane.**

Clinical Features

- Hiatus hernia is closely related to advanced age and obesity.
- **Type I or sliding hiatus hernia** is associated with **GERD** and is usually diagnosed in the presence of reflux symptoms.
- **Paraesophageal hernia**, especially when large, presents more with **obstructive symptoms:**
  - o Dysphagia, odynophagia.
  - o Early satiety.
  - o Epigastric pain.
  - o Postprandial chest pain.
  - o GI bleeding can result from mucosal ischemia or mechanical ulceration of the gastric mucosa.
  - o Mass effect of hernia contents in the chest can cause respiratory symptoms such as shortness of breath.

Complications

1. Esophagitis.
2. **Aspiration pneumonitis:** Due to recurring reflux.
3. **Obstruction or strangulation:** Occurs in large hernias, due to volvulus of stomach.

Investigations

1. **Barium swallow:** Provides the most accurate image of the gastroesophageal anatomy.
2. **Endoscopy.**
3. **Manometry.**
4. **Ambulatory pH monitoring.**
5. **CXR** and **CT scan** may show an intrathoracic gas bubble or fluid level.

Treatment

A. **PPIs** are used to treat symptoms of GERD.

B. **Surgical Repair**
   - **Laparoscopic approach** is preferred over open approach.
   - Regardless of the approach, there are 4 key steps to a paraesophageal hernia repair:
     1. **Reduction of the hernia contents** back to the abdominal cavity.
     2. **Complete excision of the hernia sac from the posterior mediastinum.**
     3. **Mobilisation of the distal esophagus to achieve a minimum of 3 cm of intra-abdominal esophageal length.**
     4. An **anti-reflux operation, i.e., fundoplication.**

[5] Plummer Vinson syndrome. *Dec 13*

- Also known as Paterson-Brown-Kelly syndrome, sideropenic dysphagia.
- It is a rare disease.

Pathophysiology

- Possible mechanisms include:
  - o Iron and nutritional deficiencies.
  - o Genetic predisposition.
  - o Autoimmunity.

Clinical Features

- Mainly affects middle aged women.
- Cervical esophageal web (usually in post-cricoid region):
  - o Causes dysphagia.
  - o Both the proximal and distal surfaces of the web are lined by squamous mucosa.

- This predisposes to cervical esophageal cancer.
- Iron deficiency anemia:
  - Koilonychia.
- Angular cheilitis, stomatitis.

Treatment

- Iron therapy.
- Diet modification.
- Endoscopic dilatation of cervical web.

[5] Stricture of esophagus. *Dec 19*

- A stricture means a narrowing of the esophagus.

Causes

- GERD, also known as reflux or peptic strictures.
- Caustic or corrosive injuries.
- Esophageal surgery or anastomotic strictures, e.g., esophagectomy, esophagogastrostomy.
- Cancer of esophagus, i.e., malignant strictures.
- Radiation therapy, when the mid-esophagus is included in the radiation field.
- Esophageal injury.
- Eosinophilic esophagitis.
- Prolonged nasogastric tube intubation.
- Congenital esophageal stenosis.
- Drugs: Tetracycline, doxycycline, potassium chloride, quinidine, NSAIDs, alendronate.
- Blistering skin lesions:
  - Cicatricial pemphigoid.
  - Epidermolysis bullosa.
- Lichen planus.
- Crohn's disease (rare cause).
- Extrinsic compression of esophagus by mediastinal lymphadenopathy mimics an intrinsic esophageal stricture.

Clinical Features

- **Site of stricture:**
  - Near GEJ – peptic strictures.
  - Lower esophagus – prolonged Ryle's tube.
  - Mid-esophagus – prolonged Ryle's tube, radiation therapy, eosinophilic esophagitis.
  - Upper esophagus – blistering skin diseases, eosinophilic esophagitis.
  - Any part – corrosives, lichen planus.
  - Dysphagia.
- **Features of the underlying disease:**
  - Regurgitation, water brash in GERD.
  - History of corrosive/lye ingestion, previous surgery, radiation therapy for lung cancer, NGT intubation, drugs intake.
  - The associated skin lesions are key to diagnosis of esophageal strictures in blistering skin diseases and lichen planus.
  - Weight loss and other features of carcinoma esophagus.

Investigations

- Barium esophagram:
  - Cancer of esophagus may show rat's tail or an apple-core like stricture.
- Endoscopy ± biopsy.

Treatment

- Endoscopic stricture dilation is undertaken for benign conditions:
  - To restore normal swallowing, a stricture should be dilated to at least 16 mm.
- Reflux strictures:
  - Dilatation.
  - Long-term treatment with a PPI.
  - Anti-reflux surgery (laparoscopic fundoplication) may be considered in younger and fitter patients.
- In patients with corrosive injuries with very long or multiple strictures, esophageal replacement is usually required, i.e., esophagectomy is done and the colon may have to be used as the replacement conduit (because of associated gastric damage, the stomach is not used).

[3] Barrett's esophagus. *March 22*

- **Definition:** It is defined as the proximal migration of columnar epithelium (salmon-coloured mucosa) in the lower esophagus extending > 1 cm above the gastroesophageal junction.

- It is a known complication of GERD.

Risk Factors

- Chronic GERD symptoms (> 5 years).
- Age > 50 years.
- Smoking.
- Central obesity.
- M > F.

Pathology

- **Long standing acid and alkaline reflux** can result in **histologic change of** the **distal esophageal mucosa** from its **normal squamous epithelium to a columnar epithelium.**
- This histologic alteration is **called intestinal metaplasia or Barrett's esophagus.**
- Patients with Barrett's have an **increased risk of dysplasia.**
- When dysplasia is present, there is an **increased risk** for development **of adenocarcinoma** of the esophagus.

Clinical Features

- Vast majority of patients with Barrett's are asymptomatic.
- Patients may give a history of GERD:
  - o Heartburn, i.e., burning sensation behind the sternum.
  - o Regurgitation or water brash, i.e., flow of refluxed gastric content into the mouth or hypopharynx.
  - o Epigastric pain.
  - o Dysphagia.

Investigations

- **Endoscopy:**
  - o Appears as velvety-red 'tongues' of mucosa that extend cephalad from the GEJ.
  - o High definition white light endoscopy including narrow band imaging is used to assess the mucosal and vascular pattern of the Barrett's segment.
  - o Chromoendoscopy.
- **Biopsy** is taken via endoscopy as per **Seattle protocol.**

Treatment

A. Treatment of Underlying GERD

- **Drugs:**
  - o PPI (proton pump inhibitors), e.g., Panto-prazole.
  - o H2 receptor antagonists, e.g., Ranitidine.
  - o Antacids.
- Anti reflux surgery, e.g., Nissen's fundoplication.

B. Resection of Barrett's

- In patients with **high grade dysplastic Barrett's esophagus, without suspicion of invasive cancer**, the epithelium can be ablated or resected. This aims to **completely eradicate all intestinal metaplasia** and can be done by:
  - o Photodynamic therapy.
  - o Radiofrequency ablation.
  - o Cryotherapy.
  - o EMR – Endoscopic Mucosal Resection.
  - o ESD – Endoscopic Submucosal Dissection.

C. Surgery

- **Esophagectomy** should be considered if there is **adenocarcinoma which is T1b or higher**.

[10] Describe pathophysiology, clinical features and management of carcinoma esophagus. ***March 21***

[10] Enumerate causes of dysphagia. Write about aetiopathology, investigations and management of carcinoma esophagus. ***Oct 20***

[10] Describe the aetiology, pathology and management of carcinoma esophagus. ***Dec 19***

CARCINOMA ESOPHAGUS

- Squamous cell carcinoma is the most common type in India.
- Adenocarcinoma is the most common type in the West.

Types/Classification

- Squamous cell carcinoma.
- Adenocarcinoma.

- **Rare types:**
  - o Melanoma.
  - o Small cell carcinoma.
- **Secondaries:** Bronchogenic carcinoma.

Aetiology

Factor (s)	SCC	Adenocarcinoma
Smoking	+++	+
Alcohol	+++	-
Hot beverages	+	-
N-nitroso containing food (e.g., pickled vegetables)	+	-
Chewing betel nut	+	-
Drinking yerba mate	+	-
Dietary deficiency of fresh green vegetables, fruits and vitamins	+	-
Low socioeconomic status	+	-
Fungal toxin or virus	+	-
H/o radiation to mediastinum	+	+
Lye corrosive stricture	+	-
History of upper aerodigestive malignancy	+++	-
Plummer-Vinson syndrome	+	-
Achalasia	+	-
Obesity	-	++
GERD	-	+++
Barrett's esophagus	-	++++

Pathology

- Both squamous cell and adenocarcinoma develop from dysplastic mucosa.
- Most adenocarcinomas are mucin producing with intestinal type features.
- Site of esophagus affected:
  - o SCC – Upper ⅓rd and middle ⅓rd.
  - o Adenocarcinoma – Lower ⅓rd and GEJ.
- Both cell types may directly infiltrate adjacent organs.
- Esophageal wall has a rich network of submucosal lymphatics, and therefore longitudinal submucosal spread of cancer is common.
- Lymph node metastases can involve the cervical area, the mediastinum as well as the perigastric/celiac axis.
- Distant hematogenous spread: Non regional lymph nodes, lungs, liver, brain and bones.
- Peritoneal mets is an important mode of spread for adenocarcinoma of the GEJ, but is rare for SCC.

Clinical Features

- Age: 50-70 years.
- M > F.
- The most common symptom is progressive dysphagia: first to solids, then to liquids, then to water and then to the patient's own saliva. This is related to increasing luminal obstruction by the cancer.
- Anorexia.
- Weight loss.
- Odynophagia.
- Symptoms of regurgitation.
- Hoarseness of voice indicates involvement of recurrent laryngeal nerve.
- Aspiration.
- Choking and cough on drinking water are typical of fistulation between the esophagus and the airway. There may be associated hemoptysis as well.
- Blood loss: Adenocarcinoma > SCC; if chronic, it can lead to iron deficiency anemia.
- Acute GI bleeding can occur, though it is rarely severe, except for aortoesophageal fistula, which usually presents with a smaller sentinel bleed followed by massive bleeding that is invariably fatal.
- Poor prognosis: This is because patients present late. Patients with early disease have no symptoms and the cancer tends to metastasize early.

Investigations

1. **Barium swallow:**
   - Apple core or rat's tail appearance is seen.
2. **Endoscopy:**
   - Will visualize the tumor.
   - Biopsies or brush cytology can be taken to confirm the diagnosis.
   - Chromoendoscopy using Lugol's iodine, narrow band imaging endoscopy can also be used.
3. **Endoscopic ultrasound (EUS):**
   - It is the only imaging modality able to distinguish the various layers of the esophageal wall.
   - Used for staging.
   - Can accurately assess infiltration to adjacent structures.

4. **EUS guided FNAC:**
   - Can be used to obtain cytological proof of involved lymph nodes.
5. **CT scan:**
   - Used to assess local invasion and distant spread.
6. **FDG-PET scan:**
   - Used for detecting regional and non-regional nodes, as well as distant mets.
   - Uptake by the tumor may have some prognostic value and is useful in predicting histological response and outcome.
7. **Laparoscopy:**
   - Laparoscopic staging is useful in adenocarcinomas, but not in SCC.
   - Should be reserved for patients in whom confirmation of metastatic disease that is not otherwise obtainable is essential in deciding on treatment.
8. **Bronchoscopy:**
   - Can assess airway involvement by the tumor.

Treatment

- Principles of treatment depend on the disease stage and physiological reserve of the patient.

A. Endoscopic Treatment

- Early cancers are amenable to curative endoscopic treatment:
  1. Endoscopic mucosal resection (EMR).
  2. Endoscopic submucosal dissection (ESD).
- Used for treatment of T_{1a}.

B. Surgery

- The primary indication for surgical resection is for potential cure.
- Indicated in patients whose tumors are confined to the esophageal wall and only limited local/regional disease is found.
- Used for treatment of T_{1b}, T_2, N_0 .
- Surgical procedures usually performed are:
  1. **Left thoracoabdominal approach.**
  2. **Right thoracotomy:**
     - o Also known as Ivor Lewis procedure or Lewis Tanner procedure.
     - o **It is a 2 phase esophagectomy:** Laparotomy followed by a right thoracotomy.
  3. **Mc Keown esophagectomy:**
     - o **It is a 3 phase esophagectomy:** Right thoracotomy followed by laparotomy, followed by neck incision.
  4. **Left thoracic resection or Sweet esophagectomy.**
  5. **Transhiatal esophagectomy or Orringer esophagectomy:**
     - o Cervical and abdominal approach.
     - o Gastric conduit is delivered to the neck for cervical anastomosis.
  6. **Minimally invasive approaches:**
     - o VATS (Video Assisted Thoracoscopic Surgery), laparoscopy or robotic techniques.

C. Multimodality Treatment

- Indicated for $\geq T_3$, N+.
- Neoadjuvant chemotherapy or neoadjuvant chemoradiotherapy is more popular than adjuvant therapy.
- Immunotherapy is also used.
- **Drugs used:** Cisplatin, carboplatin, 5-FU, taxanes.

D. Palliation

- **SEMS** or **Self-Expanding Metallic Stent** is a simple and effective means to relieve dysphagia.

CAUSES OF DYSPHAGIA

A. Esophageal Obstruction

- Peptic strictures.
- Schatzki ring.
- Malignancy.
- Benign neoplasm.
- Foreign body.

B. Esophageal Motility Disorders

- Ineffective esophageal motility.
- Diffuse esophageal spasm.

- Hypercontractile or 'jackhammer' esophagus.
- Fragmented peristalsis.
- Achalasia cardia.

OTHER IMPORTANT TOPICS

PER-ORAL ENDOSCOPIC MYOTOMY (POEM)

- It involves creation of a long esophageal myotomy using a flexible GI endoscope.
- After incising the esophageal mucosa, a tunnel is created in the esophageal wall, circular muscle is divided to a point distal to the LES and the esophageal mucosal opening is closed with clips.
- If done properly, it is as effective as laparoscopic Heller's myotomy.
- **Uses:**
  - o Achalasia cardia.
  - o Distal esophageal spasm.
  - o Hypercontractile esophagus.

39

Stomach and Duodenum

ANATOMY AND PHYSIOLOGY OF STOMACH

[5] Blood supply and lymphatic drainage of stomach. ***June 14***

Blood Supply of Stomach

Arterial Supply

- The stomach has an arterial supply on both the greater and lesser curves.
- There are 4 main arteries to the stomach:
  1. **Left gastric artery**
     - o Arises from the coeliac trunk and divides into an ascending (esophageal) branch and a descending branch.
     - o It is closely apposed to the lesser curvature, which it supplies along with the cardia.
  2. **Right gastric artery**
     - o Arises from the common hepatic artery.
     - o Divides into a number of branches to the stomach (and duodenum) along the lesser curvature and anastomoses with the left gastric artery.
  3. **Right gastroepiploic artery**
     - o Arises from the gastroduodenal artery (which itself arises from the hepatic artery).
     - o It anastomoses with the left gastroepiploic vessel with which it forms an arcade supplying the greater curvature.
  4. **Left gastroepiploic artery**
     - o Arises from the splenic artery.
     - o Contributes to the arterial arcade along the greater curvature.
     - o The splenic artery also gives 5-7 small branches (called short gastric arteries) which supply the fundus.

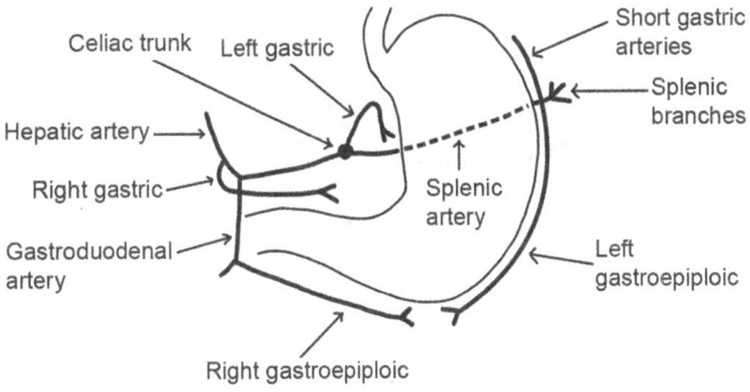

Figure 1: Blood supply of stomach

Venous Drainage

- In general, the veins accompany the arteries. Those along the lesser curvature drain into the portal vein and those along the greater curvature drain into the splenic vein.

Lymphatic Drainage of Stomach

- Understanding the lymphatic drainage of the stomach is the key to understanding radical surgery for gastric cancer.
- The lymphatics of the antrum drain into:
  - o **Superiorly:** Right gastric lymph nodes.
  - o **Inferiorly:** Right gastroepiploic lymph nodes and subpyloric lymph nodes.
- The lymphatics of the pylorus drain into:
  - o **Superiorly:** Right gastric suprapyloric nodes.
  - o **Inferiorly:** Subpyloric lymph nodes situated around the gastroduodenal artery.
- Efferent lymphatics from suprapyloric lymph nodes converge on the para-aortic nodes around the celiac axis.
- Efferent lymphatics from the subpyloric lymph nodes pass to the main superior mesenteric lymph nodes situated around the origin of the superior mesenteric artery.
- Lymphatics vessels related to the cardia communicate freely with those of the esophagus.

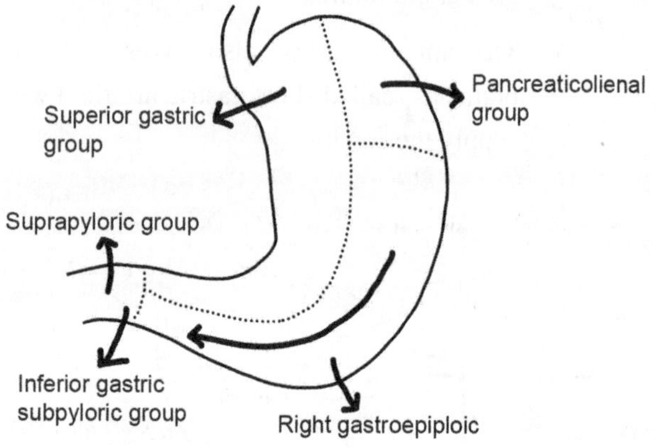

Figure 2: Lymphatic drainage of stomach

PEPTIC ULCER DISEASE

[5] Helicobacter pylori. ***Dec 18***

[3] Helicobacter pylori. ***July 23***

- It is a **Gram-negative, microaerophilic, spiral** (helical) bacterium usually found in the stomach.
- Infection with *H. pylori* **may be the most common human infection.**

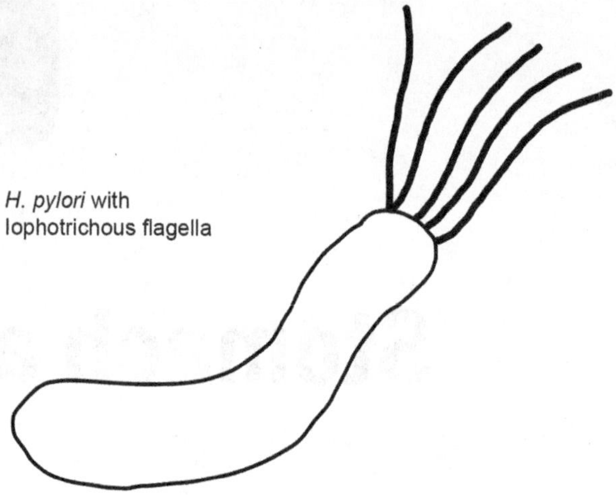

Figure 3: *Helicobacter pylori*

Conditions Associated with *H. Pylori*

1. Chronic gastritis (type B).
2. Peptic ulcer disease.
3. Gastric cancer, i.e., gastric adenocarcinoma.
4. Gastric MALT lymphoma.
5. Gastric diffuse large B cell lymphoma.

Epidemiology

- Infection with *H. pylori* may be the most common human infection.
- Incidence of infection **increases with age.**
- Most infections are **acquired in childhood.**
- Possibility of infection is **higher in low socio-economic** groups.
- Means of spread has not been identified, but the organism can occur in faeces and **faeco-oral spread** seems most likely.

Pathogenesis

1. Obligate urease activity

H. pylori hydrolyses urea

↓

Ammonia is produced (strong alkali)

↓

Stimulates antral G cells to release gastrin, i.e., **hypergastrinemia**

↓

Gastric acid hypersecretion

2. Infection with *H. pylori* leads to **disruption of the gastric mucous barrier** by the enzymes produced by the organism and induces inflammation in the gastric epithelium.
3. Some strains of *H. pylori* produce **cytotoxins**, notably the **Cag A and Vac A** products.
4. *H. pylori* is now classified by the WHO as a **class 1 carcinogen.**

Diagnosis

1. **C^{13} and C^{14} breath tests.**
2. **Rapid urease test**, is performed on gastric biopsies, which are taken endoscopically.
3. **Modified Giemsa stain and Warthin-Starry silver stain** are used to identify *H. pylori.*
4. **Culture media:** Brucella agar or Columbia agar.
5. Previous or current infection with the organism may also be detected **serologically.**
6. **Faecal antigen tests.**

Treatment

- The profound hypochlorhydria produced by **PPIs combined with antibiotics** is effective in eradicating the organism.
- **Commonly used eradication regimens include a PPI and two antibiotics such as metronidazole and amoxicillin.**
- Very high eradication rates can be achieved with combinations that **include the antibiotic clarithromycin.**

> [10] Describe the aetiology, clinical features, investigations and management of peptic ulcer disease. ***March 24***
>
> [10] Describe the aetiopathogenesis, clinical features, investigations and management of peptic ulcer disease. Add a note on gastric outlet obstruction. ***June 14***
>
> [5] Peptic ulcer. ***August 22, June 16***
>
> [5] Complications of duodenal ulcers. ***March 22, June 13***
>
> [3] Complications of peptic ulcer. ***March 21, July 15***

- **Definition:** Peptic ulcers are **erosions in the GI mucosa that extend through the muscularis mucosae.**

Acute v/s Chronic

- In the past, much distinction was made between acute and chronic peptic ulcers, however, this difference can sometimes be difficult to determine clinically.
- It is probably best to consider that there is a **spectrum of disease from the superficial gastric and duodenal ulceration, frequently seen at endoscopy, to deep chronic penetrating ulcers.**

Sites for Peptic Ulcers

- Common sites for peptic ulcers are:
  1. First part of duodenum.
  2. Lesser curvature of stomach.
  3. On the stoma following gastric surgery.
  4. Esophagus.
  5. Adjacent to a Meckel's diverticulum containing ectopic gastric epithelium.
- In general, the ulcer **occurs at a junction between different types of epithelia**, in the epithelium least resistant to acid damage.

Aetiopathogenesis

- Peptic ulcers are caused by **decreased defensive factors, increased aggressive factors or both.**
- Most ulcers are caused by ***H. pylori* infection or NSAID use.**

A. Defensive (or Protective) Factors

- Mucosal bicarbonate secretion.
- Mucous production.
- Adequate blood flow.
- Growth factors.
- Cell renewal.
- Endogenous prostaglandins.

B. Damaging (or Aggressive) Factors

- *Helicobacter pylori* infection.
- NSAIDs.
- Alcohol.
- Smoking.
- Hydrochloric acid secretion.

- Pepsins.
- Duodenal reflux of bile.
- Ischemia.
- Hypoxia.
- Gastrinoma (Zollinger-Ellison syndrome).

Clinical Features

- **Duodenal ulcers are more common** than gastric ulcers.
- **Duodenal ulcer:** M > F.
- **Gastric ulcer:** M = F.
- Gastric ulcers are more common in low socio-economic status, as *H. pylori* is more prevalent.
- **Pain:**
  - o The **most common symptom is mid epigastric abdominal pain** that is usually well localized.
  - o Pain is generally tolerable.
  - o **Gastric ulcers: Eating precipitates the pain.**
  - o **Duodenal ulcers: Eating may sometimes relieve the discomfort.**
  - o Pain is normally **intermittent** rather than intractable.
  - o Pain is **periodic**, i.e., symptoms may disappear for weeks or months only to return again. This periodicity may be related to the spontaneous healing of the ulcer.
  - o Pain is **worse during** periods of emotional **stress.**
  - o When pain becomes constant, this suggests that there is deeper penetration of the ulcer.
  - o Referral of pain to the back means penetration into pancreas.
  - o Diffuse peritoneal irritation is the result of free perforation.
- **Vomiting:**
  - o It is not a notable feature unless stenosis has occurred.
- **Alteration in weight:**
  - o Weight loss, or sometimes, weight gain may occur.
  - o Patients with gastric ulceration are often underweight, but this may precede occurrence of the ulcer.

Clinical Features of Complications

A. Bleeding

- May be chronic and presentation with **microcytic anemia** is not uncommon.
- Acute presentation is with **hematemesis and melena.**

B. Obstruction

- Gastric outlet obstruction can occur in **duodenal ulcers or in patients with type II or III gastric ulcers.**

C. Perforation

Gastric Ulcers

- The **most common complication of gastric ulcer is perforation.**
- **The most common site of gastric ulcer perforation is along the anterior aspect of lesser curvature.**

Duodenal Ulcers

- Anterior duodenal ulcers perforate.
- Posterior duodenal ulcers bleed.

D. Fistula Formation

- Spontaneous gastrocolic fistulas may occur with benign gastric ulcers.

E. Malignancy

Gastric Ulcers

- Associated with malignancy.
- It is **difficult to differentiate between gastric carcinoma and a benign ulcer.**
- A benign appearing gastric ulcer may actually be malignant and an ulcerated gastric cancer may mimic a benign ulcer.

Duodenal Ulcers

- Malignancy is extremely rare.

Investigations

A. Gastroduodenoscopy

- Visualizes the entire stomach and duodenum (first and second part).
- A 'U' manoeuvre is carried out to inspect the incisura, lesser curve and GEJ.
- Biopsy can be taken:

- o To rule out malignancy.
- o **Rapid Urease Test (RUT)** kits are commercially available which can be used on the biopsy specimen to diagnose the presence of ***H. pylori.***
- o Sample can be stained with routine hematoxylin-eosin stains or special stains (e.g., silver, Giemsa, Genta) to diagnose *H. pylori.*
- o Histology can also assess the severity of gastritis.
- o Attention should be given to the pylorus to note whether there is any prepyloric or pyloric channel ulceration, and also whether it is deformed, which is often the case with chronic duodenal ulceration.
- o In the duodenum, care must be taken to view all of the first part and the endoscope advanced into the second part.

B. Urea Breath Test

- Non-invasive.
- Carbon labelled urea breath test is based on the ability of *H. pylori* to hydrolyze urea as a result of its production of urease.

C. Stool Antigen Can Diagnose *H. pylori.*

D. Serology Can be Used to Diagnose *H. pylori.*

E. Upper GI Radiography:

- In a duodenal ulcer, barium can be demonstrated within the ulcer crater.
- Useful to determine the location and depth of penetration of the ulcer and the extent of deformation from chronic fibrosis.

Treatment

A. Medical Treatment

a. Antacids:

- Reduce gastric acidity by reacting with HCl, forming a salt, and raising the gastric pH.
- Magnesium and aluminium salts are used.

b. Sucralfate:

- Sucrose polymerises and binds to the ulcer crater to produce a protective coating that can last for 6 hours.
- Helps in mucosal healing.

c. H_2 receptor antagonists:

- Famotidine, Ranitidine, Cimetidine.
- Decrease the production of HCl by inhibiting the H_2 receptors on parietal cells.

d. Proton pump inhibitors:

- Most potent drugs which decrease the production of HCl.
- Irreversibly bind and inhibit the H^+-K^+ ATPase on the parietal cell.

e. Treatment of *H. pylori* infection, i.e., eradication therapy:

- Eradication therapy is now routinely given to patients with peptic ulceration.
  1. **Bismuth quadruple therapy** = PPI + bismuth + tetracycline + metronidazole.
  2. **Clarithromycin triple therapy** = PPI + clarithromycin + amoxicillin ***or*** PPI + clarithromycin + metronidazole.
  3. **Concomitant regimen** = PPI + clarithromycin + amoxicillin + metronidazole.
- If *H. pylori* is the main aetiological factor (essentially in patients not taking NSAIDs), then complete eradication of the organism will cure the disease.
- Eradication therapy has no role in patients with NSAID associated ulcers.

B. Surgical Procedures for Peptic Ulcer

- Elective surgeries for peptic ulcer disease have become rare as medical therapy has improved.
- The goal for operative ulcer therapy is as follows:

Duodenal Ulcers

- **To exclude acid from the duodenum.**
- This is done by:
  - o **Diversion of acid** away from the duodenum.
  - o **Reducing the secretory potential** of the stomach.
- These can be accomplished by:
  - o Removing vagal stimulation via **vagotomy.**
  - o Removing gastrin-driven secretion by performing an **antrectomy.**

- o Decreasing the number of parietal cells with a **subtotal gastrectomy.**
- o **Combination** procedure.

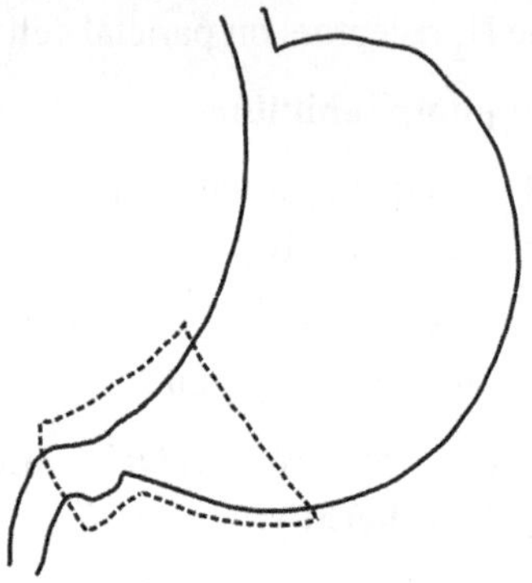

Figure 4: Antrectomy

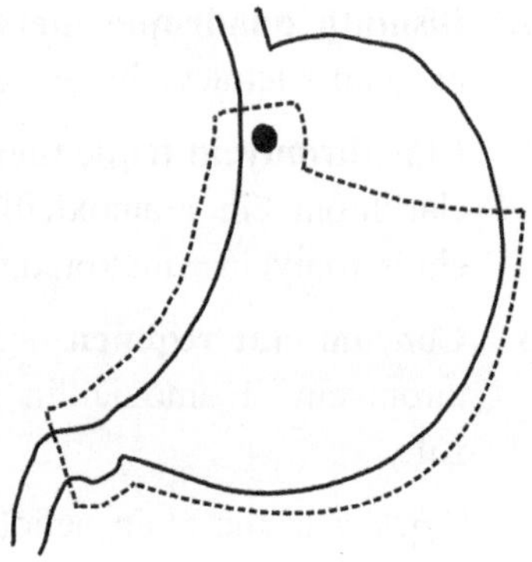

Figure 5: Subtotal gastrectomy

Gastric Ulcers

- In contrast to surgery for duodenal ulcer, where the principal objective is to reduce duodenal exposure to gastric acid, in gastric ulcer surgery **the ulcer is usually excised so that malignancy can then be confidently excluded.**
- The standard operation is the **Billroth I.**

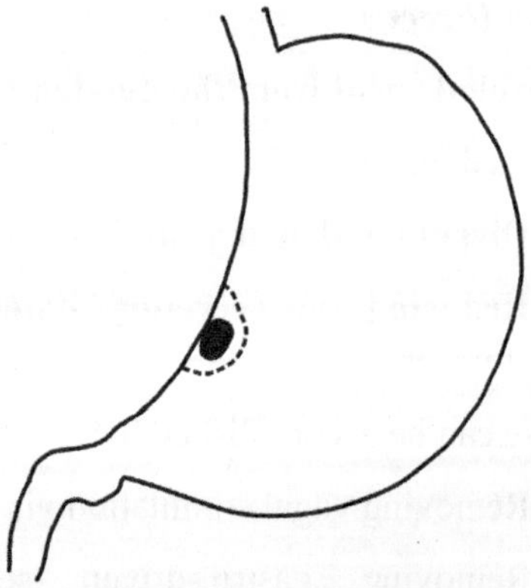

Figure 6: Ulcer excision

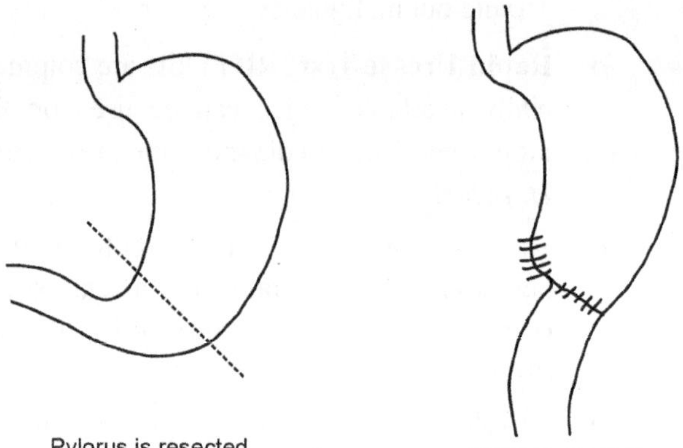

Figure 7: Billroth I

GASTRIC OUTLET OBSTRUCTION

- Gastric Outlet Obstruction (GOO) refers to a condition where there is a blockage preventing stomach contents from passing into the duodenum.
- The 2 most common causes of GOO are gastric cancer and pyloric stenosis secondary to peptic ulceration.
- With the decreasing incidence of peptic ulceration, GOO should be considered malignant, unless and until proven otherwise.

Causes

- **Peptic ulcer disease:** Ulcers can cause swelling and inflammation, leading to obstruction.
- **Gastric cancer:** Tumours in the stomach can grow and block the outlet.
- **Pancreatic cancer:** Tumours near the duodenum can compress and obstruct the gastric outlet.
- **Gallstones:** Large gall stones can migrate into the duodenum and cause obstruction.
- **Duodenal strictures:** Narrowing of the duodenum due to inflammation or scarring.
- **Foreign bodies:** Ingested objects can sometimes obstruct the gastric outlet.
- **Functional pyloric stenosis**
- **Congenital or infantile hypertrophic pyloric stenosis**
- **Crohn's disease:** Can lead to strictures in the GIT, including near the stomach outlet.
- **Infections:** Rarely, infections or parasitic infestations can cause obstruction.
- **Post-surgical iatrogenic adhesions.**

Pathophysiology

- **Acute inflammation** of the duodenum or pylorus can lead to mechanical **obstruction, because of edema.**
- **Chronic inflammation** leads to recurrent episodes of injury and healing, ultimately leading to **fibrosis, scarring and stenosis** of the outflow tract.
- The **stomach can become massively dilated** in this setting and lose its muscular tone.

Clinical Features

- In benign GOO, there is usually a **long history of peptic ulcer disease.**
- History of **vomiting** which is characteristically of **undigested food and is non-bilious.**
- Weight loss.
- Early satiety.
- Anorexia.
- Patient appears unwell and dehydrated.
- Features of the underlying disease.

Metabolic Effects of GOO

- Vomiting HCl results in **hypochloremic alkalosis**.
- Initially, the urine has a low chloride and high bicarbonate content, reflecting the primary metabolic abnormality.
- As vomiting continues, **dehydration progresses**, and more profound metabolic abnormalities arise, partly related to renal dysfunction.
- With time, the patient becomes progressively hyponatremic and more profoundly dehydrated.
- Because of the dehydration, **sodium is retained and potassium and hydrogen ions are excreted**.
- This results in the **urine becoming paradoxically acidic and hypokalemia ensues**.
- **Alkalosis leads to a lowering in the circulating ionized calcium** and tetany can occur.
- **End result: Hypokalemic, hypochloremic, metabolic alkalosis with paradoxical aciduria**.

Investigations

A. Lab tests

- CBC
- Electrolytes
- Renal Function Tests
- Liver Function Tests

B. Imaging

- Upper GI series or barium meal
- CT scan
    - o Identifies the cause of obstruction, such as tumours or external compression.
    - o Evaluates extent of obstruction.

C. Upper GI endoscopy

- Esophagogastroduodenoscopy.
- Can directly visualise the obstruction and even identify its cause (e.g. peptic ulcer, tumour).
- Biopsies of suspicious lesions or tissues can be taken.
- Also has a therapeutic role as it can treat the obstruction by dilation or stenting.

D. Additional tests

- Gastric Emptying Studies can help diagnose functional causes of obstruction.
- Endoscopic Ultrasound (EUS) is useful for identifying the nature of the obstruction (e.g., tumour invasion).

Treatment

- Involves two things:
    1. **Correcting the metabolic abnormalities.**
    2. **Dealing with the mechanical obstruction.**
- Patient should be **rehydrated with IV isotonic NS with potassium supplementation.**
- Replacing the sodium chloride and water allows the kidney to correct the acid-base abnormality.
- Metabolic abnormalities may be less if the obstruction is due to malignancy, as the acid-base disturbance is less pronounced.
- Stomach should be emptied using a wide bore tube.
- A large NGT may not be sufficiently large to deal with the contents of the stomach, and it may be necessary to pass an orogastric tube and lavage the stomach until it is completely emptied.
- This allows investigation with endoscopy and contrast radiology.
- **Biopsy of the area around the pylorus is essential to exclude malignancy.**

- Early cases may settle with conservative treatment, as edema around the ulcer diminishes as the ulcer is healed.
- Traditionally, **severe cases are treated surgically, usually with a gastroenterostomy rather than a pyloroplasty.**
- **Endoscopic treatment with balloon dilatation** may be most useful in early cases and may have to be repeated several times.
- A **duodenal stent insertion** may be considered in patients with unresectable malignancy.

[3] Hourglass stomach. ***Feb 23***

- It is due to **cicatricial contracture around a saddle-shaped, lesser curve ulcer**.
- In extreme cases, the stomach is divided into 2 compartments, united by a channel which barely admits a pencil.

Clinical Features

- F >>> M.
- Symptoms become constant and periodicity is lost.
- Vomiting is more frequent.
- Weight loss.

Investigations

- Barium meal.
- Endoscopy.

Treatment

- Billroth I gastrectomy, with removal of the 2nd pouch and the isthmus.

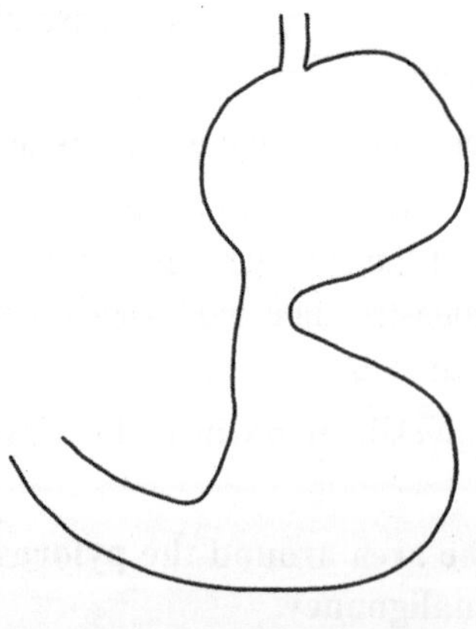

Figure 8: Hourglass stomach

TEAPOT STOMACH

- Also known as **handbag stomach.**
- **Cicatrisation around a long-standing gastric ulcer** often causes **shortening of the lesser curvature**, thus producing the teapot deformity of the stomach.
- Presents with signs and symptoms of **pyloric stenosis.**
- **Investigations:** Barium meal, endoscopy.

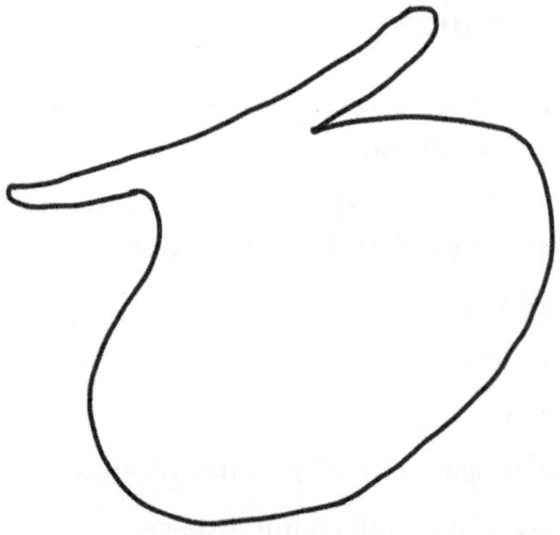

Figure 9: Teapot stomach

[3] Vagotomy. ***March 22***

SURGICAL TREATMENT OF PEPTIC ULCER

Duodenal Ulcer

- The **goal of surgery** in duodenal ulcers is **to exclude acid from the duodenum**. This is done by:
  - o **Diversion of acid** away from the duodenum.
  - o **Reducing the secretory potential** of the stomach.

A. Gastrectomy Based Procedures

- Gastrectomy in the form of either Billroth I or Billroth II/Polya is performed.
- **Billroth I gastrectomy:** The lower half of the stomach is removed, and the cut stomach is anastomosed to the first part of the duodenum.
- **Billroth II/Polya gastrectomy:** Two-thirds of the stomach is removed, the duodenal stump is closed and the stomach is anastomosed to the jejunum. This diverts the gastric secretions away from the duodenum.

- There is no elective role for these procedures in the treatment of duodenal ulcer, but the safer Polya procedure is occasionally needed in the management of complex ulcer disease presenting as an emergency.

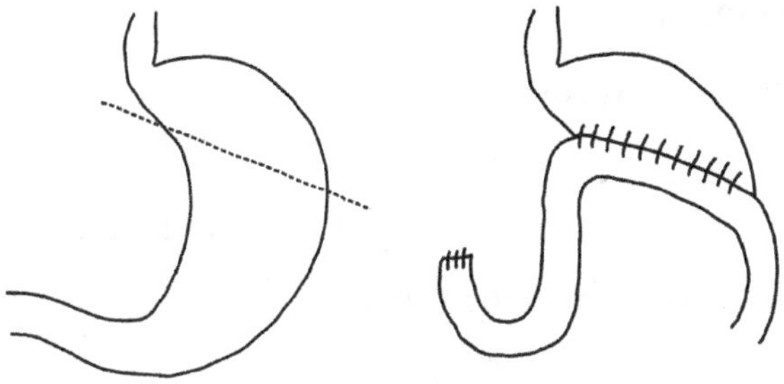

Figure 10: Billroth II or Polya gastrectomy

B. Vagotomy

- Vagotomy, i.e., sectioning of the vagus nerve decreases peak acid output by ~ 50%, whereas vagotomy + antrectomy decreases peak acid output by ~ 85%.

1. Truncal Vagotomy

  - Performed by **division of the left and right vagus nerves above the hepatic and celiac branches**, just above the GEJ.
  - Some from of **drainage procedure is usually done** along with truncal vagotomy to avoid gastric stasis. This is because pyloric relaxation is mediated by vagal stimulation, and a **vagotomy without a drainage procedure can cause delayed gastric emptying**, e.g., Heineke-Mikulicz pyloroplasty.
  - **When the duodenal bulb is scarred, a Finney pyloroplasty or Jaboulay gastroduodenostomy** may be a useful alternative.
  - Significant scarring or inflammation may necessitate a **gastrojejunostomy**.
  - Truncal vagotomy can also be **combined with antrectomy.**

- **Selective Vagotomy**
  - **Divides the main right and left vagus nerves** just distal to the celiac and hepatic branches.
  - Pyloric drainage procedure is also performed.
- **Highly Selective Vagotomy**
  - Also known as parietal cell vagotomy or proximal gastric vagotomy.
  - **Divides only the vagus nerves supplying the acid producing portion of the stomach** within the corpus and fundus.
  - Preserves the vagal innervation of the gastric antrum and pylorus, so there is **no need for routine drainage procedures.**

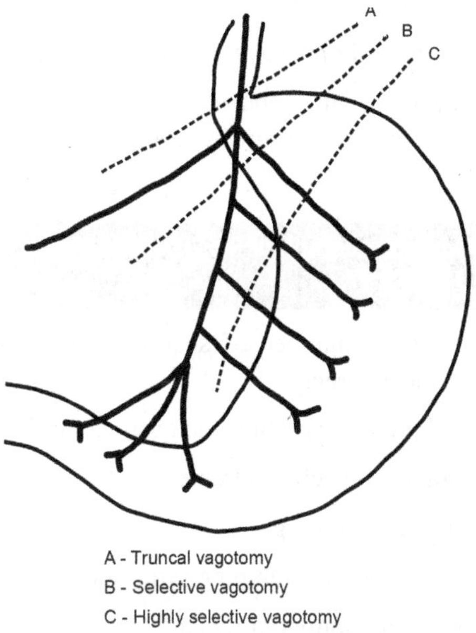

Figure 11: Types of vagotomy

C. Gastrojejunostomy

- It is an alternative drainage procedure to pyloroplasty.
- Jejunum is anastomosed to the posterior, dependent wall of the stomach.

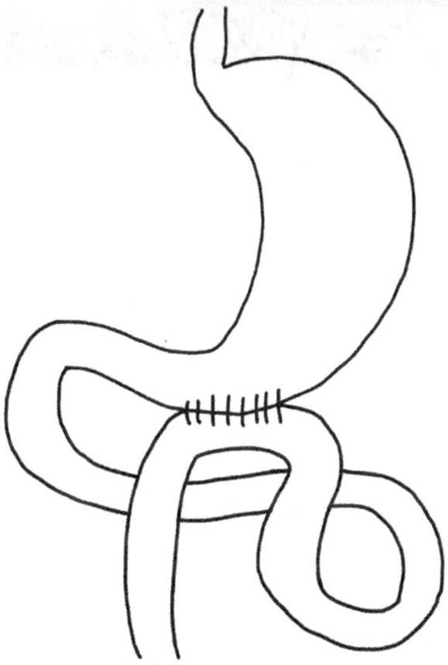

Figure 12: Gastrojejunostomy

Gastric Ulcer

- In contrast to surgery for duodenal ulcer, where the principal objective is to reduce duodenal exposure to gastric acid, in gastric ulcer surgery **the ulcer is usually excised so that malignancy can then be confidently excluded.**
- **The standard operation is the Billroth I.**
- However, as with duodenal ulceration, such surgery is now performed only for complications of gastric ulcer.

[3] Mention complications of peptic ulcer surgery. ***Dec 15***

- There are a number of sequelae/complications of peptic ulcer surgery:
  1. Recurrent ulceration and gastrocolic fistula.
  2. Small stomach syndrome.
  3. Bilious vomiting.
  4. Early and late dumping syndrome.
  5. Post vagotomy diarrhoea.
  6. Malignant transformation.
  7. Nutritional disorders (weight loss, vitamin deficiencies).
  8. Gallstones.
- These sequelae principally follow from the more destructive operations that are now seldom performed.

[3] Bleeding peptic ulcer. ***Dec 19***

Risk Factors

- Older age group.
- NSAID use.
- *H. pylori.*

Clinical Features

- Patients with upper GI bleeding from peptic ulcer disease can present with **hematemesis, melena or both.**

Investigations

- Upper GI endoscopy is used to visualize the lesion.
- The lesion can be categorized using the **Forrest classification**.
- **Blatchford and Rockall scoring system** is used to grade the severity of bleeding.

Treatment

A. Medical Treatment

- Limited efficacy.
- **Drugs:** H_2 antagonists, PPIs, tranexamic acid.
- Treatment of *H. pylori.*

B. Therapeutic Endoscopy

- Can achieve hemostasis in 70% of cases.
- **Combination of adrenaline injection with heater probe and/or clips.**
- **Argon laser** can also be used to achieve hemostasis.
- Therapeutic endoscopy is not effective in patients who are bleeding from large vessels.

C. Angioembolization

- Indicated in patients where the source of bleeding cannot be identified or in those who rebleed after endoscopy.
- **Angiography with transcatheter embolization** is used.

D. Surgical Treatment

- Patients with the following findings on endoscopy are candidates for surgical treatment:
  - o Visible vessel in the ulcer base.
  - o Spurting vessel.
  - o An ulcer with a clot in the base.
  - o In general, a patient who has required > 6 units of blood transfusion needs surgical treatment.
  - o Oversewing of bleeding vessel (usually the gastroduodenal artery) with a three-point U stitch technique.

[5] Clinical features and management of perforated peptic ulcer. ***June 19***

[3] Pneumoperitoneum. ***March 21***

- Perforation is a complication of peptic ulcer disease.

Risk Factors

- NSAID use.
- *Helicobacter pylori* infection.
- Stressful lifestyle.

Sites of Perforation

- Anterior surface of duodenum (most common).
- Anterior surface of stomach, usually near the lesser curvature or the pyloric antrum.
- Rarely, an ulcer on the posterior wall of the stomach perforates into the lesser sac.

Pathogenesis

- The gastric or duodenal contents escape through the perforation into the general peritoneal cavity, resulting in peritoneal irritation (called **peritonism**). This causes pain.
- The **peritoneum reacts to this chemical irritation by secreting peritoneal fluid copiously** and this gives relief of pain for a short time.
- This stage of reaction lasts from 3-6 hours, and is followed by **diffuse bacterial peritonitis**.
- Usually, the symptoms of perforation occur with dramatic suddenness.

Clinical Features

- A patient who may have a **history of peptic ulceration**, develops **sudden onset severe generalized pain abdomen** (due to the irritant effect of gastric acid on peritoneum).
- **Bacterial peritonitis supervenes** over a few hours, usually accompanied by a deterioration in the patient's condition.

On Examination

- Patient is in a state of **shock,** with tachycardia.
- **Pyrexia** is observed few hours after the event.
- Patient **lies still**, as even the slightest movement causes pain.
- **Per abdomen:**
  - o **Board like rigidity.**
  - o Does not move with respiration.
  - o Sufficient gas may escape to reduce or even **obliterate liver dullness** in the mid axillary line.
  - o **Pelvic tenderness** may be elicited on rectal examination.

Investigations

1. **Plain X-rays:**
   - **Chest X-ray is the investigation of choice** to detect pneumoperitoneum.
   - Erect X-ray of abdomen also shows pneumoperitoneum.
   - Free **gas under diaphragm** is seen.
   - **Rigler sign or double wall sign:** Gas outlines both sides of the bowel wall, i.e., gas within the bowel's lumen and gas within the peritoneal cavity.
   - **Cupola sign:** On supine X-ray of abdomen, lucency is seen overlying the lower thoracic vertebral bodies.
   - **Continuous diaphragm sign:** Diaphragm can be seen continuously across the midline.
   - **Leaping dolphin sign.**
2. **CT scan:**
   - Accurately detects and localizes bowel perforation.
3. **Upper GI study with water soluble contrast medium *or* small bowel follow through with oral contrast:**
   - Can be useful for confirmation of an equivocal appearance on CT.

Treatment

The treatment is initial resuscitation followed by surgery:

A. Resuscitation

- NPO.
- IV fluids.
- Analgesics.
- Antibiotics.

B. Open Surgery

- **Exploratory laparotomy** is performed, usually through an upper midline incision.

- The most important component of the operation is a **thorough peritoneal lavage** to remove all of the fluid and food debris.
- **Duodenal perforation:**
    - o **Perforations < 1 cm** can be **closed primarily** and **buttressed** with a well-vascularized **omentum.**
    - o For larger perforations or ulcers with fibrotic edges that cannot be brought together without tension, a **Graham patch repair** with healthy omentum is performed.

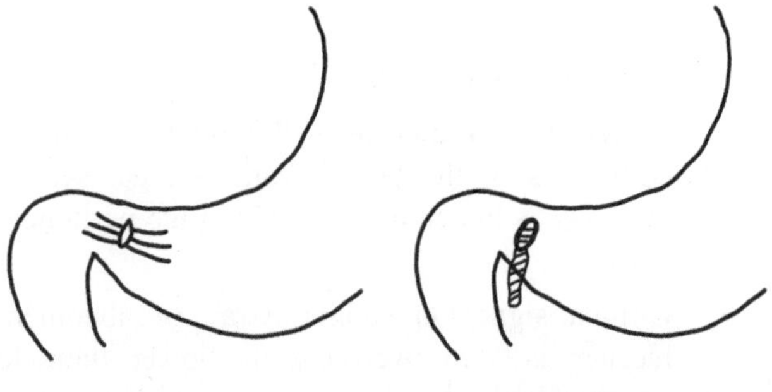

Figure 13: Graham omental patch

- Gastric ulcers should, if possible, be excised and closed, so that malignancy can be excluded.
- For patients with massive duodenal or gastric perforation in whom simple closure is impossible, a **distal gastrectomy with Roux-en-Y reconstruction** is the procedure of choice.

C. Laparoscopy

- Can be done if the expertise is available.

D. Post-Op

- Stomach is kept empty post operatively by Ryle's tube to promote healing in the residual ulcer.
- PPI.
- *H. pylori* eradication is mandatory.

[5]	Congenital Hypertrophic Pyloric Stenosis. ***Sept 21***
[3]	Ramstedt operation. ***March 22***
[5]	Electrolyte abnormalities in Congenital Hypertrophic Pyloric Stenosis. ***March 21***
[5]	Infantile Hypertrophic Pyloric Stenosis. ***Dec 16***

- Also known as infantile hypertrophic pyloric stenosis.
- It is a **disease of neonates and infants,** starting between 2 and 6 weeks of age.

Aetiopathogenesis

- Boys > girls.
- First born male infants are at highest risk.

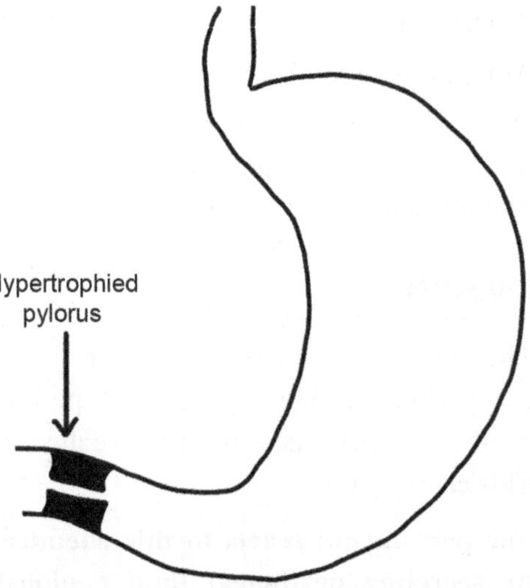

Figure 14: Hypertrophied pylorus in congenital hypertrophic pyloric stenosis

Hypertrophy of the circular muscle of the pylorus
↓
Constriction and obstruction of the gastric outlet
↓
Non-bilious, projectile vomiting

- Although the exact cause is unknown, a lack of nitric oxide synthase in pyloric tissue has been implicated.
- Maternal family history.

Clinical Features

- Most common between the ages of 2 and 8 weeks.
- Infants present with progressively worsening, **non-bilious emesis** that is **projectile** in nature.
- Immediately **after vomiting**, the baby is often very **hungry.**
- **Constipation** is usually present, and when stool is passed, it is small and dry.
- Loss of weight.
- Failure to thrive.

On Examination

- Visible peristalsis.
- After the child has been fed, **peristaltic waves may be seen passing from left to right** across the upper abdomen.
- Palpation of the pyloric '**olive**' tumour in the epigastrium is pathognomonic.
- The hypertrophied pylorus is best felt in a relaxed (feeding) baby.

Metabolic and Electrolyte Abnormalities

- Persistent vomiting leads to loss of hydrochloric acid, which results in hypochloremic alkalosis.
- Initially, the urine has a low chloride and high bicarbonate content, reflecting the primary metabolic abnormality.
- As vomiting continues, dehydration progresses and more profound metabolic abnormalities arise, partly related to renal dysfunction.
- With time the patient becomes progressively hyponatremic and more dehydrated.
- Because of the dehydration, sodium is retained and potassium and hydrogen ions are excreted.
- This results in the urine becoming paradoxically acidic and hypokalemia ensues.
- Alkalosis leads to a lowering in the circulating ionized calcium, and tetany can occur.
- **End result: Hypokalemic, hypochloremic, metabolic alkalosis with paradoxical aciduria.**

Investigations

- **USG:** In the presence of functional gastric outlet obstruction, the following findings are diagnostic:
  - o Pyloric muscle thickness > 3 - 4 mm.
  - o Pyloric muscle length > 15 - 18 mm.

Treatment

A. Correction of Metabolic and Electrolyte Abnormalities

- Resuscitation with IV fluids establishes an adequate urine output, which in turn, restores acid-base balance.
- Child is kept NPO and the stomach is emptied with a 8 - 10 Fr nasogastric tube.
- Correction may take 24 - 48 hours.
- 0.9% NS with 0.15% KCl in 5D given at 6-7.5 ml/kg/hr provides maintenance and corrects the abnormalities, i.e.:
  - o 0.9% Normal Saline (NS).
  - o 0.15% Potassium Chloride in 5% Dextrose.
- As the chloride defect is replaced, the kidneys correct the pH.

B. Surgery

- **Ramstedt's pyloromyotomy** is performed:
  - o Laparoscopically.
  - o Open surgery – through a supraumbilical or RUQ incision.
- A pyloric serosal incision is made, and deepened to cut the muscularis propria, leaving an intact submucosa.
- Incision must extend onto the stomach. It is usually made from the duodenal fornix to the gastric antrum. Short incisions cause an early recurrence.

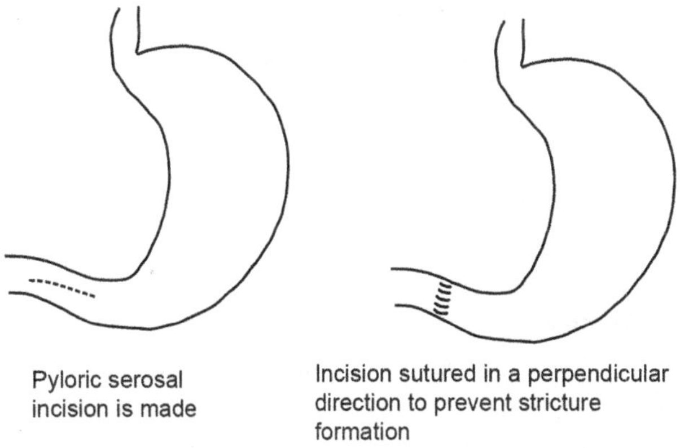

Figure 15: Ramstedt pyloromyotomy

C. Post-op Care

- IV fluids are continued until oral feeds are re-established within 24 hours.

CA STOMACH

[10] Discuss clinical features, pathology and management of carcinoma of stomach. ***June 19***

[3] Modes of spread of Ca stomach. ***Dec 18, July 18, June 13***

[10] Carcinoma stomach – aetiopathogenesis, diagnosis and management. ***June 17***

[10] Discuss causes, pathology, clinical features and management of carcinoma of stomach. ***July 15***

- It is one of the **most common causes of cancer death.**
- Outlook is generally poor, owing to the advanced stage at presentation.

Aetiology

It is a **multi-factorial disease**. The factors associated with increased risk for developing stomach cancer are as follows:

A. Nutritional

- Low fat or protein consumption.
- Salted or smoked meat, fish.
- High nitrate consumption (N-nitroso compounds).
- Obesity.
- High complex carbohydrate consumption.
- Deficiency of anti-oxidants.

B. Environmental

- Lack of refrigeration.
- Poor drinking water (e.g., contaminated well water).
- Smoking.
- Alcohol.
- Dust ingestion from a variety of industrial processes.

C. Medical

- Prior gastric or peptic ulcer surgery. This is thought to be related to bile reflux and intestinal metaplasia.
- *H. pylori* and Epstein-Barr virus infection.
- Atrophic gastritis.
- Gastric adenomatous polyps.
- Pernicious anaemia.
- Prior abdominal irradiation.

D. Genetic

Site Affected

- The most common site for gastric cancer in the West is **proximal stomach.**
- There is an increase in the incidence of carcinoma in the proximal stomach, **particularly the GEJ.**

Pathology

A. Lauren Classification

- The most useful clinicopathological classification of gastric cancer is the Lauren classification.
- In this system, there are principally two forms of gastric cancer:
  1. Intestinal gastric cancer.
  2. Diffuse gastric cancer (often with signet ring cells).

INTESTINAL	DIFFUSE
Tumour resembles a carcinoma elsewhere in the tubular GIT	Infiltrates deeply into the stomach
Forms polypoid tumours or ulcer	Does not form obvious mass lesions but spreads widely in the gastric wall
Probably arises in areas of intestinal metaplasia	—
Better prognosis	Worse prognosis

B. Gastric Cancer Can Be Divided into Early Gastric Cancer and Advanced Gastric Cancer

EARLY

- Defined as cancer limited to the mucosa and submucosa with or without lymph node involvement.
- The **Japanese classification**, further divides early gastric cancer into the following types:
  - o **Type 1 and 2:** Involves only mucosa.
  - o **Type 3:** Involves submucosa also.
    1. Protruded.
    2. Superficial:
       a. Elevated.
       b. Flat.
       c. Depressed.
    3. Excavated.

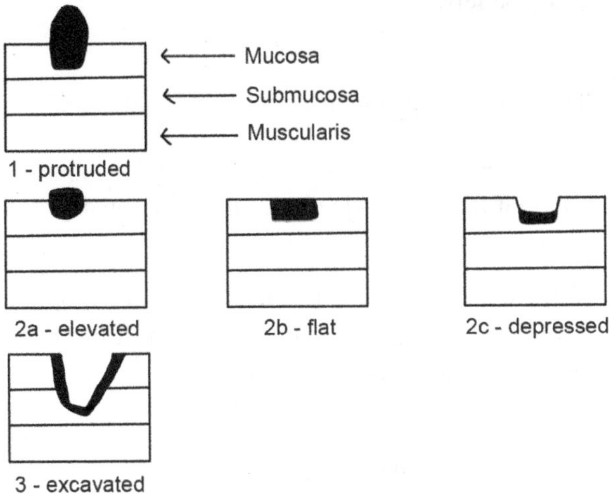

Figure 16: Japanese classification of gastric cancer

ADVANCED

- Involves the muscularis.
- The macroscopic appearance of advanced gastric cancer has been classified by **Bormann** into 4 types:
  1. Polypoid.
  2. Fungating.
  3. Ulcerative.
  4. Diffuse/Linitis plastica.

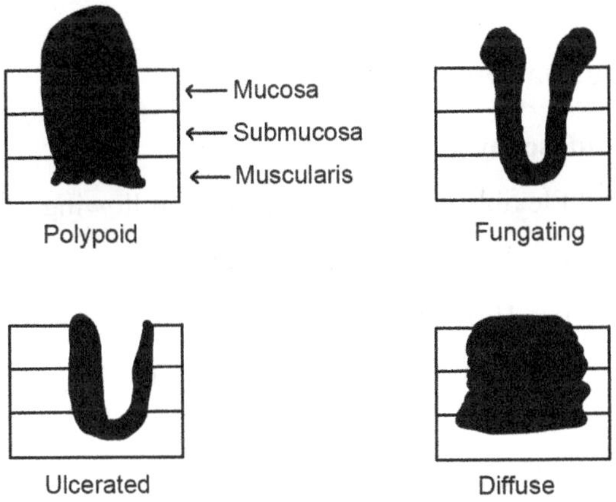

Figure 17: Bormann classification of gastric cancer

Staging

- TNM staging is widely used.
- All gastric tumours whose epicentre is within 5 cm of GEJ and extend into esophagus are classified as esophageal cancers and are staged according to the esophageal staging system.
- Tumours whose epicentre is within 5 cm of GEJ, but do not extend into the esophagus, and all other gastric cancers, are staged using the gastric staging system.
- **Tx:** Primary tumour cannot be assessed.
- **T0:** No evidence of primary tumour.
- **Tis:** Carcinoma *in situ*: Intraepithelial tumour without invasion of the lamina propria, high-grade dysplasia.
- **T1:** Tumour involves lamina propria, muscularis mucosa or submucosa.
  - o **1a:** Tumour invades lamina propria or muscularis mucosa.
  - o **1b:** Tumour invades submucosa.
- **T2:** Tumour invades muscularis propria.
- **T3:** Tumour involves subserosa.
- **T4:** Tumour perforates serosa (visceral peritoneum) or invades adjacent structures.
  - o **4a:** Tumour perforates serosa.
  - o **4b:** Tumour invades adjacent structures.
- **Nx:** Regional lymph nodes cannot be assessed.
- **N0:** No regional lymph node metastasis.
- **N1:** Metastasis in 1 or 2 regional lymph nodes.
- **N2:** Metastasis in 3–6 regional lymph nodes.
- **N3:** Metastasis in $\geq$ 7 regional lymph nodes.
  - o **3a:** Metastasis in 7–15 regional lymph nodes.
  - o **3b:** Metastasis in $\geq$ 16 regional lymph nodes.
- **M0:** No distant metastasis.
- **M1:** Distant metastasis.
- Involvement of non-regional intra-abdominal lymph nodes such as retropancreatic, mesenteric and para-aortic groups is considered to be distant metastasis (M1).
- Involvement of the liver or the presence of peritoneal seedlings is also staged as M1.

Spread of Carcinoma Stomach

A. Direct Spread

- Tumour penetrates the muscularis, serosa and ultimately adjacent organs such as the pancreas, colon and liver.

B. Lymphatic Spread

- This is by both permeation and emboli to the affected tiers of lymph nodes.
- May be extensive.
- **Troisier's sign: Tumour appears in the left supraclavicular lymph nodes.**
- Diffuse type of gastric cancer (as per Lauren's classification) spreads via the submucosal and subserosal lymphatic plexus and penetrates the gastric wall at an early stage.
- Unlike malignancies such as breast cancer, nodal involvement does not imply systemic dissemination.

C. Blood Borne Metastases

- **Occurs first to the liver** and subsequently to other organs, including lungs and bone.
- Uncommon in the absence of nodal disease.

D. Transperitoneal Spread

- It is a **common mode of spread once the tumour has reached the serosa** of the stomach.
- Indicates incurability.
- Tumours can manifest anywhere in the peritoneal cavity and commonly gives rise to **ascites.**
- Advanced peritoneal disease may be palpated either abdominally or rectally as a tumour 'shelf' (called **Blumer's shelf**).
- Ovaries may sometimes be the only site of transcoelomic spread (called **Krukenberg's tumour**).
- Tumours may spread via the abdominal cavity to the umbilicus (called **Sister Mary Joseph's nodule**).
- Transperitoneal spread of gastric cancer can be **detected most effectively by laparoscopy** and cytology.

Clinical Features

- Men > women.
- Incidence increases with age.
- Unfortunately, early gastric cancer **has no specific features to distinguish it from benign dyspepsia and a high index of suspicion is therefore necessary.**
- The clinical features of advanced gastric cancer are usually obvious.
- Early satiety.
- Bloating.
- Distension of abdomen.
- Vomiting.
- Tumour frequently bleeds, resulting in iron deficiency anemia.
- Gastric outlet obstruction leads to dysphagia, epigastric fullness or vomiting, which in turn causes metabolic alkalosis.
- Asthenia.
- Significant weight loss due to anorexia.
- Non metastatic effects of malignancy are seen. These features result from the effects of the tumour on thrombotic and hemostatic mechanisms, e.g., **Trousseau's sign** (phlebothrombosis of superficial veins of leg, deep vein thrombosis).
- Metastatic symptoms:
  - o Obstructive jaundice due to secondary deposits in the liver.
  - o Ascites from carcinomatosis of the peritoneum
  - o Krukenberg's tumours.
  - o **Troisier's sign:** Enlarged lymph node in left supraclavicular fossa.

Investigations

A. Endoscopy

- Flexible endoscopy allows the following:
  - o Visualisation of tumour.
  - o Biopsy can be taken.
  - o Can help treat patients with obstruction or bleeding.

B. Endoscopic Ultrasound

- It gives the following information:
  - o Provides the most accurate evaluation of the **depth of tumour** invasion.
  - o Assessment of **perigastric lymph node** involvement.
  - o Can sometimes identify **involvement of surrounding organs** or the presence of ascites.

C. CT Scan

- Of chest, abdomen and pelvis with oral and IV contrast agents is **mandatory to evaluate metastatic disease.**

D. PET-CT Scan

- Can detect **occult mets.**
- Done in patients who are being considered for neoadjuvant chemotherapy.

E. Staging Laparoscopy.

Treatment

A. Neoadjuvant Chemotherapy

- **FLOT regimen is used:** 5-fluorouracil, leucovorin, oxaliplatin, taxanes (docetaxel).
- **ECF regimen was used earlier:** Epirubicin, cisplatin, 5-fluorouracil.

B. Surgery

- **Complete resection of the gastric tumour with a wide margin of normal stomach** is the standard of care for resection with curative intent.
- Extent of resection depends on the location of the tumour in the stomach and size of the tumour:

 1. **Total gastrectomy**
    - o Stomach is removed en bloc, including the tissues of the entire greater omentum and lesser omentum.
    - o Gastrointestinal continuity is reconstituted by means of a roux loop, i.e., an esophagojejunostomy.
    - o Extent of lymph node dissection:
      - ♦ **D1:** Involves removal of the perigastric nodes.
      - ♦ **D2:** Involves clearance of the major arterial trunks.
 2. **Subtotal gastrectomy**
    - o Proximal stomach is preserved.
    - o Indicated for tumours in the distal stomach.
    - o Preferred reconstruction is to use a roux loop.
    - o Billroth II reconstruction can also be used.
 3. **Palliative surgery**
    - o In patients with significant symptoms of either obstruction or bleeding, palliative resection is appropriate.

C. Other Treatment Modalities

- Because of the failure of radical surgery to cure advanced gastric cancer, other treatment modalities are used. These are palliative:

 1. **Palliative radiotherapy**
    - o Routine use of radiotherapy is controversial and not recommended.
    - o Radiotherapy has a role in the palliative treatment of painful bony mets.
 2. **Palliative chemotherapy**
    - o ECF or FLOT regimens are generally used.
    - o Trastuzumab is also used.

OTHERS

[3] Zollinger-Ellison Syndrome. *March 22*

- Also known as gastrinoma.
- **Definition:** It is a condition that includes:

 1. **Fulminating ulcer diathesis in the stomach, duodenum or atypical sites.**
 2. **Recurrent ulceration** despite adequate therapy.
 3. Non-β islet cell tumours of the pancreas (**gastrinoma**).

Aetiopathology

- May be either sporadic or associated with MEN-1 (which is autosomal dominant).
- Tumours are most commonly found in the **gastrinoma triangle of Passaro**:
  - o Junction of the cystic duct and CBD, superiorly.
  - o Junction of second and third parts of duodenum, inferiorly.
  - o Junction of neck and body of pancreas, medially (essentially the superior mesenteric artery).

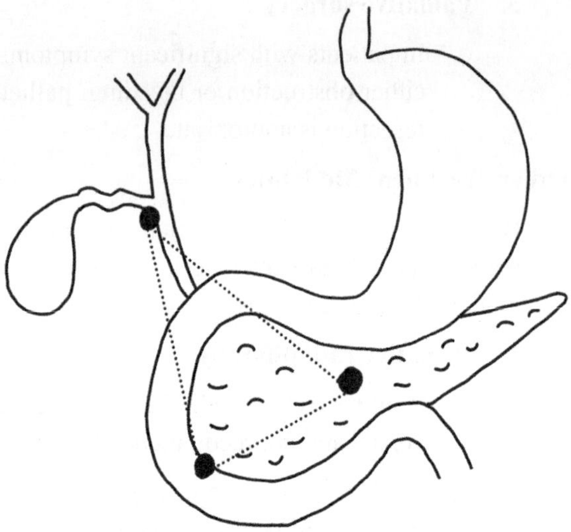

Figure 18: Triangle of Passaro

- In sporadic disease, tumours are mostly located in the duodenum and are small (< 5 mm) and multiple. These **arise in the G cells** found in Brunner's glands.
- In **MEN -1**, all tumours are in the **duodenum.**
- In the **pancreas**, it occurs especially in the **head**.
- Patients with pancreatic tumours have a worse prognosis than those with primary tumours in the duodenum.

Clinical Features

- > **90%** of patients with gastrinomas have **peptic ulcer disease**, often multiple or in unusual sites.
- **Abdominal pain from either peptic ulcer disease or GERD is the most common symptom.**
- **Diarrhoea** is another common symptom, caused by the large volume of gastric acid secretion.
- Many patients have a history of high **alcohol** use, which may be a **risk factor**.
- Majority of tumours have metastasized by the time of presentation.

Investigations

- **Fasting serum gastrin:**
  - o It is the cornerstone of diagnosing ZES.
  - o **If elevated, the gastric pH is measured.**
- **Gastric pH:**
  - o If pH is <2 and fasting serum gastrin is > 10-fold elevated, the diagnosis is confirmed.
- **Secretin provocation test** can be used.
- Once a diagnosis is confirmed, **all patients are screened for MEN-1** (biochemical and genetic).

Localization Studies

- **Indications:**
  - o Indicated only after a diagnosis of ZES has been confirmed.
  - o Indicated because the tumors are often small and multiple.

1. **Ga^{68} – labelled SSAs with PET-CT.**
2. **SRS or Somatostatin Receptor Scinti-graphy.**
3. **EUS or Endoscopic Ultrasound.**

Treatment

A. Surgery

- All tumors with sporadic gastrinoma without metastases should be **excised.**
- During excision, **peritumoral lymph nodes should be sampled** for histological assessment.
- In **MEN-1/gastrinoma**, surgery is not recommended for patients with tumors < 2 cm.
  - o Tumors > 2 cm are enucleated.
  - o Parathyroidectomy reduces gastric acid secretion.
- Palliative resection of liver mets may be beneficial.

B. Medical

- **PPI** therapy is the management of choice.
- Even after surgical excision, most patients require continued medical treatment.
- For patients with advanced locoregional disease or mets, **PPI + somatostatin analogues** is the first line treatment.
- In refractory cases, locoregional ablative therapy such as **radiofrequency ablation or chemoembolization** may be effective.

[5] GIST. *July 18*

- GISTs are the most common mesenchymal neoplasms of the GIT.

Cells of Origin

- They are distinct tumours **derived from the interstitial cells of Cajal**, which is a GI pacemaker cell.

Site

- May arise in any part of the GIT, but **half are found in the stomach**.

Aetiology

- Almost universally associated with a mutation in the tyrosine kinase C-KIT oncogene (**CD-117**).
- Mutation in platelet derived growth factor receptor alpha (**PDGFRA**).

Pathology

- Express **CD-117 and CD-34.**
- Size and mitotic index are the best predictors of metastases.
- Peritoneal and liver mets are most common.
- Spread to lymph nodes is extremely rare.

Clinical Features

- M = F.
- Small GISTs of the stomach are probably quite common and remain unnoticed.
- Larger tumours present with nonspecific gastric symptoms:
  - o Early satiety.
  - o Bloating.
  - o Vague abdominal pain.
- **Bleeding can occur** and is generally in the form of **melena** or, less frequently, **frank hematemesis.**
- Tumour rupture with **intra-abdominal hemorrhage** is uncommon.
- Many patients remain **asymptomatic** and tumours are discovered incidentally at the time of another surgery or during imaging performed for other indications.

Investigations

- **Endoscopy:**
  - o Biopsy can also be taken.
  - o Because the mucosa overlying the tumour is normal, endoscopic biopsy can be **uninformative unless the tumour has ulcerated**.
- **Targeted biopsy by endoscopic ultrasonography.**
- CT of the abdomen and pelvis with oral and IV contrast is used to assess for metastatic disease.
- MRI is preferred in patients who cannot receive IV contrast or for rectal GISTs.
- Immunohistochemical staining for CD117, CD34 and PDGFRA are used to confirm the diagnosis.

Treatment

A. The Mainstay of Treatment is Complete Surgical Resection

- Smaller tumours can be treated by **wedge excision.**
- Larger tumours may require a **gastrectomy or duodenectomy**, but lymphadenectomy is not required.
- Tumours which are even more larger may require **multivisceral resection.**
- Resection of mets.

B. Targeted Therapy

- GISTs are sensitive to the tyrosine kinase antagonist Imatinib.
- Can be used in the neoadjuvant or adjuvant setting.

[3] Troisier's sign. *Dec 17*

- Troisier's sign represents an **enlargement of a left sided supraclavicular lymph node**.
- The enlarged node is called **Virchow's node** or Troisier node or Virchow-Troisier node.

Associations

1. Carcinoma stomach.
2. Cancer of esophagus and intestines.
3. Cancers of urogenital system.
4. Cancers of CBD, gallbladder.
5. Hepatocellular carcinoma.
6. Ca pancreas.
7. Ca lung.

Anatomical Location

- It is located in the **supraclavicular fossa**, deep to the platysma and clavicular head of the sternocleidomastoid muscle.
- Near the **junction of the thoracic duct and the left subclavian vein.**

Route of Spread

- **Tumour embolization via the thoracic duct** usually leads to the enlargement of left supraclavicular lymph node.

Clinical Importance

- It **indicates inoperability.**
- Patients with enlarged Virchow's node are usually given palliative care.

[5] Upper GI bleed. *Dec 18*

- **Definition:** Upper GI bleed refers to **bleeding that occurs from proximal to the ligament of Treitz.**
- Upper GI bleed is the **most common presentation of gastrointestinal bleeding**, i.e., it is more common than lower GI bleed.

Causes

1. **Peptic Ulcers**
    - It is the most common cause of upper GI bleed.
    - Duodenal > gastric > esophageal.
2. **Erosions**
    - It is the 2nd most common cause.
    - Esophageal > gastric > duodenal.
3. **Esophageal Varices**
    - Associated with liver cirrhosis and portal hypertension.
4. Mallory-Weiss syndrome.
5. Dieulafoy lesions.
6. Tumours.
7. GAVE or gastric antral vascular ectasia.
8. Aortoenteric fistula.
9. Crohn's disease.
10. Hemosuccus pancreaticus.

Treatment

- **Endoscopy is both diagnostic and therapeutic:**
    - o **Band ligation**
    - o **Stapling.**
    - o **Argon plasma coagulation.**
- **Indications for surgery:**
    1. Hemodynamic instability despite vigorous resuscitation.
    2. Failure of endoscopic techniques to arrest hemorrhage.
    3. Recurrent hemorrhage after initial stabilisation.
    4. Shock associated with recurrent hemorrhage.
    5. Continued slow bleeding with a transfusion requirement of > 3 units/day.

[5] Trichobezoar of stomach. *Dec 13*

- Also known as hairballs, Rapunzel syndrome.
- It is a collection of hair in the stomach.
- It is an unusual condition.

Aetiopathology

- It is caused by the **ingestion of hair**, which remains undigested in the stomach.
- It can give rise to **gastroduodenal ulceration** leading to hematemesis, perforation, peritonitis or obstruction.
- Usually associated with an **underlying psychiatric disorder.**
- Patients **may also have underlying gastric dysmotility issues,** such as prior gastric surgery, gastroparesis or gastric outlet obstruction.

Clinical Features

- Is almost **exclusively seen in young girls** with an underlying psychiatric disorder.
- The patient usually has **long hair** and has a **habit of chewing or sucking on the hair.**
- Early satiety.
- Pain.
- Nausea/vomiting.

- Weight loss.

Investigations

- **Endoscopy** confirms the diagnosis and is the investigation of choice.
- X-rays or CT scan can show a bezoar as a mass or filling defect within the stomach.

Treatment

- Removal of the trichobezoar via **gastrotomy**.

40

Bariatric Surgery

[MCQ] Conditions associated with severe obesity are the following except: ***CBME March 24***

A. Type 2 diabetes mellitus

B. Polycystic ovary syndrome

C. Hypertension

D. Hypothyroidism*

CONDITIONS THAT ARE ASSOCIATED WITH SEVERE AND COMPLEX OBESITY

- Type 2 diabetes.
- Hypertension.
- Dyslipidemia.
- Obstructive sleep apnea.
- Arthritis and functional impairment.
- Gastroesophageal reflux disease.
- Non-alcoholic fatty liver disease/non-alcoholic steatohepatosis.
- Polycystic ovary syndrome.
- Clinical depression.
- Various cancers, in particular endometrial cancer.

[3] Write a note on metabolic surgeries.
CBME June 24

TYPES OF BARIATRIC SURGERIES OR METABOLIC SURGERIES

- The phrases 'metabolic' or 'diabetes' surgery are increasingly being used in conjunction with, or instead of, 'bariatric surgery' owing to the highly effective way that surgery improves the metabolic syndrome, with weight loss being a welcome additional effect.
- Type 2 diabetes is part of the 'metabolic syndrome', which includes high blood pressure, dyslipidemia and polycystic ovary syndrome.
- There are 2 primary mechanisms by which metabolic surgeries act:
  1. Caloric restriction, called restrictive surgeries.
  2. Nutrient malabsorption, called malabsorptive surgeries.

Type of surgery	Restrictive	Malabsorptive
Vertical banded gastroplasty (historical)	++++	0
Lap adjustable gastric banding	++++	0
Laparoscopic sleeve gastrectomy	++++	+
Roux-en-Y gastric bypass	++++	+++
Biliopancreatic diversion/duodenal switch	++	++++

Restrictive Surgeries

- Vertical banded gastroplasty (historical).
- Lap adjustable gastric banding.
- Laparoscopic sleeve gastrectomy.
- Roux-en-Y gastric bypass.

Malabsorptive Surgeries

- Biliopancreatic diversion.
- Duodenal switch.

OTHER IMPORTANT TOPICS

DEFINITIONS OF OVERWEIGHT AND OBESITY

Adult weight status	BMI (kg/m^2)
Normal	18.5–24.9
Overweight	25.0–29.9
Class 1 obesity	30.0–34.9
Class 2 obesity	35.0–39.9
Class 3 obesity	≥40.0

41

Small Intestine

[5] Meckel's diverticulum. *August 22, July 23*

[3] Meckel's diverticulum. *Sept 21*

- **Definition:** Meckel's diverticulum is a **persistent remnant of the vitellointestinal duct**.

Description

- It is found on the **anti-mesenteric side of the ileum.**
- **Congenital diverticulum.**
- It is a **true diverticulum**, therefore contains all three layers of the bowel wall.
- Has its **own blood supply.**

Rule of 2s

- Present in 2% of the population.
- Located 2 feet proximal to the ileocecal valve.
- 2 inches long.
- Contains 2 types of ectopic mucosa: Gastric and pancreatic.

Clinical Features

- Vast majority are **asymptomatic.**
- May present in the following ways:
  1. **Hemorrhage:**
     - If gastric mucosa is present, peptic ulceration can occur and present as painless dark rectal bleeding or melena.
  2. **Diverticulitis:**
     - Presents like appendicitis, although if perforation occurs, the presentation may resemble a perforated duodenal ulcer.
  3. **Intussusception:**
     - It can be the lead point for ileo-ileal or ileo-colic intussusception.
  4. **Chronic ulceration:**
     - Pain is felt around the umbilicus (as the diverticulum is of midgut in origin).
  5. **Intestinal obstruction:**
     - A band between the apex of the diverticulum and the umbilicus (also part of the vitello-intestinal duct) may cause obstruction directly, or by predisposing to the development of a volvulus around it.
  6. **Perforation**

Investigations

1. **Sodium ^{99m}Tc-pertechnetate scintigraphy:**
   - **It is the single most accurate diagnostic test.**
   - The ^{99m}Tc-pertechnetate is preferentially taken up by the mucus-secreting cells of gastric mucosa and ectopic gastric tissue in the diverticulum.
   - Accuracy can be improved by the use of drugs such as cimetidine.
   - When the tests come negative, but Meckel's is still suspected, other tests are used.

2. **Barium contrast imaging.**
3. **Mesenteric arteriography.**
4. **Double balloon endoscopy.**

Treatment

- When **incidentally found** in the course of abdominal surgery, a Meckel's diverticulum can safely be **left alone**, provided it has a wide mouth and is not thickened.
- Whenever there is doubt, it can be **resected**. There are 2 ways of doing so:
  1. Resecting the diverticulum and suturing the defect at its base.
  2. By performing a limited small bowel resection with anastomosis.

[5] Aetiology of ileal perforation. *Oct 20*

Causes

- **Inflammatory bowel disease (Crohn's disease, ulcerative colitis):**
  - o These lead to inflammation and ulceration in the intestinal wall, which may eventually progress to perforation.
- **Intestinal obstruction:**
  - o Can cause increased pressure, leading to perforation.
  - o Especially seen in closed loop.
- **Appendicitis:**
  - o Can cause perforation that affects the surrounding structures, including the ileum.
- **Blunt trauma to abdomen.**
- **Meckel's diverticulum:**
  - o If it contains gastric mucosa, it can cause perforation of adjacent ileum.
- **Foreign body ingestion.**
- **Ischemia:** Tumours, vascular anomalies.
- **Infections:** Typhoid, TB.
- **Iatrogenic:**
  - o Complications from previous abdominal surgeries.
- **Tumours.**

Clinical Features

- Pain abdomen.
- **Bacterial peritonitis** supervenes over a few hours, usually accompanied by a deterioration in the patient's condition.

On Examination

- Patient is in a state of **shock**, with tachycardia.
- Pyrexia.
- Patient lies still, as even the **slightest movement causes pain.**
- **Per Abdomen:**
  - o Board like rigidity.
  - o Abdomen does not move with respiration.
  - o Obliteration of liver dullness.

Investigations

1. **Plain X-ray:**
   - Chest X-ray, erect X-ray of abdomen.
   - Air under diaphragm is seen.
   - Rigler sign or double wall sign.
   - Cupola sign.
2. **CT scan.**

Treatment

It is **initial resuscitation followed by surgery.**

A. **Resuscitation**
   - NPO.
   - IV fluids.
   - Analgesics.
   - Antibiotics.

B. **Open Surgery**
   - **Exploratory laparotomy** is done, followed by a thorough **peritoneal lavage.**
   - Surgical options are:
     1. **Primary closure:**
        - o Done in small perforations which are detected early.

2. **Bowel resection and anastomosis:**
   - o Affected portion of ileum is resected and healthy ends of ileum are anastomosed.
   - o Performed when damaged area of ileum cannot be repaired primarily and the remaining ileum is healthy.
3. **Temporary loop ileostomy:**
   - o Indicated when the bowel is unhealthy (e.g., inflamed) such that anastomosis won't take.
   - o The stoma is closed after an interval which allows the underlying pathology to heal.

[5] Peutz-Jeghers syndrome. *Dec 14*

- It is an **autosomal dominant hereditary cancer syndrome.**

Causes

- **Mutation** of the **STK-11/LKB-1 gene** located on **chromosome 19p.**
- **Autosomal dominant** mode of inheritance.

Components/Clinical Features

- Small (1 or 2 mm), **brown or black spots located in the circumoral region of the face, buccal mucosa, forearms, palms, soles, digits and perianal area**.
- Multiple **hamartomatous polyps:** Jejunum and ileum > rectum and colon > stomach.
- **Most common symptom is recurrent colicky abdominal pain**, usually the result of intermittent intussusception. These patients complain of lower abdominal pain + palpable mass.
- **Hemorrhage** as a result of autoamputation of the polyps may occur:
  - o Most commonly manifested by anemia.
  - o Acute life threatening hemorrhage is rare.
- **Malignancy** may occur at the following sites:
  - o Small intestine.
  - o Stomach.
  - o Pancreas.
  - o Ovary.
  - o Lungs.
  - o Uterus.
  - o Breast.

HPE

- Polyps are due to an **overgrowth of the muscularis mucosa.**

Investigations

- **Screening** programs consist of the following:
  - o Upper GI endoscopy.
  - o Lower GI endoscopy.
  - o Mammogram/breast MRI.
  - o Pap smear.
  - o Endoscopic ultrasound/MRCP + CA 19-9.

Treatment

- **Asymptomatic polyps > 1 cm should be removed endoscopically** to decrease future complications such as bleeding and intussusception.
- **Surgery:**
  - o **Indications:** Obstruction and bleeding.
  - o **Goal of surgery is to remove the affected segment, preserving as much bowel as possible.**
- **Intervention may require:**
  - o Push enteroscopy.
  - o Combined laparoscopy/laparotomy with endoscopy may be necessary as these small bowel polyps may not be visualized by other means.

42

Large Intestine and Rectum

[5] Hirschsprung's disease. ***Dec 17, Dec 12***

[3] Hirschsprung's disease. ***August 22, Sept 21***

- **Definition:** Aganglionated distal colon/rectum, characterized by an absence of ganglion cells in the myenteric (Auerbach's) and submucosal (Meissner's) plexus.

Aetiology

- M>F.
- Family history.
- Associated with Down's syndrome.
- **Genes:** RET, EDNRB, EDN-3.

Pathogenesis

Migration of neural-crest derived intestinal neurons is affected. **(Neurocristopathy)**

↓

Aganglionosis

↓

Thickened nerve trunks in the distal bowel

- Aganglionosis extends from:
  - o Anus to sigmoid colon (most common).
  - o Anus to proximal colon.
  - o Anus to terminal ileum.
- Aganglionic bowel fails to relax, causing a **functional obstruction.**
- A **transition zone** lies between dilated, proximal, normal bowel and narrow, distal aganglionic bowel.

Clinical Features

- **Neonatal Hirschsprung's** presents with:
  - o Delayed passage of meconium.
  - o Abdominal distension.
  - o Bilious vomiting.
- Those with missed diagnoses of Hirschsprung's may present **later in life** with a **chronic history of abdominal distension and constipation.**

Complications

- **Enterocolitis is the most common cause of death** in patients with uncorrected Hirschsprung's disease.

Investigations

- **Rectal biopsy:**
  - o Gold standard.
  - o Commonly done bedside using a suction rectal biopsy kit.
- **Contrast enema:**
  - o May show the narrow aganglionic segment, a cone and dilated proximal bowel.

Treatment

- The initial treatment is to establish fecal passage:
    - o Rectal/bowel washouts is tried first.
    - o If this fails, a stoma is fashioned using frozen section histopathology to identify ganglionic bowel.
- The only curative treatment of Hirschsprung's is **excision of the entire aganglionic segment + bringing ganglionic bowel to the anus.**
- There are various definitive procedures which can do so:
    - o Swenson.
    - o Duhamel.
    - o Soave.
    - o Transanal pull through operations.

[10] Discuss the aetiology, clinical features and management of prolapse rectum. ***June 19***

[5] Prolapse rectum. ***March 21, Oct 20, July 18, Dec 15***

- Also known as procidentia.
- **Definition:** It is a circumferential, full-thickness intussusception of the rectal wall.

Causes/Risk Factors

- Age > 40 years.
- F > M.
- Prior pelvic surgery.
- Chronic straining and constipation.
- Chronic diarrhea.
- Vaginal delivery.
- Multiparity.
- Pelvic floor dysfunction and/or anatomic defects.
- Neurologic diseases/injuries.
- Psychiatric diseases that require medications which cause constipation.

Pathophysiology

- Prolapse **often commences as an intussusception** of the rectum, which descends to protrude outside the anus.
- The process **starts** with the **anterior wall** of the rectum, where the **supporting tissues are weakest**.

Clinical Features

- Age:
    - o Complete prolapse is **uncommon in children** but **may occur as a result of malnutrition.**
    - o In **adults**, it can occur at any age, but is **more common in the elderly.**
- F > M.
- Discomfort due to the prolapsed tissue.
- Majority of patients complain of **fecal incontinence** (passive or urge incontinence).
- Incontinence with drainage of mucus or blood.
- History of constipation.
- Pudendal neuropathy with a prolonged pudendal nerve terminal motor latency.
- **Constipation or obstructed defecation**, i.e., feeling of an incomplete rectal evacuation during defecation; is particularly seen in patients with intra-rectal prolapse.
- In women, it is commonly associated with other pelvic organ prolapse.

On Examination

- It is > 4 cm and commonly as much as 10-15 cm in length.
- Rectal prolapse has concentric folds.
- On palpation between the finger and thumb:
    - o Complete prolapse feels much thicker than mucosal prolapse.
    - o Consists of a double thickness of the entire wall of the rectum.
- Any prolapse > 5 cm in length will contain anteriorly, between its layers, a pouch of peritoneum.
- When large, the peritoneal pouch may contain small intestine or bladder.
- Anal sphincter is characteristically patulous and gapes widely on straining, to allow the rectum to prolapse.

Complications

- Rectal ulceration.
- Bleeding.
- Incarceration, with ischemia and necrosis of the rectum.

Investigations

- Patient is examined in left lateral decubitus or in sitting or squatting position during straining.
- Patient may be asked to take a 'selfie' at home to document the prolapse.
- Proctoscopy.
- Fluoroscopic or MRI defecography.
- Colonoscopy.
- Colonic transit study.
- Endoanal ultrasound.

Treatment

A. Non-Operative Management

- Prolapse associated symptoms of constipation and fecal incontinence can be palliated with medical treatment, in order to improve quality of life.
- Adequate fluid intake, fibre supplements and stool softeners can treat constipation.
- Sugar or salt can be used topically to reduce rectal mucosal edema and facilitate reduction of the prolapsed tissue.
- Enemas and suppositories help with defecation.

B. Operative Repair

- Surgery is required for full-thickness rectal prolapse, and the operation can be performed via a perineal or abdominal approach.

Perineal Approach

- **Advantages of perineal approach:**
  - o Minimal post-op pain.
  - o Early mobility.
  - o Low morbidity.

1. Thiersch's operation

- A steel wire or silastic tape is placed around anal canal.

2. Delorme's operation

- Circumferential stripping of rectal mucosa + plication of underlying muscle.

3. Altemier's procedure

- Full-thickness resection + hand-sewn coloanal anastomosis.

Abdominal Approach

- Can be done via open or laparoscopic surgery.
- **Principle:** To fix the rectum in its normal anatomical position:

1. **Inserting a sheet of polypropylene mesh between the rectum and the sacrum.**
2. **Hitching up the rectosigmoid junction with a Teflon sling to the front of the sacrum.**
3. **Simply suturing the mobilized rectum to the sacrum using 4-6 interrupted non-absorbable sutures, called 'sutured rectopexy'.**
4. **Sutured rectopexy + resection rectopexy.**
5. **Laparoscopic ventral mesh rectopexy.**

- **Advantages of abdominal route:**
  - o Lower rate of recurrence.

[5] Colonic diverticulosis. *August 22*

COLONIC DIVERTICULA

- **Definition:** Diverticula of the colon are acquired herniations of colonic mucosa, protruding through the circular muscle at the points where the blood vessels penetrate the colonic wall.

Aetiology

- Diverticular disease is a consequence of a refined Western diet, deficient in dietary fibre.
- Collagen structure gets altered with ageing.

Pathophysiology

1. Hypertrophy of the muscular layers of the colon wall.
2. Narrowed lumen.
3. Disordered colonic motility

↓

Localized high pressure zones

↓

Mucosa herniates through the circular muscle at the points where blood vessels penetrate the bowel wall (i.e., areas of weakness)

- Classically formed on the mesenteric side of the colonic wall.
- Sigmoid colon is most commonly involved.
- Sometimes, the entire large bowel is involved, from the caecum to the rectosigmoid junction.

- Rectum is generally not affected as it has an extra layer of muscle.
- **Diverticulosis:**
  - o Primary stage of the disease.
  - o Related to **muscular incoordination and spasm**, resulting in **increased segmentation** and **intraluminal pressure.**
  - o This leads to **diverticulum formation.**

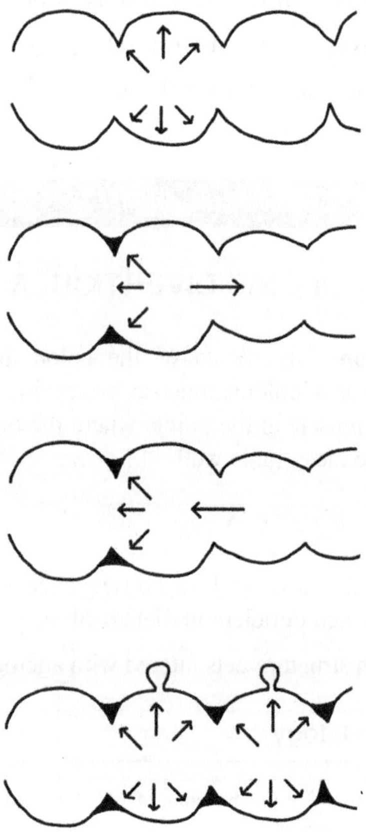

Segmentation of the colon

Figure 1: Segmentation of the colon in diverticulosis

Clinical Features

- Majority of patients with diverticulosis are asymptomatic.
- Distension.
- Flatulence.
- Sensation of heaviness in the lower abdomen.
- Excessive colonic segmentation can cause severe colicky pain in the left iliac fossa.
- Pain waxes and wanes very fast.

Complications of Diverticular Disease

1. **Diverticulitis**
   - Recurrent periodic inflammation and pain.
2. **Perforation**
   - Leading to general peritonitis or local (pericolic) abscess formation.
3. **Intestinal obstruction**
   - Due to progressive fibrosis causing stenosis.
4. **Hemorrhage**
   - Diverticulitis may present with profuse colonic hemorrhage.
5. **Fistula formation**
   - Vesico-colic, vagino-colic, entero-colic, colo-cutaneous.

Investigations

- **CECT scan**
  - o Can identify diverticula as well as its complications.
- **Colonoscopy**
  - o Usually avoided for 6 weeks after an acute attack for fear of causing perforation.
- **Barium enema**
  - o Was used earlier.

Treatment

A. Medical

- High fibre diet.
- Bulk forming laxatives.
- Antispasmodics.
- IV antibiotics and bowel rest in the case of diverticulitis.

B. Surgical

- Surgical treatment is rarely, if ever, appropriate for diverticular disease in the absence of complications.
- Hartmann's procedure is often the safest option in an emergency sitting.
- Primary anastomosis (with or without proximal diversion) can be considered in selected patients.
- Elective resection may be considered for recurrent attacks or complications.

[3] Solitary rectal ulcer. ***June 17, June 14***

SOLITARY RECTAL ULCER SYNDROME

- It is a rare chronic benign disorder.

Aetiology

The cause is **multifactorial** and includes:
1. Internal rectal prolapse
2. Abnormal/paradoxical contraction of the puborectalis muscle

↓

Trauma and compression of the anterior rectal wall on the upper anal canal, during straining and defecation

↓

Mucosal ischemia

↓

Ulceration

Clinical Features

- Young adults (30-40 years).
- F > M.
- Rectal bleeding.
- Prolonged excessive straining.
- Incomplete defecation/tenesmus.
- Mucous discharge.
- Perineal and abdominal pain.
- Constipation.

On Examination

- Ulcer on the anterior wall of the rectum, situated 6-8 cm from the anal verge.
- May heal, leaving a polypoid appearance.
- Intra-rectal prolapse.

Differential Diagnosis

- Rectal cancer.
- Inflammatory Bowel Disease, particularly Crohn's.

Investigations

1. **Proctography**
   - May also indicate accompanying rectal intussusception or anterior rectal wall prolapse.
2. **Biopsy**
   - It is confirmatory.

Treatment

A. Medical

- Patient education.
- High fiber diet.
- Stool softeners.
- Bulking laxatives.
- Avoidance of straining and/or anal digitations.
- Minimizing time on the toilet.
- Sucralfate.
- Corticosteroids.
- Mesalamine enemas.
- Re-coordination of defecation using biofeedback therapy.

B. Surgical

- The various surgical options are:
  1. **Local excision of the ulcer.**
  2. **Treatment of the rectal prolapse.**
     - o Trans-anal stapled resection of the intussusception (STARR procedure).
     - o Re-suspension of the rectum by abdominal rectopexy.
  3. In rare cases, **rectal excision** may be required **with or without stoma.**

[3] Colostomy. ***March 21, Dec 19***
[3] Types of colostomy. ***Dec 16, Dec 13***

COLOSTOMY

- A colostomy is a planned opening made in the colon to divert feces and flatus through the abdominal wall, where they can be collected in an external appliance.
- Exteriorisation of the large intestine is called a stoma.

Indications for Colostomy Formation

1. To protect a distal anastomosis or allow healing, away from the fecal flow.
2. Following resection, when anastomosis is unsafe or not possible.
3. To relieve obstruction when resection is not feasible.
4. To reduce disease activity (e.g., Crohn's disease).
5. To allow alternative bowel control (incontinence).

TYPES

Depending on Duration

1. **Temporary.**
2. **Permanent.**

Depending on the Way it is Fashioned

1. **Loop colostomy:**
   - A mobilised loop of colon is brought out onto the anterior abdominal wall
   - It is temporary.
   - If there is resolution of the indication for which the temporary stoma was constructed, the colostomy can usually be closed without recourse to a laparotomy.
2. **End colostomy:**
   - Permanent stoma.
   - Formed after an abdominoperineal excision of the rectum or as part of a Hartmann's procedure.
3. **Double-barrelled colostomy:**
   - Also known as Paul-Mikulicz stoma.
   - Occasionally, when resection of a segment of colon has occurred but the patient is too ill to undergo a safe reanastomosis, it is possible and appropriate to bring up both ends of the bowel to the abdominal wall.

Complications of Stoma

- Skin irritation.
- Prolapse.
- Retraction.
- Ischemia.
- Stenosis.
- Parastomal hernia.
- Bleeding.
- Fistulation.

[10] Describe the clinical features, investigations and management of carcinoma colon. ***Dec 18***

[10] Carcinoma rectum – pathology, clinical features and management. ***Dec 17***

[3] Duke's staging for carcinoma rectum. ***August 22, March 21, Dec 15***

COLORECTAL CANCER

- It is one of the most common causes of cancer death in the West.
- **Rectum: 1/3rd** of the total colorectal cancers.

  Colon: 2/3rd.
- Most large bowel cancers arise from left colon: **Rectum > sigmoid.**

Aetiology

- **Adenoma-carcinoma sequence:**
  - o Most colorectal cancers are thought to develop from adenomatous polyps through a sequence of genetic mutations influenced by environmental factors.
  - o **Genes involved: APC, K-RAS, p53.**
- Associated with **high intake of red meat** and particularly **processed meat products (containing haem and N-nitroso compounds).**
- **Dietary fibre has a protective effect:**
  - o Increased roughage is associated with reduced colonic transit times that in turn reduce exposure of the mucosa to dietary carcinogens.
- **Smoking** and **alcohol** increases risk.
- **High magnesium** and **calcium** intake may be **protective.**
- **Anti-oxidants** such as **vitamin E** and **selenium** are **protective.**
- **Inflammatory bowel disease** increases the risk.
- **Cholecystectomy** marginally increases the risk of **right sided colon cancer.**
- Prostaglandin inhibitors, particularly aspirin, is protective.

Molecular Subtypes

- There are 4 Consensus Molecular Subtypes (CMS):
  - o **CMS 1**: Microsatellite instability (MSI) occurs sporadically, particularly in right-sided tumours.
  - o **CMS 2**: WNT and MYC signaling activation.
  - o **CMS 3**: Metabolic dysregulation.
  - o **CMS 4**: Transforming growth factor beta activation.

Pathology

- Macroscopically, the growth takes one of four forms:
  1. **Annular:** Produces obstructive symptoms.
  2. **Tubular:** Produces obstructive symptoms.
  3. **Ulcerating:** Present with bleeding.
  4. **Cauliflower:** Present with bleeding.
- **Microscopically: Columnar cell adenocarcinoma.**

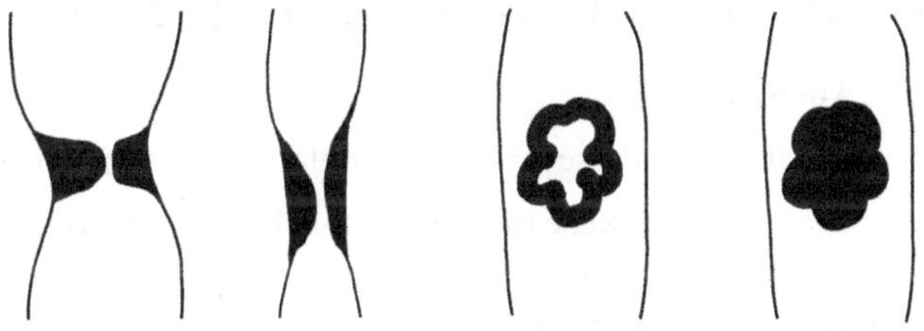

Figure 2: Types of colon cancer

Spread

A. Local Invasion, i.e., Direct Spread

- May be longitudinal or radial.
- May be retroperitoneal (ureter, duodenum) or intraperitoneal.

B. Lymphatics

- Involvement of the lymph nodes by tumour, progresses from those closest to the bowel along the course of lymphatics to central nodes.

C. Hematogenous

- Most commonly to the liver via by the portal vein.
- 2nd most common: Lungs.

D. Transcoelomic Spread

- Can spread from the serosa of the bowel or via subperitoneal lymphatics to other structures within the peritoneal cavity; including peritoneum, ovary and omentum.

Staging

1. **Duke's staging**
   - Originally described for rectal tumours but has been adopted for colon cancer also.
2. **TNM staging**
   - It is more detailed than Duke's staging and is regarded as the international standard.
3. **Astler-Coller staging.**

Duke's Staging

- **A**: Invasion of but not breaching the muscularis propria ***or*** the growth is limited to the rectal wall.
- **B**: Breaching the muscularis propria but not involving lymph nodes ***or*** the growth extends to the extra-rectal tissues, but without mets to the regional lymph nodes.
- **C**: Lymph nodes involved ***or*** there are secondary deposits in the regional lymph nodes.
  - o **C1**: Local pararectal lymph nodes alone are involved.
  - o **C2**: Nodes accompanying the supplying blood vessels to their origin from the aorta are involved.
- **D** : Widespread metastases.

Clinical Features

- Colorectal cancers usually occur in patients >50 years age:
  - o If it occurs earlier, it is usually part of a syndrome and is familial.
- M > F.
  - o But the incidence is increasing in women.

Carcinoma of Left Colon

- The main symptoms are those of increasing **intestinal obstruction**, because of the following reasons:
  - o Tumours are of the stenosing variety.
  - o Faecal content is relatively solid.
  - o Lumen of the bowel is comparatively narrow.
- **Pain:**
  - o Usually intestinal colic.
  - o If it becomes a constant ache, it suggests inoperability or pericolitis.

- **Alteration of bowel habit:**
  - o Patient has increasing attacks of constipation.
  - o Because of the increasing use of purgatives or because of irritation by the scybala causing excessive secretion of mucus above the constricting neoplasm, attacks of constipation are followed by diarrhea.
- **Palpable lump.**
- **Distension:**
  - o Lower abdominal distension can be seen, which, just like the pain, is relieved by passing flatus.

Carcinoma of the Sigmoid

- Follows the general pattern as that of descending colon, but there are differences.
- **Pain is usually colicky** from the beginning.
- **Tenesmus:**
  - o Feeling of the need for evacuation may result in tenesmus accompanied by the passage of mucus and blood, especially in the early morning.
- **Bladder symptoms:**
  - o Not unusual and in some instances, they herald colovesical fistula.

Carcinoma of the Rectum

- **Bleeding per rectum:**
  - o Earliest and most common symptom.
  - o Bleeding is bright red in colour and painless.
  - o Can be mixed with stools or be separate in the toilet bowl.
- **Tenesmus:**
  - o Patient experiences a sensation of needing to evacuate the rectum but is unable to pass stools.
  - o Early symptom.
  - o Almost invariably present in patients with tumours of the lower half of the rectum.
  - o Patient may endeavour to empty the rectum several times a day (called spurious diarrhoea), often with the passage of flatus and a little blood-stained mucus ('bloody slime').
- **Alteration in bowel habit:**
  - o Tendency to more frequent defecation and the passage of looser stool.
  - o Early morning bloody diarrhea.
  - o Although a change to looser stools is more common, patients with a stenosing carcinoma at the rectosigmoid junction may complain of increasing constipation.
- **Pain:**
  - o It is a late symptom.
  - o Colicky pain is present in obstructive tumours of the rectosigmoid.
  - o Advanced cancers may infiltrate the sacral plexus, giving rise to severe, intractable pain.
- **Weight loss.**

Carcinoma of Transverse Colon

- **May be mistaken for a carcinoma of the stomach** because of the position of the tumour together with the **anemia** and **lassitude** that it causes.

Carcinoma of Caecum and Ascending Colon

- **Anemia:**
  - o It is usually severe and unyielding to treatment.
  - o This is because tumours in this location are of the ulcerative type and bleed.
- **Mass in the right iliac fossa.**
- Caecal carcinoma is sometimes discovered unexpectedly at operation for acute appendicitis or for an appendicular abscess that fails to resolve.
- On rare occasions, appendix is inflamed, or even gangrenous, from destruction to its lumen by the carcinoma.
- Rarely, a papilliferous growth may be the lead point for an **intussusception.**

Investigations

A. Screening

- Colon cancer is suited to screening as the prognosis is better, the earlier stage the disease is diagnosed; and polypectomy allows the prevention of cancer development.
- These tests aim to detect occult fecal blood:
  - o Guaiac-based test, which detects peroxidase like activity of fecal hematin.
  - o Fecal immunochemical test.
- Flexible sigmoidoscopy is also used.

B. Colonoscopy

- It is the investigation of choice if colorectal cancer is suspected.
- Entire length of the colon and caecum, up to the terminal ileum is examined.
- Biopsy can be taken.
- Synchronous polyps or carcinomas can also be detected.

C. Double Contrast Barium Enema

- Was used earlier.
- No longer used.

D. Virtual Colonoscopy

- CT colonography.
- Can pick up polyps ≤ 6 mm.
- Non-invasive.

E. CECT Scan

- Used as a diagnostic tool in patients with a palpable abdominal mass.
- CT of the thorax, abdomen and pelvis is the standard means of staging colorectal cancer.

F. MRI

- Is used for staging rectal cancer.

Treatment of Colon Cancer

A. Surgical Treatment

Pre-op preparation:

- Pre-op mechanical bowel preparation + pre-op oral antibiotics reduces surgical site infection, anastomotic leak, post-op ileus, reoperation and even mortality.
- Stoma marking and counselling is also done.

Goal of surgery:

- To remove the primary tumour and its draining locoregional lymph nodes.
- **Margins should be free, colon cancer:** 5 cm.
- Anastomosis must be constructed without any tension.

Carcinoma of the caecum or ascending colon:

- **Right hemicolectomy.**
- **Complete mesocolic excision, with removal of the lymphovascular supply** of the resected colon with flush ligation of the ileocolic and right colic vessels at their origin from the superior mesenteric artery.
- Mesentery of the distal 10 cm of the ileum and the mesocolon as far as the proximal 1/3rd of the transverse colon is divided.
- **Anastomosis between ileum and transverse colon.**

Carcinoma of transverse colon and splenic flexure:

- **Extended right hemicolectomy.**
- **Splenic flexure** is also excised.
- Whole **transverse mesocolon** is excised.

Carcinoma of descending and sigmoid colon:

- **Left hemicolectomy.**
- The inferior mesenteric artery below its left colic branch, together with the related paracolic lymph nodes, is included in the resection by ligating the inferior mesenteric artery close to its origin (high tie).
- Tension free **anastomosis** is done, **between transverse colon and rectum.**
- **If the anastomosis is below the peritoneal reflection the rectum, a temporary diverting stoma** may be fashioned proximally, usually by formation of a loop ileostomy.

Obstructing colon cancers:

- **Goal:** Relief of obstruction, resection of ischemic or non-viable bowel and resection of the tumour.
- **Left-sided obstruction: Hartmann's** is done if primary anastomosis is unsafe.
- **Right-sided obstruction:** A primary **ileocolic anastomosis** can be performed safely; but for patients with a high risk of anastomotic failure, a diversion stoma is done.

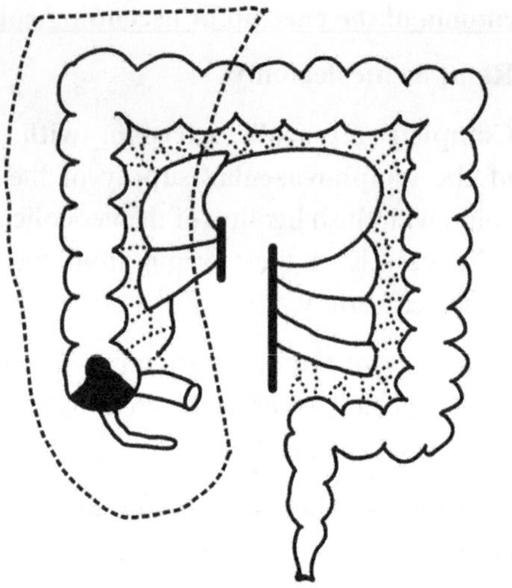

Figure 3: Area to be resected when growth is in the caecum

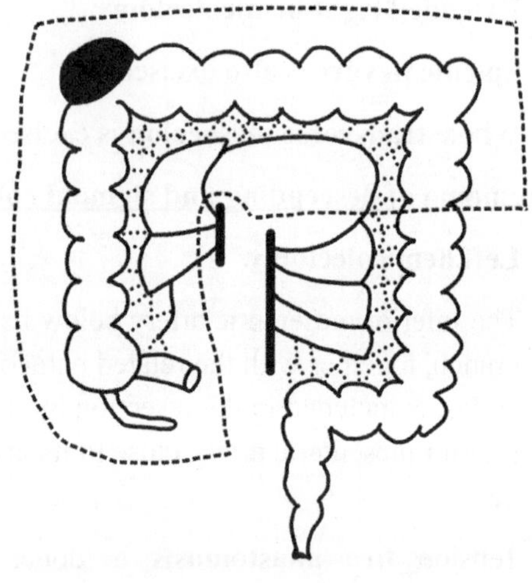

Figure 4: Area to be resected when growth is in the hepatic flexure

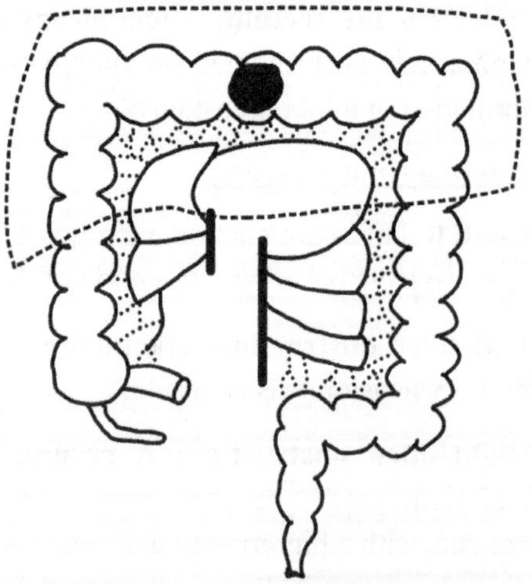

Figure 5: Area to be resected when growth is in the transverse colon

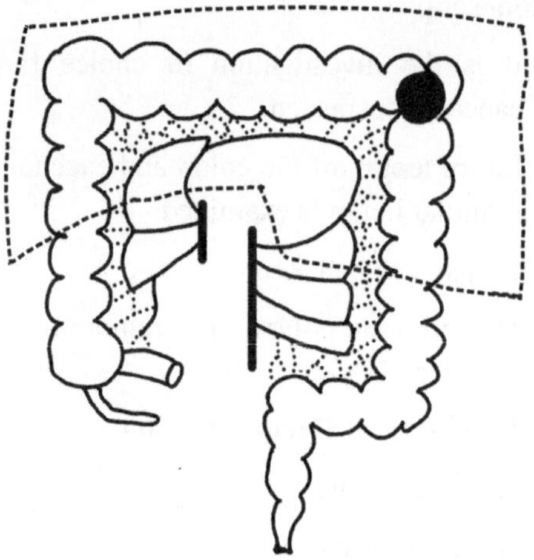

Figure 6: Area to be resected when growth is in the splenic flexure or proximal part of descending colon

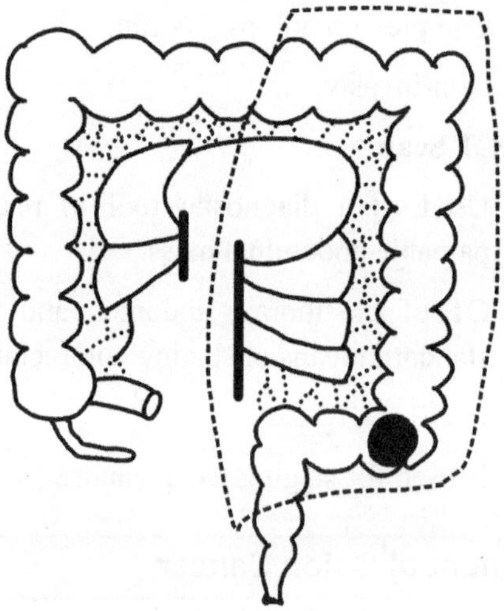

Figure 7: Area to be resected when growth is in the pelvic colon

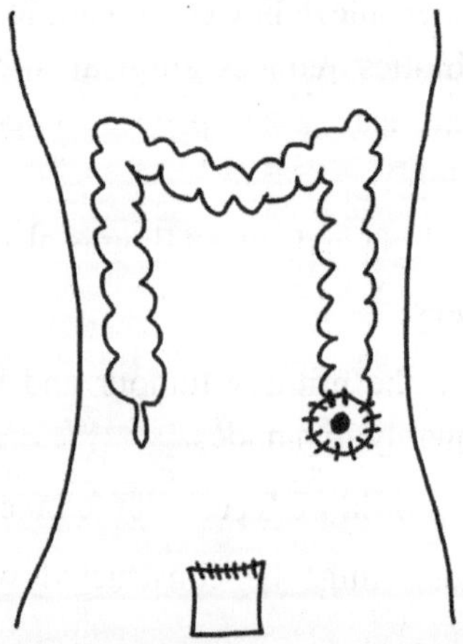

Figure 8: Hartmann's procedure

B. Adjuvant Chemotherapy

- It is indicated in patients with **node-positive colon cancer, i.e., stage III/Dukes C.**
- **FOLFOX:** Folinic acid, 5-fluorouracil, oxaliplatin.
- **CAPOX:** Capecitabine, oxaliplatin.
- **FOLFIRI:** Folinic acid, 5-fluorouracil, irinotecan.
- **FOLFOXIRI:** Folinic acid, 5-fluorouracil, oxaliplatin, irinotecan.

C. Colorectal Cancer with Liver Mets

- Liver mets can be resected.

Treatment of Rectal Cancer

A. Neo-Adjuvant Therapy

- **Neo-adjuvant radiotherapy (NART) or neo-adjuvant chemoradiotherapy (NACTRT) is used in locally advanced tumours**, i.e., tumours which invade a neighboring structure or threaten to breach the circumferential resection margin.
- **Aim is to downstage the cancer** and increase the chances of a complete resection with clear oncological margins.

B. Surgery

- Surgical excision of tumour is the mainstay of curative therapy.

Principles of surgery

- Radical excision of the rectum, together with the mesorectum and associated lymph nodes, i.e., TME or **Total Mesorectal Excision.**
- When radical excision is possible, the aim should be **to restore gastrointestinal continuity and continence by preserving the anal sphincter whenever feasible.**
- **Anterior resection (a sphincter saving operation)** is usually possible for tumours whose lower margin is ≥ 2 cm above anorectal junction.
- It involves **high proximal ligation of the inferior mesenteric lymphovascular pedicle.**
- The **distal margin should be ≥ 1 cm.**

Types of surgery for Ca rectum

- The level of anterior resection is named depending on the level of the colorectal anastomosis:

1. **High anterior resection**
   - o Colorectal anastomosis is above the peritoneal reflection.
2. **Low anterior resection**
   - o Colorectal anastomosis is below the peritoneal reflection.
3. **Ultra-low anterior resection**
   - o Colorectal anastomosis is at the level of pelvic floor or puborectalis.

- In the past, **removal of the rectum and anus with a permanent colostomy (abdominoperineal resection)** was often required for tumours. This is a non-sphincter saving procedure and is rarely done nowadays, because the introduction of stapled anastomosis and chemoradiotherapy downstaging has enabled many more patients to be treated by a sphincter saving procedure.

Choice of surgery

- The choice of surgery depends on the location of the cancer:

1. **Early T1 and T2 cancers:**
   - o Organ preserving surgical techniques are preferred
   - o This means that the rectum is not excised, but full-thickness excision of the cancer is done using TEMS (Transanal Endoscopic Micro Surgery).
2. **Rectosigmoid cancers and those in the upper 1/3rd of rectum:**
   - o High anterior resection is done.
3. **Tumours in middle and lower 1/3rd of rectum:**
   - o LAR, i.e., low anterior resection is done.
   - o Gastrointestinal continuity is restored via a straight low coloanal anastomosis or a colopouch-anal anastomosis.
   - o In cancers situated below the peritoneal reflection, it is usual practice to defunction the anastomosis with a temporary stoma because of the higher risk of anastomotic leak.
4. **Some tumours of the lower 1/3rd of rectum:**
   - o APR or abdominoperineal resection is still required for some tumours of the

lower 1/3rd of rectum that are unsuitable for a sphincter saving procedure.

5. **Elderly and frail patients:**
   - o Hartmann's operation is done in elderly and frail patients in whom there is concern about poor anal sphincter function and post-op incontinence or the viability of an anastomosis.
   - o Colorectal excision follows the same principles as the other procedures, but the rectal stump is stapled closed and the proximal colon exteriorised as a permanent end colostomy.
6. **Pelvic exenteration:**
   - o When carcinoma of the rectum has spread to contiguous organs, a more radical operation known as pelvic exenteration can remove these structures en bloc.

C. Adjuvant Therapy

- Radiotherapy and chemotherapy are both used.
- Chemotherapy drugs and regimens are the same as for colon cancer.

D. Palliation

- Considered in the presence of widespread mets:
  - o Endoluminal stenting.
  - o External beam radiotherapy.
  - o Palliative colostomy.

OTHER IMPORTANT TOPICS

ADENOMATOUS POLYPS OF COLON

- Also known as neoplastic polyps, since all adenomas have a malignant potential.
- The term 'polyp' is a clinical description of any protrusion of the mucosa.
- It encompasses a variety of histologically different tumours.
- Polyps can occur singly, synchronously in small numbers or as part of a polyposis syndrome.
- Adenomatous polyps are the most common polyps with malignant potential.
- The most common adenomatous polyps are tubular adenomas, and they are frequently pedunculated.

Types of Adenomatous Polyps

A. On the Basis of Histology

1. **Tubular:**
   - Characterized by branched tubular glands on histology.
   - Most common subtype.
2. **Villous:**
   - Have long finger-like projections of the surface epithelium.
3. **Tubulovillous:**
   - Have features of both types.

B. On the Basis of Morphology

1. Sessile.
2. Pedunculated.

Risk of Malignancy

- The risk of malignancy is dependent on:
  - o Histology.
  - o Morphology.
  - o Size.
- Tubular adenomas have the lowest risk, with increasing risk as villous features predominate.
- Tubular adenomas are generally pedunculated.
- Villous adenomas are generally sessile.
- Sessile and particularly depressed lesions have more malignant potential than pedunculated lesions.
- The risk of malignant change increases with size, almost one-third of large (>3 cm) colonic adenomas will have an area of invasive malignancy.

Investigations

- **Colonoscopy**
  - o Size is assessed.
  - o Morphology.
- **Biopsy/HPE**
  - o Pit pattern.
  - o Biopsy should not be taken if referral for endoscopic mucosal resection or endoscopic submucosal dissection is being considered.

Treatment

1. **Colonoscopic resection:**
   - The polyp can be resected colonoscopically if it is considered appropriate and safe.
   - Various techniques are available:
     - o Hot or cold snare polypectomy is done for smaller pedunculated lesions.
     - o Larger polyps or sessile polyps may require infiltration of saline into the underlying muscularis mucosa to raise the polyp before snare resection.
     - o EMR or endoscopic mucosal resection.
     - o ESD or endoscopic submucosal dissection.
   - The area of the polyp should be tattooed to facilitate later endoscopic or laparoscopic localisation of the site of the polyp (especially if malignancy is suspected).
   - Failure of submucosal injection to elevate a polyp is suggestive of malignancy.
   - A biopsy should not be taken if referral for endoscopic mucosal resection or endoscopic submucosal dissection is being considered.
   - EMR and ESD carry a risk of colonic perforation and should only be performed by an experienced endoscopist.
   - Rectal adenomas may also be treated by endoscopic or transanal resection.

2. **Surgery:**
   - Polyps that cannot be removed via colonoscopy are referred for surgery.
   - Sessile polyps with a central depression that do not elevate adequately with saline injection (non-lifting sign) are at increased risk for perforation with endoscopic removal and at higher risk of harbouring neoplasia and are commonly referred for surgical removal by **segmental colectomy.**

Polyp Surveillance

- The need for follow-up and frequency of surveillance colonoscopy is dependent on:
  - o Polyp morphology.
  - o Number of polyps.
  - o Size of polyps.
  - o Age of the patient.
  - o Comorbidities.
  - o Family history.
  - o Accuracy and completeness of the index test.
- These factors allow polyps to be divided into low, intermediate and high risk.
- **High risk polyps:**
  - o ≥ 2 premalignant polyps, including at least one advanced colorectal polyp (defined as a serrated polyp ≥10 mm in size *or* containing any grade of dysplasia *or* as an adenoma ≥10 mm in size *or* containing high-grade dysplasia).
  - o ≥ 5 premalignant polyps.

43

Inflammatory Bowel Disease

[5] Ulcerative colitis. *March 22, Dec 18*

[3] Ulcerative colitis. *Oct 20*

- It is an **inflammatory bowel disease.**
- It is a **chronic condition** that is **confined to the large intestine.**

Aetiology

- The overall **incidence is steadily increasing worldwide** and is linked to:
  - o Improved public hygiene.
  - o Industrialization.
  - o Western diet.
  - o Genetic predisposition.
  - o Environmental factors that trigger abnormal immune responses that lead to intestinal inflammation.

Pathology

- UC is characterised by **mucosal inflammation of the large bowel, *always involving the rectum* (proctitis) and extending to involve varying degrees of more proximal colon (colitis).**
- When the entire colon and rectum are involved (**pancolitis**), some patients may also have a degree of '**backwash ileitis**', in which there is secondary inflammation in the terminal ileum.
- It is a chronic condition that tends to be **relapsing and remitting.**
- Early relapse and persistent disease **within the first 2 years of diagnosis** are both predictors of a **severe disease course.**

HPE

- Atrophy and distortion of the crypts.
- Irregularity of the mucosal villi.
- Marked infiltration of plasma cells within the deep lamina propria (basal plasmacytosis).
- Mucus depletion.
- Pseudopolyposis.
- Irregular mucosal swelling called **dysplasia associated lesions or mass (DALMs)** are highly predictive of coexisting carcinoma.
- Stricturing is very unusual and should prompt urgent assessment because of the possibility of coexisting carcinoma.

Clinical Features

The clinical presentation depends on extent of disease:

a. If inflammation is confined to rectum (proctitis):

- Rectal bleeding.
- Tenesmus.
- Mucous discharge.
- Disease often remains confined to rectum, usually with a benign course.

b. When colon is involved (colitis):

- Bloody diarrhea.
- Urgency.

c. **Severe and/or extensive colitis:**

- Anaemia.
- Hypoproteinemia.
- Electrolyte disturbances.
- Pain is unusual.
- Systemic illness:
  - o Malaise.
  - o Loss of appetite.
  - o Fever.
- Children with poorly controlled colitis may have impaired growth.
- The more extensive the disease, the more likely are extraintestinal manifestations to occur.

Investigations

A. Endoscopy

- Rigid proctoscopy, flexible sigmoidoscopy or colonoscopy.
- Can detect proctitis, colitis:
  - o Mucosa is hyperemic.
  - o Bleeds on touch.
  - o Purulent exudate may be present.
- When there has been remission and relapse:
  - o Regenerative mucosal nodules or pseudo-polyps.
  - o Tiny ulcers may be seen that appear to coalesce.
- Colonoscopy is contraindicated in severe acute colitis because of the risk of colonic perforation.
- Biopsy can also be taken.

B. Radiology

- Plain X-ray abdomen:
  - o May demonstrate toxic megacolon.
- CT scan:
  - o Significant thickening of colonic wall.
  - o Inflammatory stranding in colonic mesentery.

Treatment

A. Medical Treatment

a. **5-Amino salicylic acid (5-ASA) derivatives:**

- First line treatment.
- Given topically (per rectum) or systemically.
- COX inhibitors.
- It does not get degraded before reaching the colon.
- Used as a single agent:
  - o To treat ulcerative proctitis.
  - o As maintenance therapy following induction of remission.

b. **Corticosteroids**

- **Drugs:** Prednisone, hydrocortisone.
- Used either topically or systemically.
- Widespread anti-inflammatory action.
- Used in combination with 5-ASA derivatives to induce remission of symptoms.

c. **Immunosuppressants/Thiopurine:**

- **Drugs:** Azathioprine (it is a prodrug which is metabolised to 6-mercapto purine), Cyclosporine.
- Both drugs are immunosuppressants and inhibit cell mediated immunity.
- Used to maintain remission stage: These are a 'steroid-sparing' class of drugs that are usually begun once patients are placed on steroids and perhaps have been unsuccessful in weaning off steroids.

d. **Monoclonal antibodies:**

- Drugs: Infliximab, Adalimumab
- Both are TNF-α antagonists, which has a central role in inflammatory cascades.

B. Nutritional Support

- Patients with moderate nutritional impairment will require nutritional supplementation.
- Severely malnourished patients may require enteral tube or even IV feeding.
- Anaemia, hypoproteinemia and electrolyte, vitamin and metabolic bone problems must all be addressed.
- Nutritional optimisation improves surgical outcomes.

C. Surgery

- Indications for surgery are as follows:
  - o Severe or fulminating disease failing to respond to medical therapy.

- o Chronic disease with anemia, frequent stools, urgency and tenesmus.
- o Steroid dependent disease where remission cannot be maintained without substantial doses of steroids with harmful side effects.
- o Intolerance or side effects of medical therapy required to control the disease, e.g., steroid psychosis, azathioprine induced pancreatitis.
- o Growth retardation in children or adolescents.
- o Neoplastic change: Patients who have severe dysplasia or carcinoma.
- o Associated sclerosing cholangitis.
- o Extraintestinal manifestations.
- o Rarely, severe hemorrhage or stenosis causing obstruction.

- The procedures done are:

a. **Emergency:**

- o The safest procedure is **subtotal colectomy and end ileostomy**

b. **Elective:**

- o The following operations are available:
  1. **Subtotal colectomy and ileostomy.**
  2. **Proctocolectomy and permanent end ileostomy.**
  3. **Restorative proctocolectomy with ileal pouch-anal anastomosis.**
  4. **Subtotal colectomy and ileo-rectal anastomosis.**

[5] Mention extraintestinal manifestations of ulcerative colitis. *Dec 15*

- The extraintestinal manifestations of ulcerative colitis are as follows:

1. **Arthritis:**
   - o It is typically an asymmetrical large joint polyarthropathy which affects knees, ankles, elbows and wrists.
2. **Sacroiliitis.**
3. **Ankylosing spondylitis.**
4. **Sclerosing cholangitis.**
   - o This can progress to cirrhosis and hepatocellular failure.
5. **Cholangiocarcinoma.**
6. **Erythema nodosum.**
7. **Pyoderma gangrenosum.**
8. **Uveitis.**
9. **Episcleritis.**

[5] Crohn's disease. *Dec 19, June 16, July 15, July 23*

[3] Crohn's disease. *Aug 22, June 14*

- Also known as **regional enteritis.**
- It is an **inflammatory bowel disease.**
- It is characterised by a chronic **full-thickness inflammatory process that can affect any part of the GIT from the lips to the anal margin.**

Aetiology

- Not understood completely.
- Involves a complex interplay of genetic and environmental factors.
- **Infectious agents:**
  - o *Mycobacterium paratuberculosis.*
  - o Enteroadherent *Escherichia coli.*
- Highly refined diet, food additives, preservatives.
- High levels of sanitation in childhood.
- Smoking increases the relative risk of Crohn's and is an exacerbating factor after diagnosis.
- **Genetic factors:** NOD2/CARD15.
- Family history.
- Alterations in the gut microbiome, with generally decreased microbial diversity.

Pathogenesis

- Increased **gut mucosal permeability** leads to **increased passage of luminal antigens** that induces a **cell-mediated inflammatory response.**
- Pro-inflammatory cytokines (**IL-2 and TNF**) **are then released.**
- Associated with a **defect in suppressor T-cells.**

Pathology

- It **may affect any portion of the GIT from mouth to anus.**

- The **terminal ileum is the most commonly affected segment** of bowel, often occurring in combination with other areas of disease.
- More **proximal small bowel is less frequently involved.**
- **Perianal lesions** are **common.**
- Fibrotic thickening of the intestinal wall with narrowing (**stricturing**) of the lumen.
- Fat wrapping is seen (**encroachment of mesenteric fat** around the bowel).
- There is usually **dilated bowel just proximal to the stricture.**
- There are **deep mucosal ulcerations with linear or serpiginous (snake like) patterns** in the strictured area itself.
- Edema between ulcers gives rise to a characteristic **cobblestone appearance of the mucosa.**
- The **transmural inflammation (a pathognomonic feature of Crohn's)** may lead to segments of bowel becoming adherent to each other and to surrounding structures, forming inflammatory masses with mesenteric abscesses and fistulation into adjacent organs.
- **Serosa** is usually **opaque**, with **thickening of the mesentery** and **enlarged mesenteric lymph nodes.**
- It is characteristically discontinuous, with inflamed areas separated by apparently normal intestine, so called **skip lesions.**

HPE

- **Focal areas of chronic inflammation involving all layers** of the intestinal wall with **lymphoid aggregates.**
- **Non-caseating giant cell granulomas** are pathognomonic, and are most commonly seen in anorectal disease.
- **Multifocal arterial occlusions** are found in thickened muscularis propria.
- Nerve cell hyperplasia.
- Deep, fissuring ulceration within affected areas.
- There may be completely normal areas immediately next to areas of severe inflammation.

Clinical Features

- The clinical presentation depends on the pattern of disease:
    - May present acutely with ileal inflammation and symptoms and signs resembling those of acute appendicitis.
    - Free perforation of the small intestine resulting in a local or diffuse peritonitis.
    - May rarely present with acute severe colitis.
- **Small bowel Crohn's disease often presents with:**
    - Bouts of abdominal pain.
    - Mild diarrhea.
    - A tender mass may be palpable in the right iliac fossa.
    - Intermittent fever.
    - Anemia.
    - Weight loss.
    - After months of repeated attacks characterised by acute inflammation, the affected area of intestine undergoes stenosis along with fibrosis, causing chronic obstructive symptoms.
    - As the disease progresses, transmural fissuring, intra-abdominal abscesses and fistulae may develop.
    - Children developing the illness before puberty may have retarded growth and sexual development.
- **Fistulation:**
    - May occur into adjacent loops of bowel (entero-enteric or interloop fistulae).
    - Ileosigmoid fistulation causes profuse diarrhea.
    - Enterovesical (into the urinary bladder).
    - Into the female genital tract (rectovaginal fistula).
    - Into the duodenum.
    - Enterocutaneous fistula.
- **Colonic involvement presents with symptoms of colitis and proctitis:**
    - Bloody diarrhea.
    - Tenesmus.
    - Mucous discharge.
- **Perianal problems:**
    - Large, edematous and inflamed skin tags.
    - Fissures.
    - Superficial ulcers are relatively painless.

- o Deep cavitating ulcers are painful and can cause perianal abscesses and fistulae.
- o Dense, fibrous stricturing (stenosis) at the anorectal junction.
- o Incontinence.

Investigations

A. Serologic Markers

- pANCA or perinuclear anti-neutrophil cytoplasmic antibody.
- BPI or bactericidal/permeability increasing protein.
- Lactoferrin.
- Cathepsin G.
- Elastase.
- ASCA or anti-Saccharomyces Cereivisiae antibody.
- Anti-C Bir 1 or outer membrane porin of flagellin.
- Omp C - IgG or outer membrane porin of *E coli.*

B. Blood Tests

- CBC may show anemia.
- Active inflammatory disease is usually associated with low serum albumin, magnesium, zinc and selenium.
- CRP and ESR correlate with disease activity.

C. Stool Markers

- Calprotectin.
- Lactoferrin.

D. Endoscopy (Colonoscopy, Upper GI Endoscopy, Enteroscopy)

- The earliest findings are aphthous ulcers, surrounded by a rim of erythematous mucosa.
- Skip lesions.
- Cobblestone appearance.
- Stricturing.
- Deep longitudinal ulcers.
- Biopsy should be taken to exclude malignancy.

E. Radiology

- CT enterography or MR enterography show the following:
  - o Bowel damage.
  - o Transmural thickening.
  - o Intestinal strictures.
- **High resolution USG:**
  - o Inflamed and thickened bowel loops.
  - o Fluid collections and abscesses.
- **CT scan with oral contrast:**
  - o Fistulae.
  - o Intra-abdominal abscesses.
  - o Bowel thickening or dilatation.
- **MRI:**
  - o Perianal disease.
- **Contrast X-rays:**
  - o Long lengths of narrowed terminal ileum called string sign of Kantor.
  - o Fistulae between adjacent bowel loops and organs.

Treatment

Medical Treatment

A. Corticosteroids

- Used to treat acute flares.
- **Oral drugs:** Prednisone.
- Steroid enemas.

B. Aminosalicylates

- 5-ASA agents are used to treat colonic symptoms.

C. Antibiotics

- May be used to treat an inflammatory mass or abscess.
- Ciprofloxacin, metronidazole.
- A confirmed abscess should be treated by percutaneous drainage and/or surgery.

D. Immunomodulators

- Used for maintenance therapy.
- Azathioprine (6-mercapto purine), cyclosporine.
- Inhibit cell mediated immune responses.

E. Monoclonal Antibodies

- Infliximab, adalimumab.
- Used for induction as well as maintenance of remission.

- Anti-TNFα activity.
- Newer drugs such as vedolizumab and etrolizumab prevent leukocyte migration, preferentially in the GIT.

Nutritional Support

- Oral supplementation, enteral tube, parenteral nutrition.
- Correct anemia, hypoproteinemia, dyselectrolytemia, vitamin and mineral deficiencies.

Endoscopy

- Balloon dilation of fibrostenotic strictures.
- Contraindicated in inflamed or ulcerated strictures because of the risk of perforation.

Surgery

The surgical options depend on the pattern of disease.

1. **Ileo-caecal resection**
   - It is done with a primary anastomosis between ileum and ascending or transverse colon.
   - Ileostomy without primary anastomosis is indicated if the patient is unwell, has active infection or is nutritionally depleted.
2. **Segmental resection**
   - Of short segments of small or large bowel strictures.
3. **Colectomy and ileorectal anastomosis**
   - When only colon is involved, and rectum and anus are spared.
4. **Subtotal colectomy and ileostomy.**
5. **Temporary loop ileostomy**
   - Done in patients with acute distal Crohn's, allowing remission and later restoration of continuity or in patients with severe perianal or rectal disease.
6. **Panproctocolectomy**
   - Done with a permanent ileostomy.
   - In patients with severe colonic and anal involvement.
7. **Strictureplasty**
   - Heineke-Mikulicz technique.
   - Finney technique.

Treatment of Perianal Crohn's Disease

- Drainage of abscess.
- **Fistulae:** Setons, fistulotomy, advancement flaps, Ligation of Intersphincteric Fistulous Tract (LIFT).
- **Monoclonal antibodies:** Infliximab, adalimumab.

OTHER IMPORTANT TOPICS

CROHN'S DISEASE v/s ULCERATIVE COLITIS

PARAMETER	CROHN'S DISEASE	ULCERATIVE COLITIS
Symptoms and signs		
Diarrhoea	Common	Common
Rectal bleeding	Less common	Almost always
Abdominal pain (cramps)	Moderate to severe	Mild to moderate
Palpable mass	At times	No (unless large cancer)
Anal complaints	Frequent (>50%)	Infrequent (<20%)
Radiologic findings		
Ileal disease	Common	Rare (backwash ileitis)
Nodularity, fuzziness	No	Yes
Distribution	Skip lesions	Rectum, extending proximally and continuously
Ulcers	Linear, cobblestone, fissures	Collar-button
Toxic dilation	Rare	Uncommon
Proctoscopic findings		
Anal fissure, fistula, abscess	Common	Rare
Rectal sparing	Common (50%)	Rare (5%)
Granular mucosa	No	Yes
Ulceration	Linear, deep, scattered	Superficial, universal

44

Intestinal Obstruction

SMALL BOWEL OBSTRUCTION/ INTESTINAL OBSTRUCTION

[10] Discuss aetiology, clinical features and management of small bowel obstruction. ***August 22, Dec 15***

[10] Describe briefly aetiology, clinical features and management of acute intestinal obstruction. ***Sept 21***

[10] Describe the aetiology, clinical features and management of small bowel obstruction. ***Dec 18***

[10] Discuss the clinical features, investigations and management of small bowel obstruction. ***June 13***

[10] Discuss causes, pathophysiology, clinical features and management of acute intestinal obstruction. ***Dec 12***

[5] Acute intestinal obstruction. ***Dec 15***

[3] Mention the causes of intestinal obstruction. ***July 15***

- Intestinal obstruction is a **common surgical emergency** and because of its serious nature, it demands early diagnosis and speedy relief.

Causes/Types

Intestinal obstruction may be broadly classified into 2 types:

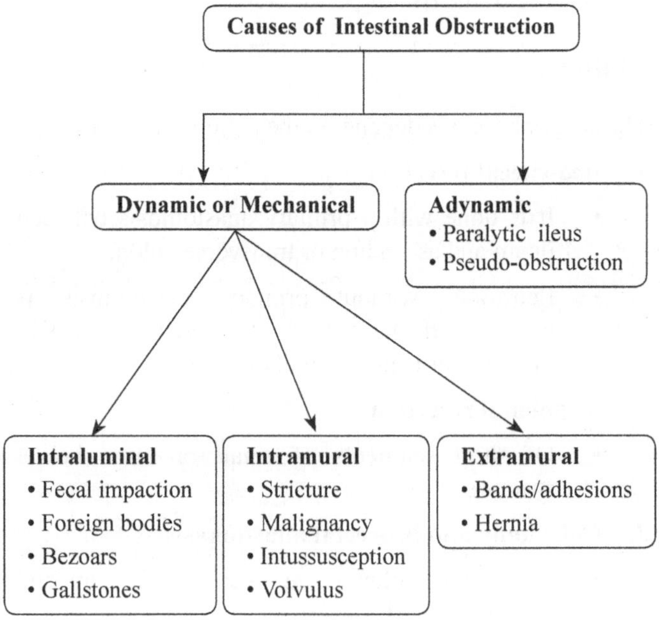

A. Dynamic or Mechanical Obstruction

- **Peristalsis is present** and it is **working against a mechanical obstruction**.
- It may occur in an acute or a chronic form.
- The mechanical obstruction may be in the lumen, in the wall or outside the wall.

a. Intraluminal:

- o Fecal impaction.
- o Foreign bodies.
- o Bezoars.
- o Gallstones.

b. **Intramural:**
   - o Stricture.
   - o Malignancy.
   - o Intussusception.
   - o Volvulus.

c. **Extramural:**
   - o Bands/adhesions (this is the **most common cause of intestinal obstruction**).
   - o Hernia.

B. Adynamic Obstruction

- There is no mechanical obstruction.
- Peristalsis is absent or inadequate.
- **Causes:**
  - o Paralytic ileus.
  - o Pseudo-obstruction.

Pathophysiology

- Irrespective of aetiology or acuteness of onset, in dynamic (mechanical) obstruction:
  - o The **bowel proximal** to the obstruction **dilates.**
  - o The bowel **below** the **obstruction exhibits normal peristalsis and absorption until it becomes empty and collapses.**
- Initially, proximal peristalsis is increased in an attempt to overcome the obstruction.
- If the obstruction is not relieved, the bowel continues to dilate; **ultimately** there is a reduction in peristaltic strength, **resulting in flaccidity and paralysis.**
- The distension proximal to an obstruction is caused by two factors:
  1. **Gas:**
     - o Bacterial overgrowth produces gas.
     - o Majority of the gas is made up of nitrogen (90%) and hydrogen sulphide.
  2. **Fluid:**
     - o Consists of various digestive juices: Saliva – 500 ml + bile – 500 ml + pancreatic secretions – 500 ml + gastric secretions – 1000 ml. This is over a period of 24 hours.
- These accumulate in the gut lumen as **absorption** by the obstructed gut **is retarded.**
- **Dehydration and electrolyte loss** are therefore due to:
  - o Reduced oral intake.
  - o Defective intestinal absorption.
  - o Losses as a result of vomiting.
  - o Sequestration in the bowel lumen.
  - o Transudation of fluid into the peritoneal cavity.
- In simple intestinal obstruction the blood supply is intact, whereas in strangulated intestinal obstruction the blood supply is decreased or absent.

Clinical Features

- The diagnosis of dynamic intestinal obstruction is based on the **classic quartet** of symptoms:
  1. Pain abdomen.
  2. Distension.
  3. Vomiting.
  4. Absolute constipation or obstipation.

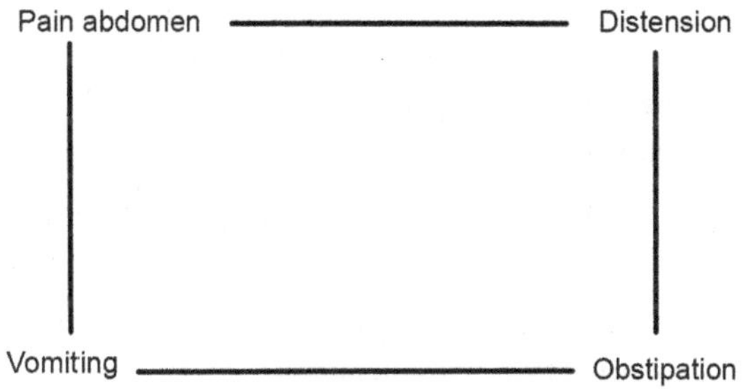

Figure 1: Quadrad of intestinal obstruction

- **Pain:**
  - o It is the **first symptom.**
  - o Occurs suddenly and is **usually severe.**
  - o **Colicky** in nature.
  - o Usually centered on the umbilicus (small bowel) or lower abdomen (large bowel).
  - o With increasing distension, the colicky pain is replaced by a more diffuse constant pain.
  - o The development of **severe pain suggests strangulation**, especially if it is continuous.

- **Vomiting:**
  - o The more distal the obstruction, the longer the interval between the onset of symptoms and the appearance of nausea and vomiting.
  - o In **small bowel** obstruction the vomitus contains **digested food.**
  - o In **large bowel** obstruction the vomitus contains **feculent material.**
- **Distension:**
  - o The degree of distension is dependent on the site of obstruction and is **greater, the more distal the lesion.**
  - o **Visible peristalsis** may be present in thin patients which can sometimes be provoked by flicking the abdominal wall.
- **Absolute constipation or obstipation:**
  - o Neither feces nor flatus is passed.
  - o It is a cardinal feature of intestinal obstruction.
  - o Some patients may pass flatus or faeces after the onset of obstruction as a result of the evacuation of the distal bowel contents.
- **Dehydration:**
  - o Seen most commonly in small bowel obstruction **because of repeated vomiting and fluid sequestration**.
  - o Dry skin and tongue, sunken eyes, oliguria, hypovolemic shock.
  - o Blood **urea** level and **hematocrit rise**, giving a secondary polycythemia.
- **Pyrexia** in the presence of obstruction indicates:
  - o The onset of ischemia..
  - o Intestinal perforation.
  - o Inflammation or abscess associated with the obstructing disease.
- **Localized abdominal tenderness** indicates impending or established **ischemia**.
- The development of peritonism or **peritonitis** indicates impending or established infarction and/or **perforation**.
- **Bowel sounds:**
  - o **High pitched bowel sounds** are present in the vast majority of patients with intestinal obstruction.
  - o Bowel sounds **may be scanty or absent** if the obstruction is longstanding and the **small bowel has become inactive**.
  - o The presence of normal bowel sounds means that there is no intestinal obstruction.
- In all cases of suspected intestinal obstruction, the **hernial orifices must be examined.**

Investigations

A. X-ray Abdomen

- Erect X-rays are no longer routinely obtained and the **radiological diagnosis is based on a supine abdominal film**. An erect film may be subsequently requested when further doubt exists.
- Dilation of bowel loops is seen on supine X-ray. The various threshold levels for bowel dilation are:
  - o Small bowel: 3 cm
  - o Caecum: 12 cm
  - o Proximal large bowel: 9 cm
  - o Distal large bowel: 6 cm
- Obstructed small bowel is characterized by straight segments that are generally central and lie transversely.
- **No/minimal gas is seen in the colon.**
- **Jejunum** is characterized by its **valvulae conniventes**, which completely pass across the width of the bowel and are regularly spaced, giving a **'concertina' or ladder effect**.

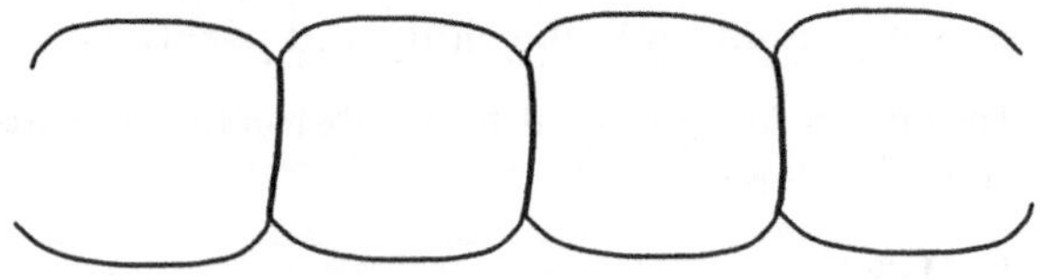

Figure 2: Valvulae conniventes

- The **distal ileum is featureless.**
- A distended caecum appears as a rounded gas shadow in the right iliac fossa.
- **Large bowel** (except for caecum) **shows haustral folds**, which are spaced irregularly, do not cross the whole diameter of the bowel and do not have indentations placed opposite one another.

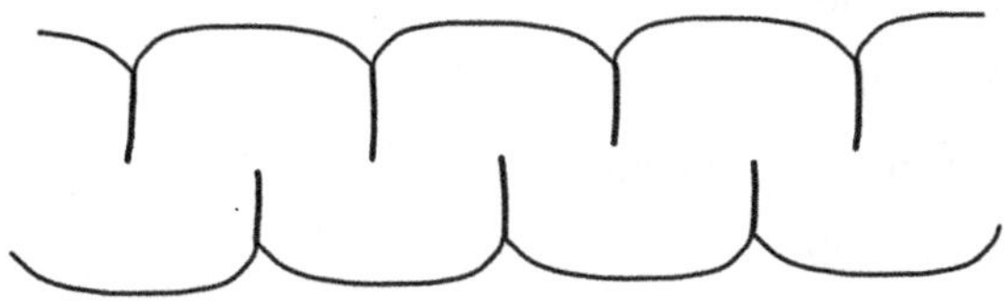

Figure 3: Haustral folds

- Small bowel fluid levels may be seen on an erect X-ray:
  - o In adults, **2 inconstant fluid levels**: One at the duodenal cap and the other in the terminal ileum, may be regarded as normal.
  - o During the obstructive process, **fluid levels** become more conspicuous and **more numerous** when paralysis has occurred.
  - o In the small bowel, the **number of fluid levels is directly proportional to the degree of obstruction and to its site**, the number increasing the more distal the lesion.
- Low colonic obstruction does not commonly give rise to small bowel fluid levels unless advanced.
  - o High colonic obstruction may do so in the presence of an incompetent ileocecal valve.
- **Colonic obstruction** is usually associated with a **large amount of gas** in the **cecum.**

B. CT Scan

- Highly accurate.
- Now used very widely.
- Can demonstrate the cause.
- Proximal dilation with distal compression is seen.

Treatment

A. Gastrointestinal Drainage via A Nasogastric Tube

- Nasogastric decompression is achieved by the passage of a non-vented (Ryle) or vented (Salem) tube.
- Normally placed on free drainage with 4-hourly aspiration but may be placed on continuous or intermittent suction.

B. Fluid and Electrolyte Replacement

- The basic biochemical abnormality in intestinal obstruction is **sodium and water loss**.
- Therefore, the **appropriate replacement is Hartmann's solution or normal saline**.
- The volume required varies and should be determined by clinical, hematological and biochemical criteria.

C. Relief of Obstruction

D. Surgical Treatment

- It is necessary for most cases of intestinal obstruction but **should be delayed until resuscitation is complete**, provided there is no sign of strangulation or evidence of closed loop obstruction.
- **Indications for early surgical intervention:**
  1. Obstructed external hernia.
  2. Intestinal strangulation.
  3. Obstruction in a virgin abdomen.
- If there is complete obstruction, but no evidence of intestinal ischemia, it is reasonable to defer surgery until the patient has been adequately resuscitated.
- Where obstruction is likely to be secondary to adhesions, **conservative management may be continued for up to 72 hours in the hope of spontaneous resolution.**
- If the site of obstruction is unknown, adequate exposure is best achieved by a **midline laparotomy** incision. Assessment is directed to:
  - o The site of the obstruction.
  - o The nature of the obstruction.
  - o The viability of the gut.
- **Operative decompression** should be performed whenever possible.
- The simplest and safest method is to insert a large bore orogastric tube and to **milk the small bowel contents in a retrograde manner** to the stomach for aspiration.
- The **type of surgical procedure required will depend upon the cause** of obstruction:
  - o Division of adhesions or adhesiolysis.
  - o Excision.
  - o Bypass.
  - o Proximal decompression or stoma formation.

[5] Post-op adhesions. *Oct 20*

- Post-op adhesions are the **most common cause of intestinal obstruction.**
- It is an **extramural dynamic cause** of intestinal obstruction.

Causes

1. **Acute inflammation:** Sites of anastomoses, reperitonealisation of raw areas, trauma, ischemia.
2. **Foreign material:** Talc, starch, gauze, silk.
3. **Infection:** Peritonitis, tuberculosis.
4. **Chronic inflammatory conditions:** Crohn's disease.
5. **Radiation enteritis.**

Pathogenesis

- Adhesions start to **form within hours of abdominal surgery.**
- In the **early post op period,** the onset of such a mechanical obstruction may be **difficult to differentiate from paralytic items.**
- Any source of peritoneal irritation results in local **fibrin** production, which **produces adhesions** between apposed surfaces.
- **Early fibrinous adhesions may disappear when the cause is removed or they may become vascularized and be replaced by mature fibrous tissue.**
- Post-op adhesions giving rise to intestinal obstruction **usually involve the lower small bowel** and less commonly the large bowel.

Prevention of Adhesions

- Factors that may limit adhesion formation include:
  - o Good surgical technique.
  - o Washing of the peritoneal cavity with saline to remove clots.
  - o Minimizing contact with gauze.
  - o Covering anastomoses and raw peritoneal surfaces.

Clinical Features

- Pain abdomen.
- Distension.
- Vomiting.
- Absolute constipation.
- Dehydration.
- Hypovolemic shock.
- High pitched bowel sounds are present in the vast majority of patients with intestinal obstruction. Bowel sounds may be scanty or absent if the obstruction is longstanding and the small bowel has become inactive.

Investigations

- X-ray abdomen: erect, supine.
- CECT abdomen.

Treatment

- Patient is initially treated conservatively, provided there are no signs of strangulation.
- Should rarely continue conservative treatment for >72 hours.
- At operation, **divide only the causative adhesion(s) and limit dissection.**
- **Repair serosal tears; invaginate (or resect) areas of doubtful viability.**

[3] Paralytic ileus. *Dec 19*

[5] Paralytic ileus. *July 15*

[5] Causes of paralytic ileus. *July 23*

- **Definition:** Paralytic ileus **may be defined as a state in which there is failure of transmission of peristaltic waves secondary to neuromuscular failure, i.e., in the myenteric (Auerbach's) and submucous (Meissner's) plexuses.**
- It is a type of **adynamic intestinal obstruction**, i.e., there is no mechanical obstruction *but* peristalsis is absent or inadequate.

Types/Causes

Paralytic ileus can be of the following types:

1. **Postoperative:**
   - A degree of ileus usually occurs after any abdominal procedure and is **self-limiting**, with a variable duration of 24-72 hours.

- Post-op ileus may be **prolonged** in the presence of **hypoproteinemia or metabolic abnormality**.

2. **Infection:**
   - Intra-abdominal sepsis may give rise to localized or generalized ileus.
3. **Reflex ileus:**
   - This may occur following fractures of the spine or ribs, retroperitoneal haemorrhage or even after the application of a plaster jacket.
4. **Metabolic:**
   - Uremia and hypokalemia are the most common contributory factors.

Clinical Features

- Paralytic ileus takes on a clinical significance if, **72 hours after laparotomy:**
  - o There has been **no return of bowel sounds** on auscultation.
  - o There has been **no passage of flatus**.
- Abdominal **distension becomes more marked** and drum like (tympanitic).
- Distension causes an increase in pain from the abdominal wound.
- **Colicky pain is not a feature.**
- In the absence of gastric aspiration, there is **effortless vomiting** of large volumes of dirty fluid.
- There may be **respiratory distress** from the abdominal distension.
- Pulse rate increases.
- Prolonged distension increases the **risk of wound dehiscence.**
- **Bowel sounds:**
  - o **High pitched tinkling note**, 'like bells at evening pealing'.
  - o Occurs **every 10-30 seconds.**
  - o It is distinctive of paralytic ileus.
  - o It is not because of peristalsis, but is **due to the overflow of fluid from one distended loop to another.**

Investigations

- Paralytic ileus is a clinical diagnosis:
  - o **X-ray Abdomen:**
    - a. Supine film – Dilated gas filled bowel loops.
    - b. Erect film – Multiple air fluid levels.
  - o Renal function tests.

Treatment

- Specific treatment is **directed towards the cause**, but the following general principles apply.
- If a **primary cause** is identified, then it **must be treated.**
- Restriction of oral intake by keeping the patient **NPO**.
- Gastrointestinal distension must be relieved by **decompression.**
  - o Nasogastric tube or Ryle's tube.
  - o Flatus tube.
- Close attention to **fluid and electrolyte balance** is essential.
- There is no convincing evidence for the use of prokinetic drugs to treat post-op adynamic ileus.
- If paralytic ileus is prolonged, a **CT scan will demonstrate any intra-abdominal sepsis or mechanical obstruction** and therefore guide any requirement for laparotomy.
- The decision to take a patient back to theatre is always difficult.
- The need for a re-laparotomy becomes increasingly likely the longer the bowel inactivity persists, particularly if it lasts for > 7 days or if bowel activity recommences after surgery and then ceases.

[5] Intussusception. *March 21, June 19, Dec 16, June 14, Feb 23*

[3] Types and causes of intussusception. *June 17*

- **Definition:** Acute intussusception occurs when **one portion of the gut invaginates into an immediately adjacent segment**. Almost invariably, it is the **proximal into the distal.**

Causes

- Almost **90% of cases are idiopathic** but an **associated upper respiratory tract infection or gastroenteritis may precede the condition.**
- **Hyperplasia of Peyer's patches** in the terminal ileum may be the **initiating event.**
- Weaning.
- Loss of passively acquired maternal immunity.

- **Common viral pathogens**
- **Lead point** causing intussusception is common after the age of 2 years:
  - o Meckel's diverticulum.
  - o Polyp (e.g., Peutz-Jeghers syndrome).
  - o Duplication.
  - o Henoch-Schönlein purpura.
  - o Appendix.
  - o Submucosal lipoma.
  - o Other tumours.

Pathology

- An intussusception is composed of **3 parts:**
  1. The entering or inner tube (**intussusceptum**).
  2. The **returning or middle tube.**
  3. The sheath or outer tube (**intussuscipiens**).
- The part that advances is called the apex, the mass is the intussusception and the neck is the junction of the entering layer with the mass.

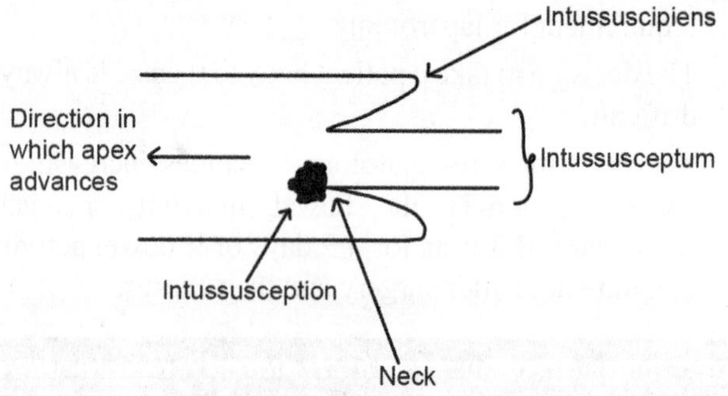

Figure 4: Parts of intussusception

Types

- Intussusception may be anatomically defined according to the site and extent of invagination:
  - o Ileo-ileal.
  - o **Ileo-colic (most common in children).**
  - o Ileoileo-colic.
  - o **Colo-colic (most common in adults).**
  - o Multiple.
  - o Retrograde.
  - o Others.
- The **degree of ischemia is dependent on the tightness of invagination**, which is usually greatest as it passes through the ileocecal valve.

Clinical Features

- It is seen **most commonly in children**, with a peak incidence between 5 and 10 months of age.
- When seen in **older children (>2 years) and adults**, it is associated with a pathological **lead point.**
- M > F.
- The classic presentation is with **episodes of screaming and drawing up of the legs** in a previously well, male infant.
- Attacks **last for a few minutes** and **recur** repeatedly.
- During attacks the child appears pale and **between episodes** may be **listless**.
- Vomiting may or may not occur initially, but becomes noticeable and bile stained with time.
- **Red currant jelly stool**, i.e., containing blood and mucus.
- **In extensive ileocolic or colocolic intussusception, the apex may be palpable or even protrude from the anus.**
- Unrelieved, peritonitis may result secondary to gangrene.

On Examination

- Examination should be undertaken between episodes of colic without disturbing the child.
- Abdomen is not distended initially.
- A **lump that hardens on palpation** may be present.
- Sausage shaped lump with concavity towards umbilicus.
- **Sign of Dance:** Feeling of emptiness in the right iliac fossa.

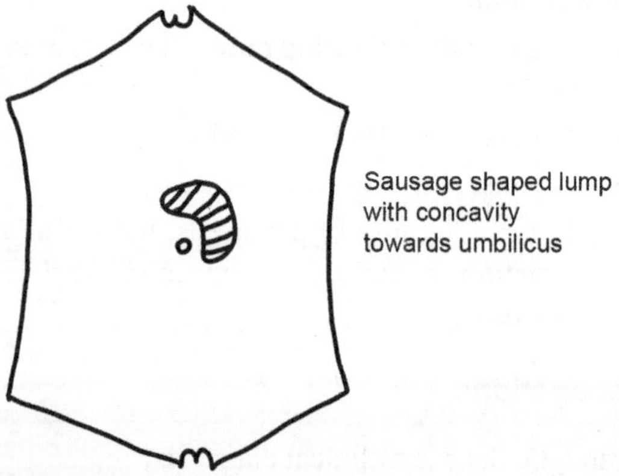

Figure 5: Clinical examination of intussusception

Investigations

1. **X-ray**
   - Evidence of small or large bowel obstruction.
   - In ileocolic cases, cecal gas shadow is absent.
   - A soft tissue opacity is often visible in children.
2. **Barium enema**
   - May be used to diagnose the presence of an ileocolic intussusception.
3. **USG**
   - Has a high diagnostic sensitivity in children.
   - **Doughnut appearance** of concentric rings.
4. **CT scan**
   - It is the **most accurate** imaging method to confirm intussusception.
   - **Target or sausage shaped soft tissue mass with a layering effect is seen.**
   - **Mesenteric vessels within the bowel lumen** are also typical.

Treatment

a. **Nasogastric drainage.**

b. **Resuscitation with IV fluids.**

c. **Broad spectrum antibiotics.**

d. **Non-operative reduction:**
   - Can be attempted using an air or barium enema.
   - Recurrence is common after non-operative reduction.

e. **Surgery:**
   - Required when radiological reduction has failed or is contraindicated.
   - Following laparotomy, **reduction is achieved by gently compressing the most distal part of the intussusception towards its origin**.

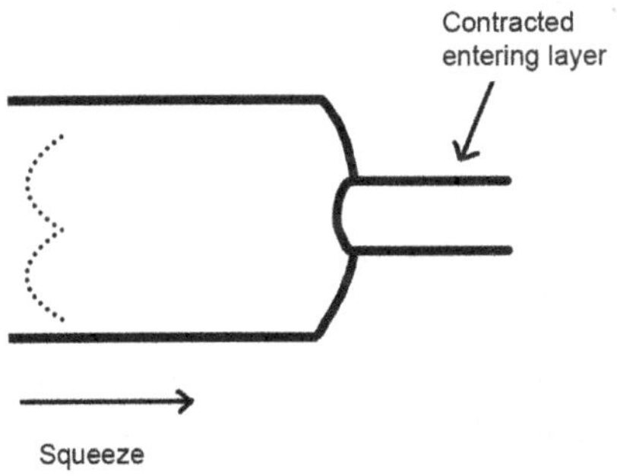

Figure 6: Method of reducing an intussusception

- Viability of the whole bowel should be checked carefully.
- An irreducible intussusception or one complicated by infarction or a pathological lead point requires **resection and primary anastomosis**.

[3] Nasogastric tube. *Dec 14*

- A nasogastric tube is a flexible, hollow tube that is inserted through the nose and down the nasopharynx, oropharynx, hypopharynx and esophagus into the stomach.
- It is made of silicone, polyurethane or polyvinyl chloride.
- It is available in various sizes/diameters.

Uses

1. **Decompression** of stomach/upper GIT in a case of intestinal obstruction.
2. **Enteral feeding** (in patients who are unable to eat or swallow).
3. Gastric **lavage** (in cases of poisoning).
4. It helps **regain gastric tone.**
5. To **administer drugs.**
6. **Diagnostic purposes** (to collect gastric contents for analysis).
7. **Prevents aspiration** of gastric contents into lungs, in patients who have difficulty swallowing.
8. **Pre-op preparation**, e.g., before gastrectomy.

VOLVULUS

[10] Aetiopathogenesis of sigmoid volvulus and write in detail about the management. *July 18*

[5] Volvulus of sigmoid colon. *March 22, Oct 20, Dec 18, Dec 17, Dec 15*

[3] Coffee bean appearance. *June 14*

[3] Causes of sigmoid volvulus. *Dec 13*

- **Definition:** A sigmoid volvulus is a **twist of the sigmoid colon and the mesentery that supplies it.**
- It is the **most common volvulus.**

Predisposing Factors

- Band of adhesions (Peridiverticulitis).
- Overloaded pelvic colon, i.e., chronic constipation.

- Long pelvic mesocolon.
- Narrow attachment of pelvic mesocolon.
- Pelvic mass.
- Pregnancy.
- Fiber rich diet.

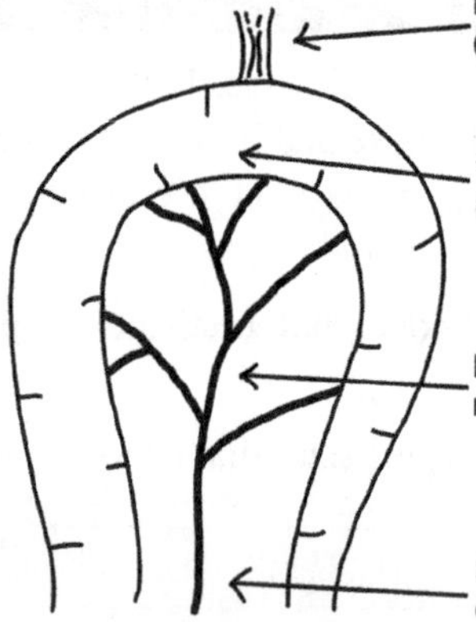

Figure 7: Predisposing causes of sigmoid volvulus

Pathogenesis

- The loop may **rotate half a turn**, in which event **spontaneous rectification** sometimes occurs.
- After the loop has **rotated 1½ turns**, the **veins** involved in the torsion **are compressed and the loop becomes greatly congested**.
- If it **rotates > 1½ turns**, the blood supply is cut off entirely and the **loop becomes gangrenous**.
- Rotation nearly always occurs in an **anticlockwise direction**.

Clinical Features

- Patients tend to be elderly and institutionalized.
- M > F.
- There is often a **history of acute attacks** of left sided abdominal pain, probably due to a partial volvulus, that untwists itself and is followed by the passage of large quantities of flatus and faeces.
- Sudden onset.
- **Severe abdominal pain**, which often starts while the patient is straining at stool.
- **Abdominal distension** soon follows:
  - o In no other condition does extreme abdominal distension occur so quickly.
  - o If the patient is examined 2 or 3 hours after the commencement of the attack, the distension is mainly left sided.
  - o In a matter of 6 hours, the whole abdomen becomes distended.
- Hiccough and **retching** occurs early.
- **Vomiting** occurs late.
- Constipation is absolute (**obstipation**), i.e., neither stools nor flatus is passed.
- Severe pain is a warning sign of ischemia.
- It is associated with:
  1. **Chronic neurological conditions:** Parkinson's disease, multiple sclerosis, pseudobulbar palsy.
  2. **Medications from chronic psychiatric conditions:** Chronic schizophrenia.

Investigations

1. **CT scan:**
   - It is the **mainstay of diagnosis.**
   - A large gas filled loop is seen, which lacks haustra and forms a closed-loop obstruction.
   - **Whirl sign:** Twisting of the mesentery and mesenteric vessels.
   - **X marks the spot sign:** Crossing loops of bowel are seen at the site of the transition.
2. **Plain X-ray of abdomen:**
   - Shows a large, dilated loop of the colon, often with a few gas fluid levels.
   - Rectal gas shadow is absent.
   - **Coffee bean sign:**
     - o Also known as **kidney bean** sign or **bent inner tube** sign.
     - o It is a radiological finding of plain X-ray of abdomen which is typically seen in sigmoid volvulus.
     - o The thick 'inner wall' represents the double wall thickness of apposed loops of bowel, with thin outer walls due to single wall thickness.
     - o The **apex of the dilated colon points into the right upper quadrant**.

Treatment

A. Non-Operative Decompression

- The initial management of sigmoid volvulus is non-operative decompression.
- This is done using either a rigid sigmoidoscope or a colonoscope.
- Direct vision allows assessment of mucosal viability and derotation.
- If derotation is successful, a well lubricated flatus tube should be inserted proximal to the point of torsion and left for 2-5 days.
- After successful derotation, elective interval sigmoid resection with primary anastomosis should be performed due to the high rate of recurrence.
- Bloody bowel contents or discoloured mucosa suggests ischemia and the need for urgent surgery.
  - o Attempted derotation in this situation should be abandoned as it could lead to circulatory collapse and death.

B. Surgery

1. **Resection of the volvulus followed by stoma formation:**
   - This is the **treatment of choice.**
   - **Hartmann's procedure:**
     - o The volvulus is resected.
     - o The proximal end is brought out as an end stoma.
     - o The distal rectal stump is oversewn.
   - **Paul Mikulicz double barreled stoma:**
     - o The volvulus is resected.
     - o Both the proximal and distal ends are brought out in the stoma.
   - When there is evidence of gangrene, it may be wise to ligate the mesenteric vessels before untwisting the volvulus to theoretically avoid the systemic release of ischemic toxins.
2. **Resection with primary anastomosis:**
   - Less commonly practiced.
   - Can be performed safely when the bowel is deemed to be absolutely healthy.

C. Percutaneous Endoscopic Colostomy

- This is an alternative to surgical resection in very unfit patients.
- A colonoscope is used to place a drainage tube through the abdominal wall into the sigmoid to fix the bowel in an untwisted position.

[5] Volvulus neonatorum. *Dec 19*

- It is a twisting or axial rotation of a portion of bowel about its mesentery, in neonates.
- It is a surgical emergency.

Causes

1. Malrotation of the gut.
2. Congenital bands or adhesions.
3. Genetic/familial predisposition.

Clinical Features

- Abdominal distension.
- Vomiting.
- Absolute constipation (obstipation).
- Bloody stools indicates tissue damage or compromised blood supply to intestines.
- Irritability.
- Lethargy.
- Poor feeding.
- Hyperperistaltic bowel sounds are heard initially; later the abdomen becomes silent.

Complications

- Peritonitis.
- Shock.

Pathogenesis

- Luminal obstruction is seen when there is >180° torsion.
- Vascular occlusion in mesentery is seen when there is >360° torsion.
- Bacterial fermentation adds to distension.
- Increasing intraluminal pressure impairs capillary perfusion.

- Mesenteric veins become obstructed as a result of the mechanical twisting; thrombosis results and contributes to ischemia.

Investigations

- X-ray abdomen.
- USG.
- Barium contrast studies.
- CT abdomen.
- MRI abdomen.

Treatment

- Nasogastric decompression.
- IV fluids.
- **Exploratory laparotomy:**
  - o Resection of diseased segment + anastomosis.
  - o Resection + stoma.

45

Appendix

[10] Describe the clinical features, management and differential diagnosis of acute appendicitis. ***Dec 19***

[10] Describe the clinical features and management of acute appendicitis. ***July 18***

[10] Discuss aetiology, pathology, clinical features and management of acute appendicitis. ***July 15***

[5] Acute appendicitis. ***August 22***

ACUTE APPENDICITIS

- The incidence of appendicitis had risen in the first half of the last century, but has also fallen dramatically in the past 30 years.

Aetiology

- **Decreased dietary fibre** and increased consumption of **refined carbohydrates**.
- **Race:** More common in **Whites.**
- **Social status:** More common among the **upper and middle classes.**
- **Obstruction of lumen of appendix**: Obstructing agent is usually a faecolith or a stricture; very rarely: foreign body, roundworm, threadworms or pin worms.
- **Distal obstruction of colon:** Usually an obstructing right colon carcinoma.
- Abuse of **purgatives.**
- **Bacteriology: Mixed infections.**
  - o **Gram (-):** *Escherichia coli, Pseudomonas aeruginosa, Klebsiella pneumoniae, Citrobacter, Enterobacter.*
  - o **Gram (+):** *Enterococcus, Streptococcus.*

Pathophysiology

- Acute appendicitis can cause infection of the peritoneal cavity in two ways:
  1. By perforation.
  2. By transmigration of bacteria through the appendicular wall.
- The greater omentum tries to wall off the spread of peritoneal invasion.
- There are two types of acute appendicitis:
  1. Non-obstructive or catarrhal.
  2. Obstructive.

Non-Obstructive or Catarrhal Appendicitis

- Inflammation usually starts in the mucous membrane, less often in the lymph follicles and can terminate in one of the following ways:
  - o Resolution.
  - o Ulceration.
  - o Suppuration.
  - o Fibrosis.
  - o Gangrene.

Inflammation starts in the mucosa

↓

Infection reaches the loose submucous tissues

↓

Appendix becomes turgid, dusky red and hemorrhages occur into the mucosa

↓

Artery gets occluded by inflammation or thrombosis

↓

Vascular supply of distal appendix is compromised

↓

Gangrene of the tip occurs

- Progresses slowly, so protective barriers are formed and the resulting peritonitis is localized.
- After resolution of the acute attack, fibrosis usually occurs and therefore a shrunken tip is the classical finding in recurrent appendicitis.

Obstructive Acute Appendicitis

- More common than non-obstructive.

Obstruction in the
(a) Lumen: Faecolith, foreign body or parasites
(b) Wall: Inflammatory, direct occlusion by a carcinoma of the cecum
(c) Outside the wall: Adhesions and kinking

↓

Due to obstruction, the products of inflammation become pent up

↓

Inflammation rapidly progresses and results in gangrene or perforation

- Faecolith is the most common cause of obstruction.
- Since it progresses rapidly, there is no time for protective barriers to form and early widespread peritonitis occurs.

Risk Factors for Perforation of Appendix

- Extremes of age.
- Immunosuppression.
- Diabetes mellitus.
- Faecolith obstruction.
- Pelvic appendix.
- Previous abdominal surgery.

Clinical Features

- **Age:** Relatively rare in infants and becomes increasingly common in childhood and early adult life, reaching a peak incidence in teens and early 20s. After middle age, the risk of developing appendicitis is quite small.
- **Sex:**
  - o Before puberty: M=F.
  - o Teenage and young adults: M:F = 3:2.
  - o > 25 years: M=F.
- **Migrating abdominal pain:**
  - o Patient initially complains of central abdominal or periumbilical pain (due to involvement of visceral peritoneum) which then migrates to the right iliac fossa (due to irritation of parietal peritoneum).
  - o Central abdominal pain is colicky in nature, whereas the pain in the right iliac fossa is constant.
- Atypical presentations include pain that is predominantly parietal or predominantly visceral and poorly localized.
- Atypical presentation is more common in the elderly.
- An inflamed appendix in the pelvis may cause suprapubic discomfort and tenesmus.
- Tenderness may thus be elicited only on rectal examination.
- Central abdominal pain is associated with anorexia, particularly in children.
- Nausea ± vomiting.
- Coughing or sudden movement exacerbates the right iliac fossa pain.
- Pyrexia.
- Tachycardia.

Signs in Acute Appendicitis

- **Muscle guarding over Mc Burney's point** (junction of lateral 1/3rd and medial 2/3rd of a line joining ASIS with umbilicus).

- **Finger pointing sign:** Patients point with a finger to the site of maximum pain, i.e., Mc Burney's point.
- **Rovsing sign:** Deep palpation of the left iliac fossa causes pain in the right iliac fossa.
- **Psoas sign:** If the inflamed appendix lies on the psoas muscle, it goes into spasm and the patient will lie with the right hip flexed for pain relief.
- **Obturator sign:** If an inflamed appendix is in contact with the obturator internus, flexion and internal rotation of the hip will cause pain in the hypogastrium.
- **Cutaneous hyperesthesia** may be demonstrable in the right iliac fossa.

MANTRELS or Alvarado Score

- Acute appendicitis is essentially a clinical diagnosis.
- The Alvarado or MANTRELS score is the most widely used scoring system which assists in diagnosis.

  Migratory right iliac fossa pain: 1.

  Anorexia: 1.

  Nausea and vomiting: 1.

  Tenderness in the right iliac fossa: 2.

  Rebound tenderness: 1.

  Elevated temperature: 1.

  Leucocytosis: 2.

  Shift to left: 1.

  Total = 10.
- Interpretation of Alvarado score:

  ≤ 4: Normal.

  5-6: Equivocal.

  7-8: Probable appendicitis.

  9-10: Very probable.

Investigations

1. **Ultrasound:**
   - More useful in children and thin adults.
   - Aperistaltic, non-compressible, dilated appendix (>6 mm diameter) is suggestive of acute appendicitis.
2. **CECT or contrast enhanced CT scan:**
   - More accurate than USG.
   - Radiation exposure with its carcinogenic effects are a concern.
   - Low dose protocols, which reduce the radiation dose to the patient by upto 80% are gaining popularity.
   - Especially useful in patients in whom there is diagnostic uncertainty, e.g., older patients, where acute diverticulitis, intestinal obstruction and neoplasm are the likely DD.

Treatment

A. Operative Management

- The traditional treatment for acute appendicitis is appendicectomy.
- There should be no unnecessary delay.
- All patients, particularly those most at risk of serious morbidity, benefit by a short period of intensive pre-op preparation.
  - o IV fluids.
  - o Foley's catheterization is needed only in the very ill.
  - o **Antibiotics:** IV metronidazole and 3rd generation cephalosporins. A single pre-op dose of antibiotics reduces the incidence of post-op wound infection. When peritonitis is suspected, therapeutic IV antibiotics to cover gram-negative bacilli as well as anaerobic cocci should be given.
  - o Antipyretics/analgesics.
- Performed under GA with the patient supine.
- Either an open or laparoscopic approach.
- After anaesthesia the right iliac fossa should be palpated for a mass.
- If a mass is palpable, a conservative approach may be adopted.

Open Appendicectomy

- Incisions used:
  - o **Grid iron incision** is most widely used.
  - o **Lanz incision** is more cosmetic.
  - o When the diagnosis is in doubt, particularly in the presence of intestinal obstruction, a lower midline abdominal incision is preferred.
- The appendix is present at the convergence of taeniae coli.

- Appendix is controlled with a Babcock or Lane's forceps.
- Mesoappendix is clamped in artery forceps, divided and ligated.
- Appendix is crushed and ligated at its base and then divided.
- Appendiceal stump may or may not be inverted.

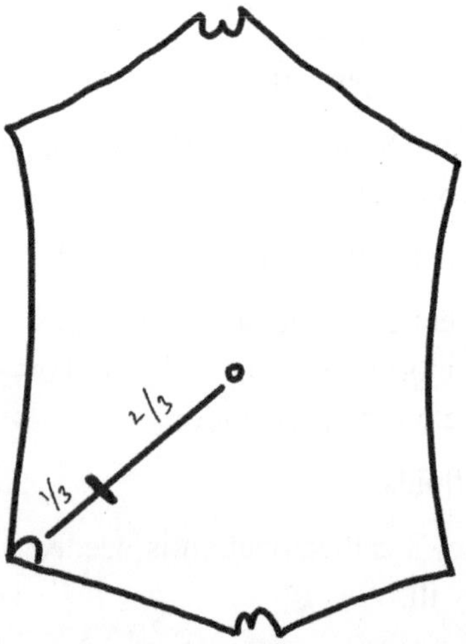

Grid iron incision for appendicitis, at right angles to a line joining the anterior superior iliac spine and umbilicus, centred on McBurney's point

Figure 1: Grid iron incision

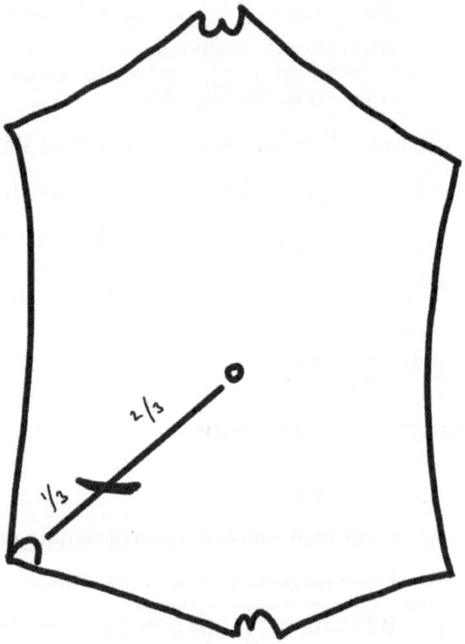

Transverse or skin crease (Lanz incision)

Figure 2: Lanz incision

B. Non-Operative or Conservative Management

- While surgery remains the standard teaching, there is an emerging body of literature to support a trial of conservative management in patients with uncomplicated (absence of appendicolith, perforation or abscess) appendicitis.
- Keep patient NPO.
- IV antibiotics: Metronidazole, 3rd generation cephalosporins, ertapenem.
- This approach may be considered in the well patient with limited signs or those with high operative risk (multiple comorbidities).

[10] Discuss the differential diagnosis of lump in right iliac fossa. Discuss the management of appendicular mass. ***Dec 16***

[5] Management of appendicular mass. ***Sept 21***

[5] Appendicular mass. ***Dec 18, Dec 17***

[3] Appendicular mass. ***Oct 20***

[3] Differential diagnosis of right iliac fossa mass. ***Dec 12***

[3] Ochsner - Sherren regimen. ***Feb 23***

[3] Differential diagnosis for right iliac fossa mass. Enumerate components of Ochsner - Sherren regimen. ***CBME March 24***

[10] Enumerate the differential diagnosis of a right iliac fossa mass. How do you manage a patient with an appendicular mass? ***CBME June 24***

APPENDICULAR LUMP

- Also known as appendicular mass, peri-appendicular phlegmon.
- On day 3 after an attack of acute appendicitis, a tender mass can frequently be felt in the right iliac fossa.
- Sometimes, the mass may even be situated in the pelvis.
- The mass is composed mainly of the greater omentum, oedematous caecal wall and oedematous portions of the small intestine. In its midst, is a perforated or otherwise inflamed appendix.
- By day 4 or 5, the mass becomes more circumscribed.
- As the rigidity of the overlying musculature passes off, its periphery can be defined clearly and should be outlined with a skin marker.

- During the ensuing days (day 5-10), one of two things will happen:
  1. The swelling either becomes larger, and an appendicular abscess results; or
  2. It becomes smaller, and subsides slowly as the inflammation resolves.

Differential Diagnosis of An Appendicular Mass

1. Carcinoma of caecum.
2. Crohn's disease.
3. Ovarian carcinoma.
4. Parametritis.
5. Actinomycosis.
6. Tuberculosis.
7. Twisted ovarian cyst.
8. Mesenteric lymphadenitis.

Investigations

- USG.
- CECT.

Treatment

- If an appendicular mass is present and the condition of the patient is satisfactory, the treatment is conservative, i.e., **Ochsner-Sherren regimen.**
- This decision is based on the fact that nature has already localised the lesion and surgery at this time is difficult, bloody and dangerous.
- It may be impossible to find the appendix and occasionally a faecal fistula may form.
- **Components of Ochsner-Sherren regimen:**
  a. The limits of the mass should be marked with a skin marker and it should be regularly examined to look for changes in the size of the mass.
  b. Temperature and pulse rate should be recorded every 4th hourly.
  c. IV antibiotics.
  d. Patient should be kept NPO and IV fluids given. An input/output chart is maintained.
- Clinical improvement is usually evident within 24-48 hours.
- Criteria for stopping conservative treatment:
  - o A rising pulse rate.
  - o Increasing or spreading abdominal pain.
  - o Increasing size of the mass.
- Clinical deterioration or evidence of peritonitis is an indication for early laparotomy.
- If the lump resolves, the patient should be discharged and called for an interval appendicectomy after 6-12 weeks.

[3] Appendicular abscess. *March 22*

- An appendicular abscess refers to a **localized collection of pus** that forms in the abdomen or pelvis as a **sequelae of acute appendicitis.**

Aetiopathogenesis

- In **non-obstructive acute appendicitis**, the inflammation usually commences in the mucosa and as it progresses to involve the submucosa, it **can sometimes terminate in suppuration,** i.e., abscess formation.
- In **obstructive appendicitis**, the products of inflammation become pent up in the appendix. These **contents can sometimes suppurate**, and if the appendix undergoes a perforation or gangrene formation, the **contents leak out and results in abscess formation.**
- An **appendicular mass can also sometimes suppurate** giving rise to abscess formation.
- **Causative bacteria:** *Escherichia coli, Pseudomonas aeruginosa, Klebsiella pneumoniae.*
- The location of the abscess depends on the position of the appendix. Thus, the **most common site is in the lateral part of the iliac fossa (extension of retrocecal suppuration). The 2nd most common site is in the pelvis.**

Clinical Features

These are the same as that of acute appendicitis:

- Migratory pain (from peri-umbilical to RIF).
- Anorexia.
- Nausea and vomiting.
- Tenderness in right iliac fossa.
- Rebound tenderness in right iliac fossa.
- **Variable pyrexia.**

Investigations

1. **USG:**
   - Diagnoses acute appendicitis, mass as well as collection of pus.
2. **Contrast enhanced CT scan:**
   - Has a higher accuracy than USG.
3. CBC may show **leukocytosis.**

Treatment

1. **Percutaneous drainage of the abscess:**
   - Done **under radiological guidance (USG, CT or fluoroscopy)** by an interventional radiologist.
2. **Surgery:**
   - **Lavage ± appendicectomy.**
   - Toileting of the right iliac fossa and pelvis is done.
   - This is followed by appendicectomy, if it is feasible.
   - **If appendicectomy is not feasible (due to lump formation), a drain is placed and the patient is asked to come for an interval appendicectomy.**
3. **Interval appendicectomy:**
   - The patient is asked to come **after 6 weeks**, as by this time, the inflammation would have resolved.
   - There are 2 reasons for doing an interval appendicectomy:
     a. Chances of recurrent appendicitis.
     b. The appendix might harbor an underlying malignant pathology.

[5] Carcinoid tumour. ***March 21***

[3] Carcinoid tumour. ***June 19***

- Also known as appendiceal neuroendocrine neoplasms (**ANENs**), neuroendocrine tumours (**NETs**).
- They are the **most common primary tumours of the appendix**.
- They occur throughout the GIT, most commonly in the appendix, ileum and rectum (in decreasing order of frequency).

Pathology

- **Cells of origin: Subepithelial neuroendocrine cells of appendix.** In the bowel, it arises from **Kulchitsky cells** at the base of **intestinal crypts of Lieberkuhn.**
- Small, well-circumscribed lesions.
- Majority are located in the **tip of the appendix.**
- **Immunohistochemistry: Synaptophysin and chromogranin A.**
- Can be either benign or malignant.
- **Size** is the best initial **predictor of malignant behaviour and metastatic potential.**
- Spreads to the regional lymph nodes, liver.

Classification

Tumors are classified as grade 1-3 according to their proliferative capacity (determined by the Ki-67 index and mitotic rate).

Clinical Features

- F > M.
- Age: 40-50 years.
- **Most patients are asymptomatic.**
- Patients may present with symptoms due to a mass.
- Symptoms of metastasis (**carcinoid syndrome**).
- May produce dense fibrosis in the surrounding tissues, resulting in distortion and scarring of the bowel and associated mesentery.

Investigations

1. **CECT scan.**
2. **MRI of the abdomen:**
   - These are done to rule out regional or distant metastatic disease.
3. **Octreotide scanning (somatostatin receptor scintigraphy):**
   - Used to assess the extent of disease preoperatively.
4. **Serum chromogranin A** is a tumour marker and especially used for post-op follow-up.

Treatment

The treatment and prognosis of NETs depends upon their grade, tumour size and the extent of tumour invasion.

a. **Size ≤ 1 cm:**
   - Appendicectomy with excision of the mesoappendix.

b. **Size 1–2 cm:**
   - **If the Ki-67 index is low (<30%):** Appendicectomy with excision of the mesoappendix.
   - **If the Ki-67 index is high (>30%):** Right hemicolectomy.

c. **Size > 2 cm:**
   - Right hemicolectomy + regional lymphadenectomy.

[5] Carcinoid syndrome. *Dec 13*

- Seen with **neuroendocrine or carcinoid tumours** of midgut (e.g., small intestine) **with liver mets.**

Pathophysiology

- Carcinoid tumours in the GIT, especially the **small intestine**, secrete **excess serotonin (5-HT)** which is rapidly metabolised by the liver.
- In the presence of **liver mets**, it **secretes serotonin into the inferior vena cava, avoiding hepatic first-pass metabolism.**
- This leads to symptoms of **serotonin excess**, known as **carcinoid syndrome.**
- Seen in 20–30% of patients with liver metastases.
- **Other vasoactive peptides** that are produced by NETs: **Histamine, prostaglandins and kallikrein.**

Clinical Features

- Sweating.
- Flushing, characteristically induced by alcohol.
- Reddish-blue cyanosis.
- Bronchospasm leading to asthmatic attacks.
- **Hedinger syndrome:** Restrictive cardiomyopathy secondary to fibrotic right heart valvular disease (pulmonary and tricuspid stenosis, tricuspid regurgitation).
- Diarrhea.
- Borborygmi.

Investigations

- **Serotonin levels** in the **blood.**
- **Urinary serotonin** levels.
- **CECT and MRI of abdomen** are done to rule out regional or distant metastatic disease.
- **Octreotide scanning (somatostatin receptor scintigraphy)** is used to assess the extent of disease preoperatively.

Treatment

A. **Medical Therapy**
   - Somatostatin analogs (e.g., **octreotide, lanreotide**) inhibits the release of serotonin and other vasoactive substances.
   - **Telotristat** inhibits tryptophan hydroxylase, which is involved in the synthesis of serotonin.

B. **Surgical Therapy**
   - Same as carcinoid tumour.
   - Select cases of liver mets can be surgically resected.

OTHER IMPORTANT TOPICS

ANATOMY OF THE APPENDIX

- The vermiform appendix is present only in humans, certain anthropoid apes and the wombat.
- Blind muscular tube with mucosal, submucosal, muscular and serosal layers.
- **Positions of appendix:**
   - o Retrocecal - most common.
   - o Pelvic - 2nd most common.
   - o Others - para-cecal, sub-cecal, pre-ileal, post-ileal.
- The position of the base of the appendix is constant, being found at the confluence of the 3 taenia coli of the cecum.
- At operation, the taenia coli helps the surgeon to locate the appendix.

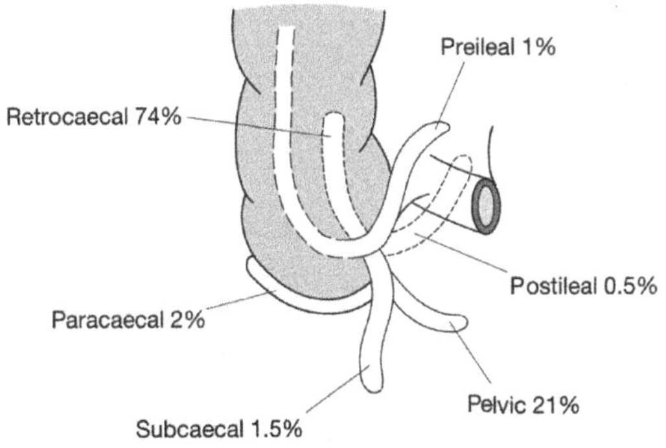

Figure 3: Positions of appendix

- The appendicular artery, which is a branch of the ileocolic artery gives blood supply to the appendix. An accessory appendicular artery may also be present.

DIFFERENTIAL DIAGNOSIS OF ACUTE APPENDICITIS

A. Children

- Gastroenteritis.
- Mesenteric adenitis.
- Meckel's diverticulitis.
- Intussusception.
- Henoch-Schönlein purpura.
- Lobar pneumonia.

B. Adults

- Regional enteritis.
- Ureteric colic.
- Perforated peptic ulcer.
- Torsion of testis.
- Pancreatitis.
- Rectus sheath hematoma.

C. Adult Female

- Mittelschmerz.
- Pelvic inflammatory disease.
- Pyelonephritis.
- Ectopic pregnancy.
- Torsion/rupture of ovarian cyst.
- Endometriosis.

D. Elderly

- Diverticulitis.
- Intestinal obstruction.
- Colonic carcinoma.
- Torsion appendix epiploicae.
- Mesenteric infarction.
- Leaking aortic aneurysm.

46

Anus

[5] Hemorrhoids. *Dec 16, June 14*

Definition: Hemorrhoids are symptomatic enlargements of the internal hemorrhoidal venous plexus.

Cause

- Upright posture of humans.
- Absence of valves in the portal venous system.
- Raised abdominal pressure.
- Pregnancy.
- Straining during defecation/constipation.

Pathogenesis

- The internal hemorrhoidal venous plexus constitutes the submucosal component of the anal cushions that are important in sealing the anal canal.
- Shearing forces lead to:
    - Mucosal trauma (bleeding).
    - Caudal displacement of anal cushions (prolapse).
    - This in turn leads to impaired venous drainage, progressive venous engorgement, local stasis and transudation of fluid (pruritus).
- With time, fragmentation of the supporting structures (a normal consequence of ageing but perhaps accelerated in those with hemorrhoids) leads to loss of elasticity of the cushions such that they no longer retract following defecation.

Clinical Features

- Bleeding is the earliest symptom.
    - Nature of the bleeding is characteristically separate from the motion and is seen either on the paper on wiping or as a fresh splash in the pan.
    - Bleeding is rarely sufficient to cause anemia.
    - Bleeding is usually painless.
- Pruritus is common due to irritation of skin by mucus discharge.
- Patient rarely complains of pain.
- Internal hemorrhoids are classically present in the 3, 7 and 11 o'clock positions (with the patient in lithotomy position).
- Secondary hemorrhoids may develop between the primary positions.
- External hemorrhoids refer to venous channels of the inferior hemorrhoidal plexus deep in the skin surrounding the anal verge.

Classification

- There are 4 degrees of hemorrhoids:
    - **1st degree:** Only bleeding.
    - **2nd degree:** Prolapse but reduces spontaneously.
    - **3rd degree:** Prolapse but has to be manually reduced.
    - **4th degree:** Permanently prolapsed.

Complications

- Strangulation and thrombosis.
- Ulceration.

- Gangrene.
- Portal pyemia.

Investigations

- It is a clinical diagnosis.
- Proctoscopy.
- Colonoscopy is indicated in patients > 40 years of age to exclude colorectal malignancy.
- Examination under anesthesia.

Treatment

A. Improve Bowel and Defecatory Habits

- Patient is asked to consume a high fibre diet.
- Adopt a defecatory position to minimize straining.

B. Laxatives, Stool Softeners, Bulking Agents

- Lactulose syrup.
- Psyllium husk.
- Liquid paraffin.
- Milk of magnesia.

C. Creams

- Can be applied at night and before defecation.
- Phlebotonics (plant based flavonoid extracts), e.g., euphorbia prostrata extract.
- Synthetic compounds, e.g., calcium dobesilate.
- These may reduce capillary permeability and increase lymphatic drainage.

D. Injection Sclerotherapy

- Submucosal injection of 5% phenol in arachis oil or almond oil.
- The sclerosant is injected into the apex of the pedicle and not into the hemorrhoid itself.
- The aim is to cause fibrosis that obliterates the vascular channels and to produce a scar that supports prolapsing anorectal mucosa.
- Indicated in patients with first or second degree internal hemorrhoids whose symptoms are not improved by conservative measures.

E. Rubber Band Ligation

- Barron's bander is used to slip tight elastic bands onto the base of the pedicle of each hemorrhoid.
- Band is applied above the dentate line as below the line, it can cause intense pain.
- Band causes ischemic necrosis of the piles, which sloughs off and may be associated with bleeding.
- The resulting fibrosis supports the remaining anal cushions.
- Indicated in patients with first or second degree internal hemorrhoids whose symptoms are not improved by conservative measures.

F. Surgery

- The indications for hemorrhoidectomy are as follows:
  - o 3rd and 4th degree hemorrhoids.
  - o 2nd degree hemorrhoids that have not been cured by non-operative treatments.
  - o *Mixed hemorrhoids*, when the external hemorrhoid is well defined.
  - o Bleeding causing anemia.
- Hemorrhoidectomy can be performed via the following techniques:

  1. **Open technique:**
     - o Also known as Milligan-Morgan operation.
     - o Hemorrhoid is identified, dissected, transfixed and excised.
     - o The mucosal defect is left open to heal by secondary intention.
  2. **Closed technique:**
     - o Also known as Ferguson operation.
     - o Hemorrhoid is identified, dissected, transfixed and excised.
     - o Anal mucosal defect is closed with a continuous suture.
  3. **Stapled technique:**
     - o Stapled hemorrhoidopexy, also known as PPH (procedure for prolapse and hemorrhoids).
     - o A circular stapling device is used to excise a cylinder of mucosa and submucosa (together with the vessels within) above the dentate line while simultaneously stapling the mucosal ends together.
  4. **Transanal hemorrhoid artery ligation (HAL):**
     - o Transanal doppler guided ligation of those vessels feeding the hemorrhoidal masses with or without suture mucopexy.

[3] Fissure in ano. ***March 21, Dec 19***

[5] Management of fissure in ano. ***June 13***

- Also known as anal fissure.
- **Definition:** It is a longitudinal ulcer in the anoderm of the distal anal canal, which extends proximally from the anal verge towards, but not beyond the dentate line.

Aetiology

- Frequently seen in the **posterior midline** because of the following reasons:
  - o Shearing forces act at this site during defecation.
  - o Less elastic anoderm.
  - o Increased density of longitudinal muscle extensions in this region of the anal circumference.
- **Anterior anal fissures** are more common in women and may arise following vaginal delivery.
- **Ectopic site anal fissures** could be due to sexual assault.
- **Other causes:**
  - o Crohn's disease.
  - o TB.
  - o STDs – syphilis, chlamydia, chancroid, lymphogranuloma venereum, herpes simplex virus.
  - o Kaposi's sarcoma.
  - o B-cell lymphoma.
  - o Squamous cell carcinoma.

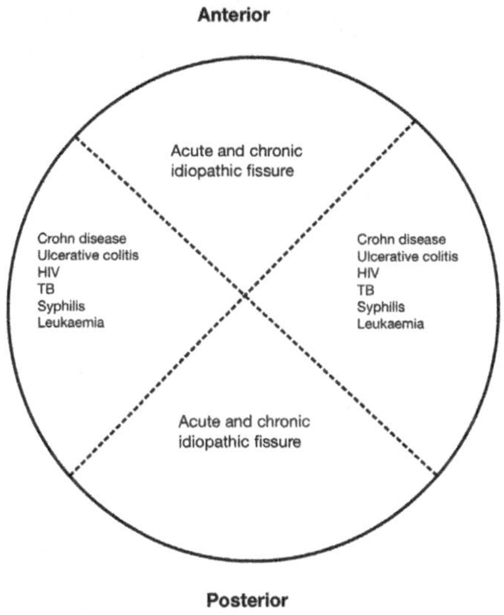

Figure 1: Location and causes of anal fissures

Pathogenesis

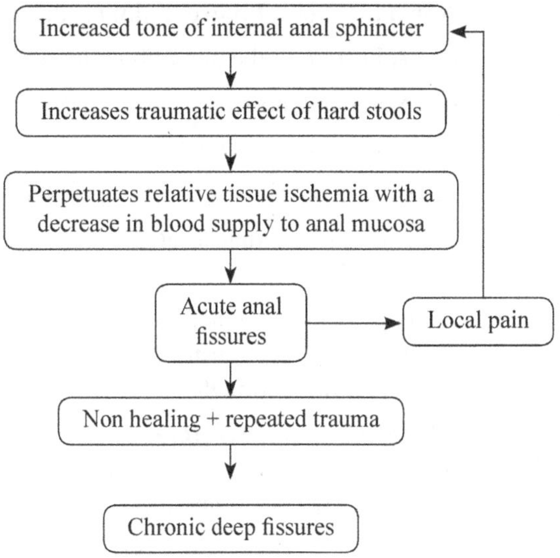

Clinical Features

- Can affect any age, but most common in young adults.
- **Acute anal fissures:** Complains of **severe anal pain during defecation**, which usually resolves only to recur at the next evacuation.
- A trace of **fresh blood is noticed in the pan after defecation** or on the tissue after wiping (bright red blood).
- A fissure that is not in the midline or one that has atypical features, should raise the suspicion of a specific aetiology.
- Complains of mucous discharge.
- May complains of itching.
- History of constipation.

On Examination

- Ulcer which is usually in the midline of the anal canal.
- Chronic fissures have the following characteristics:
  1. Hypertrophied anal papilla internally.
  2. Sentinel tag externally.
  3. In between the two, there is an indurated anal ulcer where the fibres of internal sphincter are exposed.

Treatment

A. Conservative Management

- Conservative management results in the healing

of almost all acute fissures and the majority of chronic fissures.

- **Normalisation of bowel habits** is done by:
  - o Add fibre to the diet to bulk up the stool.
  - o Stool softeners.
  - o Adequate water intake.
- **Warm sitz bath** helps to relieve sphincter spasm.
- Topical **local anaesthetics** (lignocaine 2%) relieve pain.
- Patients who have normal bowel function but strain excessively during defection benefit from **anorectal biofeedback.**
- **Chemical sphincterotomy**, i.e., drugs which induce internal sphincter (smooth muscle) relaxation by topical application:
  1. Glyceryl Trinitrate 0.2 % (nitric oxide donor).
  2. Diltiazem 2% (calcium channel blocker).
  3. Botulinum toxin 10-100 U (injected into the internal sphincter).

B. Operative Measures

1. **Lateral internal sphincterotomy (LIS):**
   - Internal sphincter is divided away from the fissure itself, usually either in the right or the left lateral positions.
   - External tags can be excised.
   - **Complications:** Hemorrhage, hematoma, bruising, perianal abscess, fistula, incontinence.
2. **Fissurectomy:**
   - Involves excising the fibrotic edge, curettage of the base and excision of the sentinel tag and/or anal papilla.
   - Done if there are contraindications to LIS.
   - Frequently combined with an advancement flap anoplasty.
3. **Anal advancement flap:**
   - Considered in those with an increased risk of altered continence following LIS, especially in postpartum women and those with normal or low resting anal pressures.
   - After fissurectomy, an inverted house-shaped flap of perianal skin is carefully mobilised on its blood supply and advanced without tension to cover the fissure.

[5] Ischiorectal abscess. *March 21, Dec 17, June 17, Feb 23*

- It is a type of anorectal abscess.

Causative Organisms

- *Escherichia coli, Staphylococcus aureus, Bacteroides, Streptococcus, Proteus.*

Cause

- The abscess commences as an infection of an anal gland.
- Penetration of rectal wall (e.g., by a fish bone).
- Blood borne infection.
- Extension of a cutaneous boil.
- Underlying rectal disease: Neoplasm, Crohn's disease.

Pathogenesis

- The **cryptoglandular theory of intersphincteric anal gland infection** holds that: pus, which travels along the path of least resistance, may spread laterally across the external sphincter to form an ischiorectal abscess.
- The fat which fills the ischiorectal fossa is particularly vulnerable because it is poorly vascularized.
- The **ischiorectal fossa communicates with** its counterpart of the **opposite side** via the post sphincteric space, and can therefore involve the contralateral fossa.
- If there is an internal opening into the anal canal, a **horseshoe abscess** develops which envelops the whole of the posterior part of the circumference of the anal canal.

Clinical Features

- M>F.
- Painful, throbbing swelling in the anal region.
- Fever.
- Tender, brawny induration palpable on the corresponding side of the anal canal and the floor of the fossa.

Investigations

- It is a clinical diagnosis.
- In case of diagnostic dilemma, the following can be done:
  - o USG.
  - o MRI.
  - o Examination under anesthesia.
  - o Sigmoidoscopy.
  - o Proctoscopy.

Treatment

- Incision and drainage through the perineal skin.
- A cruciate incision is made over the most fluctuant point.
- Skin edges are excised to deroof the abscess.
- Although drainage must be ensured, skin preservation is important and wide excision of otherwise healthy tissue should be avoided.
- If an underlying fistula is found, a loose draining seton may be passed.
- IV antibiotics.

[5] Fistula in ano. ***August 22, Sept 21, Dec 18***

[3] Fistula in ano. ***June 14***

[3] Classify fistula in ano. ***Dec 17, Dec12***

[3] Mention the types of fistula in ano. ***Dec 14***

[3] Goodsall's rule. ***Sept 21, July 18, Dec 16, July 15, July 23***

[MCQ] Goodsall's rule is applicable for: ***CBME June 24***

A. Fissure in ano B. Fistula in ano*

C. Hemorrhoids D. Pilonidal sinus

- Also known as anal fistula.
- **Definition:** It is a chronic abnormal communication extending from the anorectal lumen (the internal opening) to an external opening on the skin of the perineum or buttock (or rarely, in women, to the vagina).

Causes

- The majority are idiopathic or cryptoglandular.
- Crohn's disease.
- Tuberculosis.
- Lymphogranuloma venereum.
- Actinomycosis.
- Rectal duplication.
- Foreign body.
- Malignancy.

Pathology

- It usually results from an anorectal abscess which burst spontaneously or was opened inadequately.
- The fistula continues to discharge and, because of constant reinfection from the anal canal or rectum, rarely closes permanently without surgical aid.
- It is lined with granulation tissue.

Types/Classification

A. Park's Classification

- Classifies fistulae on the basis of the relation between the primary track to the external sphincter.
  1. **Inter-sphincteric fistula (Type I)**
     - o The fistula tract passes through the internal anal sphincter muscle and is confined within it.
  2. **Trans-sphincteric fistula (Type II)**
     - o The fistula tract traverses both the internal and external sphincter muscles.
  3. **Supra-sphincteric fistula (Type III)**
     - o The fistula tract starts within the anal canal, extends upwards between the internal and external sphincters, and then curves around the external sphincter before exiting through the perianal skin.
  4. **Extra-sphincteric fistula (Type IV)**
     - o The fistula tract passes outside the sphincter complex.

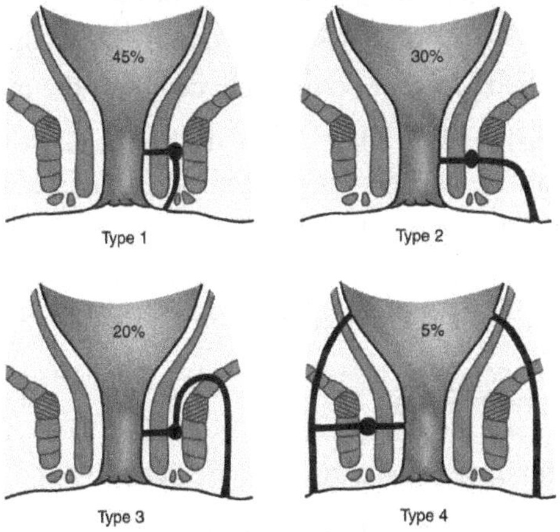

Park classification of fistula-in ano: Type 1, intersphincteric; Type 2, Trans-sphincteric; Type 3, Suprasphincteric; and Type 4, Extrasphincteric

Figure 2: Park's classification

B. American Gastroenterology Association Classification

a. **Simple fistula:**
   - Low (superficial or low inter-sphincteric or low trans-sphincteric tract).
   - Single external opening.

b. **Complex fistula:**
   - High (high inter or trans-sphincteric tract).
   - Extra or supra-sphincteric tract.
   - Presence of abscess or collection.
   - Anovaginal fistula.
   - Anal stricture.

- Inter-sphincteric and trans-sphincteric fistula are the most common.

Clinical Features

- Persistent seropurulent discharge that irritates the skin in the neighbourhood and causes discomfort.
- Often the history dates back for years, and a history of anorectal sepsis may be present.
- So long as the opening is large enough for the pus to escape, pain is not a symptom, but if the orifice is occluded pain increases until the discharge erupts.
- Frequently, there is a solitary external opening, usually situated within 3.75 cm of the anus, presenting as a small elevation with granulation tissue pouting from the mouth of the opening.
- Sometimes, superficial healing occurs, pus accumulates and an abscess re-forms and discharges through the same opening, or a new opening.
- Thus, there may be ≥2 external openings, usually grouped together on the right or left of the midline.
- Occasionally, when both ischiorectal fossae are involved, an opening is seen on each side, in which case there is often intercommunication between them.
- There is induration of the skin and subcutaneous tissue around the fistula.

Goodsall's Rule

- It can be used as a guide to predict:
  1. The course of the fistula track.
  2. The location of the internal opening.
- Fistulas with an external opening in the anterior half of the anus typically track in a radial fashion directly into the anal canal.

  Exception: If the external opening is >3 cm from anal verge, it curves posteriorly to open at the midline.
- Fistulas with an external opening in the posterior half of the anus often tracks in a curvilinear fashion to a posterior midline internal opening.

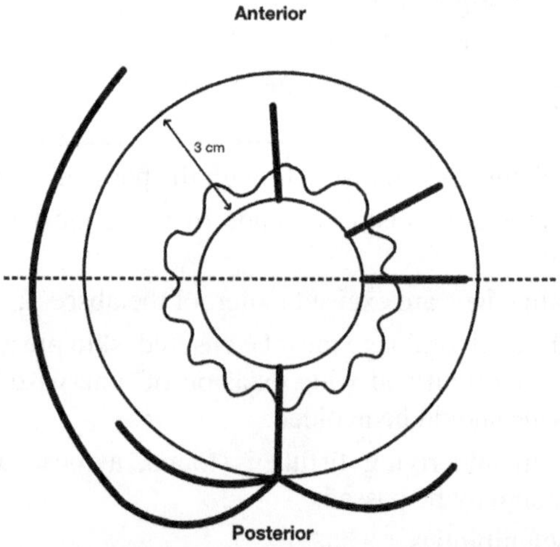

Figure 3: Goodsall's rule

Investigations

- Proctoscopy
- MRI is the gold standard. It can demonstrate secondary extensions, which may be missed at surgery and cause persistence.
  - o Fistulography.
  - o CT scan is especially useful if an extra sphincteric fistula is suspected.

Treatment

1. **Fistulotomy**
   - It involves division of all structures lying between the external and internal openings.
   - Applied mainly to intersphincteric fistulas and transsphincteric fistulas involving <30% of the external sphincter.
2. **Fistulectomy**
   - It involves coring out of the fistula, usually by diathermy.
   - The entire fistulous track is excised.

3. **Setons:**
   - Loose setons are tied such that there is no tension upon the encircled tissue; there is no intent to cut the tissue.
   - Tight or cutting setons are placed with the intention of cutting through the enclosed muscle.
   - The seton should be non-absorbable, non-degenerative and comfortable.
   - Loose setons are most commonly used before 'advanced' techniques (fistulectomy, advancement flap, cutting seton) while sepsis resolves and secondary extensions heal as part of a staged fistulotomy.
4. **Ligation of Intersphincteric Fistula Tract or LIFT:**
   - It involves disconnection of the internal opening from the fistula tract at the level of the intersphincteric plane.
   - It is a sphincter saving procedure.
   - It maintains continence.
5. **Advancement flaps:**
   - It preserves both anatomy and function.
6. **Biological agents:**
   - An ideal biological agent seals the fistula tract and allows ingrowth of healthy tissue to replace it.
7. **VAAFT or Video Assisted Anal Fistula Treatment.**
8. **FiLaC or Fistula tract Laser Closure.**

[5] Pilonidal sinus. ***Dec 14, Dec 12***

[3] Pilonidal sinus. ***Oct 20, June 19, June 17, Dec 16, Dec 15***

- **Definition:** The term pilonidal sinus describes a condition found in the natal cleft overlying the coccyx, consisting of one or more, usually non-infected, midline openings, which communicate with a fibrous track lined by granulation tissue and containing hair lying loosely within the lumen.

Aetiology

- **Congenital theory** is considered obsolete.
- The **acquired theory** is favoured because of the following reasons:
  - o Interdigital pilonidal sinus is an occupational disease of hairdressers.
  - o Age of appearance is older than expected of a congenital lesion.
  - o Hair follicles are rarely present in the walls of the sinus.
  - o Pointed hair ends are directed towards the blind end of the sinus.
  - o Mostly affects hirsute men.
  - o Recurrence is common, even though adequate excision of the track is carried out.

Pathogenesis

Shed/broken hairs collect in the natal cleft.

↓

Buttock friction + shearing forces

↓

1. Hair drills through the midline skin.
2. Infection in relation to a hair follicle allows hair to enter the skin by suction.

↓

Subcutaneous, chronically infected, midline track, i.e., PRIMARY PILONIDAL SINUS.

- Secondary tracks may spread laterally, which may emerge at the skin as granulation tissue-lined, discharging openings.
- The sinus track runs cephalad.
- Carcinoma arising in chronic pilonidal disease is very rare.

Clinical Features

- M > F.
- Usually occurs after puberty, but before 30 years of age.
- Dark haired individuals > soft blonde haired individuals.
- Complains of intermittent pain, swelling and discharge at the natal cleft.
- History of repeated abscesses that have burst spontaneously, or have been incised.
- Primary sinus may have one or many openings, all of which are strictly in the midline between the level of

the sacrococcygeal joint and the tip of the coccyx.

Differential Diagnosis

- Hidradenitis suppurativa.
- Complex anal fistula.
- Osteomyelitis with draining skin sinuses.
- Infective conditions: TB, actinomycosis.

Treatment

A. Acute Exacerbation (Abscess)

- Abscess should be drained through a small longitudinal incision made over it and away from the midline.
- Curettage of granulation tissue and hair.

B. Chronic Pilonidal Sinus

- Following procedures are done:
  1. Laying open of all tracks ± marsupialisation.
  2. Excision of all tracks ± primary closure.
  3. Excision of all tracks + closure, by a means which avoids a midline wound (tension free closure).
- **Limberg flap:** rhomboid excision + closure by a rotational flap.
- **Z-plasty.**
- **Karydakis flap:** off midline excision + closure by an advancement flap.
- **Bascom's procedure:**
  - o Incision is made lateral to the midline to gain access to the sinus cavity.
  - o Hair and granulation tissue are removed.
  - o Excision and closure of midline pits.
  - o Lateral wound is left open to heal by secondary intention.

C. Post-Op Elimination of Hair

- Shaving.
- Depilation.
- Laser removal.

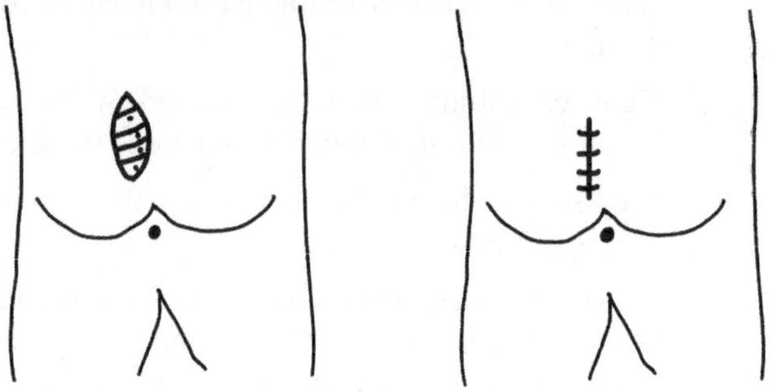

Figure 4: Karydaki's operation

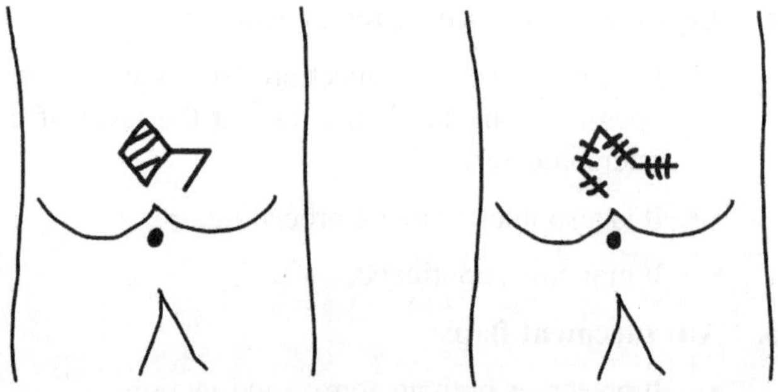

Figure 5: Limberg flap

[3] Watering can perineum. *Feb 23*

- This refers to the condition where there are **several external openings in the perineum because of multiple complex fistula tracts.**
- Because of so many openings, it resembles a watering can.
- The **perineum may become densely fibrotic, rigid** and is **covered with multiple discharging openings.**
- **Causes:**
  - o Crohn's disease.
  - o Tuberculosis.
  - o Tight strictures with periurethral abscess.
- **Investigations:** MRI.
- **Treatment:** Draining setons.

47

Urinary Symptoms and Investigations

[5] List the differential diagnosis for haematuria and elaborate on investigations. *CBME March 24*

[3] Causes of haematuria. *Dec 18, Dec 16*

HAEMATURIA

- Haematuria occurs when there is blood in the urine.
- It is now classified as visible haematuria (VH) or non-visible haematuria (NVH).
- The older terminology was macroscopic (or frank or gross) haematuria and microscopic (or dipstick) haematuria.
- Enquiry should be made about the timing of the blood in relation to the urinary stream:
  A. **Initial:** Urethral pathology.
  B. **Throughout the stream:** Bladder or upper tracts.
  C. **Terminal:** Bladder neck or prostate pathology.
- History of degree of haematuria and its frequency should also be taken.

Causes

A list of potential causes for haematuria can be rapidly generated by considering TIN or Trauma, Infection and Neoplasm at all levels of the urinary tract from kidney to urethra.

A. Blood Dyscrasias

- Purpura.
- Sickle cell trait.
- Anticoagulants.

B. Kidneys

- Infarct.
- Injury.
- TB, filariasis.
- Stones.
- Focal and glomerular nephritis.
- Tumours: Renal cell carcinoma, transitional cell carcinoma, Wilms' tumour.

C. Ureters

- Stone in ureter.
- Neoplasm of ureter.

D. Urinary Bladder

- TB.
- Cystitis.
- Tumours.
- Bilharziasis.
- Stone.
- Jogger's haematuria.

E. Prostate

- BPH.
- Carcinoma prostate.

F. Urethra

- Neoplasm.

Investigations

- Haematuria requires detailed investigation in almost all cases, except young women with a proven UTI.

1. **Urine routine and urine C/S:**
   - o A midstream specimen is examined for infection.
   - o Cytological examination of a urine specimen for cancer cells.
   - o Presence of RBCs, WBCs help identify a UTI.
   - o Presence of casts help identify stones.
2. **USG KUB.**
3. **Flexible cystoscopy:**
   - o If UTI is ruled out as a cause for the haematuria, then a renal ultrasound scan and a flexible cystoscopy are the minimum investigations that are done in any patient with haematuria.
   - o If no aetiology can be identified on lab and imaging studies, cystoscopy is mandatory.

[3] Indications for Intra Venous Urography. ***Dec 16, June 16***

INTRAVENOUS UROGRAPHY

- It is used for the radiological examination of the urinary tract.

Technique

- The contrast (sodium diatrizoate) is injected into a suitable forearm vein.
- It travels the vasculature to reach the kidneys where it is filtered by the glomerulus.
- A series of X-ray films are then taken as it travels from the glomerulus in the kidneys to the urinary bladder. At the end of the study, the patient is asked to micturate and a final film is then taken of the bladder area.

Advantages

- Easily available.
- Lower cost.
- Lower radiation exposure.

Disadvantages

- Provides lesser information than a CT scan.
- It is tedious to perform.
- Contrast substance is allergenic and may cause anaphylaxis.
- It is dependent on renal function as the contrast agent needs to be excreted.

Indications

- IVU is rarely performed if CT is available. However if a CT IVU demonstrates delayed excretion due to obstruction, a delayed radiograph following CT IVU can identify the site of obstruction.
- Indications are as follows:
  1. Ureteric obstruction: severity, site and cause, e.g., urolithiasis.
  2. Synchronous or metachronous upper tract tumour: detailed evaluation of pelvicalyceal and ureteral morphology in patients with bladder transitional cell carcinoma.
  3. Papillary necrosis.
  4. Anatomical variations such as horseshoe kidney.
  5. Course of the ureters.
  6. Renal function.

[3] Mention the indications for cystoscopy. ***Dec 14***

CYSTOSCOPY

- A cystoscope is an instrument which visualizes the urethra and bladder.

Types

1. **Flexible cystoscopy:** Done under LA, used for diagnostic purposes.
2. **Rigid cystoscopy:** Done under GA, used for therapeutic purposes.

Hardware

- Telescopes with different fields of view are available (0°, 12°, 30° and 70° lenses are commonly used).
- Cystoscopy requires a urology stack consisting of a camera, monitor, light source, electrocautery and insufflator.

Uses

A. Diagnostic

- Flexible cystoscopy is used for diagnostic purposes:
  - a. **Haematuria**
    - o It helps identify any abnormalities in the bladder or urethra that may cause bleeding (infection, neoplasm).
  - b. **Recurrent UTIs**
    - o It can diagnose any underlying anatomical abnormalities that could be contributing to the infections.
  - c. **Obstruction**
    - o E.g., bladder stones, tumours or strictures.
  - d. **Urinary incontinence**
    - o It can identify factors which contribute to urinary incontinence.
  - e. **Trauma**
    - o To evaluate extent of damage and plan treatment.
  - f. **Biopsy**
    - o From urothelium in suspected malignancies.
  - g. **Bladder cancer**
    - o Diagnosis and monitoring.

B. Therapeutic

- Rigid cystoscopy is preferred but, flexible cystoscopy can also be used for smaller procedures.
  - a. Insertion/removal of ureteric stents.
  - b. Diathermy/laser ablation of small bladder lesions.
  - c. Removal of stones from bladder and urethra.
  - d. Control of bleeding within the bladder by cauterization.
  - e. Removal of foreign bodies.
  - f. Treatment of urethral strictures by dilation or other procedures.
  - g. BOTOX injection to help manage an overactive bladder.

OTHER IMPORTANT TOPICS

ANURIA

- Anuria is defined as the complete absence of urine production for 12 hours.
- Oliguria on the other hand, is when the amount of urine produced in a day is < 300 ml.

Causes

- Renal failure is traditionally divided into 3 types:
  1. Pre-renal.
  2. Renal.
  3. Post-renal or obstructive.

Pre-Renal Anuria

- Hypovolemia due to dehydration.
- Blood loss.
- Sepsis.
- Cardiogenic shock.
- Anesthesia: epidural and spinal anesthesia cause hypotension.
- Prolonged hypoxia due to any cause.

Renal

- Drugs: aminoglycosides, cephalosporins, diuretics, NSAIDs.
- Nephrotoxic poisons.
- Contrast media.
- Pre-eclampsia and eclampsia.
- Myoglobinuria (Crush syndrome).
- Incompatible blood transfusion.
- Disseminated intravascular coagulation.

Post-Renal or Obstructive

1. Calculi

- Renal calculus disease is the most common cause of acute obstruction leading to anuria.
- The patient is likely to have unilateral renal colic against a background of non-function of

the contralateral kidney, often due to previous surgery or pre-existing obstruction by calculus.

2. **Pelvic malignancy**
   - Carcinomas arising from the urinary bladder, prostate, cervix, ovary or rectum can all lead to obstruction of one or both ureters.
3. **Iatrogenic/surgery**
   - Due to damage to both ureters during a surgical procedure.
4. **Retroperitoneal fibrosis.**
5. **Bilharzia or Schistosomiasis may lead to ureteric fibrosis and stenosis.**
6. **Crystalluria**
   - Uric acid crystalluria can develop in patients receiving chemotherapy for leukemia or lymphoma unless they are given prophylactic treatment with allopurinol.

Pathophysiology

- The maintenance of renal function and urine production depends upon perfusion of the kidneys with oxygenated blood.
- If there is reduced renal blood flow or hypoxia, it impairs renal function.
- This precipitates acute renal failure, resulting in anuria.
- Renal failure caused by acute tubular necrosis progresses through **3 recognisable phases:**
  1. **Oliguria.**
  2. **The diuretic phase.**
  3. **Recovery.**
- The diuretic phase traditionally occurs between the 8th and 10th day but may be delayed as long as 6 weeks.
- Glomerular filtration recommences but tubular function takes longer to recover.
- In most patients the diuretic phase is followed by the recovery phase, but some never recover and will need renal replacement therapy if they are to survive.
- Factors that influence the outcome of acute renal failure include:
  - o Need for artificial ventilation.
  - o Need for inotropic support.
  - o Presence of jaundice.
- Acute Renal Failure has a significant mortality rate.

Clinical Aspects

A patient with anuria is approached in the following sequential manner:

a. **Is urine being produced?**
   - Anuria is diagnosed only after confirming that the urinary bladder is empty. This is done by doing a USG which confirms the absence of urine in the urinary bladder.
   - If even a small amount of urine is present, the bladder should be catheterized and the urine sample investigated for:
     - o Specific gravity.
     - o Presence of casts (implying a renal cause).
     - o Presence of myoglobin.
     - o C/S.

b. **Is there an obvious pre-renal cause?**
   - Clinical examination.
   - Assessment of vital signs.
   - Input and output balance.
   - Measurement of arterial oxygen concentration.

c. **Is there ureteric obstruction?**
   - USG shows some degree of ureteric dilatation and hydronephrosis.
   - A plain X-ray of the abdomen should be checked for calculi.

d. **What drugs have been given recently?**
   - If a drug is thought to be responsible for renal impairment, it should obviously be withdrawn unless its use is vital.

e. **Is this a progression to Chronic Renal Failure?**
   - The presence of shrunken kidneys on USG, normochromic anemia and hypertension suggest progression to a chronic state even if a previous history of renal failure is not available.

Treatment

A. **Initial Treatment**
   - Aimed at prompt restoration of the circulating volume deficit and correction of tissue hypoxia.
   - For patients with hypovolemia or sepsis, inotropic support with dopamine may improve cardiac efficiency and increase renal blood flow.
   - If urine production is not promptly restored, furosemide can be tried (but the drug itself may be nephrotoxic).

- Mannitol may be used as a plasma expander and osmotic diuretic.
- The aim is to achieve the best possible BP, with a CVP of 7–9 cm H_2O.
- 100% oxygen may be needed.
- If these measures fail, acute tubular necrosis has supervened.

B. Treatment of Oliguric Phase of ATN

- Excess fluid loads must be avoided.
- Fluid input is restricted to match the reduced output + insensible losses (500–800 ml per 24 hours depending on ambient conditions).
- Abnormal losses due to vomiting, nasogastric aspiration, diarrhea or fistulae will be monitored and replaced.
- A hyperkalemic acidosis is the characteristic metabolic abnormality of the oliguric phase of renal failure.
- Correction of the metabolic acidosis with IV bicarbonate is not always advisable.
- Rising serum potassium is life threatening and requires effective intervention:
    - A calcium resonium enema is the simplest remedy.
    - This ion-exchange resin can also be administered orally but is unpalatable.
    - Cautious use of IV dextrose and insulin should be considered if ion exchange fails.
    - Urgent dialysis may be necessary.

C. Treatment of Diuretic Phase of ATN

- During the diuretic phase, a heavy loss of sodium and potassium can be expected, and fluid and electrolyte requirements must be carefully judged.
- In most patients the diuretic phase is followed by the recovery phase, but some never recover and will need renal replacement therapy to survive.

D. Treatment of Acute Renal Failure

- Nutritional support with enteral feeding or TPN.
- Swabs taken from the nose and throat, sputum specimens and urine, if available, should be sent for culture. If antibiotics are required, they should be non-nephrotoxic.
- Meticulous recording of fluid balance.
- Renal support is given in the form of:
    - Peritoneal dialysis.
    - Hemodialysis.
    - Hemofiltration.
- Obstructive renal failure may require:
    - Percutaneous nephrostomy.
    - Insertion of a J-stent.

ANTEGRADE PYELOGRAPHY

- Also known as antegrade urogram.
- It is the percutaneous puncture of a dilated renal collecting system.

Method

- It is done by the interventional radiologist.
- Under fluoroscopic or ultrasound guidance, an 18 G needle, 15 cm long should be passed into a dilated calyx or pelvis.
- It is better to pass the needle into a dilated calyx rather than pelvis as there will be a better seal around the needle track and less danger of puncturing large hilar vessels.
- Temporary drainage can also be provided by a small plastic catheter introduced through the needle, which will be subsequently removed.
- The catheter now acts as a nephrostomy tube.
- Contrast medium is introduced through the nephrostomy.
- X-rays are taken.

Indications

- Can be helpful when retrograde studies are prevented by obstruction at the extreme lower end of the ureter.
- The most common indication is the placement of a nephrostomy tube to drain an obstructed infected kidney.
- To provide access for percutaneous nephrolithotomy.

Disadvantages

- Invasive.
- Requires the expertise of an interventional radiologist, so it is not easily available.
- Dye is injected which can cause allergic reactions, anaphylaxis.

48

Kidney and Ureter

CONGENITAL DISEASES

[3] Horseshoe kidney. ***June 19***

[5] Embryology, clinical features and management of horseshoe kidney. ***CBME June 24***

- This is the **most common renal fusion anomaly.**

Embryology

- The **lower poles of both kidneys are fused** such that the **isthmus lies at the level of L4-L5 vertebrae.**
- This causes **failure to ascend and rotate** so that the renal pelvis faces anteriorly and vertically with the malrotated calyces pointing posteromedially.
- The vascular supply is variable.
- The **ureter may insert high on the renal pelvis, causing pelviureteric junction obstruction.**

Clinical Features

- M > F.
- Most horseshoe kidneys are asymptomatic and detected incidentally.
- They are however **prone to become diseased because the ureters are angulated** as they pass over the fused isthmus. This produces **urinary stasis and consequently, infection and stones.**
- PUJO.
- Associated with an increased incidence of **genital anomalies.**
- The **incidence of Wilms' tumour is higher** in horseshoe kidney.

Investigations

- It has a **flower vase appearance on IV urography**.

Treatment

- Asymptomatic patients can be left alone.
- The **only indication for dividing the isthmus is during surgery for abdominal aortic aneurysm.**

HYDRONEPHROSIS

[10] Describe the clinical features and management of hydronephrosis. ***March 22***

[10] Discuss causes, pathology, clinical features and management of hydronephrosis. ***Dec 15***

[3] Dietl's crisis. ***Sept 21, Feb 23***

[3] Mention the causes for unilateral hydronephrosis. ***July 15***

- **Definition:** Aseptic dilatation of the whole or part of the kidney/urinary tract.
- It is due to a partial or intermittent obstruction to the outflow of urine.

Causes of Unilateral Ureteric Obstruction

A. Extramural Obstruction

- Tumour from adjacent structures, e.g., carcinoma of the cervix, prostate, rectum, colon or caecum.

- Idiopathic retroperitoneal fibrosis.
- Retrocaval ureter.

B. Intramural Obstruction

- Congenital stenosis, physiological narrowing of the pelviureteric junction leading to pelviureteric junction obstruction.
- Ureterocele and congenital small ureteric orifice.
- Inflammatory stricture following removal of ureteric calculus, repair of a damaged ureter or TB infection.
- Neoplasm of the ureter or bladder cancer involving the ureteric orifice.

C. Intraluminal Obstruction

- Calculus in the pelvis or ureter.
- Sloughed papilla in papillary necrosis (especially in diabetics, analgesic abusers and those with sickle cell disease) may obstruct the ureter.

Causes of Bilateral Hydronephrosis

- Bilateral hydronephrosis is usually the result of urethral obstruction, but the lesions described above may occur on both sides.
- When due to lower urinary obstruction, the cause may be:

A. Congenital

- Posterior urethral valves.
- Urethral atresia.

B. Acquired

- Benign prostatic enlargement.
- Carcinoma of the prostate.
- Post-op bladder neck scarring.
- Urethral stricture.
- Phimosis.

Clinical Features

Unilateral Hydronephrosis

- F > M.
- Right > left.
- Mild pain or dull aching in the loin.
  - o Often accompanied with a sensation of dragging heaviness.
  - o It is made worse by excessive fluid intake.
  - o Kidney may be palpable.
- Attacks of acute renal colic may occur with no palpable swelling .
- Intermittent hydronephrosis or **Dietl's crisis:**
  - o A swelling in the loin is associated with acute renal pain. Some hours later, the pain is relieved and the swelling disappears when a large volume of urine is passed.
- Antenatal detection in the foetus by USG.

Bilateral Hydronephrosis

- **From lower urinary obstruction:**
  - o Symptoms of bladder outflow obstruction predominate.
  - o Kidneys are unlikely to be palpable.
- **From bilateral upper urinary tract obstruction:**
  - o Rare compared with unilateral lesions.
  - o E.g., idiopathic retroperitoneal fibrosis, idiopathic pelviureteric junction obstruction.
- **From pregnancy:**
  - o Physiological dilatation of ureters and renal pelves.

Investigations

A. USG

- Non-invasive.
- Can diagnose PUJO in utero.

B. IVU or Intravenous Urography

- Used only if there is significant function in the obstructed kidney.
- Extra-renal pelvis is dilated.
- Minor calyces lose their normal cupping and become clubbed.
- If level of obstruction is in doubt, take follow-up films 36 hours after contrast has been injected. Contrast slowly diffuses to fill the obstructed system down to the blockage.

C. Isotope Renography

- Best test to confirm obstructive dilatation of the collecting system.

- DTPA or MAG-3 (labelled with ^{99m}Tc, a gamma ray emitter) is given IV. Its passage through the kidneys is tracked by a gamma camera.
- ^{99m}Tc-DTPA is cleared from a normal kidney but stays in the renal pelvis on the obstructed side.

D. Whitaker Test

- A percutaneous puncture of the kidney is made and fluid is infused at a constant rate with monitoring of intrapelvic pressure. An abnormal rise in pressure confirms obstruction.

E. Retrograde Pyelography

- Confirms the site of obstruction immediately before corrective surgery.

Treatment

- The indications for surgery are:
  - o Bouts of renal pain.
  - o Increasing hydronephrosis.
  - o Evidence of parenchymal damage.
  - o Infection.
  - o Mild cases should be followed by serial USG scans and should be operated upon if dilatation is increasing.
- The surgical options are:
  1. Pyeloplasty.
  2. Endoscopic pyelolysis.
  3. Nephrectomy.

Anderson-Hynes Pyeloplasty

- Upper 1/3rd of ureter and renal pelvis are mobilised.
- Ureter is dismembered from the renal pelvis.
- Redundant renal pelvis is excised.
- A new pelviureteric junction is reconfigured.
- A ureteric stent is inserted to splint the anastomosis.

Endoscopic Pyelolysis

- Endoscopic options to correct pelviureteric junction obstruction are:
  - o Retrograde balloon dilatation.
  - o Incision of the pelviureteric junction using a hot wire over a balloon.
  - o Laser incision.
  - o Percutaneous pyelolysis from above.

Nephrectomy

- Considered when the kidney has lost most of its function.
- An obstructed kidney is worth preserving if it is contributing >20% of total renal function.

UROLITHIASIS

[10] Enumerate aetiopathology, clinical features and investigations for renal calculi. Write about management of staghorn calculus. ***August 22***

[10] Enumerate the causes of renal calculi and its management. ***Dec 17***

[5] Renal calculus. ***Dec 14, March 24***

[5] Ureteric calculi. ***Feb 23***

[5] Staghorn calculus. ***Dec 19***

[3] Types of urinary calculi. ***July 23***

[3] Mention types of renal calculi. ***Dec 15***

[3] Mention types of urinary calculi. ***Dec 16, June 16, July 15***

[3] Extracorporeal Shock Wave Lithotripsy. ***March 22***

[3] PerCutaneous Nephro Lithotomy. ***Dec 19***

Epidemiology

- The modern world is witnessing a steady increase in the incidence of renal calculi.
- However, the incidence of bladder stones has declined progressively because of a reduction in poverty and improvement in basic nutrition.

Causes

A. <u>Non-modifiable Factors Associated with Stone Formation</u>

a. Age

- **Men:** Peak incidence is 30-60 years.
- **Women:** Bimodal peak in the third decade (20-30 years) and the post-menopausal period.

b. Gender: M > F.

c. **Ethnic origin:**
- More common in Whites.

d. **Family history:**
- Patients with a positive family history are 2.5 times more likely to develop stone disease.
- E.g.:
  - o Cystinuria.
  - o Type I renal tubular acidosis.
  - o Primary hyperoxaluria.
  - o Xanthinuria.
  - o 2, 8 – dihydro adeninuria.

B. **Modifiable Factors Associated with Stone Formation**

a. **Environmental factors**
- People living in hot and arid regions such as the desert or tropical areas have a higher incidence due to increased perspiratory fluid loss.

b. **Drugs**
- Predispose to stone formation through metabolic effects.
- E.g., corticosteroids, chemotherapeutic agents, acetazolamide, allopurinol, thiazides.

c. **Dietary excess**
- Rhubarb, spinach, tea, cocoa, chocolate, pepper increase urinary oxalate.

C. **Other Causes**
- Primary hyperparathyroidism.
- Prolonged immobilization: Bone resorption causes hypercalcemia and hypercalciuria.
- Milk alkali syndrome.

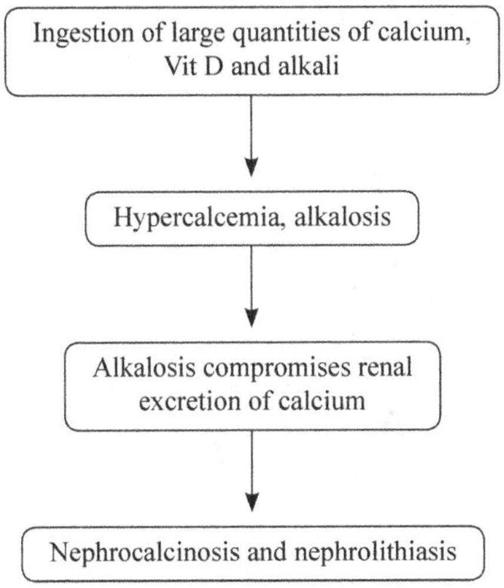

- Sarcoidosis: Non-caseating granulomata produce 1,25 – dihydroxy cholecalciferol.
- Disseminated neoplastic disease.
- Cushing's disease.
- Hyperthyroidism.
- Hyperuricosuria:
  - o Gout.
  - o Myeloproliferative disorders after cytotoxic treatment.
  - o Dietary purine and protein excesses.
  - o Inflammatory bowel disease.
  - o Ileostomies.
- Idiopathic calcium urolithiasis.
- Obstruction and stasis.
- Medullary sponge kidney.
- Urinary diversion.

Pathogenesis

- Stone formation results from a cascade of events that occur during and after urine formation.
- When the concentration of culprit salts such as calcium and oxalate overwhelm inhibitory factors, e.g., citrate, potassium, magnesium, Tamm-Horsfall mucoproteins, pH changes; they precipitate into crystals.
- These crystal nuclei may be washed off with the flow of urine or they may anchor onto sites like renal papillae to form Randall's plaques.
- Variations in urinary pH may also facilitate or inhibit stone growth.
  - o Acidic pH precipitates the formation of uric acid stones.
  - o Alkaline pH precipitates the formation of calcium phosphate stones.
- Stasis of urine also promotes new stone formation.

Normal Anatomical Narrowings of The Ureter

- There are 5 narrowings where a stone can lodge:
  1. Ureteropelvic junction.
  2. Ureter crossing the bifurcation of common iliac artery.
  3. Ureter in close relation to the vas deferens or broad ligament.

4. Ureter entering the bladder wall.
5. Ureteric orifice.

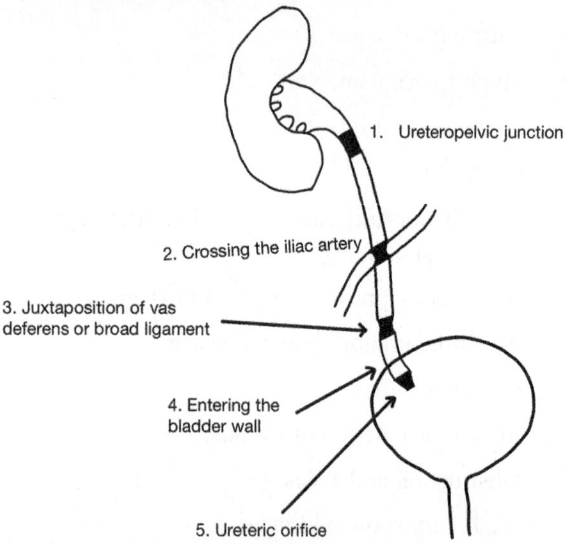

Figure 1: Normal anatomical narrowings of ureter

Types of Stones

A. Oxalate Stones

- It is the most common type of urinary tract stone.
- Also known as mulberry stone.
- Calcium oxalate stones.
- Usually single.
- Radiopaque.
- Covered with sharp projections which cause the kidney to bleed and altered blood is precipitated on the surface of the stone.
- Because of its rough surface, it gives rise to symptoms when comparatively small.
- Dihydrate stones are more common than monohydrate and is less hard.
- Factors predisposing to its formation:
  - o Hypercalciuria.
  - o Hypercalcemia.
  - o Hyperoxaluria.
  - o Hyperuricosuria.
  - o Hypocitraturia.
- Hypercalciuria is the most common metabolic abnormality and occurs as a result of dysregulation of calcium transport at various sites, including the intestine, bone or kidney.
- **Primary hyperparathyroidism** is the most common disease associated with hypercalcemia and stones

Increased PTH

↓

1. Increased bone resorption
2. Increased synthesis of 1,25 - dihydroxy vitamin D3

↓

Increased intestinal absorption of calcium

↓

Hypercalcemia, hypercalciuria

- Hyperuricosuria causes uric acid crystal formation, over which calcium oxalate crystals aggregate.

B. Phosphate Stones

- Pure calcium phosphate stones are rare.
- Common forms seen are:
  - o Apatite - seen with infection.
  - o Brushite - seen with distal RTA.

C. Infection Stones

- These are struvite and apatite stones.
- Certain bacteria such as *Proteus, Klebsiella, Serratia* or *Enterobacter* produce urease.

$$\text{Urea} \xrightarrow{\text{Urease}} CO_2 + NH_4$$

i.e., alkalinisation of urine

- Staghorn calculi are infection stones that grow in a branching pattern, taking the form of the pelvicalyceal system.

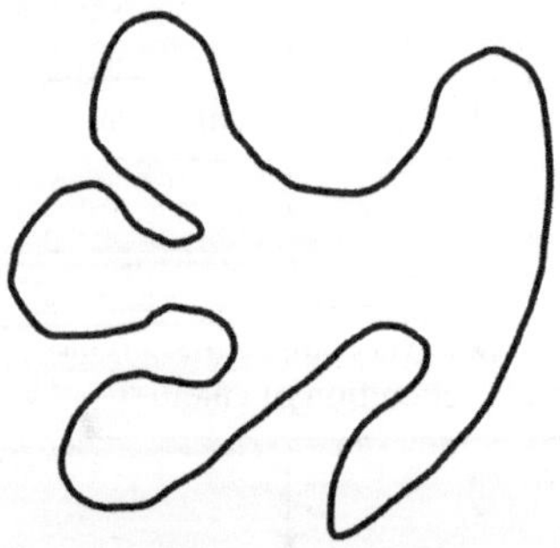

Figure 2: Staghorn calculus

- Struvite calculi are triple phosphate calculi which contain calcium phosphate with ammonium magnesium phosphate.
- Can become very large before clinical detection.
- Cause significant morbidity, which includes loss of renal function owing to chronic infection and obstructive uropathy.
- Complete clearance of a staghorn calculus is necessary, as residual fragments after treatment can cause rapid recurrence and persistence of bacteriuria.
- Long-term chemoprophylaxis is mandatory for a few months after successful removal of infection calculus.
- These are smooth and dirty white in colour.
- Because it is smooth, a phosphatic calculus gives rise to few symptoms until it has attained a large size.
- It is neither radiolucent nor as radiopaque as cystine and oxalate calculi, but is seen on X-rays because of its size rather than its density.
- The calcium content in the stone makes it radio-paque.

D. Uric Acid Stones

- Caused by hyperuricosuria.
- In acidic urine: Uric acid precipitates into crystals.
- In alkaline urine: Uric acid remains soluble.
- Hard, smooth and usually multiple.
- Contain calcium oxalate crystals which renders them radiopaque.

E. Cystine Stones

- Cystinuria is due to decreased reabsorption of cystine from proximal tubules.
- Cystine is insoluble even at physiological pH and worsens with increasing acidity.
- Very hard stones (due to the presence of disulphide bonds) and as a result do not fragment with shock wave lithotripsy.
- Usually multiple.
- Radio-opaque.
- May assume a cast of the renal pelvis and calyces.

Clinical Features

- M > F.
- 30-50 years.
- **Acute ureteric colic:**
  - o 3-5 mm calculi are responsible for acute ureteric colic.
  - o Very severe agonizing pain.
  - o Pain radiates from loin to groin and to the scrotum/labium.
  - o Never radiates to the back of the leg.
  - o Sudden in onset.
  - o Causes the patient to draw up their knees and roll about in pain.
  - o Often accompanied by vomiting and profuse sweating.
  - o An attack of colic rarely lasts > 8 hours.
  - o It is often due to a stone entering the ureter, but also occurs when a stone in the renal pelvis temporarily blocks the pelviureteric junction.
  - o Caused by hyperperistalsis of the ureteric musculature against the obstructing stone.
- **Renal pain:**
  - o Caused by distension of the renal capsule.
  - o Felt as a constant, gnawing pain in the loin/renal angle.
  - o It is often worse on movement, particularly on walking upstairs.
- **Strangury:**
  - o It is the passage of a few drops of urine, often blood stained, after painful straining.
  - o May occur if the stone is in the intramural ureter.
- **Hematuria:**
  - o Non-visible hematuria (detected on urine routine or dipstick) frequently accompanies the pain.
  - o Visible hematuria can also be seen, but it is rare.
  - o As a rule, hematuria occurs in small amounts (enough to render the urine 'smoky') during or after an attack of pain.
- **Pyuria:**
  - o Stones lead to an increase in the number of WBC's in the urine even in the absence of infection.
- **Quiescent calculus:**
  - o Some stones lie dormant for a long period, during which time there is progressive destruction of the renal parenchyma, and uremia may be the first indication.
  - o Secondary infection usually supervenes.

- **Calculuria:**
  - o Described as sand or gravel accompanying urine.
  - o Lower ureteric stones close to or lodged at the ureterovesical junction can cause symptoms of urgency and frequency.
- Malaise and weight loss can occur in longstanding infection stones or as a manifestation of renal failure.
- High grade fever with chills suggests an underlying UTI and should be considered an emergency.
- Incidentally detected asymptomatic stones are increasingly diagnosed because of the widespread use of imaging.

On Examination

- During an attack of ureteric colic there is rigidity of the lateral abdominal muscles.
- Percussion over the kidney produces a sharp stab of pain.
- Tenderness of the kidney on bimanual palpation.

Complications

- **Calculous anuria:**
  - o Bilateral obstructing ureteric stones or ureteric calculi in a solitary kidney can present with anuria.
- **Infectious complications:**
  - o Pyelonephritis.
  - o Pyonephrosis.
  - o Renal abscess.
  - o Septicemia.
- **Chronic renal failure:**
  - o Recurrent episodes of infection and obstruction cause nephron loss which results in chronic renal failure.
- Xanthogranulomatous pyelonephritis.
- Pyeloenteric or cutaneous fistulae.

Differential Diagnoses for Ureteric Colic

- Clot colic: caused by anticoagulation therapy, hemophilia, vascular tumours.
- Papillary necrosis: caused by diabetes, NSAIDs, sickle cell anemia.
- Acute appendicitis.
- Ectopic pregnancy.
- Ovarian torsion.
- Acute intestinal obstruction.
- Abdominal aortic aneurysm.
- Malingering.

Investigations

a. NCCT KUB

- Non-contrast CT of Kidney Ureter Bladder is the investigation of choice to diagnose renal calculi (both radiolucent and radiopaque).

b. Plain X-ray KUB

- Done to assess if the stone(s) are radio-opaque and if plain X-rays can be used in the follow up of a patient who is expected to pass a stone spontaneously.

c. USG KUB

- First line imaging investigation.
- Stones classically produce an acoustic shadow.
- Can be used for insertion of percutaneous nephrostomy in an obstructed renal collecting system.

d. CBC

- There is leukocytosis in case of a supervening infection.

e. Urine tests

- Majority of patients have pyuria which may be sterile pyuria or due to infection.
- Crystals are seen.
- pH of urine is important.
- C/S identifies the causative organisms in a case of infection and also tells about the antibiotic sensitivity.

f. Blood for C/S

- Sent in patients suspected of sepsis.

g. Renal function tests

- Blood urea, serum creatinine, eGFR (estimated Glomerular Filtration Rate) are done to monitor the functional status of the kidneys.

h. Metabolic evaluation

- Serum levels of calcium, phosphorus and uric acid are done to rule out hypercalcemia, hypophosphatemia and hyperuricemia.

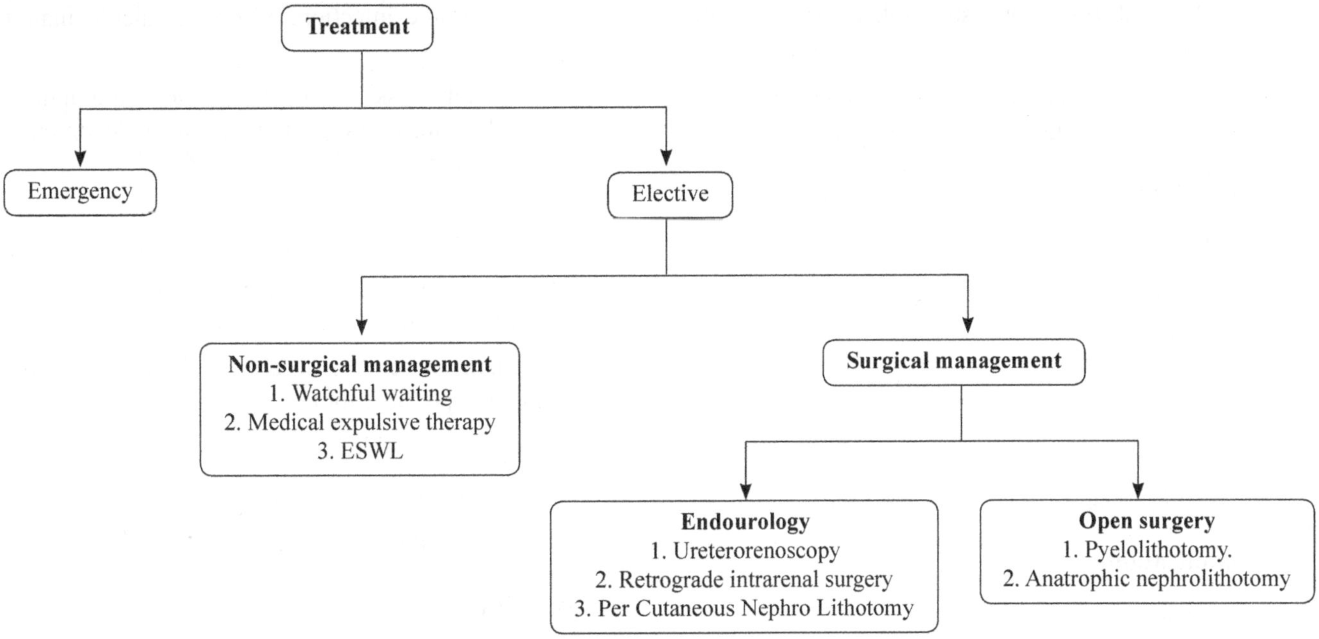

Treatment

The management of urinary tract stones can be subdivided depending on whether the patient presents in the emergency or elective setting.

Emergency

- Small stones (< 5 mm), especially in the distal ureter, are likely to pass spontaneously and are therefore just observed with analgesics.
- Drug of choice for pain: NSAIDs and paracetamol. Anti-spasmodics are not necessary to alleviate pain.
- If the patient is clinically unstable, initial stabilization in ICU is done.
- If pain does not reduce with analgesics, or if the patient shows features of sepsis or urinary obstruction, emergency urinary decompression is indicated:
  1. Ureteric stenting.
  2. Per Cutaneous Nephrostomy (PCN).
- In the absence of infection, removal of stones may be possible by ureteroscopy.

Elective

A. Non-Surgical Management

a. Watchful waiting

- Indications are:
  1. Small calculi < 5 mm in size.
  2. Non-obstructive calculi.
  3. Asymptomatic.
  4. Lower pole renal calculi.
  5. Preserved renal function.

b. Medical expulsive therapy

- Tamsulosin is an $\alpha 1$ adrenergic blocker that causes smooth muscle relaxation of the distal ureteric muscle.
- Tamsulosin can be used for:
  - o Distal ureteric stones > 5 mm.
  - o To assist passage of fragments following Shock Wave Lithotripsy.

c. Extra-corporeal Shock Wave Lithotripsy (ESWL)

- It is a non-invasive method to treat stones on an outpatient basis.

Mechanism of action

- The stone is localized using either fluoroscopy or ultrasound or both.
- Shock waves/acoustic pulse waves are generated and focused on the stones.
- Stone fragmentation occurs as a result of:
  - o Mechanical stress caused directly by the energy transmitted by the shockwaves.
  - o Indirectly by the collapse of bubbles.

- The small fragmented stones then pass out in the urine.
- Efficacy reduces with an increasing number of stones and volume of stone burden.

Indications

1. Renal calculi.
2. Stones ≤ 1.5 cm.

Contraindications

1. Obesity.
2. Pregnancy.
3. Patients taking oral anti-coagulants.

Complications

1. Arrhythmias.
2. Infection:
   - Prophylactic antibiotics are used to prevent infection as stones are often colonized by bacteria.
3. Cystine stones are hard and relatively resistant to ESWL
4. Hematuria, parenchymal hemorrhage, peri-renal hematoma.
5. Steinstrasse or 'street of stones'.
   - Occurs when the stone burden is high or when the stones are hard.
   - Means a row of closely gathered stone fragments that line the distal end of the ureter.
   - These stones are usually asymptomatic and pass spontaneously.
   - May sometimes cause obstruction, requiring surgical intervention.
   - 'Clinically insignificant residual fragments' are residual stone fragments of ≤ 4 mm after treatment, that pass spontaneously.

B. Surgical Management

- Indications are:
  - o Failure of medical management.
  - o Impaired renal function.
  - o Chronic infection: Staghorn calculi, matrix calculi.
  - o High risk occupations or geographical locations: Pilots, long distance locomotive drivers, sailors.
  - o Patient preference.
- Choice of therapy depends on multiple factors such as surgical fitness, body habits and stone characteristics.
- General principle is to choose the least invasive method possible for that particular stone.
- Options available are:
  1. Endourology.
  2. Open surgery.

Endourology

- It is the preferred method of treatment.
- **Advantages:**
  - o Minimally invasive.
  - o Technological advancements in instrumentation.
  - o More efficient energy sources for stone fragmentation.
- Current energy sources are: Pneumatic, ultrasound or laser lithotripsy.
- Type of energy source used, depends on the type of surgery and stone characteristics.
- Available options are:
  - o Ureterorenoscopy (URS).
  - o Retrograde intrarenal surgery (RIRS).
  - o Per Cutaneous nephrolithotomy (PCNL).

a. Ureterorenoscopy (URS)

- Long thin scopes are used to remove ureteric and renal stones.
- Energy sources, graspers and baskets are used.
- Types: Semi-rigid or flexible.
- A semi-rigid URS is usually used with a pneumatic lithotripter or laser energy device.
- Dormia stone-catching basket is used if the stone is < 6 mm and in the distal ureter.

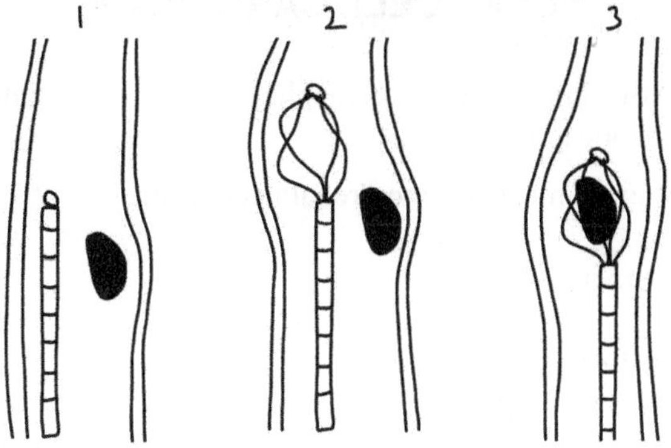

1) Basket introduced past stone
2) Opened
3) Enclosing stone, ready for withdrawal

Figure 3: Dormia basket

- Can also be used in patients with bleeding disorders, with only a moderate increase in complications.

Complications

- Ureteric perforation.
- Ureteric avulsion.
- Retropulsion.
- Injury to ureteric mucosa leading to strictures.

b. Retrograde intrarenal surgery (RIRS)

- It is slimmer and more flexible than URS.
- Thinner fibres allows for retrograde access to the kidney via the ureteric orifice.
- Laser is used as an energy source for stone fragmentation.
- It avoids the morbidity associated with PCNL.
- Indications:
    - o Renal stones < 2 cm.
    - o Lower pole calculi.
    - o Obesity.
    - o Musculoskeletal deformities (e.g., kypho-scoliosis).
    - o Renal anomalies (horseshoe kidney or pelvic kidney).
    - o Bleeding diathesis.

c. Percutaneous nephro lithotomy (PCNL)

- It involves removal of renal stones by creating a track between the skin and the pelvicalyceal system.

Mechanism

- Patient is placed in prone position.
- Stone is localized using fluoroscopy or ultrasound.
- The posterolateral calyx is commonly chosen for entry.
- A tract is established into the renal collecting system.
- The tract is dilated using a series of dilators.
- A working sheath is placed in the tract.
- Stone is fragmented using ultrasound + pneumatic + laser energy.
- Fragments are successfully removed by irrigation.
- A nephrostomy tube is left in the kidney for 24 - 48 hours.

Indications

- Renal stones > 2 cm.
- Lower pole renal stones with anatomy that is unfavourable for ESWL.
- Failed ESWL or RIRS for renal calculi.
- Staghorn calculi.

Contraindications

- Pregnancy.
- Untreated UTI.
- Bleeding diathesis.
- Current anticoagulation.

Complications

- Bleeding (severe bleeding may require selective angioembolisation).
- Infection.
- Pleural violation (in cases of supracostal puncture).
- Extravasation of urine due to rupture of the collecting system.
- Retained stone fragments.

Miniaturised PCNL

- Involves the use of smaller access tracks.

- Standard PCNL: Access track is > 28 Fr.
- In miniaturised PCNL: < 22 Fr.
- Most useful in patients with a smaller stone burden and in children.

Open Surgery

- It is reserved for complex and infected stones with anatomical abnormalities.
- Options available are:
    - o Pyelolithotomy.
    - o Anatrophic nephrolithotomy.

Prevention of Recurrent Stones

- Fluid intake of > 2.5 litres/day.
- Reduce intake of animal protein and salt.
- Dietary calcium should not be restricted.
- Supplemental calcium, if necessary, should be taken at meal times.

[MCQ] A 35-year male presented with complaints of lower abdominal pain referred to the tip of the penis, with haematuria at the end of micturition. On examination, hypogastric tenderness is present, with no guarding or rigidity. Ultrasound showed vesicular calculi. Urine culture and sensitivity showed high growth of *Proteus mirabilis*. Which of the following types of stone could it be? ***CBME June 24***

A. Uric acid stone B. Oxalate stone
C. Cystine stone D. Triple phosphate*

Answer: The growth of *Proteus mirabilis* indicates that the urine is infected and stones seen in infection are struvite stones or triple phosphate stones.

RENAL TUMOURS

[10] Causes of hematuria. Describe in detail the clinical features, investigations, management of renal cell carcinoma. ***June 16***

[5] Renal cell carcinoma. ***July 23***

[5] Hypernephroma. ***Dec 17, July 23***

[3] Paraneoplastic syndromes in renal cell carcinoma. ***Feb 23***

RENAL CELL CARCINOMA

- Also known as hypernephroma, Grawitz tumour, adenocarcinoma.
- It is the most common renal neoplasm.

Aetiology

A. Familial

- vHL syndrome (von Hippel Lindau) is the most common familial syndrome associated with RCC.

B. Sporadic

- Cigarette smoking.
- Obesity.
- Hypertension.
- Diuretics.
- Occupational exposure to petrochemicals and dyes.
- ARCD (Acquired Renal Cystic Disease) in patients on long-term hemodialysis.

Clinical Features

- Median age at presentation is 64 years.
- M : F = 2 : 1.
- Asymptomatic presentation is the most common presentation of RCC as the majority of diagnoses result from incidental detection.
- **Classic triad:** Flank pain + hematuria + palpable mass.
- Most common presenting symptom is hematuria.
- Clot colic may be seen after hematuria.
- **Constitutional symptoms:** Fever, malaise, weight loss.
- **Advanced disease:**
    - o Bilateral lower limb edema.
    - o Recent onset non-reducing right sided varicocele owing to thrombus in the IVC.
- **Metastatic symptoms:**
    - o Most common site of mets is the lung and is classically described as cannon ball mets.
    - o Lung mets: Complaints of persistent cough, hemoptysis.

  - o May occasionally present as pathological fractures (bone mets).
- **Paraneoplastic syndromes:**
  - o Elevated ESR is the most common paraneoplastic syndrome.
  - o Erythrocytosis.
  - o Hypertension.
  - o Anemia.
  - o Hypercalcemia.
  - o Persistent pyrexia may sometimes be the only symptom, is because of absorption of necrotic material and disappears after nephrectomy.

Grading

Fuhrman grading system

- It is the most widely used grading system for clear cell RCC.
- Defines 4 nuclear grades (1-4) in order of increasing nuclear size, irregularity and nucleolar prominence.

Leibovich score

- It is a prognostic score assigned following nephrectomy.
- Runs from 0 to 11 and is based on the tumour's stage, grade, size, involvement of lymph nodes and the presence of tumour necrosis histologically.

Pathology

- Cells of origin: Renal tubular epithelial cells (proximal convoluted tubule).
- Clear cell RCC is the most common subtype.
  - o Clear appearance of cytoplasm is due to accumulation of glycogen and lipids.
- Slow growing tumours.
- Bulge out of the renal contour.
- Most are solitary, but bilateral and multiple tumours are found in familial RCC.
- Prognosis of ccRCC varies, depending on various histopathological features, such as nuclear grading.
- ccRCC may be associated with loss of chromosome 3p and a mutated vHL gene.

Spread

- Directly, invading the perinephric tissue through the capsule.
- Can extend into the renal vein as a tumour thrombus.
- Vein wall invasion is associated with poor prognosis.

Staging

- I : Tumour < 7 cm and limited to the kidney.
- II : Tumour > 7 cm and limited to the kidney.
- III : Tumour in the major veins or adrenal gland with intact Gerota's fascia **or** regional lymph nodes are involved.
- IV : Tumour beyond Gerota's fascia.

Prognostic Factors

- Poor prognostic factors are:
  - o Tumour size.
  - o Venous invasion.
  - o Renal capsular invasion.
  - o Adrenal involvement.
  - o Lymph node involvement.
  - o Presence of tumour thrombus in the renal vein or IVC.

Diagnosis

<u>Radiological Investigations</u>

A. Triphasic CECT

- It is the investigation of choice for diagnosis and staging.
- Provides additional information on:
  - o Function of opposite kidney.
  - o Primary tumour extension.
  - o Venous involvement.
  - o Enlargement of regional lymph nodes.
  - o Status of adrenal glands.
  - o Intra-abdominal metastatic disease.

B. MRI

- Provides similar information to CT.
- Detects tumour infiltration into the vein wall and the level of thrombus.

C. CXR

- Should be done in all cases.
- Shows cannon ball mets.

D. Bone Scan

- Necessary in a patient with elevated alkaline phosphatase, bone pain or hypercalcemia.

Laboratory Investigations

- CBC, ESR, creatinine, LFT, LDH, corrected serum calcium, coagulation markers, urine analysis.
- Increased alkaline phosphatase should prompt further investigation to rule out liver and skeletal mets.
- LDH is useful in risk stratification of metastatic disease.

Treatment

A. Nephron Sparing Surgery

a. Partial nephrectomy:

- **Indications are:**
  - o Tumour < 4 cm.
  - o Well selected tumours 4-7 cm.
  - o Bilateral tumours.
  - o Tumours in solitary kidneys.
  - o Pre-existing renal dysfunction.
- **Complications are:**
  - o Hematuria.
  - o Perirenal hematoma.
  - o Urinary fistulas.
  - o Acute renal impairment.
  - o Infection.

b. Cryoablation

c. Radiofrequency ablation:

- Both ablation techniques are indicated in high risk patients (elderly, multiple comorbidities) with small renal tumours.

d. Bench surgery and autotransplantation:

- Is performed for larger tumours in a solitary kidney.

e. Active surveillance:

- It is indicated in elderly patients.

B. Radical Nephrectomy

- It is the gold standard treatment for localized disease.
- Classical radical nephrectomy = removal of the entire kidney enclosed in Gerota's fascia + perirenal fat + i/l adrenal gland + regional lymphadenectomy.
- Adrenal gland can be spared if there is no involvement on CT/MRI.
- Lymphadenectomy is indicated only in high risk patients with large primary tumours and enlarged lymph nodes.

C. Surgical Management of Inferior Vena Cava Thrombus

- Renal tumours are associated with IVC tumour thrombus in some cases, and the thrombus may extend as far as the right atrium.
- Thrombus extending to the retrohepatic or suprahepatic segment of the IVC requires full mobilization of the liver.
- Thrombus extending to the right atrium may require cardiopulmonary bypass and circulatory arrest.

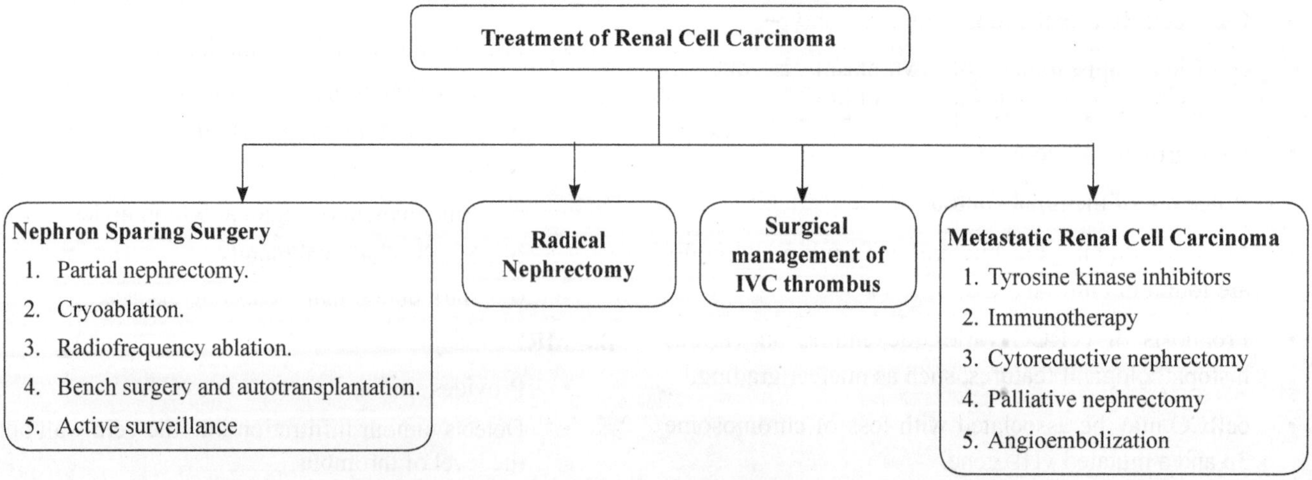

D. **Treatment of Metastatic RCC**

a. **Tyrosine kinase inhibitors**
   - Sunitinib, pazopanib.

b. **Immunotherapy**
   - RCC is an immunogenic tumour and therefore responds to immunotherapy.
   - **1st generation:** Interleukins and interferons.
   - **Targeted therapy:**
     - o Immune checkpoint inhibitors.
     - o Anti-programmed death 1/programmed death ligand-1 inhibitors.

c. **Cytoreductive nephrectomy**
   - Beneficial in good and intermediate risk patients.

d. **Palliative nephrectomy**
   - **Indications:**
     - o Intractable hematuria.
     - o Pain.
     - o Symptomatic paraneoplastic syndrome.

e. **Angioembolization**
   - Performed in medically unfit patients with intractable hematuria.

E. **RCC is radiotherapy resistant** and there is no role for radiotherapy in the treatment of RCC.

[3] Wilm's tumour. *March 22*
[5] Wilm's tumour. *March 21, June 17*

WILMS' TUMOUR

- Also known as nephroblastoma.
- It is the **most common tumour of childhood.**
- It is a malignant renal tumour **derived from embryonal cells.**

Aetiology

- Mutation in the Wilms' tumour suppressor gene (WT_1).
- Familial.

Pathology

- The tumour has **mixed elements derived from the embryonic nephrogenic tissue**, namely:
  - o Blastemal or undifferentiated tissue.
  - o Epithelial tubules.
  - o Stroma.
- Tumour can **extend into the renal vein and vena cava.**
- It metastasizes to **lymph nodes and lungs.**

Clinical Features

- Bilateral in only 5% of cases.
- The typical presentation is a child aged between 1 and 4 years of either gender with a large, palpable abdominal mass that may cross the midline.
- Hematuria.
- Hypertension.
- Fever.
- Weight loss.
- Pain is relatively uncommon.
- The large **tumour can rupture and present as an acute abdomen.**

Differential Diagnosis

- Neuroblastoma.
- Congenital mesoblastic nephroma.
- Renal cell carcinoma.
- Clear cell sarcoma.
- Rhabdoid tumour.

Investigations

a. **USG**
   - **Confirms the renal origin** and solid nature of the mass.

b. **CECT.**

c. **MRI .**
   - **CECT and MRI are necessary to stage the disease.**
   - The tumours usually infiltrate the kidneys and normal **renal parenchyma is compressed at the periphery around the tumour – called claw sign.**

d. **CT chest.**
   - The **lung is the most common site of distant mets.**

Treatment

- **Nephrectomy** + adjuvant or neo-adjuvant **chemotherapy**.
- **Chemotherapy regimens**
  - o VA: Vincristine + Actinomycin D.
  - o VAD: Vincristine + Actinomycin D + Doxorubicin.
  - o CD: Cyclophosphamide + Doxorubicin.

OTHER IMPORTANT TOPICS

CLASSIFICATION OF RENAL NEOPLASMS

A. Benign

1. Oncocytoma.
2. Angiomyolipoma.
3. Juxtaglomerular cell tumour.

B. Malignant

1. **Renal cell carcinoma:**
   - Clear cell carcinoma.
   - Papillary carcinoma (Type I and II).
   - Chromophobe carcinoma.
   - Collecting duct carcinoma.
   - Medullary carcinoma.
2. Urothelial carcinoma of renal pelvis or upper tract transitional cell carcinoma or upper tract urothelial cancer.
3. Wilms' tumour or Nephroblastoma.

RENAL TRAUMA

- Kidneys are retroperitoneal structures which are relatively fixed by their vascular pedicles.
- Kidneys are protected by:
  - o Perinephric fat.
  - o Strong posterior abdominal wall muscles.
  - o Lower rib cage.
- Renal trauma is usually a part of polytrauma.

Cause/Mechanism of Injury

- Blunt trauma > penetrating trauma.
- **Common modes of injury:**
  - o Head on collisions in RTA.
  - o Falls from height.
  - o Contact sports.
- Sudden, rapid deceleration can cause avulsion injury to the ureters at the PUJ or renal pedicle.
- Penetrating injuries cause direct tissue disruption and are usually associated with adjacent organ injuries.

Grades of Renal Injuries

- There are 5 grades with increasing severity.
- **Grade 1**
  - o Contusion or non-enlarging subcapsular perirenal hematoma.
  - o No laceration.
- **Grade 2**
  - o Superficial laceration < 1 cm: Does not involve the collecting system, therefore there is no evidence of urine extravasation.
  - o Non-expanding perirenal hematoma confined to retroperitoneum.
- **Grade 3**
  - o Laceration > 1 cm: Does not involve the renal pelvis or collecting system, therefore there is no evidence of urine extravasation.
- **Grade 4**
  - o Laceration extends to renal pelvis, which therefore causes urinary extravasation.
  - o Injury to main renal artery or vein with *contained* hemorrhage.
  - o Segmental infarctions without associated lacerations.
  - o Expanding subcapsular hematomas compressing the kidney.
- **Grade 5**
  - o Shattered kidney.
  - o Avulsion of renal hilum: Devascularisation of kidney due to hilar injury.
  - o Ureteropelvic avulsions.
  - o Complete laceration or thrombus of the main renal artery or vein.

Clinical Features

- Superficial bruising may be present, but is rare.
- Local pain and tenderness in the loin.
- **Hematuria:**
  - o Gross or microscopic hematuria is pathognomonic of renal trauma.
  - o Cardinal sign of a damaged kidney.
  - o Can sometimes be seen hours after the accident.
  - o Profuse hemorrhage may be followed by clot colic.
- **Severe delayed hematuria:**
  - o Sudden profuse hematuria occurs between the 3rd day and the 3rd week after the accident in a patient who appears to be progressing favourably.
  - o It is due to a clot becoming dislodged.
- **Meteorism:**
  - o It is abdominal distension which is seen about 24-48 hours after the accident.
  - o Caused by a retroperitoneal hematoma implicating splanchnic nerve.
- Shock + microscopic hematuria should arouse suspicion of renal injury.
- Even a slight flattening of the normal contour of the loin should arouse suspicion of renal injury.

Investigations

CECT with IV contrast:

- Investigation of choice.
- Gives information on the following:
  - o Type and extent of renal injury.
  - o Parenchymal laceration: Its depth and extension into the pelvicalyceal system.
  - o Extent of urinary extravasation.
  - o Status of the contralateral kidney.
  - o Other abdominal injuries.
- Effectively stages renal pedicle injuries.
- Arterial occlusion manifests as rim enhancement of the normal renal contour.

Indications of CECT

- Abdominal trauma with gross hematuria.
- Microscopic hematuria with hypotension (systolic BP < 90 mm Hg).
- Rapid deceleration injury.
- Children with microscopic hematuria (> 5 RBCs per hpf).
- All penetrating injuries.

Treatment

- Conservative management with close surveillance is sufficient in the majority of cases of isolated renal trauma.
- The treatment of lower grade injuries, sometimes including grade 4 injuries, is as follows:
  - o Bed rest.
  - o Antibiotics in case of penetrating injuries.
  - o Serial hemoglobin estimation.
  - o Reimaging is usually done after 2 - 4 days in cases of:
    - ♦ Falling hemoglobin levels.
    - ♦ Fever.
    - ♦ Expanding flank mass.
- Persistent urinary leak can be managed with an internal DJ stent or PCN.
- Indications for emergency surgical exploration:
  - o Expanding or pulsatile retroperitoneal hematoma.
  - o PUJ avulsion.
  - o Renal pedicle injury.
  - o Hemodynamic instability.
- Surgical options are:
  1. **Renorrhaphy**
     - o Surgical repair of a laceration or injury to the kidney.
     - o Renal parenchyma is sutured to control bleeding and restore structural integrity.
     - o Aims to preserve as much kidney tissue and function as possible.

2. **Partial nephrectomy**
   - o Removal of the devitalised portion of the kidney.
3. **Total nephrectomy**
   - o Entire kidney is removed.
   - o Indicated in grade 5 or shattered kidney.
4. **Perinephric packing**
   - o Gauze packs are placed around the injured kidney to control bleeding.
   - o Used as a temporary measure in severely injured kidneys until definitive surgery can be performed.

49

Urinary Bladder

[5] Ectopia vesicae. *Feb 23*

- Ectopia vesicae is also called bladder exstrophy.
- It is a **congenital disorder** in which **failure of development of the lower abdominal wall (infra umbilical portion)** leads to an abdominal wall defect through which the **bladder is exposed.**
- **Diastasis of pubic symphysis** and **epispadias** can coexist.
- It forms part of a spectrum of conditions ranging from epispadias to bladder exstrophy or to more severe cloacal exstrophy, the so called **exstrophy-epispadias complex.**

Embryology

Failure of mesodermal ingrowth between the ectodermal and endodermal layers of the cloacal membrane.

↓

Lower abdominal wall muscles do not form.

↓

Premature rupture of cloacal membrane.
1. Epispadias.
2. Bladder exstrophy or cloacal exstrophy.

Clinical Features

- M > F.
- Exstrophy of the bladder can be associated with a spectrum of anomalies affecting the external genitalia, urinary system, bony pelvis, abdominal wall, rectum and anus.

A. Male External Genitalia

- Shortened penis (this is due to diastasis of the pubic symphysis which results in wide separation of the crural attachments, and congenital deficiency of the corporeal tissues).

B. Female External Genitalia

- Shortened, stenotic and anteriorly displaced vagina.
- Bifid clitoris.

C. Urinary System

- Incompetent bladder neck continence mechanism.
- VUR due to lack of obliquity of the vesico-ureteric junction.

D. Bony Pelvis

- Widening (diastasis) of the pubic bones due to malrotation of the innominate bones, leading to a waddling gait.
- External rotation of anterior and posterior segments of the bony pelvis, leading to outward rotation of the lower limbs.

E. Abdominal Wall

- Low-set umbilicus with a triangular shaped fascial defect of the lower abdominal wall.
- Higher incidence of indirect inguinal hernia owing to the lack of oblique muscle fibres of the inguinal canal and large internal and external inguinal rings.

E. Anorectum

- Shortened perineum and anteriorly displaced anus.
- Imperforate anus or rectal stenosis.
- Rectal prolapse.

Surgical Treatment

- **Aims of treatment:**
  1. To preserve renal function.
  2. To achieve urinary continence.
  3. To create functional and cosmetically acceptable external genitalia.
- **Staged repair:**
  - o **Neonatal period:** Bilateral iliac osteotomies with bladder exstrophy and abdominal wall closure.
  - o **6 months - 1 year:** Epispadias repair and phallic reconstruction.
  - o **5-7 years:** Bladder neck reconstruction and b/l ureteric reimplantation (to treat VUR).
- **Recent advances:** Complete primary repair of exstrophy in the neonatal period as it optimizes outcomes with fewer procedures and without a formal bladder neck closure procedure.

[3] Acute cystitis. *March 24*

- Infection of the urinary bladder is called cystitis.

Pathogenesis

- The most common route of infection is **ascending UTI.**

Contamination of vaginal and periurethral area with uropathogenic organisms originating from GIT

↓

Adherence and migration of bacteria into the urethra and bladder

↓

Bacterial internalisation into the urothelial cell

↓

Formation of:
1. Intracellular bacterial communities (IBCs).
2. Quiescent intracellular reservoirs (QIRs).

IBCs and QIRs act in a similar way to a biofilm, may remain viable for months and act as a source of recurrent UTI.

- Less common routes of infection:
  - o Hematogenous spread: Seen with *Staphylococcus aureus* and fungal infections.
  - o Direct infection from retroperitoneal abscess or inflammatory bowel disease.
- Most common organisms in uncomplicated UTI: *Escherichia coli* (85%), *Staphylococcus saprophyticus, Enterococcus faecalis, Proteus* and *Klebsiella.*
- Most common organisms in complicated UTI: *E. coli* (50%), enterococci, *S. aureus* and *Pseudomonas.*
- Successful infection depends on the bacterial virulence relative to the host defence mechanisms.

Bacterial virulence factors	Host defence mechanisms
• Adherence mechanisms (fimbrial and afimbrial) • Immune evasion (lipopolysaccharide O, capsule K) • Anti-IgA proteases, toxin production, β-lactamase • Resistance to antimicrobial bactericidal activity (alteration of antimicrobial binding sites) • Iron acquisition	• Commensal organisms (lactobacilli) • Mechanical integrity of mucous membranes • Antibacterial secretions (lysozyme, lactoferrin, IgA) • Antegrade flow of urine causing flushing effect • Tamm–Horsfall protein (binds to bacterial adhesion molecules) • Composition of urine (low pH, high urea) • Immune system integrity

Clinical Features

- Dysuria.
- Suprapubic pain.
- Urinary frequency.
- Urgency.
- Hematuria.
- Loin pain.
- Fevers.
- Nausea and vomiting.
- Examination should be performed to check for:
  - o Palpable bladder.
  - o Renal angle tenderness.
  - o Pelvic organ prolapse.
  - o Urethral diverticulum.
  - o Atrophic vaginitis.

Investigations

- Urinalysis (a dipstick test checks for the presence of red cells, white cells and nitrites).
- Urine microscopy.
- Urine C/S.
- Flow rate assessment.
- Measurement of postvoid residual volume.
- Renal tract ultrasound is done in recurrent UTI, to exclude anatomical pathology.
- Cystoscopy:
  - o Atypical symptoms.
  - o Hematuria.
  - o Features that raise suspicion of underlying pathology (e.g., bladder cancer, stones, urinary tract fistula).

Treatment

- Antibiotics based on C/S and local resistance patterns.
- Non-antimicrobial measures to prevent future UTI:
  - o Increasing fluid intake.
  - o Probiotics.
  - o Methenamine hippurate.
  - o D-mannose.
  - o Vaginal oestrogen therapy for postmenopausal women.

Treatment of Recurrent Cystitis

- Antimicrobial prophylaxis.
- Postcoital antimicrobial use for those with sex-linked infections.
- Intermittent self-start antimicrobial therapy.

OTHER IMPORTANT TOPICS

URINARY TRACT INFECTION

- UTI is the inflammatory response of the urothelium to bacterial invasion, usually associated with:
  - o **Bacteriuria:** Presence of bacteria in the urine.
  - o **Pyuria:** Presence of WBCs in the urine.
- **Sterile pyuria:**
  - o Pyuria in the absence of bacteriuria.
  - o Indicates an inflammatory response that is because of:
    - ♦ UTI.
    - ♦ Fastidious organisms (e.g., TB, gonorrhea).
    - ♦ Carcinoma *in situ* (CIS).
    - ♦ Bladder stones.
    - ♦ Other inflammatory conditions.

Classification

A. Based on the Condition of the Underlying Urinary Tract:

- **Uncomplicated:** Occurring in a healthy patient with a structurally and functionally normal urinary tract.
- **Complicated:** Occurring in a patient with an anatomical or functional urinary tract abnormality, in an immunocompromised patient or with more virulent or resistant bacteria.

Factors that suggest a complicated urinary tract infection	
Patient factors	• Functional or anatomical abnormality of the urinary tract • Sex (male gender) • Age (postmenopausal) • Pregnant • Immunosuppressed (e.g., diabetes, transplant, steroids) • Indwelling catheter
Bacterial factors	• Increased virulence (hospital-acquired infection) • Antimicrobial resistance (recent antibiotic use)

B. Based on the Number of Episodes

- **Isolated UTI:** Is one in which there has been an interval of at least 6 months between infections.
- **Recurrent UTI (rUTI):** Is defined as ≥ 2 episodes in 6 months ***or*** ≥ 3 episodes in 12 months.

C. Based on the Site of Infection

- **Urethritis:** Urethra.
- **Prostatitis:** Prostate.
- **Cystitis:** Urinary bladder.
- **Pyelonephritis:** Renal pelvis.

CARCINOMA OF URINARY BLADDER

Histological Subtypes of Bladder Cancer

1. **Transitional cell carcinoma or urothelial carcinoma (>90%)**
   - Most common subtype.
2. **Squamous Cell Carcinoma (1-7%)**
   - Occurs secondary to chronic inflammation.
   - E.g., indwelling catheter, stone, schistosomiasis.
3. **Primary adenocarcinoma (2%)**
   - Usually originates in the urachus (dome of the bladder) or in those with bowel in the urinary tract (due to reconstruction surgery), e.g., augmentation enterocystoplasty, bladder exstrophy repair.
4. **Metastatic adenocarcinoma (<1%)**
   - Colorectal, prostate, kidney, ovary.

Risk Factors

- Smoking.
- Occupational exposure to aromatic hydrocarbons:
  - o E.g. tanner, rubber, paint, dyes, gas and tar, hairdressers, plumbers, painters.
- Environmental carcinogens:
  - o E.g. arsenic in drinking water.
- Chronic inflammation of bladder:
  - o Indwelling catheter.
  - o Stones.
  - o Schistosomiasis (predisposes to squamous cell carcinoma).
  - o Recurrent infections leading to keratinising squamous metaplasia.
- Drugs:
  - o Phenacetin.
  - o Cyclophosphamide.
- Pelvic radiotherapy.

Grades

- **G1 :** Well differentiated.
- **G2 :** Moderately differentiated.
- **G3 :** Poorly differentiated.

Staging

Tis : Urothelial carcinoma in situ.

Ta : Non-invasive papillary urothelial carcinoma.

T1 : Invasive into lamina propria.

T2a : Invasive into inner half of muscularis propria.

T2b : Invasive into outer half of muscularis propria.

T3a : Microscopic invasion in peri-vesical soft tissue.

T3b : Macroscopic invasion in peri-vesical soft tissue.

T4 : Invasion into adjacent organs.

- **Non-muscle invasive bladder cancer (NMIBC):** Tis, Ta, T1.
- **Muscle invasive bladder cancer (MIBC) or locally advanced bladder cancer:** T2, T3, T4.

Clinical Features

- The most common symptom in painless gross hematuria.
- Bleeding may give rise to clot formation in the bladder and subsequent urinary retention.
- **Storage LUTS:**
  - o Frequency.
  - o Urgency.
  - o Dysuria.
  - o Recurrent UTI.
- **Advanced cases:**
  - o Flank pain.
  - o Weight loss.
  - o Pelvic or bone pain.
  - o Lower limb edema.

Investigations

A. Urine
- C/S
- Cytological examination for malignant cells.

B. CT Urography
- Gold standard.
- Assessment of nodal mets.

C. MRI of Bladder
- Can be useful in staging of primary tumour.

D. CT of Chest

- Should be performed in confirmed bladder cancer cases for complete staging.

E. Cystourethroscopy

- Flexible cystourethroscopy under local anesthesia is the mainstay of diagnosis.
- Biopsy can be taken.
- Conventional: White light cystoscopy.
- Newer methods: Narrow band imaging (NBI) and photodynamic blue light cystoscopy.

Treatment

Non-Muscle Invasive Bladder Cancer (NMIBC)

- Aims:
  - o To reduce the risk of tumour recurrence.
  - o To reduce the risk of progression to muscle invasive bladder cancer.
- TURBT followed by intravesical mitomycin C or BCG depending on the risk stratification.

A. Transurethral Resection of Bladder Tumour (TURBT)

- The initial management of bladder tumours consists of TURBT for accurate staging purposes
- Performed with a rigid cystoscope under GA.
- **For large tumours:** A standard fractionated resection of the entire tumour, including the tumour base with deep muscle.
- **For smaller solitary tumours (<3 cm):** En bloc resection of the entire tumour.
- Based on the histological grade and stage, the patient can be risk stratified:
  - o Low risk.
  - o Intermediate risk.
  - o High risk.

B. Post-Operative Mitomycin C Instillation

- An immediate post TURBT dose of mitomycin C should be instilled into the bladder.
- This reduces the risk of tumour recurrence.
- Indicated in intermediate risk tumours.

C. Intravesical BCG

- Immunotherapy in the form of intravesical BCG is indicated in high risk tumours.

D. Regular Cystoscopic Surveillance

- Low risk tumours.

Muscle Invasive Bladder Cancer (MIBC)

- There are 2 options in the management of MIBC:
  1. Neo-adjuvant chemotherapy followed by radical cystectomy and urinary diversion.
  2. Chemoradiotherapy.
- Primary surgical treatment is most commonly done.

A. Surgery: Radical cystectomy + pelvic lymph-adenectomy

- Indications:
  - o Multifocal high grade T1 tumours with carcinoma in situ.
  - o Poor bladder function.
  - o Significant hematuria.
  - o Upper tract obstruction
  - o Factors that affect successful radiotherapy, e.g. bilateral hip replacements, inflammatory bowel disease.
- Structures removal in radical cystectomy:
  - o **Males:** Urinary bladder and perivesical fat + prostate and seminal vesicles + pelvic lymph nodes.
  - o **Females:** Urinary bladder and perivesical fat + uterus, cervix, fallopian tubes and anterior vagina + pelvic lymph nodes.
- **Pelvic lymphadenectomy:** Removal of external and internal iliac lymph nodes, obturator nodes.

B. Urinary Diversion

- Alternative drainage for urine is necessary after removal of the bladder.
- There are various options for urinary diversion:
  1. **Ileal conduit**
     - o Most commonly done.
     - o A loop of ileum is isolated and then prepared on its own mesentery.
     - o Ureters are then implanted into the bowel either separately or as one plate and the ileostomy is created.
  2. **Orthotopic bladder**
     - o A pouch is created using small or large

bowel that is then anastomosed to the patient's urethra.

- o Studer pouch is widely performed.
- o Ureters are implanted into the pouch.

3. Continent cutaneous diversion (heterotopic bladder substitute)

- o Indicated in patients who require urethrectomy, or in whom the urethra is non-functional.
- o Studer pouch is created.
- o The appendix (or a separate section of ileum) is then anastomosed from the bladder to the umbilicus or right iliac fossa.
- o The patient can then intermittently catheterise this channel to drain the pouch.

4. Ureterosigmoidostomy (Mainz II pouch)

- o Sigmoid colon is detubularised and refashioned into a pouch into which the ureters are inserted.

C. Radical External Beam Radiotherapy

- Indicated in very elderly or in patients who are unfit for radical cystectomy.

50

Prostate

[5] Acute retention of urine. *June 13*

Urinary retention is defined as the inability to pass urine despite persistent effort.

Types

1. **Acute**
   - Painful inability to pass urine with relief of pain on catheterisation.
2. **Chronic**
   - Painless, elevated residual volume after passing urine.

Causes

a. **Anatomical bladder outlet obstruction**

Men

- BPH.
- Ca Prostate.
- Bladder neck stenosis.
- Urethral stricture.
- Urethral rupture (following pelvic fracture).

Women

- Urethral: Stricture, diverticulum, meatal stenosis, cancer.
- Prolapse.
- Extrinsic compression: Paraurethral cyst, pelvic mass (e.g. fibroids), gynecological malignancy.
- Iatrogenic: Anti-incontinence surgery, urethral reconstruction.

b. **Functional bladder outlet obstruction.**

Men

- Idiopathic high-tone non-relaxing external urethral sphincter.

Women

- Idiopathic high-tone non-relaxing external urethral sphincter (Fowler's syndrome).
- Dysfunctional voiding.
- Primary bladder neck obstruction.

c. **Detrusor under-activity**

- Pelvic surgery.
- Peripheral neuropathy.
- Diabetic cystopathy.
- Secondary to long-standing bladder outlet obstruction.

d. **Neurological disease**

- Detrusor-sphincter dyssynergia (any cause of suprasacral spinal cord disease) causing obstructed voiding.
- Sacral nerve lesion or cauda equina causing detrusor underactivity.

e. **Drugs**

- Anti-muscarinics or β_3 agonists.
- Sympathomimetics.
- Anaesthetics.
- Opioids.

f. **Transient causes**

- Following spinal or epidural anesthesia.
- Pain.
- Fecal impaction due to constipation.
- Blood clot secondary to hematuria.

Clinical Features

- Patient gives a history of inability to pass urine.
- Patient may complain of suprapubic pain.
- Urinary bladder is palpable and may sometimes extend up to the umbilicus.

Investigations

- It is a clinical diagnosis and requires no investigations.
- After catheterisation, patient is investigated to confirm the underlying cause.
- Urine examination to look for blood, WBCs.
- Renal Function Tests.
- USG of Kidney Ureter Bladder Prostate (KUBP) with post-void residual urine measurement.
- TRUS is done if BPH is suspected.
- A trans-rectal USG guided biopsy or transperineal template biopsy of prostate is done if malignancy is suspected.
- PSA.
- CECT of KUBP.
- MRI.
- Cystoscopy.
- Urodynamic studies.

Treatment

- The immediate treatment for urinary retention due to any cause is urethral catheterization (Foley's).
- Suprapubic catheterization is considered in patients who require long-term catheterization and in those in whom urethral catheterization is either not suitable or not possible.
- Once the bladder has been drained by means of a catheter, the underlying cause is looked for and treated accordingly.

Urinary Bladder Catheterisation

- The immediate treatment for urinary retention of any cause is *catheterisation.*
- The bladder can be catheterised in the following ways:
  1. Urethral catheterisation.
  2. Suprapubic cystostomy.
  3. Open cystostomy.

URETHRAL CATHETERISATION

- Size of catheter is expressed in the French scale and refers to the external diameter of the catheter.
- 1 Fr = 0.3 mm
- The standard catheter size for uncomplicated urethral catheterisation is:
  - o Women: 12 Fr or 14 Fr
  - o Men: 16 Fr
- In patients with urethral stricture, a smaller size catheter should be considered.
- In cases of haematuria with 'clot retention', a 22 Fr catheter is typically used to aid drainage of thick clots.
- Coudé tip catheters have a curved tip to allow easier passage past an enlarged prostate.
- Single-channel catheters consist of a single drainage channel only and are used for clean intermittent self-catheterisation as these catheters do not require an indwelling retention mechanism.
- Foley's catheter consists of 2 channels - a drainage channel and a channel for inflation of a balloon at the tip, which allows the catheter to be retained in the bladder.
- Foley's is the standard catheter used for uncomplicated cases of urinary retention.
- The 'three-way' catheter has an additional channel for bladder irrigation and is used for patients with:
  - o Haematuria
  - o Clot retention
  - o Following TURP
  - o Following bladder surgery

Technique for Urethral Catheterisation

1. Aseptic technique–handwashing, sterile gloves, sterile catheter pack.
2. Clean urethral meatus with antiseptic solution.
3. Instil lidocaine gel into the urethra and hold for 2–3 minutes.
4. In men, the penis should be held perpendicular and taught.

5. In women, the labia should be held apart to provide adequate exposure of the urethral meatus.
6. The catheter should be inserted as far as the 'hilt' of the catheter and should pass freely (the type of catheter is dependent on the indication).
7. If there is any resistance, catheterisation should be stopped and assistance sought.
8. The patient may require a Coudé tip catheter if the obstruction is thought to be a large prostate, or a cystoscopy to negotiate a false passage or stricture.
9. The position in the bladder is confirmed with the drainage of clear urine.
10. The balloon should be inflated with 10 mL of sterile water.
11. The catheter bag should then be attached.
12. Details regarding the type and size of catheter, and residual volume, should be clearly recorded.

SUPRAPUBIC CATHETERISATION

- Procedure:
  - o Should only be performed in those with a palpable bladder.
  - o Infiltration of local anaesthesia (1% lidocaine) to the skin and fascia of the suprapubic region, two finger-breadths above the pubic symphysis in the midline.
  - o Seldinger technique of insertion is the safest for percutaneous insertion.
  - o 16 Fr catheter is placed.
- Indications:
  - o Patients who require long-term catheterisation.
  - o Patients in whom urethral catheterisation is not suitable or possible.
- Risks:
  - o Bowel injury, especially in those who have undergone previous abdominal or pelvic surgery.
  - o In these patients, it should be performed under ultrasound and cystoscopic guidance.
- Contraindications:
  - o Known or suspected bladder carcinoma.
  - o Abdominal wall infection at the site of insertion.
  - o Uncorrected coagulopathy.
  - o Presence of a vascular graft in the suprapubic region.

OPEN CYSTOSTOMY

- Urinary bladder is catheterized by the open route, i.e. a laparotomy.
- Performed to safely enter the bladder and ensure that there is no bowel in the path of the catheter.
- Indications:
  - o Bladder cannot be confidently identified.
  - o Patients with extensive abdominal or pelvic surgery.

SPECIAL CONSIDERATIONS IN CHRONIC RETENTION OF URINE

- After catheterisation, patients may have a post-obstructive diuresis producing >200 mL of urine per hour for three consecutive hours.
- These patients should be managed with:
  - o Strict fluid balance monitoring.
  - o Postural blood pressure checks to detect postural hypotension.
  - o Daily serum electrolyte monitoring.
  - o May occasionally require intravenous fluid replacement to match the loss if the patient is unable to take enough orally.

[5] Lower Urinary Tract Symptoms. ***June 14***

[3] Mention Lower Urinary Tract Symptoms due to Benign Prostate Hyperplasia. ***July 15***

- In both sexes, non-specific symptoms of bladder dysfunction become more common with age, probably due to impairment.
- LUTS symptoms are as follows:

a. Voiding symptoms:
  - o **Hesitancy** (worsened if the bladder is very full).
  - o **Poor flow** (unimproved by straining).
  - o **Intermittent flow** (stops and starts).
  - o **Dribbling** (including after micturition).
  - o **Sensation of poor bladder emptying.**
  - o **Episodes of near retention.**

b. **Storage:**
   - o **Frequency.**
   - o **Urgency.**
   - o **Nocturia.**
   - o **Urge incontinence.**
   - o **Nocturnal incontinence (enuresis).**

- LUTS are **usually assessed by means of scoring systems,** which give a measure of severity and help in assessing the outcome of therapy.

[10] Discuss causes of acute retention of urine. Discuss management of Benign Prostate Hyperplasia. *March 21*

[5] Benign Prostate Hyperplasia. *Oct 20, June 19, July 18, June 16*

[3] Mention the symptoms of Benign Prostate Hyperplasia. *June 17, June 16*

[3] Symptoms of Benign Prostate Hyperplasia. *July 23*

BENIGN PROSTATIC HYPERPLASIA

- It is an **age-related condition** and occurs in men over 50 years of age. By the age of 60 years, 50% of men have histological evidence of BPH.
- It is a **common cause of significant lower urinary tract symptoms.**
- It is the **most common cause of bladder outflow obstruction in men > 70 years.**

Aetiology

1. Prostate enlarges because of **increased oestrogenic effects. With ageing, testosterone levels slowly but significantly decrease. However, levels of estrogenic steroids are not decreased equally.**
2. Secretion of intermediate **peptide growth factors** also plays a role.
3. **Metabolic syndrome.**
4. **Hereditary factors.**

Pathology

- BPH **affects both glandular epithelium and connective tissue stroma** to variable degrees.
- Typically affects the **submucous group of glands in the transitional zone,** forming a nodular enlargement.
- Eventually, this overgrowth **compresses the peripheral zone glands into a false capsule** and causes the appearance of the typical **'lateral lobes'.**
- **When BPH affects the central zone glands, a 'middle' lobe develops** that projects up into the bladder within the internal urethral sphincter.
- Sometimes, both lateral lobes also project into the bladder, so that, when viewed from within (i.e. during cystoscopy), the sides and back of the internal urinary meatus are surrounded by an intravesical prostatic collar.
- The most common lobe to be affected is the medial lobe.

Anatomical Effects

A. Urethra

- Prostatic urethra is lengthened, sometimes to twice it's normal length.
- It is not narrowed anatomically.
- Normal posterior curve is exaggerated, sometimes so much that it requires a curved catheter to negotiate it.
- When only one lateral lobe is enlarged, distortion of prostatic urethra occurs.

B. Bladder

- During cystoscopic examination:
   - o Bands of hypertrophied muscle fibres can be seen, called trabeculations.
   - o Between these hypertrophied bundles, there are shallow depressions, i.e. sacculations.
   - o Sometimes, one of the saccules (rarely 2 or more) continues to enlarge and forms a diverticulum.
- If BPH causes bladder outlet obstruction, the musculature of the bladder hypertrophies to overcome the obstruction and appears trabeculated.
- Significant BPH is associated with increased blood flow, and the resultant enlarged veins at the base of the bladder can rupture and cause hematuria.

Clinical Features

- This can be described under two broad headings – LUTS and BOO.

A. **Lower Urinary Tract Symptoms (LUTS)**

a. **Voiding symptoms:**

- **Hesitancy** (worsened if the bladder is very full).
- **Poor flow** (unimproved by straining).
- **Intermittent flow** (stops and starts).
- **Dribbling** (including after micturition).
- **Sensation of poor bladder emptying.**
- **Episodes of near retention.**

b. **Storage**

- Frequency.
- Urgency.
- Nocturia.
- Urge incontinence.
- Nocturnal incontinence (enuresis).

B. **Bladder Outflow Obstruction (BOO)**

- The primary effects of BOO on the bladder are:
  - o **Urinary flow rates decrease**: For a voided volume > 200 ml, it is <10 ml/s.
  - o **Voiding pressures increase**: It becomes > 80 cm H_2O.
- Long-term effects (complications) of BOO are:
  1. Acute retention of urine.
  2. Chronic retention.
  3. Impaired bladder emptying.
  4. Development of storage bladder symptoms.
  5. Hematuria.

DRE (DIGITAL RECTAL EXAMINATION) FINDINGS:

- Posterior surface of the prostate is smooth and convex.
- Rectal mucosa can be made to move over the prostate.
- In a very large prostate, it may not be possible to reach its cranial extreme.

Investigations

A. **Serum Prostate Specific Antigen (PSA)**

- The architecture of the prostate is altered in BPH which allows PSA to enter the blood stream and be detected by a blood test.
- **Normal:** <4 ng/ml.
- **Equivocal:** 4-10 ng/ml.
- **Suggestive of cancer:** > 10 ng/ml.
- **Diagnostic of cancer:** > 35 ng/ml.
- PSA levels are important to rule out prostate cancer.

B. **USG**

- Measures prostate size.
- **Post void residual urine** is measured.
- Transrectal ultrasound **(TRUS)** is also done.

C. **Flow Rate Measurement**

- A peak flow rate < 10 ml/s is suggestive of BOO.
- 2 or 3 voids should be recorded and the voided volume should be > 200 ml.

D. **Pressure Flow Urodynamic Studies**

- A urodynamic evaluation provides information about bladder pressure and urine flow.
- High intravesical pressure during voiding with a reduced flow rate is typically seen with BOO.

E. **Urine Examination**

- Urine is examined for glucose, leukocyte esterase and blood.
- C/S of mid-stream urine.

F. **Blood Tests**

- Complete Blood Count (CBC).
- **Renal Function Tests:** Blood urea, serum creatinine, electrolytes.

Treatment

A. **Drugs**

1. **α adrenergic antagonists.**
   - Inhibit the contraction of smooth muscle that is found in the prostate.
   - **Tamsulosin.**
   - **Quick acting** drugs.
2. **5 alpha-reductase inhibitors**
   - **Inhibit the conversion of testosterone to 1,5-dihydrotestosterone (active form).**
   - Result in a **decrease in the size of the prostate** gland.

- Needs to be taken for at least 6 months.
- Finasteride, Dutasteride.

3. **Phosphodiesterase-5 inhibitors**
   - Reduce smooth muscle tone.
   - Sildenafil, Tadalafil.

B. Surgery

- **Prostatectomy** is done.
- Prostate can be approached via different routes.

1. **Trans Urethral Resection of Prostate (TURP).**
   - o It is the **most commonly performed** procedure for the surgical correction of BOO.
   - o **Strips of tissue are cut from the bladder neck, down to the level of the verumontanum.**
   - o Cutting is performed by a **high frequency diathermy current**, which is applied across a loop mounted on the hand held trigger of the resectoscope.
   - o Chips of prostate are then removed from the bladder using an **Ellik evacuator.**
   - o **In monopolar TURP, resection is limited to 1 hour due to the risk of resorption of water if 1% glycine is used as an irrigant.**
   - o **The advent of bipolar TURP where normal saline is used as an irrigant permits resection of larger prostates.**
2. **Laser prostatectomy:**
   - o Green light laser ablates or vaporises the prostate.
   - o **HOLEP (Holmium Laser Enucleation of Prostate) enucleates the prostate.**
3. **Retropubic prostatectomy**
4. **Transvesical prostatectomy (through the urinary bladder)**
5. **From the perineum**

[5] Management of carcinoma prostate. ***Feb 23***

PROSTATE CANCER

- Carcinoma of the prostate is the most common malignant tumour in men > 65 years.

Aetiology

- Incidence increases with old age.
- Family history.

Pathology

- It usually originates in the peripheral zone of the prostate.
- The following types are seen:
  - o Microscopic latent cancer found on autopsy or at cystoprostatectomy.
  - o Tumours found incidentally during TURP or following screening by PSA measurement.
  - o Early localised prostate cancer.
  - o Locally advanced and high risk prostate cancer.
  - o Metastatic disease.
- It is an adenocarcinoma.

TNM Staging

- **T1:** Incidentally found tumours in a clinically benign gland after HPE of a prostatectomy specimen.
- **T2:**
  - o **2a:** Involves one lobe and is confined within the prostate capsule.
  - o **2b:** The cancer is in more than half of one side of the prostate gland, but not both sides.
  - o **2c:** The cancer is in both sides but is still inside the prostate gland.
- **T3:** Tumour extends through the capsule.
  - o **3a:** Unilateral or bilateral extension.
  - o **3b:** Seminal vesicle extension.
- **T4:** Tumour is fixed or invades adjacent structures other than seminal vesicles.

Spread

1. **Local spread:**
   - To contiguous structures.
2. **Hematogenous spread:**
   - Spreads most commonly to bone.

- Pelvic bones and lower lumbar vertebrae are most commonly involved.
- It is both osteoblastic and osteolytic.

3. **Lymphatic spread.**

Clinical Features

- Only advanced disease gives rise to symptoms, but even advanced disease may be asymptomatic. Symptoms of advanced disease include:
  - o Bladder outlet obstruction.
  - o Pelvic pain.
  - o Hematuria.
  - o Bone pain, malaise, arthritis, anemia or pancytopenia.
  - o Renal failure.
  - o Locally advanced disease or even asymptomatic mets, may be detected incidentally.
- Early prostate cancer is asymptomatic and may be found:
  - o Incidentally (following TURP for clinically benign disease, i.e., T1a and T1b).
  - o T1c: Because of serum PSA screening.
  - o As a nodule (T2) on rectal examination.

DRE

- Irregular induration, characteristically, stony hard with obliteration of the median sulcus, suggests carcinoma.

Investigations

1. **Trans Rectal Ultra Sound (TRUS) + prostate biopsy**
   - The classic abnormality seen on TRUS is a hypoechoic area in the peripheral zone.
   - $\geq$ 12 biopsies are taken under TRUS guidance.
2. **Prostate Specific Antigen**
   - It is a tumour marker.
   - It is neither sensitive nor specific.
   - **Levels:**

     1-4 ng/ml: Normal.

     4-10 ng/ml: Equivocal.

     > 10 ng/ml: Suggestive of cancer.

     > 35 ng/ml: Diagnostic of cancer.
3. **Multiparametric MRI**
   - Can diagnose early prostate cancer.
   - **PIRADS:** Prostate Imaging Reporting and Data System.
   - A score of $\geq$ 3 indicates malignancy.
4. **Transperineal Template Biopsies of the Prostate (TPTBP)**
   - May replace TRUS guided prostate biopsies as a first line test.
   - Used to further evaluate men with a negative TRUS-guided biopsy in whom there is a high suspicion of prostate cancer.
5. **Tests used for staging Ca prostate**
   - MRI.
   - TRUS.
   - Bone scan.
   - PET scan.

Scoring System

- Gleason score is used to grade prostate cancer.
- Two histological areas of prostate are each scored between 3 and 5.
- **Minimum score:** 6.
- **Maximum score:** 10.

Risk Factors for Metastases

- PSA level.
- Gleason grade.
- Clinical stage.

Treatment

Treatment options depend on stage of disease, life expectancy of patient and patient preference.

A. Localised Cancers

a. Radical prostatectomy:

- Should be carried out only in men with a life expectancy of > 10 years.
- It involves removal of the prostate down to the distal sphincter mechanism in addition to the seminal vesicles.

- The bladder neck is reconstituted and anastomosed to the urethra.

b. Radiotherapy:

- Given in the form of external beam radiotherapy or brachytherapy.

c. Active monitoring (surveillance).

B. Advanced Disease

- It is mainly palliative.
- Hormonal ablation remains the first line therapy.

a. Orchidectomy:

- o Removal of testes removes the source of testosterone.

b. Medical castration:

- o **LHRH agonists:** Leuprolide, Goserelin.
- o **Androgen receptor blockers:** Enzalutamide, flutamide.
- o **LHRH antagonist:** Degarelix.
- o **Androgen synthesis inhibitor:** Abiraterone, Cyproterone.

c. Chemotherapy:

- Docetaxel.

51

Penis and Urethra

[3] Hypospadias. *Sept 21*

- **Definition:** The external meatus is situated at some point on the undersurface of the penis or in the perineum.
- It is the most common congenital abnormality of the urethra.

Types

It is classified according to the position of the meatus.

A. Glanular

- Ectopic meatus is placed on the glans penis, but proximal to the normal site of the external meatus, which is marked by a blind pit.

B. Coronal

- Meatus is at the level of the coronal sulcus.

C. Penile

- Meatus is on the underside of the penile shaft.

D. Peno-scrotal

- Meatus is at the level of the penoscrotal junction.

E. Perineal

- Rare.
- Severe abnormality.
- Scrotum is bifid and the urethra opens between its two halves.
- Associated with disorders of sexual development.

Clinical Features

- Diagnosis is made on physical examination.
- There are 3 characteristic features:
  1. Ectopic ventrally located urethral meatus.
  2. Ventral penile curvature (chordee).
  3. Incomplete dorsal hood prepuce.

Treatment

- **Distal hypospadias:** Tubularised incised plate urethroplasty.
- **Proximal hypospadias with chordee:**
  - o 2 stage repair.
  - o 1st stage corrects the penile curvature and the 2nd stage repairs the urethra, called a Dennis Browne urethroplasty.
- Circumcision is contraindicated as preputial skin may be required for future repairs or revision.
- **Timing of surgery:** Before the age of 18 months.

[5] Rupture of urethra. *Sept 21*

RUPTURE OF URETHRA

- Rupture of the urethra is divided into 2 distinct classes:
  1. Rupture of bulbous urethra.
  2. Rupture of membranous urethra.

- Each is again subdivided into:
  - **Complete and incomplete**, which relates to the circumference of the urethral wall injured.
  - **Total and partial**, which relates to the thickness of the urethral wall injured.

BULBOUS URETHRA

- It is more common.

Aetiopathogenesis

- History of a **falling astride injury**, leading to blunt trauma of the perineum, e.g., injury from a man-hole cover.
- Other common causes: **Falling from a tree, cycling, skating, industrial accidents, gym accidents.**
- **Bulbar urethra is crushed upwards onto the pubic bone**, typically with significant bruising.

Clinical Features

- The triad of signs of a ruptured bulbous urethra are:
  1. Urethral hemorrhage, i.e., bleeding from urethral meatus.
  2. Perineal bruising and hematoma, typically with a butterfly distribution.
  3. Retention of urine.

Investigations

- Retrograde urethrogram.

Treatment

- A **gentle attempt** is made at **catheterization.**
- If the catheter fails to drain urine, a **suprapubic cystostomy** is performed.
- **Delayed anastomotic urethroplasty** is performed after 3 months.

MEMBRANOUS URETHRA

- Also known as extraperitoneal rupture of bladder.

Cause

- Pelvic fractures.
- Crush injuries.
- Most commonly seen after road traffic accidents.

Pathology

- The site of injury is usually the **bulbo-membranous junction.**
- **Bladder with the prostate and membranous urethra is disrupted from the bulbar urethra.**
- Displacement can be both posterior and superior.
- Injury can be partial or complete.
- Occasionally, the injury is complex with bladder neck disruption and rectourethral fistula.

Clinical Features

- Blood at the meatus.
- Urinary retention.
- If the bladder is not injured, there will be gradual distension of the bladder.
- If there is an intra-peritoneal rupture of bladder, signs of peritonitis will soon develop.
- If the rupture is extra-peritoneal:
  - Suprapubic tenderness.
  - Dullness to percussion in suprapubic area.
- Total membranous urethral injury may be associated with complete disruption of the puboprostatic ligaments with the bladder, which results in the prostate floating high up in the pelvis.
- A pelvic fracture is always present.
- Other associated injuries may be present.

Investigations

- Usually diagnosed on **FAST** or **CT scan** done during trauma management.
- **Retrograde urethrogram** is used to confirm the diagnosis.
- Complex patients may need evaluation with a **3D-CT or MRI of the pelvis.**

Treatment

- If the tear is partial, a **gentle attempt at catheterisation** is made.
- If urine does not drain, a **suprapubic cystostomy (percutaneous or open)** is performed.

- **Emergency laparotomy** is required for bladder rupture and bladder neck injuries.
- Early **endoscopic realignment** is done when the expertise is available. If endoscopic realignment is successful, some patients may not need further surgery.
- **Delayed anastomotic urethroplasty** is the treatment of choice and is performed after 3-6 months.

[3] Stricture urethra. ***March 24***

[3] Mention the causes for stricture urethra. ***June 13***

STRICTURE URETHRA

Aetiology

- The causes of penile and bulbar urethral stricture are as follows:
  1. Lichen sclerosus.
  2. Iatrogenic (post-catheter and/or instrumentation).
  3. Sexually transmitted diseases (gonorrhoea).
  4. Post-radiation.
  5. Traumatic.
  6. Idiopathic.
  7. Congenital.

Pathophysiology

- **Post-inflammatory strictures:**
  - o Have become less common after the introduction of effective antibiotic treatment of gonorrhoea.
  - o Commonly seen in bulbar urethra.
  - o Infection in periurethral glands, which persists after inadequately treated gonorrhoea.
  - o Infection spreads to cause peri-urethritis, which heals by fibrosis.
  - o Most strictures appear within 1 year of infection but may not cause difficulty in micturition until later.
- **Lichen Sclerosus (previously known as balanitis xerotica obliterans):**
  - o There can be a meatal stenosis and penile urethral stricture.
  - o It is an autoimmune condition or caused by infection.
  - o Strictures are typically long and difficult to treat.
  - o Common sites are penile or panurethral, but isolated bulbar urethral strictures are also seen.
- **Post-instrumentation strictures:**
  - o After an endoscopy or catheterisation.
  - o May affect any part of urethra.
- **Post-TURP strictures:**
  - o Seen in the submeatal area, the bulbar urethra or penoscrotal junction.

Clinical Features

- Hesitancy.
- Poor flow.
- Prolonged voiding time.
- Recurrent UTIs.
- Occasionally patients present with urinary retention.

Investigations

- Uroflowmetry.
- Urethroscopy.
- Urethrography.
- Ultrasound scanning to assess bladder emptying and to detect any upper tract dilatation.
- Urinary flow rate is typically prolonged and shows a box pattern.
- Retrograde urethrogram and micturating cysto urethrography using a water-soluble contrast medium.
- Urethroscopy is used to assess the stricture intraoperatively.

Complications

- Recurrent UTI.
- Retention of urine.
- Upper tract dilatation.
- Bladder stones.
- Periurethral abscess.

Treatment

1. **Urethral dilatation**
   - Dilatation is performed over a guidewire using serial plastic dilators.

- **Indications:**
  - o Soft and short strictures.
  - o Unfit patients.
  - o Patients refusing urethroplasty.
  - o Those with multiple failed urethroplasties.
- Dilatation rarely cures stricture and most patients require repeated dilations.

2. **Direct visual internal urethrotomy (DVIU)**
   - Performed using an optical urethrotome.
   - Stricture is incised under visual control using a cold knife passed through the sheath of a rigid urethrotome.
   - A laser fibre (holmium/thulium) can also be used.
   - Indicated for short, non-traumatic bulbar strictures.
   - Should not be used in the penile urethra or the sphincter active membranous urethra.
3. **Self-dilatation/clean intermittent catheterisation**
   - Patient inserts a small-calibre (12/14 Fr), usually disposable catheter into the urethra at regular intervals.
   - Thus, the patient dilates his own stricture.
   - But this is not a curative option.
   - Patients who are not willing to undergo urethroplasty may choose the option of self-dilatation.
4. **Urethroplasty**
   - Two types of urethroplasty: Anastomotic and augmentation.
   - **Anastomotic**
     - o Performed for bulbar urethral traumatic strictures where there is a gap in the urethra.
     - o Involves dissection of the two ends of the urethra, spatulation and anastomosis.
   - **Augmentation**
     - o Performed for non-traumatic and long strictures.
     - o Strictured segment of urethra is incised and augmented with a patch (graft).
     - o Usual choice of patch material is **buccal mucosa.**
     - o Lingual grafts can be harvested from the undersurface of the tongue.

[5] Phimosis. ***March 22, July 23***
[3] Pinhole meatus. ***Feb 23***
[3] Phimosis. ***July 18***
[3] Surgical procedures for phimosis. ***CBME June 24***

- **Definition:** Phimosis is inability to retract the foreskin of the penis.

Causes

- Physiological phimosis in young boys.
- Balanitis, e.g., balanitis xerotica obliterans.
- Posthitis.
- Lichen sclerosus.

Clinical Features

- Ballooning of the foreskin during micturition.
- Infection (balanoposthitis).

On Examination

- Pin-hole meatus.
- Rarely, patient may present to the emergency with retention of urine.

Treatment

- No treatment is necessary in physiological phimosis.
- True phimosis causing symptoms requires circumcision.
- In emergency situations, such as when catheterization is required, a dorsal slit under LA may be required.

[3] Circumcision. ***August 22, Dec 19, Dec 18***
[3] Indications of circumcision. ***Dec 17, June 17, Dec 15, July 15***

- **Definition:** Circumcision means removal of the foreskin of the penis.

Indications

- In infants and young boys, circumcision is usually performed at the request of the parents for social or religious reasons.
- True phimosis.
- Lichen Sclerosus.

- Recurrent attacks of balano-posthitis.
- Recurrent UTIs with abnormalities such as high grade vesicoureteral reflux.
- Inability to retract the foreskin for intercourse.
- Abnormally tight frenulum.

Contraindications

- Hypospadias.
- Penile curvature.
- Buried penis.

Technique

- Can be done under LA or Spinal or GA.
- Done under GA in children.
- Under anaesthesia, the prepuce is held in artery forceps and put on a gentle stretch.
- A circumferential incision in the penile skin is made at the level of the corona using a knife.
- The prepuce is then slit dorsally in the midline to within 1 cm of the corona (an alternative technique slits the prepuce first).
- This converts the foreskin into two flaps.
- When the undersurface of the prepuce has been separated from the glans, the inner layer of each flap is again marked with a pen and then incised with a second circumferential incision, leaving about 0.5 cm of the inner layer of the preputial skin.
- Cutting the remaining connective tissue completes the excision.
- Vessels should be preferably secured with bipolar diathermy or with absorbable sutures.
- The cut edges of the skin are approximated using interrupted absorbable sutures, making certain that the frenular vessels are ligated.

[3] Peyronie's disease. *March 21*

- It is a condition characterised by the presence of plaques (dense scar tissue) in the penis.

Aetiology

- Associated with Dupuytren's contracture.
- Exact cause is unknown.

Pathogenesis

- The disease has **2 phases**:
  1. Initial active phase (18-24 months).
  2. Later stable phase.
- The **exact cause is unknown**, but it probably **involves minor injury to the erect penis.**
- **Micro-hemorrhage** occurs **beneath the tunica albuginea.**
- This **heals with fibrosis**, resulting in **palpable plaques.**

Clinical Features

- **Penile deformity:**
  - o Presence of plaques causes the erect penis to bend towards the side of the plaque.
  - o Deformity is commonly dorsal (towards the abdomen).
  - o May prevent penetrative sexual intercourse.
- Palpable penile plaques inside the penis.
- Erectile dysfunction.
- Pain on erection.

Investigations

- It is usually a clinical diagnosis.
- MRI may be helpful.

Treatment

- There is no effective treatment in the active phase.
- **Surgical correction:**
  1. If the penis is of adequate length, the tunica albuginea is plicated on the side opposite to the maximum curvature. This can be done by a **Nesbit's procedure** or a **16-dot technique**.
  2. **Incision of the plaque** and a **bovine pericardial patch.**
- **Newer treatments:** Intralesional injections of collagenase clostridium histolyticum.

[5] Premalignant conditions of penis. ***March 21, Dec 13***

[3] Pre malignant conditions of penis. ***Dec 18, Dec 14***

A. Leukoplakia of glans penis

- **Treatment:** Fulguration, excision, cryotherapy, CO_2 laser ablation, photodynamic therapy.

B. PeIN or Penile Intraepithelial Neoplasia, also known as carcinoma in situ

- These are as follows:
  1. **Erythroplasia of Queyrat:** Involves glans penis and prepuce.
  2. **Bowen's disease:** Involves shaft of penis.
  3. **Bowenoid papulosis.**
- **Treatment of PeIN:**
  - o **Lesions on foreskin:** Circumcision, wide local excision.
  - o **Lesions on glans:** Glans resurfacing.
  - o Topical 5-fluorouracil cream.
  - o 5% imiquimod cream.
  - o Laser ablation with Nd-YAG, KTP-532 or CO_2.

C. Non-virus Related Penile Premalignant Lesions

1. **Cutaneous horn**
   - Treatment is by wide local excision
2. **Pseudoepitheliomatous keratotic and micaceous balanitis (PKMB)**
   - **Treatment:** Topical 5-FU, surgical excision, laser ablation, cryotherapy.
3. **Male Lichen Sclerosus also known as Balanitis Xerotica Obliterans**
   - **Treatment:** Clobetasol propionate cream.

D. Virus Related Penile Lesions

1. **Condylomata acuminata also known as genital warts, venereal warts, genital condyloma**
   - Associated with Human Papilloma Virus.
   - **Treatment:**
     - o Imiquimod 5% cream is the topical treatment of choice.
     - o Podophyllotoxin 0.5% solution or gel.
     - o Trichloroacetic acid.
     - o Cryotherapy with liquid nitrogen.
     - o Electrofulguration.
     - o CO_2 laser therapy.
     - o Surgical excision.
     - o Intralesional interferon alfa-2b.
     - o Cidofovir.
2. **Buschke Lowenstein tumour also known as Giant Condyloma Acuminatum**
   - Associated with HPV.
   - **Treatment:** Surgical excision ± skin graft reconstruction.
3. **Kaposi sarcoma**
   - Associated with Human Herpes Virus-8 and HIV.
   - Treatment depends on underlying cause and includes the following:
     - o Localized surgical excision.
     - o Partial penectomy.
     - o Radiation.
     - o Discontinuation of causative immuno-suppressants.
     - o Interferon and cytotoxic therapy.
     - o Nd: YAG laser.

[5] Carcinoma penis. ***Oct 20, Dec 19***

[5] Management of carcinoma penis. ***June 13***

- It is one of the most common cancers in South America.

Aetiology

- **Smegma** is in some way carcinogenic:
  - o Circumcision soon after birth confers immunity against carcinoma of the penis.
  - o Later circumcision does not seem to have the same benefit.
- **Human Papilloma Virus: Types 16 and 18.**
- **Lichen Sclerosus or Balanitis Xerotica Obliterans** is a risk factor.
- **Smoking.**

- **Phimosis** and **chronic balanoposthitis** are contributory factors.
- **Pre-malignant lesions.**

Pathology

- Ca penis is most commonly a **squamous cell carcinoma** arising in the **skin of the glans penis or the prepuce**.
- Types:
  - **a. Flat and infiltrating:** Starts as leucoplakia or penile intraepithelial neoplasia (PeIN).
  - **b. Warty:** Results from an existing papilloma.
- Local growth continues for months or years, before invasion and spread.
- Earliest **lymphatic spread** is to the **inguinal** and then to the **iliac nodes**.
- Distant mets are rare.

TNM Staging

T1 - Tumours confined to the skin.

T2 - Tumours invading the corpus spongiosum or the corpus cavernosum.

T3 - Tumours invade the urethra.

T4 - Tumours invade adjacent structures.

Nx - Regional lymph nodes cannot be assessed.

N0 - No regional lymph node mets.

N1 - Mets in a single, superficial, inguinal lymph node.

N2 - Mets in multiple or bilateral superficial inguinal lymph nodes.

N3 - Mets in deep inguinal or pelvic lymph node(s), unilateral or bilateral.

Mx - Distant mets cannot be assessed.

M0 - No evidence of distant mets.

M1 - Distant mets.

Clinical Features

- 90% of patients are > 40 years of age.
- The first symptoms are a mild irritation and a purulent discharge from the prepuce.
- Slow progression: By the time the patient presents, the growth is often large.
- Also, many patients present late with a fungating/ulcerative growth, either because of embarrassment or because of misdiagnosis.
- Secondary infection causes a foul, bloody discharge.
- There is little or no pain.
- Half of the patients complain of inguinal lymph node enlargement. These are either due to secondary deposits, or due to infection.
- In many cases, the prepuce cannot be retracted and it must be split in order to view the lesion.
- Untreated, the whole glans becomes a fungating and particularly foul smelling mass.
- In rare cases, the inguinal lymph nodes fungate through the skin of the groin and death of the patient can result from erosion of the femoral or external iliac vessels.

Investigations

- A **biopsy** should be performed to make the diagnosis.
- **MRI** is performed for local staging.
- **USG guided FNAC** of palpable inguinal lymph nodes:
  - o Confirms the presence of secondary deposits.
  - o Rule out reactive enlargement.
- **CECT of pelvis** can also be done to check for enlargement of iliac and pelvic lymph nodes.
- **PET-CT** may be useful among patients with clinically detected inguinal mets to define the presence of pelvic or distant mets.

Treatment

A. Treatment of the Primary Tumour

a. Organ preserving surgery

- The various options are:
  1. Limited excision.
  2. Moh's micrographic surgery.
  3. Laser ablation.
- Moh's micrographic surgery is based on sequential tissue excision under repeat microscopic control. This helps in accurately identifying the tumour margin and maximally preserves uninvolved tissues.

b. **Surgical excision**
- Mainstay of treatment.
- Traditionally, 2 cm margin of normal tissue was removed.
- However, recent guidelines are more conservative and recommend penis preserving surgery with excision of much lower margins of normal tissue.
- Tumours affecting:
  - o Glans penis – Glansectomy or partial penectomy.
  - o Advanced cases – Total penectomy + perineal urethrostomy.
- Such surgery is indicated even in advanced metastatic disease for reasons of local control.

c. **Treatment of associated enlarged inguinal lymph nodes**
- Should be delayed until at least 3 weeks after local treatment of the primary lesion.

Local treatment of the primary lesion.
↓
Give antibiotics for 3 weeks.
↓
- Enlargement caused by infection will subside.
- Does not subside.
  ↓
  USG guided FNAC.
  ↓
  Confirm the diagnosis.
  ↓
  Block dissection of both the groins.

- Management of patients where the nodes are not palpable, involves the use of sentinel lymph node biopsy followed by inguinal node dissection if SLNB is positive.
- Management of pelvic nodes is controversial:
  - o N2 – options are observation, pelvic lymphadenectomy or radiotherapy.
  - o N3 – no role for surgery.
- Chemotherapy is relatively ineffective and is currently reserved for palliation in those with metastatic disease.

OTHER IMPORTANT TOPICS

PARAPHIMOSIS

- **Definition:** When a tight foreskin has been retracted and cannot be returned, it is called paraphimosis.

Pathophysiology

The venous and lymphatic return from the glans and distal foreskin is obstructed.
↓
Both the glans and the foreskin become engorged and edematous.
↓
Results in even more pressure within the obstructing ring of prepuce.

Causes

1. Failure to replace the foreskin over the glans, after it has been retracted for catheterization.
2. In a very young child, paraphimosis is often seen after the foreskin has been traumatically reduced during an examination or sometimes by overzealous parental attempts at hygiene.

Clinical Features

- The diagnosis is apparent at a glance.
- Penile pain.
- Painful swelling of the distal foreskin and glans.

Treatment

- Ice bags.

- Gentle manual compression.
- Injection of a solution of hyaluronidase in normal saline.
- If careful manipulation fails, circumcision is done.
- A dorsal slit of the prepuce under LA may be enough in an emergency.

POSTERIOR URETHRAL VALVE

- **Definition:** Posterior urethral valves are congenital membranous folds that obstruct the lumen of the posterior urethra.

Pathogenesis

- These are membranes that have a small posterior slit within them.
- Typically present just distal to the verumontanum and cause obstruction to the urethra.
- Flap valves.
- They are obstructive to antegrade urinary flow and a urethral catheter can be passed retrogradely without any difficulty.

Clinical Features

- Seen exclusively in boys.

A. Antenatal Presentation

- Bilateral hydronephrosis.
- Dilated urinary bladder.
- Dilated posterior urethra.
- Oligohydramnios and lung hypoplasia are seen in severe cases.

B. Postnatal Presentation

- Presentation varies according to severity of obstruction.
- The more severe the obstruction, the earlier the presentation.
- Voiding dysfunction.
- Urinary tract infections.
- Bladder distension.
- Rarely, the valves are incomplete, and the patient presents in adolescence or adulthood.

Investigations

A. Antenatal

- **USG:** Dilated posterior urethra looks like a keyhole.

B. Postnatal

- **USG:** Used to assess renal cortical thickness.
- **Nuclear renography:** Checks for differential renal function.
- **Micturating cystourethrogram:** Vesicoureteral reflux is typically present.

Treatment

- Need to be detected and treated as early as possible to minimise the degree of renal failure.
- Initial treatment is by catheterization to drain the urine and decompress the bladder and upper urinary tracts.
- Definitive treatment is by endoscopic ablation of the valves.

CHORDEE

- Chordee is a fixed bending or bowing of the penis.
- **Causes:**
  - o Hypospadias.
  - o Acutely as a result of general urethritis.

Clinical Features

- Erection is grotesque and very painful.

Treatment

- Treat the underlying cause.

52

Testes and Scrotum

UNDESCENDED TESTES

[5]	Undescended testes. ***Oct 20, June 14***
[5]	Retractile testes. ***June 17***
[3]	Mention complications of undescended testis. ***Dec 12***

- Undescended testis is also called cryptorchidism.

Terms

- **Incomplete descent:** When the testis is arrested in some part of its **normal path** to the scrotum.
- **Ectopic testis:** Testis that is **abnormally placed outside this path.**

Physiological Descent of the Testes

- The testes **develop high on the posterior abdominal wall,** in the retroperitoneum, below the kidneys, at the level of **T10**.
- The testes **descend through the inguinal canal** into the scrotum.
- Descent happens **before birth**.
- In some boys, the testes reach the scrotum during the first 3 months of life, but full descent after that is uncommon.
- **Gubernaculum and processus vaginalis take part** in testicular descent.
- During descent, the testes carry their vessels, lymphatics, nerves and the vas deferens with them.

Location

- The undescended testes may be:
  a. **Intra-abdominal**
     - o Usually lying extraperitoneally just inside the internal inguinal ring.
  b. **Intracanalicular**
     - o In the inguinal canal.
     - o It may or may not be palpable.
  c. **Extracanalicular**
     - o Usually at the scrotal neck.
  d. **Ectopic**
     - o Superficial inguinal pouch (lies just inferior and medial to the superficial inguinal ring) is the most common site.
     - o **Other rarer ectopic sites:** Femoral triangle, root of penis, perineum.

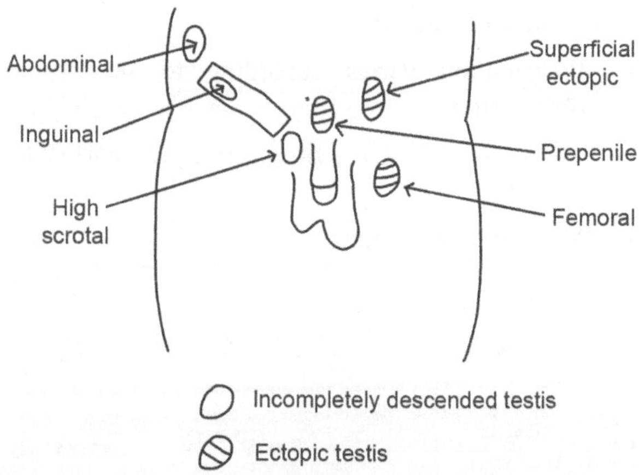

Figure 1: Undescended testis

Pathology

Gross

- Macroscopically normal in early childhood.
- By puberty it is **typically smaller** compared with its intrascrotal counterpart.

HPE

- Microscopic changes are **apparent from 1-2 years**:
  - o Loss of Leydig cells.
  - o Degeneration of Sertoli cells.
  - o Decreased spermatogenesis.
- The higher the testes, the greater the degree of histological change.
- An incompletely descended testis **tends to atrophy** as puberty approaches.

Clinical Features

- Right > left.
- Bilateral in 20% cases.
- In adults, secondary sexual characteristics are typically normal.

On Examination

- Examined in a warm room in supine position and boy should be as relaxed as possible.
- Scrotum is empty and underdeveloped.

Retractile Testis

- It is a differential diagnosis.
- During childhood, the testes are mobile and the cremasteric reflex is active.
- Because of this, any stimulation of the skin of the scrotum or thigh causes the testis to ascend and to temporarily disappear into the inguinal canal.
- When the cremaster relaxes, the testis reappears only to vanish when the scrotal skin is touched again.
- Scrotum is normal.
- Retractile testis can be gently milked from its position in the inguinal region to the bottom of the scrotum. A diagnosis of true incomplete descent should be made only if this is not possible.
- More common than true undescended testis.
- Requires no treatment.

Investigations

- USG is helpful in identifying intracanalicular testes.
- **Diagnostic laparoscopy:**
  - o **Gold standard.**
  - o Used to differentiate between the abdominal testis and a truly absent testis.

Complications

a. **Impaired fertility or infertility**
   - Reduced fertility, which may persist even after orchidopexy.

b. **Malignancy**
   - Risk of testicular cancer is higher, which persists even after orchidopexy.
   - **Most common type of testicular cancer in untreated undescended testis is seminoma.**

c. **Inguinal hernia**
   - Patients with undescended testis have a patent processus vaginalis which predisposes them to indirect inguinal hernias.

d. **Testicular torsion**
   - Undescended testis is more prone to testicular torsion, because of a developmental abnormality between the testis and its mesentery.

e. **Pain**
   - An inguinal testis is **prone to repeated trauma.**

f. **Atrophy**
   - This sometimes occurs when the testes situated in the inguinal canal is subjected to repeated trauma.

g. **Diagnostic dilemma**
   - Epididymo-orchitis occurring in a right undescended testis is impossible to differentiate from acute appendicitis.

Surgical Treatment

1. **Orchidopexy**
   - Testis and spermatic cord are mobilized and the testis is repositioned and fixed in the scrotum.

- Done **between 6 and 18 months of age.**
- For premature babies, corrected age is used to determine surgery timing.

2. **Orchidectomy**
   - Should be **considered if the incompletely descended testis is atrophic.**
   - Also done if there is suspicion of malignancy.

TORSION

[5] Torsion of testis. ***March 21, July 18***
[3] Torsion of testis. ***August 22, June 16***
[3] Mention causes of torsion testis. ***Dec 17***
[3] How to diagnose torsion testis? ***CBME March 24***

- It is a condition whereby the **spermatic cord and its contents twist in such a way that the testicular blood supply becomes compromised.**
- **If left untreated,** the blood flow to the testis ceases and the **testis dies.**

Predisposing Factors

- Torsion is **uncommon** because the normal testis is anchored and cannot rotate.
- Several abnormalities predispose to intravaginal torsion:
  1. **Bell clapper deformity or high investment of tunica vaginalis:**
     - o Typically bilateral.
     - o This is the most common cause.
  2. **Inversion of testis:**
     - o Testis is rotated so that it lies transversely or upside down.
  3. **Separation of epididymis from body of the testis:**
     - o A pedicle connects the epididymis and testis, which permits torsion to occur.

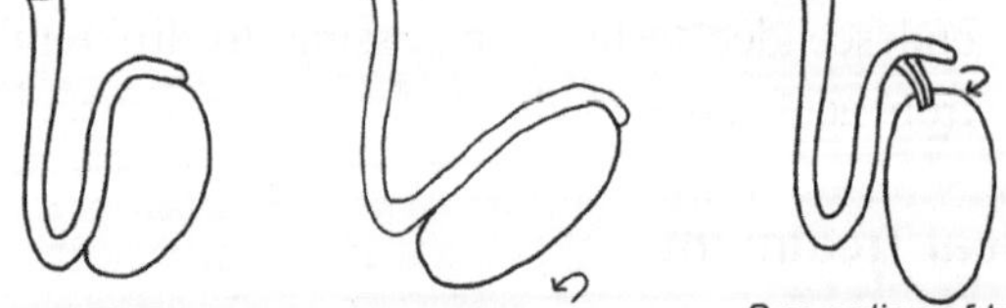

Figure 2: Predisposing factors of torsion

Pathogenesis

Mechanical, sexual or thermic stimulation of abdominal muscles (e.g. of precipitating factors: straining at stool, lifting of heavy weights, sexual activity, sport)

↓

Sudden contraction of cremasteric muscles (this is because when there is a contraction of the abdominal muscles, the cremaster also contracts)

↓

Testis is pulled upward which may cause a rotational effect on it

↓

Torsion

Factors Determining Damage to Testis

1. **Extent of the twist:**
   - **Twists of 720° cause more rapid ischemia than twists of 360° or less.**
   - 720° is two twists, whereas 360° is a single twist.
2. **Duration of the episode.**

Clinical Features

- It is a surgical **emergency.**
- Most common between 10-25 years of age.
- Sudden **agonising pain** in the groin and the lower abdomen.
- Patient feels nauseated and may **vomit.**

On Examination

- Scrotum is **swollen** and **tender.**
- **Testis** is also swollen and tender and seems **high within the scrotum.**
- **Spermatic cord** is tender and **twisted** and can be palpated above it.
- Cremasteric reflex is lost.
- Scrotal skin is usually not erythematous (but may become so with a prolonged history).
- Elevation of the testis increases the pain (**Prehn's sign**).
- There is **no fever.**

- Sometimes the testis untwists itself spontaneously without any treatment, such patients give a history of intermittent testicular pain.

Differential Diagnosis

- Epididymo-orchitis.
- Torsion of a testicular appendage.
- Mumps orchitis.
- Idiopathic scrotal edema.
- Small tense strangulated inguinal hernia.

Investigations

- **Doppler USG** can confirm the absence of the blood supply to the affected testis.

Treatment

- It is a surgical **emergency.**
- The earlier the surgery is performed, the better the prognosis.
- **Golden period for saving the testis is 6 hours.**
- If there is **any doubt about the diagnosis, urgent scrotal exploration** is indicated:
  - o Untwist the cord.
  - o If the testis is **unviable**, do an **orchidectomy.**
  - o If there is **doubt about testicular viability** after detorsion of the testis, then it should be **wrapped in a warm saline swab and observed after a few minutes.**
  - o If the testis looks viable, do an orchidopexy.
  - o **Fix the testis with 3 non-absorbable sutures** between the tunica albuginea of the testis and the scrotal raphe.
  - o **In a unilateral case, the contralateral testis should be fixed even if it is normal.** This is because the underlying predisposing abnormality is most likely bilateral.

HYDROCELE

[5] Hydrocele. ***August 22, Dec 19, Dec 15***
[3] Mention surgical procedures for hydrocele. ***July 18***
[5] Secondary hydrocele. ***Dec 14***
[3] Aetiology of hydrocele. ***June 13***
[5] Congenital hydrocele. ***Feb 23***
[3] Complications of hydrocele. ***July 23***
[5] Types and management of hydrocele. ***CBME June 24***

- **Definition:** A hydrocele is an **abnormal collection of serous fluid in a part of the processus vaginalis, usually the tunica vaginalis**. The fluid collects around the testis and occasionally along the spermatic cord.

Types

1. Congenital hydrocele.
2. Acquired hydrocele:
   i. Primary or idiopathic.
   ii. Secondary (to epididymal or testicular disease).

Aetiology

A hydrocele can form in 4 different ways:

1. By connection with the peritoneal cavity via a **patent processus vaginalis** (congenital).
2. By **excessive production of fluid** within the sac (e.g., a **secondary hydrocele**).
3. By **defective absorption of fluid (vaginal)**. This is the explanation for most primary hydroceles, although the reason why the fluid is not absorbed is not known.
4. By **interference with the lymphatic drainage** of scrotal structures.

Pathophysiology

Embryologically, the processus vaginalis is a diverticulum of the peritoneal cavity. It descends with the testis into the scrotum via the inguinal canal around the 28th week of gestation with gradual closure through infancy and childhood.

A. Communicating or Congenital Hydrocele

- A patent processus vaginalis permits flow of peritoneal fluid into the tunica vaginalis; and is associated with indirect inguinal hernia.

B. Non-Communicating or Vaginal Hydrocele

- The processus vaginalis is closed with no communication with the peritoneal cavity. Instead, fluid accumulation can be **due to excessive**

production and/or defective absorption by the tunica vaginalis, primarily because of disruption to the lymphatic drainage of scrotal structures. If idiopathic, these are called 'primary' hydroceles.

- This is the most common type of hydrocele.

C. **'Infantile Hydrocele' or 'Hydrocele of the Cord'**

- The distal end of the processus vaginalis closes correctly, but the mid portion remains patent. The proximal end may be open and communicating with the tunica vaginalis, resulting in a hydrocele of the cord.

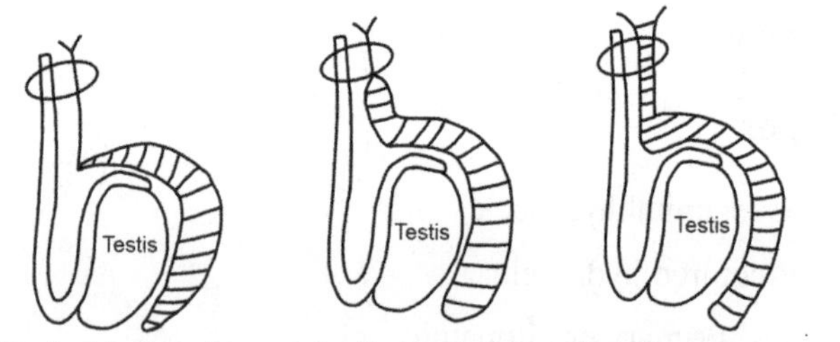

Figure 3: Types of hydrocele

Clinical Features

A. **Primary Hydrocele**

- A primary hydrocele is **seen most commonly in middle and later life**, but can also occur in older children.
- It is **usually painless** and may therefore reach a significant size before the patient presents for treatment.

On Examination:

- **Getting above the swelling** is positive, as it is a scrotal swelling. Cord and cord structures are palpable above it.
- **Testis is not palpable separately.**
- It is **transilluminant.**

B. **Secondary Hydrocele**

- Usually occurs in men > 40 years.
- A secondary hydrocele **subsides when the primary cause resolves.**

On Examination:

- Usually **lax.**
- Typically small.
- **Underlying testis is usually palpable.**

C. **Congenital Hydrocele**

- **Processus vaginalis is patent and connects with the peritoneal cavity.**
- Communication is usually too small to allow herniation of intra-abdominal contents.
- Pressure on the hydrocele does not always empty it.
- The hydrocele fluid **may drain into the peritoneal cavity when the child is lying down**; thus the hydrocele may be intermittent.
- **Ascites should be checked for**, if the swellings are bilateral.

Investigations

- A USG diagnoses a hydrocele.
- If a tumor is suspected (in case of a secondary hydrocele); the hydrocele **should not be punctured**, due to the risk of malignant needle-track implantation.

Treatment

A. **Congenital Hydrocele**

- Wait for spontaneous resolution.
- If it does not resolve spontaneously: **Herniotomy**, i.e., ligation of patent processus vaginalis.

B. **Primary or Idiopathic Hydrocele**

1. Lord's plication of sac.
2. Jaboulay's eversion of sac.
3. Aspiration of hydrocele fluid is done in patients who are unfit for surgery. It has a high recurrence rate. Injection of a sclerosant, such as tetracycline, can be effective but painful.

C. **Secondary Hydrocele**

- It subsides when the primary lesion resolves.

Complications of Hydrocele

1. **Rupture:**
   - It is usually traumatic, but may sometimes be spontaneous.
2. **Hernia of the hydrocele sac:**
   - Can sometimes occur in long standing cases.
   - Tension of fluid within the tunica causes herniation through the dartos muscle.

3. **Transformation into a hematocele:**
   - Occurs both spontaneously and as a result of trauma.
4. **Transformation into a pyocele:**
   - Due to infection.
5. **Calcification of the sac wall.**

VARICOCELE

[5] Varicocele. ***June 19, July 18, Dec 12***
[3] Varicocele. ***Dec 16, Feb 23***

- **Definition:** It is an **abnormal dilatation and enlargement of the scrotal venous (pampiniform) plexus** draining the testis.
- In some cases, the dilated vessels are cremasteric veins.

Incidence

- Occur in 15-20% of all males.
- Occur in 40% of infertile males.

Pathophysiology

- There are 3 theories:
  1. **Absence or failure of the anti-reflux valve** usually located where the testicular vein joins the left renal vein or the IVC on the right.
  2. The **'nutcracker' effect** that occurs when the left testicular vein gets trapped between the superior mesenteric artery and the aorta.
  3. **Angulation** at the junction of the left testicular vein and the left renal vein.

Causes

- Most are **idiopathic.**
- **Obstruction of the testicular vein by a renal tumour** or nephrectomy causes varicocele in later life.
- A **retroperitoneal mass** can cause an isolated right sided varicocele.
- Deep vein thrombosis.
- Renal arteriovenous malformation.
- Thrombosis of pampiniform plexus.

Clinical Features

- 90% are **left sided**. This is because the left testicular vein empties into the relatively high pressure left renal vein; whereas the right testicular vein empties into the low pressure IVC.
- Most are **asymptomatic.**
- Symptomatic varicoceles present in adolescence or early adulthood.
- Complains of a **dragging discomfort** that is worse on standing and by the end of the day.

On Examination

- Scrotum on the affected side hangs lower than normal.
- Cough impulse may be present.
- Feels like a **bag of worms.**
- In long-standing cases, the **affected testis atrophies** and is smaller and softer than the opposite side.

Classification

- **Subclinical:** Can be seen only by radiology.
- **I:** Palpable only during Valsalva manoeuvre.
- **II:** Palpable at rest, but not visible on inspection.
- **III:** Visible and palpable at rest.

Investigations

- Doppler ultrasound.

Treatment

- **1st line: Percutaneous embolisation of gonadal veins.**
- **2nd line: Surgical ligation of testicular veins.**
  - o Indications – Recurrence, if percutaneous embolisation is not possible.
- **Microsurgical varicocelectomy is the most effective method of surgical varicocelectomy.**

EPIDIDYMAL CYST

[3] Epididymal cyst. ***June 19***
[5] Epididymal cyst. ***Dec 13***

- It is a common condition.
- They are **congenital cysts**, which are usually **derived from an embryonic remnant around the epididymis** and is **filled with crystal clear fluid.**

Causes

- An epididymal cyst is due to the cystic degeneration of:
  1. Paradidymis or organ of Giraldes is the most common cause.
  2. Appendix of the epididymis (pedunculated hydatid of Morgagni).
  3. Appendix of testis (sessile hydatid of Morgagni).
  4. Vas aberrans of Haller.

Clinical Features

- Are usually found during **middle life.**
- Because of their congenital origin, they are **often bilateral.**
- They are **tense**, and they consist of an **aggregation of a number of small cysts** which on palpation feel like a bunch of **tiny grapes.**
- Usually **multiple.**
- Vary in size at presentation.
- Located posterior to and quite separate from the testis.
- **Brilliantly transilluminant with a Chinese lantern appearance.**

Investigations

- Diagnosis is confirmed by **USG.**

Treatment

- Should be **excised** if they cause discomfort:
  - o **Single large cysts:** Can be excised separately.
  - o **Recurrent or multilocular cysts:** Usually require **partial or total epididymectomy.**
- Excision interferes with the transportation of sperm from the testis on that side and may thus impair fertility.

INFECTIONS

[5] Fournier's gangrene. ***Dec 16, June 16***

- It is a form of **necrotizing fasciitis of the soft tissues of the perineum, external genitalia and perianal regions.**

Cause

- **Idiopathic** in > 50%.
- Can arise following **minor injuries** or procedures, e.g., bruise, scratch, urethral dilatation, injection of hemorrhoids, opening of a periurethral abscess.
- **Immunosuppressed,** e.g., diabetes.

Causative Organisms

- **Polymicrobial:** Mixed infection of aerobic and anaerobic bacteria.

Pathogenesis

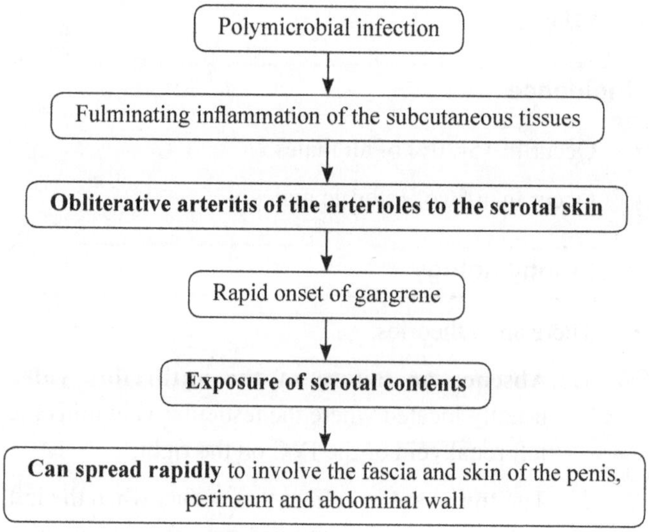

Clinical Features

- Clinical course usually progresses through the following phases:
  1. **Prodromal symptoms** of fever and lethargy for 2-7 days.
  2. **Intense genital pain is usually associated with edema** of the overlying skin; pruritus may be present.
  3. Increasing genital pain with **progressive erythema of overlying skin.**
  4. **Dusky appearance of overlying skin**; subcutaneous crepitus.

5. Obvious **gangrene** of part of the genitalia; **purulent discharge** from wounds.

- Early on, **pain may be out of proportion** to the physical findings.
- As gangrene develops, pain may subside as nerve tissue becomes necrotic.
- The greater the necrosis, the more severe the **systemic effects.**
- **Testes are exposed, but healthy.**

Investigations

- Swab for C/S.
- Tissue for C/S.
- Tissue for HPE.

Treatment

- It is a **surgical emergency.**
- **IV fluid resuscitation.**
- **Broad spectrum IV antibiotics.**
- **Extensive debridement** with wide surgical excision of dead and infected tissue.
- This is because extent of the internal necrosis is typically much greater than the external appearances suggest.
- Urinary and fecal division may be necessary.
- If patient becomes severely septic: **Supportive care in ICU.**
- Patient may require **multiple sessions of debridement.**
- Once infection has been controlled, **VAC dressing** is used as it promotes wound healing.
- **Reconstruction: Skin grafting, flap closure.**

[5] Pyocele. ***June 16***

- A scrotal pyocele is a rare urological emergency.
- **Definition:** A scrotal pyocele is a **purulent collection within the space between the visceral and parietal tunica vaginalis.**

Aetiopathogenesis

- Most commonly associated with acute epididymo-orchitis.

Clinical Features

- Subacute onset of pain and swelling, which may mimic other pathology.
- Fever may be present.

Complications

1. Fournier's gangrene.
2. Sepsis.

Investigations

- USG is the imaging modality of choice.

Treatment

- IV broad spectrum antibiotics.
- Surgical drainage.
- Some patients may ultimately require orchidectomy.

VASECTOMY

[3] Vasectomy. ***Sept 21***

[3] Complications of vasectomy. ***Dec 16, June 16, July 23***

- Vasectomy for sterilization is a **common and effective contraceptive procedure**.
- It is a surgical procedure that **involves cutting or blocking the vas deferens.**

Indications

- Performed to make the man permanently sterile.

Method

- Easily and painlessly performed under LA.
- For medicolegal reasons, **a segment of each vas has to be removed to prove** that it has been successfully divided.
- The following can be done to prevent the cut ends from rejoining:
  1. Burying the cut ends.
  2. Fascial interposition.
  3. Turning them back on themselves.

Complications

1. Spontaneous recanalization: This may restore fertility unexpectedly.
2. Testicular pain in the short-term following surgery.
3. Chronic testicular pain in the longer term, called congestion syndrome or post vasectomy pain syndrome.
4. Surgical site infection.
5. Epididymitis.
6. Bleeding or hematoma.
7. Sperm granuloma.

- The operation is **not immediately effective and contraceptive precautions should be continued until the success of the operation is confirmed by two negative semen analyses performed 12-16 weeks after surgery.**

TESTICULAR TUMOURS

[5] Classify testicular tumours. ***June 14***

- Testicular tumours are the **most common tumours in young men.**

Classification

Tumours of the testes are classified according to their predominant cellular type.

A. Germ Cell Tumours (GCTs)

i. Seminomas

- o Spermatocytic seminoma.
- o Anaplastic seminoma.

ii. Non Seminomatous Germ Cell Tumours (NSGCTs)

- o Embryonal cell carcinoma.
- o Yolk sac tumours.
- o Choriocarcinoma.
- o Teratoma.

B. Interstitial Tumours or Sex Cord-Stromal Tumours

i. Leydig cell tumours.

ii. Sertoli cell tumours.

C. Lymphomas

D. Others

- GCTs are the most common testicular tumours.
- Seminomas are the most common subtype of GCTs.

Risk Factors

1. History of testicular **maldescent or cryptorchidism:**
   - **Strongest association.**
   - Higher the testis, greater the risk.
2. History of contralateral testicular tumour or GCNIS (Germ Cell Neoplasia In Situ).
3. Family history of testicular tumours among 1st grade relatives.
4. Intratubular germ cell neoplasia.
5. History of in utero administration of DES (diethyl stilbestrol).

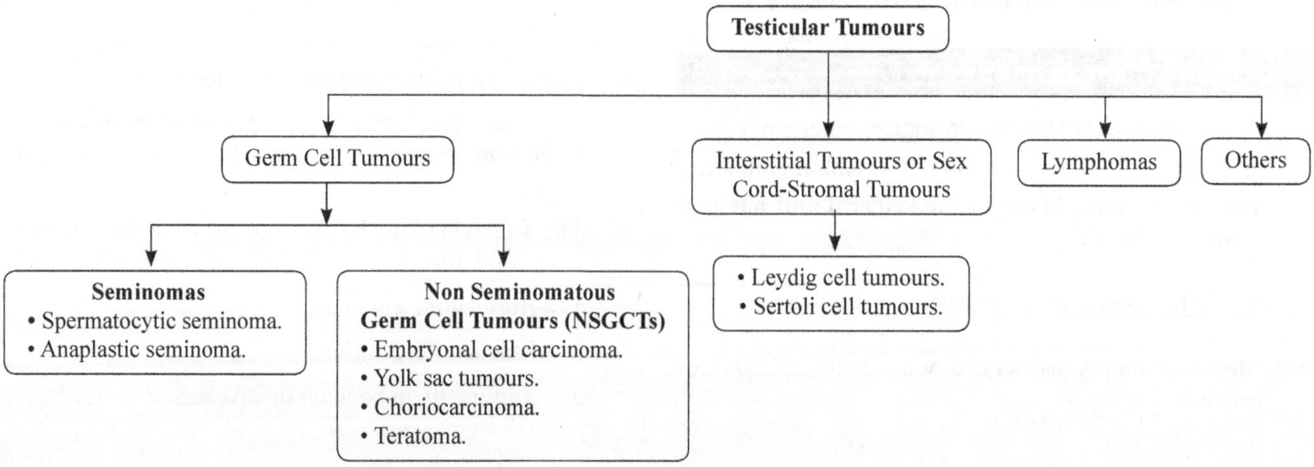

6. Klinefelter's syndrome – 47 XXY or male factor infertility.
7. Testicular feminization syndrome.

- A specific genetic marker – an isochromosome of the short arm of chr 12 (**i12p**) is pathognomonic of all types of adult GCTs as well as GCNIS.

Clinical Features

- **Age:**
    - o **Seminomas:** 30-40 years.
    - o **NSGCTs:** 20-30 years.
- Usually, the patient presents with a **painless testicular lump**.
- **Sensation of heaviness**, if testis is 2-3 times the normal size.
- Few patients experience pain.
- Some cases may simulate epididymo-orchitis.
- Rarely, some patients present with severe pain and acute enlargement of testis because of hemorrhage into the tumour.
- Rarely, predominant symptoms are of metastatic disease:
    - **a. Intra-abdominal:** Pain, mass in epigastrium.
    - **b. Lungs:** Chest pain, dyspnoea and hemoptysis.

On Examination

- **Intratesticular solid mass**, i.e., a solid testicular lump that cannot be felt separately from the testis.
- **Secondary hydrocele.**
- If epididymis is incorporated in the growth, it becomes more difficult to feel it independently.
- **Vas is never involved.**

Symptoms of Interstitial Cell Tumours

- **Leydig cell tumour masculinizes whereas a Sertoli cell tumour feminizes.**
- Most ***prepubertal*** interstitial cell tumours produce androgens, which causes the following:
    - o Sexual precocity.
    - o Prominent external genitalia.
    - o Suprapubic hair growth.
    - o Deep masculinized voice.
- Regression of these symptoms after orchidectomy may be incomplete.
- Most ***postpubertal*** interstitial cell tumours produce feminizing hormones:
    - o Gynecomastia.
    - o Erectile dysfunction.
    - o Loss of libido.
    - o Azoospermia.

Investigations

a. USG

- Mandatory test in all suspected cases of testicular tumours.
- It confirms the diagnosis.

b. Tumour markers

- The tumour markers used are:
    1. AFP or **a**lpha-**f**eto**p**rotein:
        - o Increased in NSGCTs.
        - o Never increased in seminoma.
    2. β-hCG or **b**eta **h**uman **c**horionic **g**onadotropin:
        - o Increased in germ cell tumours (both seminoma and non-seminoma).
    3. LDH or lactate dehydrogenase:
        - o Associated with high tumour burden in seminoma, i.e., it is a marker of tumour bulk.
        - o Associated with recurrence in non-seminomas.
- Tumour markers in general are increased in non-seminomatous tumours more than in seminomatous tumours.
- They are used **to monitor the response to treatment by comparing their levels before and after surgery:**
    - o If **elevated after orchidectomy**, it means the patient has **residual disease**.
    - o If **elevated after** retroperitoneal lymph node dissection **(RPLND)**, patient has **stage III disease.**

- In case of recurrence, the markers become positive earlier than X-ray studies.
- The **elevated tumour marker indicates tumour histology,** e.g., if AFP is elevated in a patient with a suspected or known seminoma it means that the tumour has non-seminomatous components as well.

c. **CXR**

- **Cannon ball appearance** is seen in lung mets.

d. **CT of chest, abdomen and pelvis**

- Detects metastases.
- Used for monitoring the response to therapy.

e. **FNAC**

- It is **contraindicated because it causes upstaging of tumour.**

Staging

Prognostic groups come under the following stages:

- **Stage I:** Non metastatic disease.
- **Stage II:** Lymph node mets.
- **Stage III:** Lymph node mets + elevated tumour markers *or* distant mets present.

TNM Staging

T_x - Primary tumour cannot be assessed.

T_0 - No evidence of primary tumour.

T_{is} - Intratubular germ cell neoplasia.

T_1 - Tumour limited to the testis and epididymis *or* tumour invasion into the tunica albuginea only.

T_2 - Involvement of tunica vaginalis.

T_3 - Tumour invades the spermatic cord.

T_4 - Tumour invades the scrotum.

N_x - Regional lymph nodes cannot be assessed.

N_0 - No regional lymph node mets.

N_1 - Mets to single or multiple lymph nodes, each < 2 cm.

N_2 - 2-5 cm.

N_3 - >5 cm.

M_x - Distant mets cannot be assessed.

M_0 - No distant mets.

M_1 - Distant mets present.

- The testes drain into the pre and para-aortic lymph nodes.
- The scrotal skin drains into inguinal lymph nodes.

Treatment

Principles of treatment of GCTs

- Treatment is **always aimed at one stage above the clinical stage.**
- **Radical inguinal orchidectomy** is the standard first line of therapy.
- **Seminomas are radiosensitive**, therefore radiotherapy is used in the treatment of seminomas.
- **Non-seminomas are radioresistant**, therefore surgery is used in the treatment of non-seminomas.
- **Chemotherapy is used in the treatment of primary tumour as well as metastatic lesions. Drugs used are bleomycin, etoposide, cisplatin.**
- Men should be offered semen analysis and sperm banking prior to interventions such as surgery and chemotherapy that may render them infertile.

A. **Seminomas**

i. **Stages I, IIA, IIB:**

- Radical inguinal orchidectomy + radiotherapy to the ipsilateral retroperitoneal, para-aortic and iliac regions.

ii. **Bulky stages II, III:**

- Radical inguinal orchidectomy + chemotherapy.

B. **Non-Seminomas**

i. **Stages I and IIA:**

- Radical inguinal orchidectomy + RPLND.

ii. **Stage IIB:**

- Radical inguinal orchidectomy + RPLND + chemotherapy.

iii. **Stage IIC and III:**

- NACT + radical inguinal orchidectomy ± RPLND.

Radical Orchidectomy

- Undertaken via an inguinal incision.
- Spermatic cord is displayed by dividing the external oblique aponeurosis and a soft clamp is placed across the cord to stop dissemination of malignant cells as the testis is mobilized into the wound.
- If there is a tumour, the cord should be doubly transfixed and divided at the level of the internal inguinal ring and the testis removed.

Principles of treatment of interstitial tumours

- 80% of the tumours are benign:
  - a. **Small tumours**
    - o Organ sparing surgery *or* conservative treatment.
  - b. **Larger tumours**
    - o High inguinal orchidectomy + multimodality treatment (if malignant).

[5] Teratoma of testis. ***March 22***

TERATOMA OF TESTIS

- Teratoma is a **non seminomatous germ cell tumour** of the testis.

Aetiology

- History of testicular maldescent or cryptorchidism.
- History of contralateral testicular tumour.
- Family history.
- Male factor infertility.

Pathology

- Teratomas consist of different tissues **derived from all 3 germ layers:** Ectoderm, endoderm and mesoderm.
- Immature components are often neuroectodermal or mesenchymal tissue.
- Mature components are often cystic with epithelial differentiation or consists of smooth muscle, connective tissue or cartilage.
- All can metastasize.

Clinical Features

- Age: 20-30 years.
- Painless testicular swelling.
- Sensation of heaviness
- Rarely, predominant symptoms are of metastatic disease.
  - o Intra-abdominal: Pain, mass in epigastrium.
  - o Lungs: Chest pain, dyspnea, hemoptysis.

Investigations

- **USG is the investigation of choice.**
- **Tumour markers:** α-fetoprotein, β-hCG, LDH.
- **CT of chest, abdomen and pelvis:** To diagnose mets.

Treatment

i. **Stages I and IIA:**
   - Radical inguinal orchidectomy + RPLND.

ii. **Stage IIB:**
   - Radical inguinal orchidectomy + RPLND + chemotherapy.

iii. **Stages IIC and III:**
   - NACT + radical inguinal orchidectomy ± RPLND.

[5] Seminoma of testis. ***Sept 21, Dec 17, July 15***

[MCQ] Which of the following is true for seminoma testis? ***CBME March 24***

A. Predominantly spreads through lymphatics*
B. Consists of a mixture of tissues
C. Secretes β-hCG
D. Spreads predominantly by blood

- Seminomas are the **most common germ cell tumour (GCT)** of testes.
- **Since GCTs are the most common tumours of testes, seminomas are also the most common overall tumours of testes.**

Aetiology

- History of testicular maldescent or cryptorchidism.
- History of contralateral testicular tumour.
- Family history.

- Intratubular germ cell neoplasia.
- Male factor infertility.
- **A specific genetic marker:** An isochromosome of the short arm of chr 12 **(i 12p)** is pathognomonic of seminoma.

Pathology

- It is a germ cell tumour.
- **Metastasizes mainly via lymphatics** and hematogenous spread is uncommon.
- Lymphatic drainage is **to para-aortic lymph nodes.**

Gross

- It has a cut surface that is homogenous and pinkish cream in color.
- It **compresses neighbouring testicular tissue.**

HPE

- Consists of **oval cells with clear cytoplasm and large, rounded nuclei with prominent nucleoli.**
- Sheets of spermatocytes are separated by a fine fibrous stroma.
- **Active lymphocytic infiltration of tumour suggests a good host response and a good prognosis.**

Clinical Features

- Age: 30-40 years.
- Painless testicular lump.
- Sensation of heaviness.
- Rarely, predominant symptoms are of metastatic disease:
  a. Intra-abdominal: Pain, mass in epigastrium.
  b. Lungs: Chest pain, dyspnea, hemoptysis.

On Examination

- Intratesticular solid mass.
- Secondary hydrocele.

Investigations

- USG is the investigation of choice.
- **Tumour markers:**
  - βhCG.
  - LDH (marker of tumour bulk).
- CT of chest, abdomen and pelvis detects mets.
- CXR shows cannon ball appearance in the presence of mets.

Treatment

- Seminomas are radiosensitive, therefore radiotherapy is used in its treatment.

  i. **Stages I, IIA, IIB:**
     - Radical inguinal orchidectomy + radiotherapy to the ipsilateral retroperitoneal, para-aortic and iliac regions.

  ii. **Bulky Stage II, Stage III:**
     - Radical inguinal orchidectomy + chemotherapy (bleomycin, etoposide, cisplatin).

53

Transplantation

[3] Principles of organ transplantation. *CBME March 24*

[3] Enumerate principles of organ transplantation. *CBME June 24*

PRINCIPLES OF ORGAN TRANSPLANTATION

Types of Donors

- Most transplant organs are from deceased donors, of which there are two types:
  1. **Donation after brainstem death (DBD)**
     - o Potential DBD donors are in an apnoeic coma that requires mechanical ventilation in ICU.
  2. **Donation after circulatory death (DCD)**
     - o **Modified Maastricht classification** is used to categorise DCD donors.
     - o **Living donation.**
     - o Limited to kidney, liver, lung and segments of small intestine.

Organ Preservation

- Transplant organs need to be stored and preserved in the period between procurement from the donor and transplantation into the recipient.
- Methods of organ preservation:
  - o Static cold storage.
  - o Hypothermic machine perfusion.
  - o Normothermic machine perfusion.
- Perfusion fluid is used to flush blood out of the microcirculation to prevent thrombosis.
- Preservation solutions have:
  - o Electrolytes.
  - o Impermeant (osmotically active molecules which prevent cellular swelling).
  - o Buffer.
- **University of Wisconsin solution** is regarded as the gold standard.

Transplant Rejection

- Allograft rejection can be divided into:
  1. **Hyperacute rejection**
     - o Due to preformed circulating donor-specific HLA antibodies or ABO antibodies.
     - o Occurs immediately after revascularisation of the donor organ.
     - o Widespread intravascular thrombosis causes infarction and loss of the graft within minutes or hours.
  2. **Acute cell-mediated rejection**
     - o Largely mediated by direct antigen presentation.
     - o Occurs in the first 3 months post transplantation.

- o Interstitial lymphocytic infiltrate is seen on biopsy.
- o **Treatment:** High-dose pulsed IV steroids, lymphocyte-depleting IV anti-thymocyte globulin (ATG).

3. **Acute antibody-mediated rejection**
   - o More serious and more difficult to treat than cell-mediated rejection.
   - o Caused by donor-specific HLA antibodies which are produced by a sensitising episode from a previous transplant, a blood transfusion or pregnancy.
   - o In the kidney, transplant biopsy shows vasculitis and complement component C4d deposition in the peritubular capillaries.
   - o **Treatment:** Plasma exchange to remove circulating antibodies, Rituximab.
4. **Chronic antibody-mediated rejection**
   - o Not well understood.
   - o Long-lived indirect antigen presentation pathway plays a role.
   - o CD4 T-cell activation also causes ongoing allograft damage.

Immunosuppression

- Challenge is to deliver sufficient immunosuppression to prevent rejection while minimising drug side effects.
- Increases the risk of both infection and malignancy.
- Immunosuppression has 2 phases:

1. **Induction**
   - o Consists of a combination of high dose IV steroids and the anti-CD25 monoclonal antibody basiliximab.
   - o Other drugs: Antithymocyte globulin, alemtuzumab.
2. **Maintenance**
   - o Triple therapy with a calcineurin inhibitor (ciclosporin or tacrolimus), an antiproliferative agent (azathioprine or mycophenolic acid) and steroids.

[3] Immunological basis of transplantation. ***CBME March 24***

IMMUNOLOGY OF TRANSPLANT REJECTION

ABO Blood Groups

- ABO antigens are expressed not only on the surface of RBCs but also on endothelial cells.
- **In all organ transplants, there must therefore be ABO blood group compatibility** between the recipient and the donor organ, using the same rules as for blood transfusion.

HLA Matching

- Allograft rejection is directed against human leukocyte antigens (HLAs), which are a group of cell surface **glycoprotein** molecules.
- HLA molecules are divided into:

1. **Class I (A, B and C)**
   - o Expressed on the surface of all nucleated cells.
2. **Class II (DR, DP and DQ)**
   - o Only expressed by antigen-presenting cells (APCs) such as dendritic cells and B lymphocytes.
   - o HLA molecules are encoded for in the **major histocompatibility complex** (MHC) on **chromosome 6.**
   - o They are highly **polymorphic**, i.e., their amino acid sequences differ widely between individuals.
   - o This **genetic variability** means that most transplant donors and recipients have different HLA profiles.
   - o Donors and transplant recipients are HLA-typed using DNA sequencing.
   - o The antigens at HLA-A, -B and -DR are together described as the **tissue type.**
   - o Level of mismatch between the HLA molecules determines the strength of the immune response.
   - o Every individual has two copies of each HLA gene and so **for each locus (A, B or DR) it is possible to have 0, 1 or 2 mismatched genes.**

- As the number of mismatches increases so does the chance of immune recognition and rejection.
- The **best matched grafts** are described as having a **mismatch of 0–0–0**, i.e., **no mismatches at A, B or DR, respectively.**
- A **completely mismatched graft** would be annotated as a **2–2–2 mismatch.**
- DR mismatches have a more powerful effect than B mismatches, and A mismatches are the least important.

Immune Response to a Transplanted Organ

- Main immune cells involved in transplant immunology are **Antigen Presenting Cells (APCs)** and **T and B lymphocytes.**
- These cell types interact by a series of specific surface molecules that are designated by CD (cluster of differentiation) numbers.
- Cell surface receptors **can only interact if they have the correct complementary 3D structures.**
- Immune response to an allograft is orchestrated by T lymphocytes.
- **When T cells encounter foreign transplant HLA antigens** they become **activated and then proliferate into clones** of cells that attack the allograft.
- Full T-cell activation requires a number of signals.
- Transplant antigen is presented to T-helper cells (CD4+) on self-MHC class II molecules by specialised APCs.
- The **class II/peptide antigen complex** is recognised by the **T-cell receptor (signal 1).**
- CD4+ T-helper cell activation also requires a co-stimulatory signal involving the interaction of pairs of molecules, one on the surface of the T cell and the other on the surface of the APC **(signal 2).**
- An example of signal 2 is the interaction of T-cell CD28 with CD80 on the APC.
- When both signal 1 and signal 2 are received, the CD4+ T-helper cell will **upregulate expression of the interleukin-2 (IL-2) receptor (CD25)** on its cell surface.
- Binding of IL-2 to its receptor causes further activation of the T cell **(signal 3).**
- The T cell will then proliferate and release more IL-2, which, in turn, leads to activation and **clonal proliferation of T-killer cells (CD8+).**
- These cytotoxic killer cells infiltrate the allograft and cause cell death by the release of molecules called perforin and granzyme.

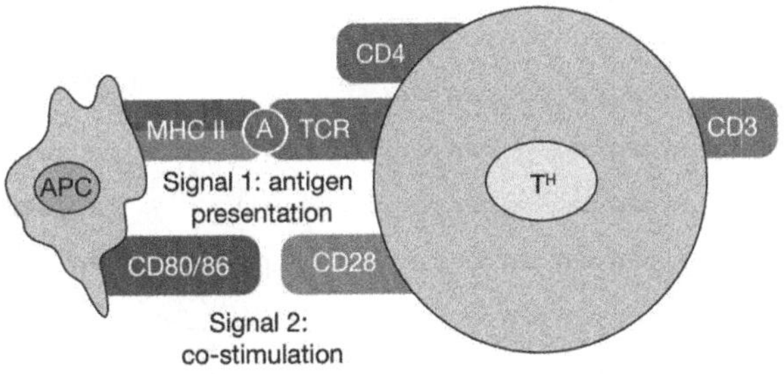

Figure 1: Interaction between an antigen-presenting cell and a CD4+ T-helper cell. A, antigen; APC, antigen-presenting cell; CD, cluster of differentiation; MHC II, major histocompatibility complex class II; TCR, T-cell receptor; TH, T-helper cell.

Antigen Presentation in Transplantation

- There are 2 main types of antigen presentation to T lymphocytes:

1. **Direct presentation**
   - Involves **donor APCs showing intact and unprocessed donor HLA** (class I or class II) molecules on their cell surface **to recipient T cells.**
   - Only occurs for the **first 6–12 weeks after transplantation** because this is the lifespan of the donor passenger APCs that are present in the allograft.
2. **Indirect presentation**
   - Performed by **recipient APCs,** which **internalise foreign donor HLA** molecules from the graft, **process them into short peptide fragments** and then **load them into the peptide groove** of recipient (self) HLA class II molecules.
   - The donor peptiderecipient HLA class II complex is then **expressed on the cell surface** and **presented to recipient T cells.**
   - Involves recipient APCs, therefore it is a **long-lived response.**

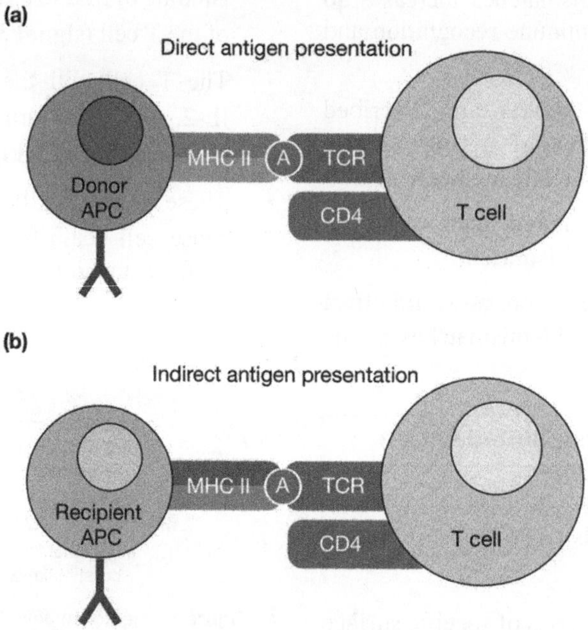

Figure 2: Direct (a) and indirect (b) antigen presentation. A, antigen; APC, antigen-presenting cell; CD, cluster of differentiation; MHC II, major histocompatibility complex class II; TCR, T-cell receptor.

54

Miscellaneous

[3] Stem cells. *March 24*

- Stem cells are undifferentiated or non-specialised cells that are able, through cell division, **to renew themselves indefinitely (self-renewal).**
- When provided with appropriate stimuli, they are also able to differentiate into one or more of the different types of specialised cells found in tissues and organs **(potency).**

Application

- For use as cell-based therapies.
- Regenerative medicine.
- Drug testing and development.
- Understanding development and disease.

Classification

A. Based on Level of Potency

- **Pluripotent:** Capable of giving rise to all cell types of the body.
- **Multipotent:** Capable of giving rise to all cell types of a particular tissue or organ.

B. Based on the Tissue from Which They are Derived

- **Early embryo:** Embryonic stem cells (ESCs)
- **Adults:** Somatic stem cells (SSCs)
- **Derived by reprogramming adult specialised cells to a pluripotent state:** Induced pluripotent stem cells (iPSCs).

Sources of Stem Cells

1. **Embryonic stem cells**
   - Derived from inner cell mass of blastocysts.
2. **Somatic stem cells**
   - Bone marrow contains hematopoietic stem cells.
   - Adipose tissue.
   - Peripheral blood contains circulating hematopoietic stem cells.
   - Specific regions of the brain contain neural stem cells.
3. **Induced pluripotent stem cells**
   - Generated by reprogramming adult cells, such as skin cells or blood cells.
4. **Umbilical cord blood stem cells**
   - Contains hematopoietic stem cells.
5. **Amniotic fluid stem cells.**

[5] Investigations of a surgical patient. *CBME March 24*

[5] Enumerate investigations in a surgical patient. *CBME June 24*

INVESTIGATIONS OF A SURGICAL PATIENT

- The aims of investigations in a surgical patient are the following:

- o To make a diagnosis.
- o To assess the general health of a patient.
- o To assess fitness for surgery.
- o For follow-up of a patient who may be receiving conservative, medical or surgical treatment.

- Investigations have evolved drastically over the years and continues to evolve.
- They can be invasive or non-invasive.
- Investigations are broadly of the following types:

A. Blood and Serum tests

- o **Complete Blood Count:** Hemoglobin, platelet count, total and differential leukocyte count.
- o **Renal Function Tests:** Blood urea nitrogen, serum creatinine, electrolytes, uric acid.
- o **Liver Function Tests:** Bilirubin (total, direct and indirect), total protein, albumin, globulin, ALP, GGT, SGOT, SGPT.
- o **Serology:** HBsAg, HCV, HIV 1 and 2.
- o **Tumour markers:** PSA, AFP, CA 19-9, CEA, β-hCG.

B. Urine Tests

- o Microscopic examination.
- o Culture/sensitivity.
- o Parasites.
- o Crystals.

C. Stool Tests

- o Occult blood.

D. Body Fluid Analysis

- o Pleural fluid.
- o Pericardial fluid.
- o CSF.

E. Imaging

- o **X-ray:** plain/contrast .
- o **USG.**
- o **CT:** plain/contrast.
- o **MRI:** plain/contrast.

F. Nuclear Medicine

- o PET-CT.
- o Sestamibi scan.

G. Assessment by Visualisation

- o Upper GI endoscopy.
- o Colonoscopy.
- o Laparoscopy.
- o Arthroscopy.

H. Tissue Diagnosis/Cytology

- o FNAC.
- o Biopsy (incision, excision, punch, etc).

I. Organ Specific

- o **Heart:** ECG, 2D ECHO, Tread Mill Test.
- o **Brain:** EEG.
- o **Arteries and veins:** Doppler, duplex, angiography.

[3] Ethics in general surgery. *CBME March 24*

[3] Describe the steps of informed written consent. *CBME June 24*

- Ethical concerns involve not only the **interests of patients,** but also the interests of **surgeons and society.**
- **Primum non nocere**: First do no harm.
- The **principle of autonomy** implies a right for patients to make their **own choices and decisions.**
- Also implies an **obligation for surgeons to permit patients to make autonomous choices** about their care.
- The **case-based paradigm** is used when two or more values or principles come into apparent conflict.
  - o **First step is to clarify the relevant principles** (e.g., autonomy, beneficence, non-maleficence, and justice) **and values at stake** (e.g., self-determination, quality of life, etc.).
  - o After identifying the principles and values that are affecting the situation, a proposed **course of action is considered.**
- **Informed consent:**
  - o It is one of the most widely established tenets of modern ethics.
  - o Adequate informed consent entails at least 4 basic elements:
    1. The surgeon documents that the **patient or surrogate has the capacity to make a medical decision.**

2. The **surgeon discloses** to the patient **details regarding the diagnosis and treatment options** sufficiently for the patient to make an informed choice.
3. The **patient demonstrates understanding** of the information disclosed before.
4. **Authorizing freely a specific treatment plan** without undue influence.

- Obtaining **informed consent** is **challenging during emergency surgery:**
  - o Emergency consent **requires the surgeon to consider if and how possible interventions might save a patient's life**, and if successful, what kind of disability might be anticipated.
  - o Surgical emergencies are one of the few instances where the **limits of patient autonomy are freely acknowledged.**
  - o Surgeons are empowered by law and ethics to act promptly in the best interests of their patients according to the surgeon's judgment.
- Informed consent in **children and minors.**
  - o They **lack the cognitive and emotional maturity** to participate fully in the process.
  - o Parents or guardians are the **surrogate decision makers.**
  - o Surgeon should strive to augment the role of decision maker.
- **Respect for patients' privacy**
  - o Patients have an autonomous right over their confidential information.
  - o The **surgeon must not disclose information revealed in the course of the treatment** to anyone else without consent.
  - o A **breach in confidentiality** is an **abuse of human dignity** and **undermines the trust between surgeon and patient.**
  - o An **exception** to surgeon-patient confidentiality is if it poses a **threat to the health and safety of others.**
  - o In some circumstances, confidentiality either must or may be breached in the **public interest, e.g., a court order, public health, legislation, etc.**

[MCQ] Post-op complications include all except: *CBME March 24*

A. Hypotension B. COPD*
C. Pneumonia D. Renal failure

POST-OP COMPLICATIONS

- Post-op complications are an **important cause of morbidity, mortality, extended hospital stay and increased costs.**
- Most patients at increased risk of developing post-op complications can be **identified during PAC using** a variety of **scoring systems.**
- Early identification of risk allows for targeted, appropriate, anticipatory and supportive medical care, which will reduce both the incidence and severity of such complications when they occur.
- **Clavien-Dindo classification:**
  - o Used to **objectively and reproducibly** measure the **impact** of surgical complications **on the outcome of the procedure.**
  - o **Graded** according to the treatment they require.
  - o Eliminates subjective bias.
  - o Prevents complications from being downgraded.
- Complications can occur throughout the post-op period and can be immediate, early or late.

System-Specific Complications

Respiratory System

- Upper airway obstruction due to laryngospasm, persisting relaxation of airway muscles, soft-tissue edema, hematoma, vocal cord dysfunction or a foreign body.
- Hypoventilation.
- Hypoxaemia.
- Atelectasis.
- Bronchospasm.
- Hypercapnia.
- Pneumonia.
- Pleural effusion.

- Pneumothorax.
- Respiratory failure.

Cardiovascular System

- Hypotension.
- Hypertension.
- Myocardial ischaemia.
- Arrhythmias.

Renal and Urinary System

- Acute kidney injury.
- Urinary retention.
- Urinary infection.

Central Nervous System

- Post-op delirium and post-op cognitive dysfunction.
- Stroke.
- Seizures.

General Post-op Complications

- Bleeding.
- Deep vein thrombosis.
- Pulmonary embolism.
- Fever.
- Wound dehiscence.
- Pressure sores.

Surgery-Specific Complications

- These are specific to the surgery that is being done.

[MCQ] Pre-op plan for better surgical outcome includes all except : ***CBME March 24***

A. Optimise patient condition

B. Informed consent

C. Document relevant information

D. No need to correct anemia*

Peri-Operative RBC Transfusion Criteria	
Hemoglobin level (g/dl)	**Indications**
< 6	Patient will benefit from transfusion
6-8	Transfusion unlikely to be of benefit in the absence of bleeding or impending surgery
> 8	No indication for transfusion in the absence of other risk factors

[5] What is surgical audit? Enumerate the steps in audit cycle. ***CBME June 24***

- Clinical audit is a process used by clinicians who seek to improve patient care.
- The process involves comparing aspects of care (structure, process and outcome) against explicit criteria and defined standards.
- Keeping track of personal outcome data and contributing to a clinical database ensures that a surgeon's own performance is monitored continuously and can be compared with a national data set to ensure compliance with agreed standards.
- There are 2 main types of audit in common practice:
  1. Single site/local audits.
  2. Multisite regional, national or international audits.

Steps of An Audit Cycle

1. Define the audit question in a multidisciplinary team.
2. Identify the body of evidence and current standards.
3. Design the audit to measure performance against agreed standards based on strong evidence. Seek appropriate advice (local audit department) and ensure institutions have agreed to undertake the audit.
4. Measure over an agreed interval.
5. Analyse results and compare performance against agreed standards.
6. Undertake gap analysis:
   a. If all standards are reached, reaudit after an agreed interval.
   b. If there is a need for improvement, identify possible interventions such as training, and agree with the involved parties.
7. Reaudit.